The Washington Manual of Oncology

Third Edition

Editors

Ramaswamy Govindan, MD
Professor
Division of Oncology
Alvin J. Siteman Cancer Center at
Washington University School of Medicine
St. Louis, Missouri

Daniel Morgensztern, MD
Associate Professor
Division of Oncology
Alvin J. Siteman Cancer Center at
Washington University School of Medicine
St. Louis, Missouri

D0967141

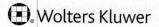

. Wolters Kluwer

Philadelphia • Baltimore • New York • London
Buenos Aires • Hong Kong • Sydney • Tokyo

Acquisitions Editor: Julie Goolsby
Senior Product Development Editor: Emilie Moyer
Production Project Manager: David Orzechowski
Manufacturing Manager: Beth Welsh
Marketing Manager: Stephanie Kindlick
Design Coordinator: Terry Mallon
Production Services: S4Carlisle Publishing Services

9 8 7 6 5 4 3 2 1

Printed in China

Library of Congress Cataloging-in-Publication Data
The Washington manual of oncology / [edited by] Ramaswamy Govindan and Daniel Morgensztern.
— Third edition.
    p. ; cm.
  Manual of oncology
  Includes bibliographical references and index.
  ISBN 978-1-4511-9347-3 (alk. paper)
  I. Govindan, Ramaswamy, editor. II. Morgensztern, Daniel, editor. III. Washington University (Saint Louis, Mo.). School of Medicine, issuing body. IV. Title: Manual of oncology.
  [DNLM: 1. Neoplasms—physiopathology—Handbooks. 2. Neoplasms—therapy—Handbooks. QZ 39]
  RC262
  616.99'4—dc23

2015000057

RRS1502

Dedicated to our colleagues in the Division of Oncology at the
Washington University School of Medicine

Preface

It has been nearly 13 years since we launched the first edition of *The Washington Manual of Oncology.* Over the past decade we have witnessed enormous progress in our understanding of molecular alterations in cancer and the use of targeted therapies and immunotherapies. Cancer care has become naturally complex and daunting. The current edition has been extensively revised to include these recent developments. Almost all the chapters have been extensively revised or rewritten. As before, this manual is written keeping the trainees in mind while also providing a quick update for the practitioners of oncology. It is our hope that you, the reader, find this manual practical, useful, and stimulating. As always, we will be very grateful to you for pointing out any inadvertent errors that have slipped all our editorial review process. Please feel free to email us with your suggestions, feedback and comments.

Ramaswamy Govindan, MD
Daniel Morgensztern, MD

Preface to the First Edition

These are exciting times in oncology. The novel imaging techniques, improved supportive care, and the availability of several new agents that have novel mechanisms of action hold considerable promise in improving the outcomes of cancer patients. In this era of information overload, it is critically important to have a practical manual that is helpful to physicians taking care of patients with cancer.

The chapters are arranged in a logical order beginning with evaluation of symptoms and proceeding in an orderly fashion through the work-up, staging, and stage-directed therapy, and finally ending with discussion on epidemiology and current focus of research. We have embarked on this first edition of *The Washington Manual of Oncology* to provide a very practical manual that is helpful to medical residents, fellows in training, nurse practitioners, and other practitioners of clinical oncology. Our plan is to publish this book in a timely fashion every two years to keep the information current and up-to-date.

Ramaswamy Govindan, MD

Acknowledgments

First and foremost, I am delighted to welcome my dear colleague, Daniel Morgensztern, as the co-editor for this edition. Dan is a terrific clinician, clinical investigator and a walking encyclopedia of Medical Oncology. His hard work, diligence, commitment and passion have truly left an indelible mark on this edition. It is no exaggeration to say that this edition would not be in your hands without Dan's help. I am truly grateful to him.

Sadly, Jonathan Pine, Senior Executive Editor at Wolters Kluwer, passed away a year ago. Jonathan had worked with me for the past 12 years. He was instrumental in guiding the production of the first two editions and initiated the process for this edition. I will miss him very much.

I want to thank the individual contributors, who are all my dear and well-respected colleagues, for their efforts. As I have found over the years, a number of individuals also work behind the scenes to produce a book. At Wolters Kluwer, Julie Goolsby, Acquisitions Editor, and Emilie Moyer, Senior Product Development Editor, were instrumental in keeping the project moving and persistent with follow-up. Julie and Emilie were kind enough to accommodate our busy schedules and remarkably patient with our delays. I am very grateful for their insight, wisdom and patience. My administrative assistant Johanna Duke is a remarkable individual. Her thoughtful, intelligent, analytical and organized approach made the editing process an enjoyable one. She is a significant contributor to the success of this edition.

I am grateful to my nursing and secretarial staff for their help while I was busy working on this project. My work was made not only easy but also pleasurable by the great environment at Washington University School of Medicine in St. Louis. I owe a particular debt of gratitude to the leadership provided by the Chief of the Division of Oncology, John F. DiPersio, MD, PhD. Even though my two children Ashwin and Akshay are now in their teen years, they continue to be adorable (most of the time). I am forever grateful to my lovely wife, Prabha, and my two children who make everything worthwhile.

Ramaswamy Govindan, MD

I thank Ramaswamy Govindan for the opportunity to collaborate as a co-editor in this remarkable manual. He is an outstanding clinician and researcher, a role model for faculty and house staff, and has been my mentor since 2004. I also thank all the authors for their excellent chapters; Emilie Moyer from Wolters Kluwer and Johanna Duke from Washington University for their tireless efforts; my parents Silvia and Felipe Morgensztern; my lovely three children Alan, David, and Michael; and my beautiful wife Marcela.

Daniel Morgensztern, MD

Acknowledgments

Contents

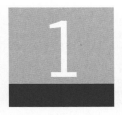

Cancer Biology— Basics of Molecular Oncogenesis

Elizabeth C. Chastain • John D. Pfeifer

I. SOURCES OF DNA DAMAGE

A. Endogenous sources of DNA damage. There are several constant, unavoidable sources of background DNA damage.

1. **Reactive oxygen species.** Reactive oxygen species (ROS) are byproducts of normal cellular metabolism and play important roles in cell signaling and homeostasis. The most common ROS include OH, NO, and peroxides. Increased environmental stress may dramatically increase ROS production, resulting in DNA damage. Collectively, these changes are known as oxidative damage and include sugar and base modifications, DNA–DNA and DNA–protein cross-links, and DNA strand breaks. ROS can also be generated by exogenous sources such as ionizing radiation, pollutants, and tobacco.

2. **Spontaneous chemical reactions.** The most common spontaneous chemical changes that alter the structure of DNA are deamination and depurination reactions, although spontaneous hydrolysis, alkylation, and adduction reactions may also occur. The mutagenic potential of the different types of reactions varies.

3. **Metal ions.** Although the evidence for DNA damage by endogenous metals is especially substantial for iron and copper, nickel, chromium, magnesium, and cadmium are also well-established human carcinogens. Metal-catalyzed reactions produce DNA adducts, resulting in a wide variety of organic compound metabolites. Metals such as arsenic, cadmium, lead, and nickel also directly inhibit DNA repair, which augments the mutagenic potential of the DNA damage they induce.

B. Exogenous sources of DNA damage

1. **Chemicals.** Although a virtually infinite number of chemicals can damage DNA, a few families of environmental and therapeutic compounds illustrate the general mechanisms involved.

    a. **Polycyclic aromatic hydrocarbons (PAHs) and related compounds.** These molecules are converted into reactive intermediate metabolites by the normal physiologic action of cytochrome P-450, a process termed metabolic activation. These reactive intermediates are responsible for DNA damage through the formation of DNA adducts. Variation in the balance between metabolic activation and detoxification influences cancer rates.

    b. **Antineoplastic agents.** Cell cycle–specific therapies include antimetabolites (i.e., 5-fluorouracil, 6-mercaptopurine, and methotrexate) that interfere with nucleotide production, and taxanes (i.e., docetaxel, paclitaxel) and vinca alkaloids, both of which disrupt microtubule formation. Cell cycle–nonspecific drugs include cytotoxic alkylating agents (i.e., cyclophosphamide, busulfan, nitrogen mustard, and thiotepa) that result in DNA damage through the formation of covalent linkages producing alkylated nucleotides, DNA–DNA cross-links, DNA–protein cross-links, and DNA strand breaks; anthracyclines (i.e., daunorubicin, doxorubicin) that inhibit topoisomerase II; and platinum-based therapies (i.e., carboplatin, cisplatin) that act primarily by causing intrastrand and interstrand cross-links.

2. **Radiation.** DNA damage caused by radiation can be classified into damage caused by ultraviolet radiation (UV light) and damage caused by ionizing radiation.

    a. **UV light.** UV-B radiation from sunlight (wavelength 280 to 315 nm) produces cyclobutane pyrimidine dimers (due to covalent bonds between adjacent thymine residues within the same strand of DNA) as well as pyrimidine (6-4) pyrimidone photoproducts (due to covalent bonds between TC or CC dimers within the same strand of DNA). Damage caused by UV-A radiation (wavelength 315 to 400 nm) is usually due to ROS-mediated mechanisms.

b. Ionizing radiation. A broad spectrum of DNA damage is caused by ionizing radiation, including individual base lesions, cross-links, and single- and double-strand breaks. Low linear energy transfer (LET) radiation (x-rays, γ-rays, electrons, and β-particles have a typical LET of less than 10 keV/μm) and high-LET radiation (protons and neutrons have a typical LET of 10 to 100 keV/μm, whereas α-particles have an LET greater than 175 keV/μm) each produce a characteristic pattern of damage.

II. TYPES OF DNA ALTERATIONS

A. Single base pair substitutions. Single base pair (bp) substitutions are among the most commonly observed mutations and may be a consequence of numerous processes, including errors in DNA replication, spontaneous chemical reactions, ROS damage, chemical mutagenesis, ionizing radiation, and failure of DNA repair mechanisms. Coding and noncoding regions are almost equally susceptible to this type of alteration.

A single bp substitution occurring within the coding sequence of a gene can lead to a significant change in the encoded amino acid, but does not cause a shift in the translational reading frame. These substitutions are classified into synonymous mutations and nonsynonymous mutations. Synonymous mutations are those in which a different codon still specifies the same amino acid and the vast majority of these changes are neutral. There are two types of nonsynonymous mutations, consisting of missense mutations (resulting in a codon that specifies a different amino acid) and nonsense mutations (production of a stop codon). The extent of disruption caused by missense mutations depends on the chemical similarities or differences between the two amino acids. Depending on the location, nonsense mutations may lead to premature termination and reduced protein function.

Single bp substitutions that occur outside the coding region of a gene can still be deleterious. Substitutions in the 5' regulatory region of a gene can alter the pattern of gene expression, and substitutions in introns, exons, or untranslated regions of a gene can affect RNA processing.

B. Gross gene deletions. There are two types of recombination events that give rise to gross gene deletions. Homologous unequal recombination occurs at homologous sequences that are not paired precisely, generally at related gene sequences or repetitive sequence elements, resulting in rejoining of homologous but nonallelic DNA sequences. Regions of repetitive sequences are especially prone to unequal crossovers and are the site of many large-scale deletions, as well as insertions, duplications, amplifications, inversions, and translocations. Nonhomologous recombination (illegitimate recombination) occurs between DNA loci that have minimal or no sequence homology.

C. Gene conversion. This type of mutation is a nonreciprocal transfer of sequence information between two loci. One of the interacting sequences (the donor or source) remains unchanged, whereas the alternative sequence (the acceptor or target) is altered by partial or total replacement by the donor sequence. Gene families with tandem repeats and clusters are particularly prone to this type of alteration.

D. Short gene deletions. The mutation rate at some microsatellites is remarkably high. Because the mutant alleles differ from the wild type by a single repeat unit without exchange of flanking markers, the proposed mechanism involves misalignment of the short direct repeats during DNA replication (due to so-called polymerase slippage).

E. Insertions. Polymerase slippage can account for short insertions just as it can for short deletions. Homologous unequal recombination between repetitive sequence elements provides a mechanism for the generation of larger insertions (which may actually be gene duplications).

F. Expansion of unstable repeat sequences. A small subset of tandem trinucleotide repeats, as well as a very limited number of longer repeats, shows anomalous behavior that causes abnormal gene expression. Repeats above a certain threshold length become extremely unstable and are virtually never transmitted unchanged from parent to child. Genes containing unstable expanding trinucleotide repeats can be grouped into two major classes: one includes genes that show very large expansions outside coding sequences, while the other class consists of genes that show modest expansion within coding sequences.

G. **Inversions.** A high degree of sequence similarity between repeats on the same chromosome may predispose to inversions by a mechanism that involves bending back of the chromatid upon itself in a process that is essentially homologous intrachromosomal recombination. Inversions not associated with significant sequence homology are apparently the result of nonhomologous recombination.

H. **Illegitimate recombination.** The RAG enzyme, responsible for the double-stranded DNA breaks that underlie the V(D)J recombination of antigen receptor genes, occasionally cuts DNA at unrelated loci that have complementary recombination signals, producing a translocation.

I. **Mitochondrial DNA damage and mutations.** Mitochondrial DNA (mtDNA) is susceptible to damage by the same processes responsible for nuclear DNA damage. ROS are an especially important source of damage, given the proximity of mtDNA to the reactive intermediates produced by the electron transport/oxidative phosphorylation of the respiratory chain. Although the types of mtDNA mutation are similar to those of nuclear DNA, the unique features of mitochondrial genetics result in an entirely different pattern of phenotype–genotype correlations.

III. **DNA REPAIR.** Only rarely does DNA repair occur through simple chemical reversal of the damage; usually, it entails excision of altered DNA followed by resynthesis. However, it is important to emphasize that many DNA alterations, including insertions, deletions, duplications, inversions, and translocations, are not targets of DNA repair pathways and are therefore highly mutagenic.

A. **Direct repair.** Human cells produce very few enzymes capable of directly reversing DNA damage. One such enzyme is O6-alkyguanine DNA alkyltransferase, produced by the O6-methylguanine methyltransferase (MGMT) gene. It removes the naturally occurring mutagenic nonnative methyl group from O6-methylguanine, restoring the base to guanine. This dealkylation reaction is significant because the altered base incorrectly pairs with thymine and hence is highly mutagenic. More recently, a set of enzymes has been discovered to catalyze the oxidative demethylation of 1-methyladenine and 3-methycytosine.

B. **Base excision repair.** A major source of DNA damage includes small chemical alterations. Base excision repair (BER) is responsible for repair of oxidized bases and alkylated bases, and is also responsible for correction of spontaneous depurination events, single-strand breaks, and some mismatched bases. While these lesions do not typically impede transcription or DNA replication, they are especially prone to produce mutations, and BER plays a crucial role in maintaining the integrity of the genome.

C. **Nucleotide excision repair.** This is the most versatile DNA repair pathway, in which the damaged or incorrect portion of a DNA strand is excised and the resulting gap is filled by repair replication using the complementary strand as a template. Lesions repaired by nucleotide excision repair (NER) typically serve as structural inhibitors to transcription and replication due to distortion of the helical conformation secondary to interference of normal base pairing.

D. **Transcription-coupled repair.** NER and BER are inefficient at repairing damage to the transcribed DNA strand of the actively expressed loci secondary to RNA polymerase II stalling at the site of the damage and sterically hindering repair. Because the stalled RNA polymerase effectively inactivates the gene, independent of whether the DNA damage would cause a mutation affecting gene function, transcription-coupled repair not only corrects DNA damage but also restores gene expression.

E. **Mismatch repair.** The mismatch repair (MMR) system corrects nucleotides mispaired by DNA polymerases within an otherwise complementary paired DNA strand. This repair mechanism can also excise small insertion/deletion loops of single-stranded DNA that result from polymerase slippage during replication of repetitive sequences or arise during recombination. The importance of this repair mechanism in maintaining genetic stability is illustrated by the observation that its absence results in mutation rates up to 1,000 times higher than normal, with a particular tendency for errors within short tandem repeats or homopolymeric stretches.

F. Translesion synthesis. The polymerases primarily responsible for replication of nuclear DNA are hampered when they encounter a chemically altered base. Translesion synthesis is a DNA damage tolerance process occurring in the vicinity of the DNA lesion that proceeds via replacement of the conventional polymerase by one or several specialized polymerases that have the ability to replicate damaged DNA. This process manages to effectively replicate damaged nuclear DNA templates despite the almost limitless diversity of DNA lesions. However, translesion synthesis polymerases display low fidelity replication of nondamaged templates, lack a proofreading function, and have flexible base-pairing properties. Hence, the capability of replicating damaged DNA through this mechanism comes at the expense of a high error rate.

G. Recombinatorial repair. Unrepaired double-strand breaks (DSBs) are highly disruptive events that interfere with proper chromosome segregation during cell division and often induce various chromosomal aberrations including aneuploidy, deletions, and chromosomal translocations. The two main DSB repair mechanisms are homologous recombination and nonhomologous end joining. Both initiate a cascade of kinase reactions that not only recruit repair factors to the site of the break, but also delay or terminate the cell cycle through DNA damage checkpoint control. The exact mechanism of cross-link repair in human cells remains unknown.

H. Defective DNA damage repair. Some of the most striking examples of hereditary cancer syndromes are due to mutations affecting genes involved in DNA repair, which emphasizes the fundamental role of repair pathways in oncogenesis.

1. Defective BER. The most direct evidence linking the role of BER in cancer comes from germline mutations in the MYH gene, which produces a glycosylase responsible for removing adenine mispaired with 8-oxoguanine or guanine. Mutations lead to recessive inheritance of multiple colorectal adenomas.

2. Defective NER. At least four photosensitivity-related syndromes have been attributed to inborn errors in NER including the autosomal recessive xeroderma pigmentosum, the brittle hair disorder trichothiodystrophy, UV sensitivity syndrome (UVSS), and a clinical disorder that combines features of both xeroderma pigmentosum and Cockayne syndrome.

3. Defective transcription-coupled repair. Inborn defects in transcription-coupled repair are associated with Cockayne syndrome.

4. Defective MMR. Defective MMR facilitates malignant transformation through the production of mutations in genes that harbor microsatellites in their coding regions, some of which have critical roles in the regulation of cell growth and apoptosis (e.g., TGFBR2 gene, which encodes the transforming growth factor β receptor II, and the BAX gene, which encodes a proapoptotic protein). Defects in MMR genes are responsible for hereditary nonpolyposis colorectal carcinoma (HNPCC). However, it is important to recognize that although microsatellite instability can be demonstrated in a variety of malignancies, in most cases the phenotype is due to somatic rather than germline mutations at MMR loci.

5. Defective translesion synthesis. Defective replication of damaged DNA due to inherited mutations in one of the translesion polymerases is responsible for xeroderma pigmentosum variant.

6. Defective double-strand break and cross-link repair. Diseases associated with impaired double-strand break repair by homologous recombination include ataxia telangiectasia, ataxia telangiectasia–like disorder, Nijmegen breakage syndrome, Fanconi anemia, familial breast–ovarian cancer syndrome, Werner's syndrome, Bloom's syndrome, and Rothmund–Thomson syndrome. Prominent clinical features shared by these diseases include radiosensitivity, genomic instability, cancer susceptibility, and immunodeficiency.

IV. VIRUSES. Several RNA and DNA viruses are associated with the development of malignancies.

A. RNA viruses. Three RNA viruses associated with malignancies include two retroviruses, human T-lymphotropic virus (HTLV-1) and human immunodeficiency virus (HIV), and the flavivirus hepatitis C virus (HCV).

1. **Retroviruses.** In general, oncogenic retroviruses can be classified into two main groups on the basis of disease-causing mechanisms. Acute transforming retroviruses are typically replication defective and cause rapid induction of tumors because they carry viral oncogenes. On the other hand, nonacute retroviruses (of which HTLV-1 is an example) are replication competent and do not carry oncogenes but rather exert their oncogenic effects by integrating within or adjacent to a cellular proto-oncogene. Retroviruses that cause immunodeficiency (of which HIV is an example) apparently promote oncogenesis only indirectly, most likely as a consequence of the immunosuppression associated with infection.

2. **Flaviviruses.** HCV infection alone is not sufficient to give rise to hepatocellular carcinoma (HCC), and oncogenesis is thought to develop as a result of the increased cellular turnover caused by long-term hepatocyte necrosis and regeneration, fibrosis, and inflammation associated with infection.

B. DNA viruses. DNA viruses from several different families have oncogenic properties.

1. **Hepadnaviruses.** Hepatitis B virus (HBV) encodes a gene (known as X) that is involved in transcriptional activation and signal transduction and has been implicated to contribute directly to tumorigenesis. Additionally, the virus can contribute to oncogenesis through direct insertional mutagenesis. However, HBV primarily promotes hepatocellular carcinogenesis indirectly, occurring most likely through increased cellular turnover caused by long-term hepatocyte necrosis and regeneration, fibrosis, and inflammation associated with infection.

2. **Herpesviruses**
   a. Epstein–Barr virus (EBV) is associated with the oncogenesis of lymphoid malignancies (including Burkitt lymphoma and classical Hodgkin lymphoma), gastric cancer, and nasopharyngeal carcinoma. The viral genome encodes more than 100 genes (including several that play a direct role in cellular transformation) and numerous microRNAs (miRNA).
   b. Kaposi sarcoma–associated herpesvirus (KSHV), also known as human herpes virus-8 (HHV-8), is associated with the development of Kaposi sarcoma, primary effusion lymphoma, and multicentric Castleman's disease. KSHV encodes many genes related to tumor development, including cyclins, inhibitors of apoptosis, and cytokines, all of which are candidates for contributing to viral oncogenesis.

3. **Papillomaviruses.** Human papillomavirus (HPV) is associated with cervical cancer, other anogenital cancers, and a subset of squamous carcinomas of the head and neck, particularly those of the oropharynx. The high-risk, cancer-associated serotypes (most commonly, HPV-16 and HPV-18) harbor two principal transforming genes, E6 and E7. The E6 protein inactivates p53, and the E7 protein interacts with the retinoblastoma (RB1) gene product. However, E6 and E7 alone are insufficient for carcinogenesis. The development of a fully transformed cellular phenotype requires alterations in a number of cellular pathways. It remains unclear why only a subset of patients infected with high-risk HPV serotypes eventually develop malignant disease.

4. **Polyomavirus.** The most recently described viral-associated malignancy is Merkel cell carcinoma, caused by Merkel cell polyomavirus (MCPyV). This rare but highly aggressive neuroendocrine skin cancer arises in elderly, immunosuppressed, and immunodeficient patients. MCPyV integrates into the host genome and may mediate oncogenesis through inactivation of the tumor suppressor pRB.

V. INDIVIDUAL GENES THAT ARE TARGETS OF ONCOGENIC MUTATIONS.
According to the clonal model of carcinogenesis, a malignant tumor arises from a single cell. This founder cell acquires an initial mutation that provides its progeny with a selective growth advantage, and from within this expanded population, another single cell acquires a second mutation that provides an additional growth advantage, and so on, until a fully transformed malignant tumor emerges. Tumor suppressor genes and oncogenes are frequent targets of mutation in this multistep process of tumor evolution.

A. Tumor suppressor genes. Normal cellular functions of tumor suppressor gene products are highly diverse, including regulation of the cell cycle, cell differentiation, apoptosis, and maintenance of genomic integrity. Dozens of tumor suppressor genes have been identified, and numerous potential candidates have been described. Many of these genes were identified by virtue of the fact that they are mutated in the germline of persons who are affected by cancer syndromes; nevertheless, for the vast majority of tumor suppressor genes, somatic mutations play a far more significant role in cancer development than do germline mutations. Tumor suppressor genes have been broadly divided into two classes, gatekeepers and caretakers.

1. **Gatekeepers.** This group directly regulates cell growth by inhibiting cellular proliferation or promoting apoptosis; familiar examples include the products of RB1, TP53, APC, NF1, NF2, WT1, MEN1, and VHL genes. Because the functions of the proteins encoded by gatekeeper genes are rate-limiting for tumor growth, tumor development occurs only when both copies of the gene are inactivated. Individuals with an autosomal dominant cancer susceptibility syndrome inherit one damaged copy, and so require only one somatic mutation to inactivate the remaining wild-type allele and initiate tumor formation. Nonetheless, inactivating mutations of both alleles of a gatekeeper are still insufficient for acquisition of a fully transformed malignant phenotype. Gatekeepers vary with tissue type, and so germline inactivation of a particular gatekeeper gene leads to only specific forms of cancer predisposition.

2. **Caretakers.** These genes are responsible for DNA repair and genomic maintenance; therefore, when inactivated by mutations, these genes indirectly facilitate oncogenesis by promoting an increased rate of mutation. Genes that encode proteins involved in DNA repair are the classic examples of caretakers, including MSH2, MLH1, PMS1, ATM, XPA through XPG, and FANCA through FNACL.

B. **Oncogenes.** The normally functioning cellular counterparts, termed proto-oncogenes, are important regulators of many aspects of cell physiology, including cell growth and differentiation. More than 75 proto-oncogenes have been identified, and their products include extracellular cytokines and growth factors (e.g., int-1 and int-2), transmembrane growth factor receptors (e.g., c-erb2/EGFR, HER2/neu, src, c-abl, c-ret, H-ras, K-ras, and N-ras), cytoplasmic kinases (e.g., BRAF), and nuclear proteins involved in the control of DNA replication (e.g., c-myc, N-myc, L-myc, c-myb).

Oncogenes represent mutated forms of proto-oncogenes, resulting in neoplastic transformation. Despite their variety, oncogenes can be divided into two general groups on the basis of the mechanism of their action. One group induces continuous or unregulated cell proliferation by inactivation of growth inhibitory signals, or by activation of growth-promoting genes, growth factors, receptors, intracellular signaling pathways, or nuclear oncoproteins. The other group immortalizes cells by rescuing them from senescence and apoptosis. Accumulated evidence from human malignancies and transgenic animal models indicates that mutation of a single oncogene is insufficient for acquisition of a fully transformed, malignant phenotype.

Only a few inherited cancer syndromes are due to germline mutations in oncogenes. Instead, most oncogene mutations are somatic and therefore associated with sporadic malignancies. For many tumor types, the involved oncogene and the type of mutation are characteristic.

VI. **INTRACELLULAR PATHWAYS THAT ARE TARGETS OF ONCOGENIC MUTATIONS**

A. **Signal transduction.** In the context of oncology, important signal transduction pathways are those that regulate cellular proliferation, differentiation, and death, often through regulation of gene transcription. Signal transduction pathways have evolved to respond to an enormous variety of stimuli and are highly interconnected to permit dynamic regulation of the strength, duration, and timing of cell responses. Many of the genes involved in signal transduction are classified as tumor suppressor genes and oncogenes.

1. **Ligands.** The various types of ligands include proteins (soluble, cell bound, and matrix), individual amino acids, lipids, gases, and soluble and polymerized nucleotides.

2. **Receptors.** Examples of cell surface receptors include receptor tyrosine kinases, serine kinases, and phosphatases; members of the Notch family; and G protein-coupled receptors. The guanylate cyclase family of receptors provides an example of related receptors that can be either membrane bound or soluble. The transcription factors that bind glucocorticoids, thyroxine, and vitamin D are examples of receptors that are located in the nucleus.

3. Signal propagation. Many ligand–receptor interactions transmit signals through small molecule second messengers, which then bind noncovalently to protein targets and affect their function. Examples of small molecule second messengers include cyclic adenosine monophosphate (cAMP), phospholipases (that generate inositol triphosphate and diacylglycerol), Ca^{2+}, and eicosanoids.

B. Regulation of the cell cycle. Cell proliferation is rigorously regulated to preserve function and integrity throughout development and adult life. Many signal transduction pathways specifically regulate promitogenic and antimitogenic proteins that control the cell cycle including the A-, B-, D-, and E-type cyclins, cyclin-dependent kinases (CDKs), and the skp, cullin, F-box containing (SCF) and anaphase-promoting complex or cyclosome (APC/C) families of protein-ubiquitin ligases. Not surprisingly, many of the genes involved in cell cycle regulation are commonly mutated or show an altered pattern of expression in a variety of human malignancies.

C. Cell cycle checkpoints. Progression through the cell cycle prior to repair of DNA damage is potentially harmful; therefore, a number of cell cycle checkpoints are employed to allow for proper DNA repair. These DNA damage checkpoints occur before S phase entry, during S phase, and before M phase entry. Additional cell cycle checkpoints include a replication checkpoint (that ensures DNA replication is complete prior to initiation of M phase), a spindle integrity checkpoint (that ensures appropriate partitioning of the chromosomes occurs before initiation of anaphase during mitosis), and a restriction checkpoint (that blocks cell cycle progression at mid-G1 phase in the absence of essential growth factors or nutrients). Loss of function of one or more of these checkpoints is a characteristic feature of many malignancies.

D. Apoptosis. Signal transduction pathways control not only cell proliferation but also programmed cell death. Apoptosis is a genetic pathway for rapid and efficient killing of unnecessary or damaged cells, which can be divided into two distinct but not mutually exclusive signaling pathways known as extrinsic and intrinsic apoptosis. Extrinsic apoptosis is elicited by the ligand-induced activation of plasma membrane proteins of the death receptor family, such as CD95/FAS and the tumor necrosis factor-α 1. Provocation of this pathway leads to downstream activation of proteolytic caspases (final effectors of the apoptotic pathway). Several cellular inhibitor of apoptosis proteins (IAPs), including cIAP1, cIAP2, and XIAP, are able to inhibit apoptosis as a result of their ability to interfere with caspase activation. Intrinsic apoptosis (also known as mitochondrial apoptosis) is regulated by the integrity of mitochondrial structure and function. If proapoptotic signals are predominant, mitochondrial membranes become permeable and release proteins such as cytochrome C, endonuclease G, Smac/DIABLO, and HTRA2 that lead to activation of caspases. In both pathways, control of apoptosis is achieved through regulation of the proapoptotic proteins BAX and BAK and the antiapoptotic proteins BCL-2, BCL-XL, and MCL-1.

Not surprisingly, there is substantial cross-talk between cellular proliferation and apoptosis pathways, often focused at various cell cycle checkpoints. Mutations or alterations in the level of expression of pro- and antiapoptotic proteins are characteristic of many human malignancies.

E. Telomere metabolism. The telomere is the nucleoprotein complex present at the end of each chromatid that functions to protect the chromosome. The enzyme telomerase catalyzes the unique reaction by which the long TTAGGG tandem repeat arrays of the telomere are synthesized. Telomerase activity is tightly controlled, although the details of the different regulatory mechanisms are not fully understood. Dysfunctions of telomerase maintenance have an important role in tumorigenesis as well as in genomic instability, since chromosomes lacking a telomere are unstable and tend to fuse with other broken chromosomes, undergo recombination, or get degraded.

VII. EXTRACELLULAR PATHWAYS THAT ARE TARGETS OF ONCOGENIC MUTATIONS

A. Angiogenesis. Tumor growth requires the development of an adequate blood supply, known as angiogenesis. Two types of angiogenesis have been described. Sprouting angiogenesis occurs through branching of new capillaries from preexisting capillaries, a process that includes degradation of the basement membrane, migration of endothelial cells in the direction of the angiogenic stimulus, endothelial cell proliferation, and capillary tube formation.

Nonsprouting angiogenesis occurs through proliferation of endothelial cells within preexisting vessels, with subsequent lumen enlargement, splitting, or fusion. It has been calculated that any increase in tumor size beyond a diameter of 0.5 mm requires angiogenesis.

Angiogenesis requires induction or elevated expression of one or more proangiogenic growth factors, coinciding with the downregulation with one or more endogenous inhibitors within the local tissue environment. The proangiogenic and antiangiogenic factors are produced by tumor cells, inflammatory cells, and adjacent normal tissue cells, and their levels are regulated by interdependent stimuli such as tissue hypoxia (mediated through the hypoxia-inducible factor-1 [HIF-1] pathway), tissue pH, and soluble growth factors. Proangiogenic molecules bind to specific receptors on endothelial cells, smooth muscle cells, and pericytes, and include members of the vascular endothelial growth factor (VEGF) family, members of the angiopoietin (Ang) family, members of the fibroblast growth factor (FGF) family, epidermal growth factor (EGF), platelet-derived growth factor (PDGF), and various chemokines. Endogenous inhibitors of angiogenesis include extracellular matrix glycoproteins (e.g., thrombospondin-1 (TSP-1), endostatin, tumstatin, canstatin), members of clotting/coagulation cascade family (e.g., angiostatin), and vasostatin (which is a fragment of calreticulin). Another recently described regulator is the Notch receptor-DLL4 signaling pathway, a system that mediates embryonic angiogenesis but appears to function as an inhibitor of tumor angiogenesis in adults.

B. Invasion and metastasis. Metastasis is the spread of cancer from the organ of origin (primary site) to distant tissues and consists of a series of interrelated steps known as the metastatic cascade. The metastatic cascade includes detachment of a tumor cell (or cells) from surrounding cells; migration through the stroma and basement membrane into the lumen of a capillary, venule, or lymphatic; intravascular survival; arrest within a capillary bed with subsequent adherence to the wall; extravasation into adjacent tissue; and proliferation with associated angiogenesis and evasion of host defenses. This cascade is dependent on numerous alterations in tumor cells including motility, cell migration, protease expression, and autocrine and paracrine growth factor expression.

1. **Cell motility.** A number of stimuli increase cell motility, including tumor-secreted molecules, local tissue microenvironment-derived factors, and growth factors. Tumor-secreted molecules generally function in autocrine loops.

2. **Cell migration.** A process central to cell migration includes diminished cell surface adhesion to produce an altered pattern of tumor cell interaction with the intercellular matrix and nonneoplastic cells. Important adhesion molecules include members of the cadherin family, members of the Ig superfamily (especially VCAM-1 and NCAM), and integrins.

3. **Proteases.** Tumor cells must produce a number of proteases that are required in order to mediate cellular changes required for migration through the extracellular matrix and connective tissue barriers. The group of proteases that has been most extensively studied is the matrix metalloproteinases (MMPs), which are inhibited by tissue inhibitors of metalloproteinases (TIMPs).

4. **Autocrine and paracrine growth factors.** Growth factors produced by transformed cells as well as nonneoplastic cells are required for many steps in the metastatic cascade. The role of nonneoplastic cells in the local tissue microenvironment is increasingly being recognized as a significant source of various growth factors.

VIII. EPIGENETIC REGULATORS. Epigenetic processes not only play important roles during development, but are also involved in maintaining tissue-specific patterns of gene expression in differentiated cells. Almost all human cancers contain substantial epigenetic abnormalities that cooperate with genetic lesions to generate a transformed phenotype. Epigenetic changes tend to arise early in carcinogenesis, often preceding somatic mutations, and allow orchestration of activation and silencing pathways.

A. DNA methylation. The addition of methyl groups to cytosine residues of CpG dinucleotides to form 5-methylcytosine is catalyzed by DNA methyltransferases (DNMTs). Methylation typically occurs within CpG-rich regions (known as CpG islands) that are often distributed in the transcriptional start sites (TSS) of regulatory regions (i.e., promoter/

enhancer regions) of genes. Increased methylation in these regions often (but not always) leads to epigenetic silencing, as often occurs for tumor suppressor genes. Additional gene expression defects linked to alterations in DNA methylation patterns involve the family of Tet methylcytosine dioxygenase proteins (TET1, TET2, and TET3) and isocitrate dehydrogenase genes (IDH1 and IDH2). Of note, hypomethylation caused by mutations in genes responsible for DNA methylation has also been suggested to play a role in several cancer types.

B. Chromatin modifiers. Active chromatin remodeling is essential for development and maintenance of normal physiologic functions, but becomes pathologically altered in cancer, leading to widespread mitotically heritable aberrations in gene expression that are characteristic of oncogenesis. The chromatin modifiers include proteins that transfer or remove acetyl or methyl modifications from histone tails, alter the position of nucleosomes along the DNA, remove nucleosomes from DNA entirely, or change the histone composition of nucleosomes in specific regions of the genome. Other proteins, known as readers, interpret these modifications and further alter local chromatin structure to either stimulate or repress gene expression.

C. RNA interference. Several classes of double- or single-stranded RNA molecules also have a role in regulation of gene expression, including short interfering RNA (siRNA), micro-RNA (miRNA), small modulatory RNA (smRNA), and long noncoding RNA (lncRNA). Also referred to as RNA interference (RNAi), RNA-mediated control of gene expression is abnormal in many malignancies.

IX. THE CANCER GENOME AND PERSONALIZED MEDICINE. Because cancer is essentially a genetic disease caused by accumulation of molecular alterations in the genome of somatic cells, advances in the knowledge of these alterations and the technologies to detect them are transforming the field of oncology. New paradigms are emerging including a shift in tumor taxonomy from histology to genetic-based, development of drugs that target specific molecular alterations, individualized treatments focused on matching patients with targeted therapy for their tumor, and the use of specific genetic alterations as highly sensitive biomarkers for disease monitoring.

A. Next-generation sequencing. Within the last decade, several next-generation sequencing (NGS) platforms have been developed that enable high-throughput DNA sequencing of large sets of genes, whole exomes, or even whole genomes from tissue samples at a reasonable cost and a short turnaround time. These NGS methods provide several advantages over traditional Sanger sequencing methods including increased sensitivity and simultaneous detection of numerous types of DNA alterations (single nucleotide variants, copy number alterations, insertions and deletions, and structural rearrangements). However, NGS approaches require very sophisticated bioinformatic analytic methods, since it is a complicated process to assemble hundreds of millions of short sequences and map them to a reference genome. With so-called deep sequence coverage, careful validation, and highly specialized bioinformatic pipelines, many groups have demonstrated that NGS can be used to guide the routine care of cancer patients.

B. "Passenger" and "Driver" mutations. At the time of diagnosis, cancer is comprised of billions of cells carrying a wide array of DNA alterations. Some of these acquired alterations have a functional role in malignant proliferation ("drivers"), but many have no functional role in tumorigenesis ("passengers").

It is becoming clear that only a minor fraction of genetic alterations are likely responsible for driving cancer evolution by providing cells a selective advantage over their neighbors. However, in many cases, passenger and driver mutations occur at similar frequencies, and proper classification remains a challenge in cancer genetics. Approaches to distinguish drivers from passengers include identification of recurrent mutations within a specific amino acid or adjacent amino acids, in a small region of a protein, or in evolutionarily conserved residues.

C. Optimizing treatment. Many large-scale studies such as The Cancer Genome Project (TCGA) and the International Cancer Genome Consortium (ICGC) have identified novel genes as potential therapeutic targets in various types of cancer. Although these studies have demonstrated that the repertoire of oncogenic mutations in several types of cancer is extremely heterogeneous, they have made it possible to define clinically relevant tumor subtypes that can be best managed with therapies tailored to the underlying specific mutations.

SUGGESTED READINGS

Bozic I, Antal T, Ohtsuki H, et al. Accumulation of driver and passenger mutations during tumor progression. *Proc Natl Acad Sci USA* 2010;107:18545–18550.

Campos EI, Reinberg D. Histones: annotating chromatin. *Annu Rev Genet* 2009;43:559–599.

Jinek M, Doudna JA. A three-dimensional view of the molecular machinery of RNA interference. *Nature* 2009;457:405–412.

Laird PW. Principles and challenges of genome wide DNA methylation analysis. *Nat Rev Genet* 2010;11:191–203.

López CA, Cleary JD, Pearson CE. Repeat instability and the basis for human diseases and as a potential target for therapy. *Nat Rev Mol Cell Biol* 2010;11:165–170.

Nguyen DX, Box PD, Massaqué J. Metastasis: from dissemination to organ-specific colonization. *Nat Rev Cancer* 2009;9:274–284.

Pfeifer JD. DNA damage, mutations, and repair. In: *Molecular Genetic Testing in Surgical Pathology*. Philadelphia, PA: Lippincott Williams & Wilkins, 2006:29–57.

Schultz DR, Harrington WJ Jr. Apoptosis: programmed cell death at a molecular level. *Semin Arthritis Rheum* 2003;32:345–369.

Weinberg RA. *Biology of Cancer*. 2nd ed. New York, NY: Garland Science Publishers, 2013.

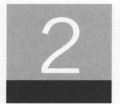

Molecular Diagnostics

Ian S. Hagemann • Christina M. Lockwood
• Catherine E. Cottrell

I. ROLE OF MOLECULAR DIAGNOSTICS. Clinical application of insights derived from molecular genetic research studies has become increasingly important in patient care. Molecular analysis is useful for diagnosis, for prognosis or predicting response to various treatment options, for monitoring minimal residual disease (treatment efficacy), for identifying predisposition to disease, and for detection of therapeutic targets in gene-specific therapy. Clinical molecular diagnostic methods have been integrated into many laboratory disciplines (Table 2-1), and published guidelines and recommendations from both professional societies and regulatory agencies have been developed to assist in the development and performance of clinical molecular pathology testing.

Molecular testing has been practiced for several decades in surgical pathology in the form of immunohistochemistry, in which antibodies are used to detect and quantify the expression of specific proteins of diagnostic, prognostic, or therapeutic importance. However, in current common usage, *molecular diagnostics* refers to the analysis of changes in nucleic acids, either DNA or RNA, and most frequently implies direct mutation testing. Genetic testing protocols can be designed to detect heritable DNA variations or, as is usually the case in neoplastic diseases, somatic or acquired DNA variations limited to abnormal cells.

At the interface of genetic disorders and acquired mutations in sporadic cancers are familial cancer syndromes. Familial cancer syndromes are inherited disorders that place patients at increased risk for particular types of tumors. Tumors resulting from a predisposition syndrome differ from their sporadic counterparts in several respects: earlier age of onset, bilateral or multifocal tumors, occurrence in multiple family members, and occurrence in more than one generation of a family. The carriers of the increased risk inherit a genetic predisposition for tumor formation as an autosomal dominant trait; this risk factor is a gene-specific germline mutation that may be screened for in DNA isolated from circulating lymphocytes (or other nontumor tissue) of affected individuals rather than tumor tissue. The characterization of the specific genes underlying familial cancer syndromes has provided important insights into the nature of many tumor suppressor genes and oncogenes. Many examples of genes that confer a hereditary predisposition to cancer have been described and include *RB1* (retinoblastoma, osteosarcoma, leukemia, and lymphoma), *TP53* (Li–Fraumeni syndrome; bone and soft tissue sarcomas, breast cancer, leukemia, and brain tumors), *BRCA1* and *BRCA2* (breast, ovarian, colon, and prostate cancers), *APC* (adenomatous polyposis coli; colon carcinoma and osteomas), *MSH2, MLH1,* and *MSH6* (hereditary nonpolyposis colorectal cancer/Lynch syndrome; colon, endometrium, ovary, and stomach cancers), *RET* (multiple endocrine neoplasia type 2 and familial medullary thyroid cancer; medullary thyroid carcinoma and pheochromocytoma), *VHL* (von Hippel–Lindau disease; renal carcinoma and pheochromocytoma), *NF1* (neurofibromatosis; neurofibroma and optic gliomas), and many others. Notably, a subset of sporadic tumors also carries mutations in these genes.

A. Specimens. Specimen requirements are dictated by type of disease and type of test (analyte and methodology). Testing for constitutional disease can generally be performed on any tissue, while testing for acquired mutations requires submission of affected tissue. Since most, but not all, molecular diagnostic techniques are currently based on polymerase chain reaction (PCR) amplification, the amount of tissue required is relatively small, and so many routine pathology specimens can be analyzed effectively.

Regardless of specimen type, two general features of the tissue sample influence molecular pathology assays. First, there must be a sufficient quantity of the specific target cell, and therefore target DNA or RNA in the sample. If testing involves a clonal tumor admixed with normal cells, or a heterogeneous tissue specimen with many different gene expression patterns, a detection threshold must be defined. Second, since the size of the nucleic acid molecules after isolation from the tissue can dramatically affect the sensitivity of the detection of specific alterations, degradation (whether due to enzymatic, heat, pH, or mechanical forces) can reduce a specimen's suitability for testing.

1. **Tissue types.** Peripheral blood, bone marrow, solid tissue biopsies, and enriched cell populations (e.g., from flow cytometry) are all adequate substrates for molecular analysis. They should be collected and transported to the molecular pathology laboratory using aseptic techniques. Transport on ice reduces cell lysis, minimizes nuclease activity, and reduces nucleic acid degradation. Specimens are stored at 4°C after receipt in the laboratory.

2. **Tissue quality.** Appropriate handling of the specimen maximizes detection limits. Hematologic specimens (peripheral blood, bone marrow) should be collected in the presence of an anticoagulant, preferably ethylenediaminetetraacetic acid (EDTA) or acid citrate dextrose (ACD). Heparin anticoagulation is discouraged, as heparin carryover after nucleic acid isolation may inhibit subsequent PCR steps. Freezing solid tissue specimens after excision also yields good preservation of nucleic acids. However, frozen whole blood or bone marrow presents distinct obstacles to the preparation of good-quality nucleic acid and should be generally avoided.

   Formalin-fixed, paraffin-embedded tissue is suitable for many molecular diagnostic tests. Fixed tissue has several advantages, two of which are that fixation dramatically inhibits nucleic acid degradation and that fixed specimens can be easily stored and transported. However, a significant limitation of fixed tissue is that the quality of extracted nucleic acids is extremely variable because all fixatives, including formalin, chemically degrade nucleic acids to a greater or lesser extent.

   Specimens sent for cytogenetic testing require special handling techniques to preserve cell viability. Specimens should be transported to the cytogenetic laboratory as soon as possible, and should be drawn in sodium heparin collection tubes in the case of hematologic samples. Solid tissues may be transported in cell culture media. Cytogenetic specimens should never be frozen, but rather handled at room temperature for short periods or with a cold pack.

3. **Tissue quantity.** Minimum sample requirements are determined by the assay methodology and the extent of target cell involvement in the tissue submitted for analysis. Genomic Southern hybridization requires approximately 5 μg of DNA (approximately 10^6 cells) per enzymatic digest for detection of single copy genomic DNA targets; hybridization signals to detect lower-molecular-weight DNA fragments (less than

TABLE 2-1	Summary of Major Methodologies for Molecular Diagnostics in Clinical Use Today					
	Specimen requirement	Variants detected	Run time	Cost	Uses	Common examples in oncology testing
Restriction fragment length polymorphism (RFLP) analysis	DNA (10 ng scale)	SNV, indels	Hours	Low	Detect polymorphisms	Factor V Leiden and prothrombin polymorphisms
Polymerase chain reaction (PCR)	DNA (10 ng scale)	SNV, indels	Hours	Low	Detect short variations	NPM1 insertion in acute myeloid leukemia
Reverse transcriptase PCR (RT-PCR)	RNA (10 ng scale)	Large indels, SV, gene expression (quantitative)	Hours	Moderate	Measure size of repeats and rearranged segments	TCRG gene rearrangement
					Detect and size translocation products	Circulating BCR-ABL transcript burden in CML
					Measure expressed transcript levels	
Southern blot	DNA (µg scale)	CNV	Days	Moderate	Size indels too large for PCR	FUS-CHOP rearrangement in liposarcoma
Karyotyping	Dividing cells	CNV, SV	Days	Moderate	Detect large-scale chromosomal abnormalities (balanced and unbalanced)	Karyotype analysis in acute myeloid leukemia
Metaphase FISH	Dividing cells	CNV, SV	24 hours	Low	Detect translocations and aneuploidy	t(15;17) in acute promyelocytic leukemia
Interphase FISH	Viable cells or fixed tissue (paraffin-embedded)	CNV, SV	24 hours	Low	Detect translocations and aneuploidy	-5/5q-, -7/7q- in acute myeloid leukemia
						ALK translocation in non–small cell lung cancer

Method	Sample	Variant types	Turnaround	Cost	Capabilities	Clinical application
Chromosomal microarray analysis (SNP)	Viable cells or fixed tissue (paraffin-embedded)	CNV, LOH	Days	Moderate	Detect whole chromosome aneuploidy, moderate size CNV (kb) and LOH (no balanced rearrangements)	*IKZF1* deletion in B-cell ALL LOH in glioblastoma (1p, 10p, 10q,19q)
Sanger sequencing	DNA (10 ng scale)	SNV, small indels	Days	Moderate	Genotype specific nucleotide positions Confirm sequence results from other methods	Germline *RET* mutation in suspected multiple endocrine neoplasia
Next-generation sequencing	DNA (100 ng scale)	SNV, indels, SV, CNV	Days	High	Genotype numerous positions simultaneously	Whole-gene sequencing of multiple actionable genes in solid tumors (*EGFR, KIT, ERBB2, KRAS*)

CNV, copy-number variant; indel: insertion/deletion; LOH, loss of heterozygosity; SNV, single-nucleotide variant; SV, structural variant.

1 kb in length) may require more DNA. PCR amplification has significantly reduced DNA requirements, and typically only 20 to 200 ng of DNA (approximately 10^3 to 10^4 cells) is needed per reaction for many applications, though multiplexed PCR may require additional DNA to equally represent all targets. The sensitivity of PCR for detection of a few target molecules in a large background of unaltered DNA molecules (1 in 10^5) is one of the principal strengths of this methodology in molecular pathology.

B. Technical versus diagnostic aspects of testing. The analytical sensitivity and specificity of a molecular genetic test may be unrelated to its diagnostic sensitivity and specificity. Several factors influence the diagnostic sensitivity and specificity of a test, including the supposition that only a subset of cases of a specific tumor may harbor a characteristic mutation, more than one genetic abnormality may be associated with a specific tumor, and more than one tumor may share the same mutation. Thus, a molecular genetic method with perfect analytical performance can have a lower sensitivity and specificity when used for diagnostic or prognostic testing of patient samples. Differences between the analytical and diagnostic levels of analysis are often overlooked even though they account for many of the confusing or seemingly conflicting results regarding the utility of diagnostic molecular genetic testing in clinical practice.

    1. Reported estimates of test performance. The experimental design of published studies regarding the utility of molecular diagnosis varies considerably. Many studies of test performance are complicated by the presence of selection bias (also called verification bias, posttest referral bias, and workup bias) or discrepant analysis (also known as discordant analysis or review bias), which hinders interpretation of the test results in the setting of routine clinical practice.

    2. Discordant cases. Cases arise in which there is a lack of concordance between the diagnosis suggested by molecular genetic findings and the morphologic diagnosis. The debate over the best approach to resolve the ambiguity presented by these cases, especially those that are presumed false positives, reflects the fundamental impact of molecular genetics on the classification of disease as well as the power of morphology as the historic standard of pathologic diagnosis by which new methods of classification are measured. Rather than arbitrarily assuming that genetic testing or morphology is superior in all cases, the most reasonable way to handle discordant cases is to acknowledge the presence of the discrepancy, and to reappraise all the clinical data, pathologic findings, and therapeutic implications. For those cases in which the diagnosis suggested by morphology and genetic testing are different, prospective clinical trials are required to assess whether stage, prognosis, and response to treatment are more accurately predicted by the molecular test than by the morphologic findings on which current staging and treatment protocols are based.

C. Single-gene versus multigene testing. Despite the fact that molecular analysis of single markers has clinical value for many neoplasms, testing focused on individual loci is a reflection of the immaturity of molecular diagnostics rather than an optimized testing paradigm. Simultaneous analysis of multiple loci will likely provide more accurate diagnostic, prognostic, and therapeutic information. Consequently, clinical use of microarray and next-generation sequencing technologies that enable evaluation of thousands of markers from individual tumor specimens will likely expand.

II. CYTOGENETICS.
A number of specific cytogenetic abnormalities uniquely characterize morphologically and clinically distinct subsets of hematopoietic malignancies and solid tumors.

A. Traditional karyotype analysis. Metaphase chromosome analysis can be performed on many different cell types, although different sample and handling procedures may be required. Inappropriate handling, as well as delay between specimen collection and culture initiation, can markedly decrease the likelihood that the sample will grow in vitro. Communication and coordination with the cytogenetics laboratory are essential.

Traditional karyotype analysis begins with a period of in vitro cell culture of the tissue sample and may be aided by the presence of mitogens to stimulate cell division. After a period of time in culture, cells undergo a process known as harvesting to produce a cell preparation suitable for downstream analysis. During the harvest, cells are exposed to a hypotonic solution, which causes cell swelling and assists in aiding proper chromosome spreading, followed by fixation using a methanol–acetic acid mixture. At times a mitotic inhibitor may be used during harvest to arrest cells in metaphase. Slides are prepared by dropping the fixed cell suspension onto a glass microscope slide, followed by staining to allow for visualization.

The most widely used staining technique is termed G-banding and relies on an enzymatic digestion (often with trypsin) followed by treatment with Giemsa or Wright's stain to band the chromosomes. Chromosome resolution and quality are variable (dependent on the cell type, as well as the mode of preparation), but karyotype analysis is most often performed with a resolution of 400 to 600 bands per haploid set of chromosomes. Analysis is performed at a band-for-band level in order to identify structural and numeric chromosome abnormalities. Routine chromosome analysis of oncology specimens (bone marrow, involved peripheral blood, and tissue) requires band-for-band analysis of 20 metaphase cells. During analysis a karyogram is generated and serves as the representative image of the chromosomal complement of the cell displayed in a standard format. A standard clinical cytogenetics report will include information about the study performed, including banding technique, number of cells counted and analyzed, and banding resolution, as well as providing an interpretation, and a karyotype described according to the International System for Cytogenetic Nomenclature (ISCN).

1. **Advantages.** The power of conventional cytogenetic analysis lies in its ability to provide simultaneous analysis of the entire genome, albeit at low resolution, without requiring any foreknowledge of the chromosomal regions involved in the disease process. In many cases, the type and/or location of the identified chromosomal abnormalities can be used to aid in diagnosis or direct prognosis.

2. **Limitations.** The clinical utility of traditional chromosome analysis is restricted by two general features of the method. First, from a technical standpoint, analysis can be performed only on viable tissue specimens that contain actively dividing cells. Second, from a sensitivity standpoint, analysis has a resolution of only approximately 3 to 4 million base pairs (Mb) at an 850-band level, and only approximately 7 to 8 Mb at a 400-band level. Consequently, traditional chromosome analysis is suited only for the detection of numerical abnormalities and gross structural rearrangements; the method does not have the sensitivity to detect small copy number alterations, small insertion and deletion events, or single-nucleotide variation.

B. **Fluorescence in situ hybridization.** Use of nucleic acid probes labeled with fluorochromes and visualized through fluorescence microscopy has revolutionized in situ hybridization for detection of abnormalities in chromosome number and chromosome structure. Fluorescence in situ hybridization (FISH) probes may be categorically described as unique sequence probes, repetitive sequence probes, or whole chromosome probes. The most commonly used probe type is that which hybridizes to unique sequence in the genome. Unique sequence probes may be used to detect changes in the copy number of a specific locus (e.g., *TP53*), or to assay for rearrangements involving a specific locus (such as *BCR-ABL* or *PML-RARA*). Repetitive sequence probes hybridize to sequences that are present in hundreds to thousands of copies, and so produce strong signals; the most widely used probes of this type bind to α-satellite sequences of centromeres. β-satellite sequences, Y-chromosome satellite sequences, and telomeric repeat sequences may also serve as FISH probe targets. Repetitive sequence probes are most useful for the detection of chromosome aneuploidy. Whole chromosome probes, also known as chromosome painting probes, consist of thousands of overlapping probes that recognize unique and moderately repetitive sequences along the entire length of individual chromosomes. Probes of this type are used to confirm the interpretation of aberrations identified by traditional karyotype analysis, or to establish the chromosomal origin of structural rearrangements that are difficult to evaluate by other approaches.

1. **Interphase FISH.** In clinical oncology testing, interphase (nuclear) in situ hybridization is the method of choice for rapid assessment of aneuploidy or gene rearrangement. Interphase FISH may be performed as a stand-alone assay, or in combination with (often prior to) chromosome analysis. There is no requirement for actively proliferating cells for interphase FISH analysis, making this technique advantageous over metaphase

FISH or chromosome analysis. The high sensitivity of interphase FISH also makes it useful for uncovering small rearrangements not detectable in standard karyotypes, as well as detecting cytogenetic alterations present in a very limited population of cells. However, only the number and relative position of the fluorochrome probe is obtained through this methodology.

Since interphase FISH analysis eliminates the need for in vitro cell culture, the technique can be used to study a broader range of cell and tissue types (and therefore a broader range of tumors) than can be evaluated by traditional karyotype analysis. This characteristic allows archival material, frequently formalin-fixed, paraffin-embedded (FFPE) specimens, to be assayed by interphase FISH.

    a. Advantages. Both repetitive sequence probes and unique sequence probes can be used for interphase FISH; concurrent hybridization with a combination of probes labeled with different fluorochromes permits simultaneous detection of two or more DNA regions of interest. Methodologic advances have made it possible to detect low copy-number gene sequences as small as 500 base pairs in length, although the efficiency of interphase FISH with small probes is quite low. Large numbers of interphase cells (200 to 500) are typically assayed per probe set allowing for low-level disease or subclonal cell populations to be detected.

    b. Limitations. Even with optimized probes, interphase FISH lacks the resolution in routine use to detect small chromosomal copy number alterations less than several hundred kb in size. Notably, this technique cannot be used to evaluate some classes of mutations that are characteristic of many sporadic tumors and familial cancer syndromes, such as single base-pair substitutions or small insertions or deletions. FISH probes for structural rearrangements such as translocations and inversions are optimized to detect the most common molecular breakpoints, and may fail to detect complex rearrangements or those with atypical breakpoints.

  2. Metaphase FISH. As with chromosome analysis, metaphase FISH requires actively dividing cells in order to obtain metaphase spreads for analysis. This technique provides additional information over interphase FISH in that the underlying structure of the chromosomes is revealed. Metaphase FISH data may be of particular use when deciphering complex chromosomal rearrangements as the probe can be visualized relative to chromosome position.

  3. Multiplex metaphase FISH and spectral karyotyping (SKY). These two related techniques make it possible to hybridize metaphase chromosome spreads with a combination of probes. Both techniques are useful for the detection of aneuploidy as well as chromosome rearrangements; in many cases, the techniques can establish the chromosomal origin of rearrangements that cannot be defined on the basis of traditional karyotype analysis.

C. Copy number-based microarray analysis

  1. Comparative genomic hybridization. Essentially a modification of in situ hybridization, comparative genomic hybridization (CGH) makes it possible to survey the genome for chromosomal deletions and amplifications. CGH was originally developed as a method to determine the relative copy number state in a tumor sample by hybridizing differentially labeled DNA derived from a tumor and a reference sample against metaphase chromosome spreads. Over time this technique evolved into array CGH, an approach that uses a microarray consisting of an ordered arrangement of DNA molecules linked to a solid matrix support. Genomic clones on the array, such as bacterial artificial chromosomes or synthesized oligonucleotide probes, serve as the substrate for the hybridization product. Array CGH relies on cohybridization of differentially labeled target DNA (patient or tumor) with that of control (reference) DNA against probes on the solid matrix. The DNA bound to each probe is quantified using a laser scanner allowing for relative copy number gains or losses between target and control samples to be determined. The resolution of array CGH is in theory limited only by the number of features in the array; commercially available arrays currently provide a resolution of under 10 kb.

  2. SNP array analysis. The methodology for copy number evaluation has further evolved to include the use of probes for single-nucleotide polymorphism (SNP) detection in the assay.

The inclusion of SNP probes is advantageous in that zygosity can be assessed, and therefore regions of the genome demonstrating a loss of heterozygosity (LOH), whether copy number-neutral or due to copy number alteration, can be defined. Also of note, SNP array analysis typically relies on the use of an in silico reference against which a target sample is compared to assess for relative copy number gain or loss; a modification that therefore only requires the target sample to be hybridized to the matrix support of the array. Chromosomal microarrays carrying probes for both SNPs and nonpolymorphic sites currently play a major role in the workup of patients with suspected constitutional disorders due to chromosomal copy number alterations. Increasingly, this methodology is being applied to oncology studies to assess the status of copy number and zygosity in a tumor sample.

    a. Advantages. Both aCGH and SNP array analysis allow for a rapid, genome-wide assessment of copy number at a very high resolution using DNA derived from fresh or fixed tissue. Whole chromosomes gains and losses, as well as smaller copy number alterations in the kilobase range are detectable. SNP array analysis also allows for an assessment of LOH.

    b. Disadvantages. Balanced rearrangements are not detectable by either methodology. Very small copy number alterations (intragenic) are often below the limit of detection of the assay.

III. TISSUE IN SITU HYBRIDIZATION. Tissue in situ hybridization for mRNA is a versatile technique but is technically demanding. The approach can be used to correlate the expression level of a specific gene with tissue changes characteristic of a disease, with a tumor's phenotype, or to monitor transgene expression in gene therapy regimens. However, even when optimized, the technique's sensitivity is below that of PCR-based methods, and the method is therefore not currently in widespread use.

IV. SOUTHERN BLOT HYBRIDIZATION. This filter hybridization method consists of DNA purification, digestion by a restriction endonuclease, size fractionation by gel electrophoresis, transfer and immobilization on a synthetic membrane made of nitrocellulose or nylon, and then hybridization to a specific nucleic acid probe. The probe is visualized by either radioisotopic or nonisotopic methods, and the location of the probe indicates not only the presence of the target sequence, but also the size of the enzyme-digested DNA fragment in which it is contained.

Southern blot hybridization has historically been used to detect genomic rearrangements characteristic of specific tumor types, but can also be used to detect different alleles of the same gene, point mutations, deletions, and insertions. Since the method is quantitative, it may provide information about gene copy number.

Southern blot hybridization has been a reliable and versatile method for sequence-specific DNA analysis, but requires at least 10 mm^3 of fresh or frozen tissue in which there has been limited DNA degradation. Although the technique was widely used for molecular analysis of tissue specimens for several decades, PCR-based methods have replaced the routine use of Southern blot hybridization for many assays because PCR-based methods have similar reliability but increased sensitivity, are usually more rapid and less cumbersome, require less tissue, and can be performed on FFPE tissue.

V. POLYMERASE CHAIN REACTION. PCR makes it possible to detect a broad range of chromosomal abnormalities, from gross structural alterations such as translocations and deletions to single base-pair mutations, in individual genes. PCR can be performed on areas of tumor (or even individual cells) macro- or microdissected from routinely prepared tissue or cytology slides, or separated by flow cytometry. This is an advantage in that PCR methods enable correlation between tissue morphology and genetic abnormalities of specific regions of tumor, specific cell populations, or even individual cells. The clinical utility of PCR is due to the wide range of template DNA that can be amplified, the technique's intrinsic extreme sensitivity, and the wide range of variations of the basic method that can be performed.

    A. Basic PCR. A PCR mixture includes the DNA sample to be assayed, a thermostable DNA polymerase, the four deoxynucleotide triphosphates (dNTPs), and short oligonucleotide primers (typically approximately 20 base pairs in length) designed to be complementary to the regions that flank the DNA sequence of interest. With each PCR cycle, the DNA region of interest is doubled, resulting in exponential amplification.

1. **Advantages.** Basic PCR (and the variations described below) has many advantages over the techniques of Southern and Northern blot hybridization that have traditionally been used to analyze specific regions of DNA and mRNA. PCR-based analysis can be completed in hours instead of days, can be applied to a wider range of tissues (including fresh, frozen, or fixed tissue), requires much less template DNA or RNA, is able to detect target DNA or RNA even when present in a background of vast excess of nontarget sequence, and is highly versatile.

2. **Limitations.** When optimized, PCR can detect one abnormal cell in a background of 10^5 normal cells, and can detect single copy genes from individual cells. However, many technical factors conspire to lower the clinical sensitivity of PCR. The most important practical limitation is degradation of target DNA or mRNA, especially when extracted from fixed tissue.

   The extreme sensitivity of PCR demands constant attention to laboratory organization and test design to avoid specimen contamination, the most troublesome technical issue. Contamination can be largely avoided by meticulous laboratory technique and maintenance, physical separation and containment of the various stages of the PCR procedure, and regular UV irradiation of laboratory workspaces and instruments to degrade any transient uncontained DNA.

   By design, PCR only analyzes the chromosomal region flanked by the primers employed. Therefore, unlike conventional cytogenetics, PCR does not survey the entire genome. Similarly, RT-PCR only analyzes the target mRNA, and provides no information about the presence of mutations or level of transcription of other related genes. Thus, design of the PCR assay is a critical factor affecting clinical sensitivity.

B. **Reverse transcriptase PCR.** In RT-PCR, mRNA is extracted from the sample and reverse transcribed into complementary DNA (cDNA). This cDNA then serves as the template in a subsequent PCR amplification. The use of RT-PCR permits straightforward amplification of the coding region of spliced, multiexon DNA sequences. This technique also permits detection of targeted translocations, including BCR-ABL.

C. **Multiplex PCR.** This approach involves the simultaneous amplification of multiple target sequences in a single reaction tube through the use of multiple primer pairs. It is used to evaluate a number of different sites for the presence of a mutation in a single reaction, and is therefore a practical screening method. The multiple sequences of interest must be widely spaced on the chromosome, or present on different chromosomes, to avoid cross-priming events.

D. **Methylation-specific PCR.** Pretreatment of the DNA sample with sodium bisulfite, which reduces unmethylated cytosines to uracil, makes it possible to evaluate the methylation status of individual CpG sites. This approach is used in tests to characterize specific gene silencing patterns that are correlated with tumor subgroups that are likely to respond to specific chemotherapeutic regimens.

E. **Quantitative PCR.** Also referred to as real-time PCR, this method permits more reliable quantification of the amount of input DNA than is possible by traditional endpoint measurement of the DNA product. Since the PCR product is quantified as the reaction progresses (i.e., in real-time) rather than after PCR completion, it avoids the potential artifacts of amplification efficiency. Quantitative PCR often provides more precise measurements of DNA or mRNA than can be achieved by filter hybridization or microarray-based methods.

   When mRNA is the substrate, quantitative RT-PCR can be used to correlate changes in gene expression with the clinical features of a disease or a specific tumor type. One example in current use is the Oncotype DX breast cancer assay (Genomic Health, Inc.; Redwood City, CA), which measures the expression of 21 genes by RT-PCR and applies a formula to calculate a recurrence score.

VI. DNA SEQUENCE ANALYSIS

A. **Direct methods of sequence analysis.** Although most molecular diagnostics involve querying DNA for sequence variants, a minority of assays involve DNA sequencing per se. Sequence data is somewhat cumbersome to integrate into a laboratory workflow, as the readout consists of alphabetic DNA sequence that requires manipulation or visual inspection to extract a test result, whereas tests with surrogate readouts, such as presence or absence of a band on an agarose gel, are more amenable to multiplexing and may be less expensive to perform. Sequencing is, however, invaluable in scenarios in which numerous different variants can occur, such as in *BRCA1* and *BRCA2* gene testing for hereditary breast–ovarian cancer.

Virtually all routine direct DNA sequence analysis is automated and performed on templates generated by the chain-termination method (Sanger sequencing). Even though these reactions require a very low quantity of template DNA, the amount of DNA present in patient specimens is seldom sufficient for analysis without a preliminary amplification step, usually PCR. The PCR-amplified template is used as input to a sequencing reaction whose product is a mixture of single-stranded DNA fragments of various lengths, each tagged at one end with a fluorophore indicating the identity of the 3´ nucleotide. These products are then resolved by capillary electrophoresis with fluorescent detection.

B. Single-nucleotide polymorphism (SNP) analysis. SNPs are common in the human genome, and once a set of SNPs is linked with an increased susceptibility to a certain disease, prognosis, or response to therapy, focused analysis of the SNPs (also known as haplotype analysis) may circumvent the need for more extensive DNA sequence analysis. More refined SNP catalogs, with identification of "tag SNPs" linked with traits of interest, will likely make systematic analysis of SNPs an important clinical tool.

C. Indirect methods of sequence analysis. Once normal and mutant alleles at a specific locus have been characterized by direct DNA sequence analysis, indirect methods can often provide enough sequence information to be of clinical utility. These indirect techniques include allelic discrimination by size, restriction fragment length polymorphism (RFLP) analysis, allele-specific PCR, single-strand conformational polymorphism (SSCP) analysis, heteroduplex analysis, denaturing gradient gel electrophoresis, cleavage of mismatched nucleotides, ligase chain reaction, the protein truncation test, and numerous variants, used either alone or in combination. These indirect methods are based on PCR and may be applied to a broad range of clinical specimens. In addition, many of the indirect methods are faster and less expensive than direct sequence analysis, and are ideally suited for screening large numbers of samples from patients.

D. Sequence analysis by microarray technology. High-density DNA microarrays have found their greatest use in hybridization-based evaluation of gene expression and as chromosomal microarrays for detection of karyotypic anomalies, but chip-based hybridization analysis is also a suitable platform for sequence analysis. Microarrays have been developed for simultaneous detection of numerous viral sequences and for genotyping multiple clinically significant positions in genes such as *CFTR* and *TP53*. Microarray-based sequencing has become less common in clinical practice as direct sequencing technologies have become more widely available.

E. Clinical next-generation sequencing. "Next-generation" sequencing (NGS) methods have revolutionized the life sciences by dramatically increasing the throughput of DNA sequencing. Many of the currently available NGS techniques have been described as cyclic array sequencing platforms, because they involve dispersal of target sequences across the surface of a two-dimensional array, followed by sequencing of those targets. The resulting short sequence reads can be reassembled de novo or, much more commonly in clinical applications, aligned to a reference genome. The Illumina (Illumina Inc., San Diego, CA), Ion Torrent (Thermo Fisher Scientific, Waltham, MA), and Roche 454 (Roche Diagnostics, Indianapolis, IN) platforms are the most widely used at present.

NGS has several attributes that are attractive in cancer testing. Since each library fragment is individually sequenced, the resulting data can resolve intratumor sequence heterogeneity, revealing the clonal structure of the tumor. NGS has the potential to detect all four of the major classes of genetic variation: single-nucleotide variants, insertions and deletions, structural variants, and copy-number variants. The technique can be performed upon DNA extracted from formalin-fixed, paraffin-embedded tissue, a commonly available specimen type. Finally, although these tests are currently not inexpensive, the cost per nucleotide sequenced is extremely low, and the cost of the test increases less than linearly with the size of the region analyzed.

Although NGS was initially developed as a research technique, it has found several prominent roles in clinical testing. Noninvasive prenatal testing (NIPT), based on analysis of cell-free fetal DNA in the maternal circulation, has resulted in a dramatic drop in invasive prenatal diagnostic procedures and is now recommended by the American College of Obstetricians and Gynecologists for women at high risk for fetal aneuploidy. NGS has also been adopted as a platform for simultaneous sequencing of multiple genes for constitutional disorders, including familial cancer syndromes. The most prominent application of NGS in clinical oncology, however, is the development of tests to detect actionable somatic variants in multiple cancer-related genes. These "cancer panels" leverage the fact that assessment of individual genes is no longer sufficient to guide selection of targeted therapies. Simultaneous detection of variants in multiple genes is potentially a more comprehensive and cost-effective approach than sequential testing of individual genes, yielding a large amount of predictive and/or prognostic data in a clinically relevant time frame.

VII. **MICROARRAY-BASED GENE EXPRESSION PROFILING.** The morphologic features of disease are essentially reflections of altered gene expression within diseased cells. Characterization of disease-specific alterations in gene expression is therefore an area of intense interest. Given the limitations of Northern blot hybridization, a variety of new methodologies have been developed to identify differentially expressed genes, of which microarray technology is the most widely used.

Microarray technology is based on the principle of nucleic acid hybridization. Fundamentally, a DNA microarray (or gene chip) employs multiple sets of DNAs or oligonucleotides complementary to the thousands of genes to be investigated, each attached at a known location on a glass or nylon membrane substrate the size of a computer chip. When RNA extracted from the clinical sample is used as the input, microarrays make it possible to rapidly measure the expression of thousands of genes in parallel. Fluorophore-labeled test (or target) RNA derived from the specimen is hybridized to the chip, and emitted light produced by laser scanning allows for quantitation of gene expression of even low-abundance transcripts.

1. **Applications.** Microarray-based techniques, although still largely experimental, are increasingly being used in clinical settings to demonstrate specific and reproducible differences in gene expression profiles that are of diagnostic utility, or that can be used to predict prognosis or response to specific therapeutic regimens. One such assay that has entered clinical use is MammaPrint (Agendia, Inc., Irvine, CA), an in vitro diagnostic multivariate index assay (IVDMIA) cleared by the FDA. The test measures expression of 70 genes on a microarray platform to classify patients into a low-risk or high-risk group.

2. **Limitations.** Microarray-based gene expression technology has until recently been applicable only to fresh or frozen tissue, but it has now been shown that it can potentially be validated in FFPE samples. Another major challenge facing microarray-based expression profiling (as well as other genome-wide techniques) is interpretation of the massive quantity of data generated by each sample tested.

VIII. **EMERGING TECHNIQUES**

A. **Pharmacogenetics.** In addition to tumor-specific genetic abnormalities, genetic variation has been estimated to account for 20% to 95% of variability in the metabolism, disposition, and effect of the drugs used to treat patients with cancer. Pharmacogenetics offers the opportunity not only to optimize the efficacy of therapy, but also to minimize toxicity. Many centers are now using prospective genotyping of a few targeted genes to guide antineoplastic treatment and dosing choices. These include thiopurine methyltransferase (TPMT) point mutations in mercaptopurine therapy for acute leukemia, thymidylate synthase enhancer region (TSER) polymorphisms in 5-fluorouracil therapy for colorectal cancer, and UDP glucuronosyl transferase (UGT1A1) promoter region variants in irinotecan therapy for metastatic colorectal cancer. Genome-wide analysis of the role of genetic variation to predict an individual patient's response to treatment with a specific drug is known as pharmacogenomics.

B. **Analysis of epigenetic modifications.** Techniques for quantitative detection of the methylation status of every human gene individually have been developed. Given the effect of epigenetic changes on gene expression, it is reasonable to anticipate that the pattern of methylation at defined sets of loci may eventually become a component of the pathologic evaluation of individual tumors. At present, no test based upon methylation is associated with clear clinical benefit.

C. **Proteomics.** This technique is focused on the analysis of patterns of protein expression rather than the analysis of nucleic acids. Methods for high-sensitivity, high-throughput evaluation of protein expression profiles have been developed—methods that make it possible to identify patterns that correlate with specific malignancies, underlying mutations, epigenetic changes, transcriptional profiles, response to drug therapy, and so on.

D. **Analysis of RNA interference.** It has recently become clear that several classes of short single-stranded or double-stranded RNA molecules that are responsible for RNA interference (RNAi) have a profound role in the regulation of gene expression. The demonstration that the profile of miRNAs (one class of small RNAs that mediate RNAi) is different in normal and neoplastic tissue, that alterations in miRNA are oncogenic, and that RNAi-based approaches can have therapeutic benefit all suggest that analysis of specific small RNA molecules, either individually or on a genome-wide basis, may in the future have an important role in the molecular evaluation of tumors.

ACKNOWLEDGMENT

The authors thank Drs. John Pfeifer and Barbara Zehnbauer, authors of the previous edition of this chapter.

SUGGESTED READINGS

Barik S. Silence of the transcripts: RNA interference in medicine. *J Mol Med* 2005;83:764–773.

Bossuyt PM, Reitsma JB, Bruns DE, et al. Towards complete and accurate reporting of studies of diagnostic accuracy: the STARD initiative. *Ann Intern Med* 2003;138:40–44.

Chen EC, Miller SA, DeRisi JL, et al. Using a pan-viral microarray assay (Virochip) to screen clinical samples for viral pathogens. *J Vis Exp* 2011;50:2536.

Cottrell CE, Al-Kateb H, Bredemeyer AJ, et al. Validation of a next-generation sequencing assay for clinical molecular oncology. *J Mol Diagn* 2014;16:89–105.

Dieffenbach CW, Dveksler GS. *PCR Primer: A Laboratory Manual.* Plainview, NY: Cold Spring Harbor Laboratory Press, 1995.

Gersen SL. *The Principles of Clinical Cytogenetics.* New York, NY: Springer, 2012.

International HapMap Consortium. A haplotype map of the human genome. *Nature* 2005;437:1299–1320.

Ladanyi M, Gerald WL. *Expression Profiling of Human Tumors: Diagnostic and Research Applications.* Totowa, NJ: Humana Press, 2003.

Lewin J, Schmitt AO, Adorjan P, et al. Quantitative DNA methylation analysis based on four-dye trace data from direct sequencing of PCR amplificates. *Bioinformatics* 2004;20:3005–3012.

Marsh S, McLeod HL. Pharmacogenomics: from bedside to clinical practice. *Hum Mol Genet* 2006;15(Spec No 1):R89–R93.

Misek DE, Imafuku Y, Hanash SM. Application of proteomic technologies to tumor analysis. *Pharmacogenomics* 2004;5:1129–1137.

Pfeifer JD. *Molecular Genetic Testing in Surgical Pathology.* Philadelphia, PA: Lippincott, Williams & Wilkins, 2006.

Pfeifer JD, Hill DA, O'Sullivan MJ, et al. Diagnostic gold standard for soft tissue tumours: morphology or molecular genetics? *Histopathology* 2000;37:485–500.

Pritchard CC, Salipante SJ, Koehler K, et al. Validation and implementation of targeted capture and sequencing for the detection of actionable mutation, copy number variation, and gene rearrangement in clinical cancer specimens. *J Mol Diagn* 2014;16:56–67.

Pritchard CC, Smith C, Salipante SJ, et al. ColoSeq provides comprehensive Lynch and polyposis syndrome mutational analysis using massively parallel sequencing. *J Mol Diagn* 2012;14:357–366.

Shaffer LG, McGowan-Jordan J, Schmid M, eds; International Standing Committee on Human Cytogenetic Nomenclature. *ISCN 2013: An International System for Human Cytogenetic Nomenclature.* Basel, Switzerland: Karger, 2013.

Spencer DH, Sehn JK, Abel HJ, et al. Comparison of clinical targeted next-generation sequence data from formalin-fixed and fresh-frozen tissue specimens. *J Mol Diagn* 2013;15:623–633.

Vogelstein B, Kinzler KW. *The Genetic Basis of Human Cancer*, 2nd ed. New York, NY: McGraw-Hill, 2002.

Wu L, Williams PM, Koch W. Clinical applications of microarray-based diagnostic tests. *BioTechniques* 2005;39:S577–S582.

3 Principles and Practice of Surgery in Cancer Therapy

Amber Traugott • Rebecca L. Aft

I. **THE CHANGING ROLE OF THE SURGICAL ONCOLOGIST IN THE 21ST CENTURY.** Early cancer therapy centered on surgical excision as the primary treatment modality for solid tumors. It was theorized that cancer spread occurred sequentially from the primary site to the regional lymph nodes and then on to distant sites. Therefore, it was hypothesized that complete local excision of all cancerous cells would lead to effective disease control. In patients with untreated cancer, median survival was frequently measured in months. Early *en bloc* resection of tumors with contiguous normal surrounding tissue and lymph nodes led to improved overall survival. As a consequence, increasingly aggressive and extensive resections of malignant tumors were performed. As the initial improvement in survival began to plateau, it became apparent that successively larger resections to obtain locoregional control of larger tumors did not necessarily translate into further survival benefit. This led to the testing and development of screening strategies and adjuvant therapies. As medical and surgical care of the cancer patient has become increasingly refined, surgeons have also been able to develop surgical approaches that decrease perioperative morbidity and mortality, while providing the same oncologic outcome. Neoadjuvant protocols are being used in many cancers to reduce the extent of resection needed to gain locoregional control of tumors, or to identify patients with aggressive tumor biology who are unlikely to benefit from surgery with curative intent. In addition, minimally invasive surgical techniques now enjoy widespread use in the surgical treatment of a wide variety of solid tumors. The current role for the surgeon in the management of patients with cancers involves a broad spectrum of surgical procedures for diagnosis, local control, cure, and palliation.

II. **DIAGNOSTIC PROCEDURES: ACQUISITION OF MATERIAL FOR DIAGNOSIS.** Once a lesion has been identified, one role of the surgical oncologist is to provide adequate material for definitive diagnosis. The method of biopsy requires consideration of the differential diagnosis, amount of tissue needed for definitive diagnosis, location of the lesion, and potential forms of treatment. It is preferable to perform biopsies of lesions at the periphery where viable tumor is located, because the cores of solid tumors may be necrotic. This also allows the pathologist to evaluate the invasion into normal tissue since some tumors (thyroid) have low mitotic rates and bland cytologic features, which are insufficient for determining malignancy. General principles for biopsy include sampling representative tissue, obtaining adequate tissue for diagnosis, procuring viable tissue, minimizing contamination of adjacent uninvolved tissues, orienting the tissue for margin analysis, and providing tissue to the pathologist in the appropriate conditions (fresh or fixed).

A. **Fine needle aspiration cytology.** Fine needle aspiration (FNA) yields a smear of single cells and aggregates for cytologic analysis. The biopsy is performed using a 22- to 25-gauge needle, which can be percutaneously guided to most anatomic sites. Imaging guidance (including endoscopic or endobronchial ultrasound [EUS/EBUS]) may be used to improve the accuracy of sampling for nonpalpable lesions or lesions in deep tissues. Although the track of the needle is theoretically contaminated with malignant cells, in practice, FNA-track metastases are rarely a clinical problem. Diagnosis is based on the cytologic features of the cells including cohesiveness, nuclear and cytoplasmic morphology, and number. An advantage of FNA is that a wide area of the tumor can be sampled. The limitations of FNA include (a) small sample size; (b) lack of information on histologic architecture that cannot distinguish between in situ and invasive tumors (breast, thyroid); (c) inability to obtain grade of tumors; and (d) interpretation of certain immunohistochemical stains. FNA can be useful for diagnosing recurrent lymphoma; however, for a primary diagnosis of lymphoma, more tissue may be required.

B. **Core needle biopsy.** Core needle biopsies yield fragments of tissue, which allow the evaluation of tumor architecture. The biopsy is performed using 14- to 16-gauge needles specifically designed for this purpose (Tru-Cut, Biopsy). Larger biopsy specimens that sample larger areas of tissue can be obtained with vacuum-assisted devices (Vicora, Mammotome). Core needle biopsies can also be combined with imaging such as mammography (stereotactic core biopsy), computed tomography (CT), or ultrasonography. A false-negative biopsy may result if the needle misses or skives (pares) the malignant tumor, which may occur with very sclerotic cancers such as in the breast. The most common complication of core needle biopsies is bleeding, and the procedure should be cautiously performed in patients with coagulopathies. In addition, masses near large vascular structures, hollow organs, or in the central nervous system (CNS) are not amenable to this procedure.

C. **Cutaneous punch biopsy.** Punch biopsies are used to obtain tissue from cutaneous lesions using 2- to 6-mm round surgical blades. A full-thickness skin specimen including subcutaneous fat is obtained. The procedure is simple to perform, with few complications, and is useful for obtaining tissue for pathologic diagnosis from suggestive skin lesions (melanoma, basal cell, or squamous cell carcinoma) that may subsequently require definitive surgical resection.

D. **Open biopsy**
1. **Incisional biopsy.** Occasionally, neoplasms are not amenable to percutaneous needle biopsy because of anatomic location, requirements for large amounts of tissue for diagnosis (sarcomas), or concern regarding sampling errors in diffuse lesions. An incisional biopsy is the most expedient method for obtaining tissue for definitive diagnosis. These procedures are usually performed in an outpatient surgical setting. A wedge of tissue large enough for accurate diagnosis is removed from the periphery of the lesion. Excellent hemostasis must be obtained to avoid hematogenous seeding. The biopsy incision should be planned such that it can be included in the tissue to be removed by subsequent definitive surgery (longitudinal for limb sarcomas) because some tumors have a propensity for seeding the biopsy incision. A biopsy site that is far removed from the potential operative incision can severely jeopardize later attempts for surgical control of the tumor or potential limb-sparing procedures and can result in a compromised surgery.
2. **Excisional biopsy.** Excisional biopsies remove the entire lesion and are best suited for small lesions, particularly when a needle biopsy is inappropriate for technical, safety, or diagnostic reasons, or where the gross architecture of the lesion impacts the diagnosis. This may be curative for small cancers (melanoma, breast cancer, sarcoma, and basal cell carcinomas). Depending on the size of the lesion and the closure required, excisional biopsies can be performed as an office-based procedure or in the operating room. All specimens should be oriented for accurate margin assessment. This allows the surgeon to resect additional tissue for inadequate or close margins.

III. **STAGING: DETERMINING THE EXTENT OF DISEASE AND RESECTABILITY.** When distant disease is suspected, most cancers can be staged with CT, positron emission tomography (PET), magnetic resonance imaging (MRI), or bone radionuclide scans. However, surgical staging procedures for melanoma, breast cancer, a subset of abdominal malignancies, and thoracic malignancies are more sensitive than currently available radiographic modalities and alter patient management in a large percentage of cases.

A. **Mediastinoscopy.** Mediastinoscopy is used for the preoperative staging of bronchogenic carcinoma and evaluation of mediastinal adenopathy. It is the most accurate method for staging mediastinal lymph nodes. The procedure is performed under general anesthesia. A transverse surgical incision is made above the sternal notch, and a mediastinoscope is inserted along the trachea. Lymph node can be biopsied from the pretracheal, subcarinal, and paratracheal node stations and examined for metastatic disease. The procedure is highly sensitive (100%) and specific (90%) in staging of bronchogenic carcinoma and has low morbidity and mortality. Endoscopic ultrasound (EUS) and endobronchial ultrasound (EBUS) can also be used to obtain needle biopsies of mediastinal lymph nodes.

Together, these techniques (EUS, EBUS, and mediastinoscopy) are important tools to help stage mediastinal lymph nodes.

B. Laparotomy. Radiographic staging and laparoscopy have largely replaced laparotomy. Laparotomy is used selectively for staging ovarian and nonseminomatous testicular cancers. The procedure is performed under general anesthesia through a midline incision. The procedure has low morbidity and short recovery. Complications include infection, bleeding, wound dehiscence, and rare events related to exploration of the intra-abdominal contents and general anesthesia.

C. Laparoscopy. Laparoscopic approaches to the staging of patients with cancer are now routine for a number of intra-abdominal malignancies (liver, pancreas, stomach, and medullary thyroid carcinoma). Laparoscopy has been shown to decrease the incidence of unnecessary laparotomies for unresectable disease in up to 70% of patients with abdominal malignancies. Diagnostic laparoscopy for staging is usually performed at the time of a planned laparotomy or laparoscopic excision with curative intent. If distant or unresectable disease is found, then an unnecessary laparotomy or extensive laparoscopic dissection is avoided. The procedure is performed under general anesthesia. Biopsies of solid organs, lymph nodes, and suggestive lesions can be obtained. When laparoscopy is combined with intraoperative ultrasonography, lesions deep in the parenchyma of an organ can be identified, as well as tumor invasion into adjacent structures, such as major blood vessels. This is especially useful in evaluation of the liver and pancreatic malignancies and may be the most sensitive imaging technique for the detection of liver metastases. The procedure has few complications and may be performed on an outpatient basis. Port-site metastasis and intra-abdominal spread by the pneumoperitoneum, although of theoretical concern, are rare (less than 1% of cases).

D. Lymphadenectomy. The location, type of cancer, and clinical evidence of nodal involvement are the major considerations in performing lymphadenectomy. Presence and extent of nodal involvement is the most accurate risk indicator of distant disease development for many cancers. In general, regional lymph nodes should be removed when the likelihood of metastases is high or if lymph nodes are found by clinical examination to be involved. If possible, regional lymph nodes should be removed at the time of the primary surgery. If a lymph node is found to exceed 3 cm in size, the tumor likely has extranodal extension and involves the perinodal fat. These lymph nodes should be resected with surrounding fat and, if of low morbidity, the adjacent nerves (i.e., intercostal brachial sensory nerve of the axilla). The survival benefit of lymphadenectomy varies from malignancy to malignancy; it is heavily influenced by the effectiveness of adjuvant chemotherapy for the cancer in question. Therefore, the goal of lymphadenectomy for all cancers is to obtain sufficient lymph node tissue to adequately stage the patient. For those cancers where lymphadenectomy improves survival, the optimal extent of resection provides the best oncologic outcome without subjecting the patient to unnecessary surgical morbidity or mortality. In some cases, such as in gastric adenocarcinoma, this ideal extent of lymphadenectomy is the subject of ongoing study and controversy. The major morbidity of regional lymphadenectomy for axillary or inguinal lymphadenectomy is limb lymphedema and injury to adjacent nerves. More extensive lymphadenectomies within the chest or abdomen can result in increased surgical mortality, as well as injury to surrounding organs or major neurovascular structures.

E. Sentinel lymph node biopsy. Sentinel lymph node biopsy (SLNB) is based on data demonstrating hierarchical lymphatic drainage occurring from the primary tumor to the first draining lymph node (sentinel lymph node [SLN]) and then to the remaining nodes in the regional lymphatic basin. Numerous studies have demonstrated that localized malignancies metastasize to the SLN before involving other nodes in the basin. Therefore, the presence or absence of metastatic disease in the SLN predicts the status of the entire regional lymphatic basin. SLNB is currently used for staging the axilla in breast cancer and regional nodal basins in melanoma. It is under investigation for a number of other malignancies (gynecologic, head, and neck). Two techniques are used for lymphatic mapping, which may be used independently or in combination. The first technique involves the injection of a radiolabeled colloid around the lesion, which is followed radiographically and/ or intraoperatively by using the gamma probe. The second technique employs blue dye (isosulfan blue, lymphazurin blue, and methylene blue), which is injected intraoperatively around the tumor and allowed to percolate through the lymphatics. In both techniques, an incision is made at the edge of the nodal basin, and the SLN is identified by tracing blue or radioactive lymphatic channels to the first blue or radioactive node. If more than one nodal basin is potentially involved, then preoperative lymphoscintigraphy may be performed to identify the draining nodal basins. In experienced hands, the procedure has very high specificity and sensitivity. The advantages of SLNB are selective lymph node dissections in those patients who would benefit most, avoiding the morbidity associated with lymph node clearance in those patients with low risk of disease, and the ability to perform immunohistochemical stains or polymerase chain reaction (PCR) to detect micrometastatic disease. Disadvantages of SLNB are related to the skill of the operator, which may result in a significant false-negative rate.

IV. SURGICAL TREATMENT. Surgical planning involves consideration of the tumor stage and location, the general health of the patient, expected morbidity and mortality of the procedure, probability of successful treatment, and the availability and effectiveness of other treatment modalities. Surgical resection of solid tumors provides excellent local control and is currently the only curative option for most solid tumors.

A. Primary resection

1. **Principles of Surgical Resection.** The primary goal of cancer surgery is the complete extirpation of local and regional disease for local control and for decreasing the risk of local recurrence. This involves removing the primary lesion with adequate margins of normal surrounding tissue to minimize the risk of local recurrence. The stage, mechanisms of local spread, morbidity, and mortality of the procedure must be taken into consideration before any surgical procedure is undertaken. In patients with metastatic disease, long-term control may not be as important as it is in patients who have localized disease, which may be surgically curable, although in these cases surgery can be palliative. Knowledge of the most common avenues of spread for the various histologic types of cancers is essential for successful local control. Depending on the cell of origin, cancers may spread mucosally, submucosally, along fascial planes, or along nerves (Table 3-1). With advances in anesthesia, minimally invasive surgical approaches, postoperative care, and reconstructive procedures, large surgical procedures can be performed safely in elderly patients and patients with multiple comorbid conditions. Intraoperatively, successful resection requires good exposure, excision of previous biopsy sites, maintaining a bloodless surgical field to visualize the extent of tumor spread, and *en bloc* resection of the tumor and surrounding normal tissue. Local recurrence or wound seeding can be theoretically minimized by minimal manipulation of the tumor, confining dissection to normal tissue, and early ligation of major feeding vessels at their origin. Complete removal of the tumors has many favorable effects, including minimizing residual disease and eliminating hypoxic, poorly vascularized cells, which are drug and radiation resistant.

2. **Premalignant lesions and prophylactic surgery.** Surgery is indicated for premalignant lesions and noninvasive cancers of the skin, mouth, cervix, colon, breast, and thyroid, although only a proportion of such lesions may progress to malignancy (Table 3-2). Several inherited disorders associated with increased cancer risk have been described. Surgery can significantly reduce cancer occurrence (Table 3-3).

B. Operative principles

1. **Anatomy.** The anatomic location of cancers is an important consideration in surgical planning. Some tumors cannot be adequately treated by surgical resection alone because of anatomic constraints, which may result in incomplete excision (nasopharynx). Residual microscopic disease after surgical resection can sometimes be treated effectively with adjuvant radiation therapy to decrease local recurrence. Those patients whose lesions are intimately involved with major blood vessels (lung/aorta) or bilaterally involve an essential organ (liver) or those with a limited life expectancy due to the natural history of the disease may not benefit from surgical resection.

TABLE 3-1	Adequate Tissue Margins for Primary Malignancy Treated with Surgery Alone

Tissue	Margin	Rationale
Melanoma		
In situ	0.5–1 cm	
<1.0 mm	1 cm	Localized
1.01–2 mm	1–2 cm	
>2.0 mm	2 cm	Increased risk of local recurrence
Sarcoma	Excise entire muscle group or 1 cm	–
Breast, invasive	1 cm	Must be combined with radiation therapy because of multifocality
Colon	2–5 cm	–
Esophagus	10 cm	Potential for extensive submucosal spread
Squamous cell carcinoma of head/neck	1 cm	May be limited by adjacent structures
Lung	Excise lobe or lung	–
Pancreas	1 mm–1 cm	Margins may be limited by surrounding vessels
Liver	1 cm	–
Basal cell carcinoma	2 mm	Very localized malignant area
Stomach	6 cm	Intramural spread

TABLE 3-2	Surgery for In Situ Disease and Atypia

Organ	Pathology	Detection method
Cervix	Atypia	Papanicolaou test
Mouth	Dysplasia	Oral examination
Gastroesophageal tract	Dysplasia (Barrett) leukoplakia	Endoscopy
Breast	In situ	Mammogram/physical examination

TABLE 3-3	Prophylactic Surgery

Disorder	Cancer risk	Surgery
Familial polyposis coli	100% risk	Colectomy
Ulcerative colitis	With dysplasia, >50% risk	Colectomy
MEN II/FMTC	100% medullary thyroid cancer (genetic screening)	Thyroidectomy
BRCA1/2	>60% breast cancer	Mastectomy

FMTC, familial medullary thyroid cancer; MEN, multiple endocrine neoplasia.

2. **Neoadjuvant therapy before resection.** If a lesion is resectable and localized at the time of diagnosis, then surgery should be performed. Large lesions or lesions invading into surrounding structures that are not initially resectable may be amenable to volume reduction with initial (neoadjuvant) chemotherapy or radiation therapy. This strategy has allowed successful but more limited, less morbid resections or function-preserving resections of many cancers (colorectal, breast, larynx, and pancreatic cancers). In addition, the response to neoadjuvant therapy is useful for monitoring response to various treatment regimens. If a pathologic complete response is possible, the surgical site should be marked with metallic clips at the time of biopsy for future identification at the time of surgery. A disadvantage of neoadjuvant therapy is the possible delay in undergoing standard curative therapy. Infrequently, a patient may have disease progression on neoadjuvant therapy, to the point where curative surgical resection is no longer possible. However, this subset of patients may have biologically aggressive disease that would have been unlikely to respond to adjuvant therapy after resection, thus increasing the risk of recurrence after surgery. Therefore, it is possible that this process selects for patients who would not have benefited from surgical resection, in terms of survival or disease-free survival.

   Preoperative radiation therapy may be used alone or in combination with chemotherapy to reduce tumor size before resection. In some cancers, such as rectal cancer, it also provides the benefit of decreased local recurrence after resection, even when given preoperatively. Advantages of preoperative radiation therapy are potentially smaller treatment fields and reduced potential seeding of the tumor during surgery. Disadvantages of preoperative radiotherapy include the resulting fibrosis, which may obscure resection margins and increase the difficulty and morbidity of the surgery. Preoperative radiation therapy renders the wound edges functionally ischemic, which may affect the type of reconstruction performed and tissue resected or result in increased wound complications. Although neoadjuvant therapy may decrease the size of the lesion, there is generally little benefit in overall survival.

C. **Extent of resection.** Extent of resection depends on the organ involved and method of local spread. Adequate margins range from 1 mm to 5 cm for cutaneous and hollow organ tumors. Resections for solid organ tumors are usually guided by the blood supply, and usually resection of a lobe (liver, lung) or the entire organ (kidney) or a partial resection (pancreas) is performed. The most efficacious method for local control and prevention of local recurrence is wide excision. This may require encompassing any biopsy incision or needle tract into the *en bloc* excision. If the malignancy is adherent to a contiguous organ, then a partial resection of the latter organ may be performed to obtain negative margins. Most solid tumors have a propensity for dissemination through local lymphatics to regional lymph nodes. If a lymph node in the draining area exceeds 3 cm in size, the tumor is likely extranodal and involves the perinodal fat. Local excision is then inadequate and *en bloc* resection of the organ, regional lymph nodes, and adjacent involved regions should be performed. To prevent seeding of tumor, the no-touch technique can be used, which includes minimal palpation of the tumor and early ligation of the blood supply to limit dislodgement of the tumor cells into the venous circulation. Although the ability of these techniques to reduce local recurrence is controversial, their theoretic value has led to widespread acceptance. If a second area of the body requires surgery at the time of tumor excision, gloves, gowns, sheets, and instruments must be changed. This further prevents transplantation of tumor to a distant site.

   If margins are positive after resection, options include further surgery, adjuvant therapy, or careful follow-up. If microscopic tumor is found at the resection margin, adjuvant postoperative radiation may be given. However, this may be associated with a higher risk of tumor recurrence, poorer cosmetic results, and more radiation complications due to the higher radiation doses required (breast, sarcoma, and head/neck cancers). These patients may benefit from re-excision of the tumor bed to achieve microscopically clear margins if this is technically feasible. In these cases, the potential morbidity and mortality of repeat surgery should be assessed.

D. **Laparoscopic and laparoscopy-assisted surgeries.** Laparoscopic or laparoscopy-assisted tumor resections are increasingly being performed worldwide, and are now standard options for curative resection in many cancers. The most common laparoscopic cancer surgery performed is colectomy. Laparoscopy-assisted distal pancreatectomies, hepatectomies, adrenalectomies, gastrectomies, esophagectomies, nephrectomies, prostatectomies, and video-assisted thoracic (VAT) lobectomies are now performed routinely for cancer surgery in appropriately selected patients. In general, laparoscopic procedures result in shorter hospital stay, less intraoperative blood loss, decreased requirement for analgesics, and earlier return to normal activities. Concerns have been raised regarding margin width and *en bloc* resection of draining nodal basins; however, studies examining these issues for colectomy have reported no significant difference. Indeed, data suggests that this holds true for other laparoscopic resection options.

V. METASTASES AND RECURRENT DISEASE

A. **Distant metastasis.** With many types of cancer, death is often the result of metastatic disease. It is often assumed that the patient with disseminated disease is not a candidate for surgical procedures. However, subsets of patients with isolated metastases are amenable to a complete surgical resection (hepatic and pulmonary) with resulting increased survival. Excisions of symptomatic metastases that cannot be treated by other means are appropriate for resection to improve quality of life (melanoma, breast, thyroid, and other endocrine cancers). This includes patients with subcutaneous metastases that present cosmetic problems and bowel metastases that cause obstruction or bleeding. Patients with multiple metastases to the lung or liver should be considered for resection if the metastases are present in only one organ system, if there is adequate normal parenchyma remaining after resection, and if the operative risk is minimal. The longer the time interval between initial diagnosis and the appearance of metastatic disease, the more likely it is that surgery will be beneficial and result in increased overall survival. Resection of a small number of pulmonary metastases from sarcoma or localized lung and liver metastases from colorectal cancers will result in increased survival for approximately 25% of patients. In breast cancer, there is emerging evidence that surgery of the breast improves overall survival in patients with metastatic disease.

B. **Resection for recurrent locoregional disease.** Local recurrence of cancer can result from incomplete excision at the initial surgery, the presence of residual cancer cells distant from the primary lesion, or second primary tumors that develop in residual normal tissue. Intensive follow-up is used to detect recurrent or persistent tumors before distant dissemination occurs. With some cancers, the presence of local recurrence may signal the presence of distant disease in a proportion of patients (approximately 50% for breast cancer). Similar surgical principles apply to resection of recurrent disease.

C. **Palliative surgery.** Significant improvement in quality of life and alleviation of symptoms can be achieved with palliative surgery, which allows patients to resume as many of their normal daily activities as possible (Table 3-4). This includes resection for

TABLE 3-4	Palliative Surgical Procedures
Presentation	**Surgical procedure**
Malignant pleural effusion	Thoracostomy tube, sclerosis
Biliary obstruction	Stent or choledochojejunostomy
Bowel obstruction, large	Diverting ileostomy or colostomy with mucous fistula, endoscopic stent placement
Bowel obstruction, small	Resection, bypass, gastrostomy tube
Bowel obstruction, duodenal	Gastrojejunostomy
Esophageal obstruction	Stent, gastrostomy tube
Locally advanced breast cancer	Salvage mastectomy

obstruction, pain, bleeding, or perforation of a hollow viscus or for hormonal effects of endocrine tumors (insulinomas, gastrinomas, and medullary thyroid cancers). As laparoscopic techniques become more common, these minimally invasive approaches may provide invaluable tools for allowing patients the ability to maximize their quality of life without the morbidity associated with open surgery.

VI. RECONSTRUCTION: FUNCTIONAL AND COSMETIC. Advances in the understanding of the tissue blood supply have allowed improvements in the coverage of surgical defects after cancer resections. Rarely are disfiguring primary closures or skin grafts the only option. Two advances have led to major changes in plastic reconstructions of cancer resections. The first was the anatomic elucidation of muscular blood supply, which allowed tissue associated with a defined vascular network to be moved to a defect within reach of its pedicle. The second advance was in the field of microsurgery, which allowed muscle flaps with the overlying subcutaneous fat and skin to be detached from their original blood supply and reanastomosed to vessels in a different anatomic area. These advances meant that multiple-stage reconstructions were no longer required to bring well-vascularized tissue into a surgical defect. This decreases the risk of postoperative wound complications and avoids delays in commencing adjuvant therapy. Currently, immediate reconstruction is frequently performed during the same surgery as an oncologic resection. With these techniques, large amounts of tissue can be reliably transplanted to fill dead spaces, pad and cover susceptible organs or structures, and provide restoration of form, function, and contour. Free and pedicled tissue transfers are used for reconstruction after surgery for the breast, mandibular area, and perineum. Commonly used donor myocutaneous flaps include the latissimus dorsi, rectus abdominis, and gracilis muscles. If bone is required, fibula-based flaps are commonly used. Flap success rate is 95%, and multiple studies have demonstrated improved quality of life with reconstruction procedures and no decrement in the ability to detect recurrence. In those patients requiring adjuvant therapy, reconstruction does not delay the time to initiation of treatment. Disadvantages of reconstruction are secondary problems at the donor site and increased operative time.

VII. ABLATIVE MODALITIES. Some patients with liver tumors, who are not candidates for surgical resection, may be able to undergo ablation treatment. Patients may not be able to tolerate surgical resection owing to their overall health status, or when the extent of surgical resection required would leave inadequate functional liver tissue remaining. This is especially a consideration in the presence of cirrhosis or chemotherapy-induced liver injury. Ablative therapies have been best studied for primary hepatocellular carcinoma, and for colorectal cancer metastases to the liver. However, limited data exists for ablation of other malignancies metastatic to the liver, including breast cancer, gynecologic malignancies, and neuroendocrine tumors. Ablation also has been studied in the treatment of primary lung and renal cancers. Generally, the evidence suggests that ablation confers a survival benefit over untreated disease or chemotherapy alone in patients ineligible for resection. In some studies, the overall survival rate may approach that of surgical resection. However, the local recurrence rate is generally inferior to surgical resection, and multiple treatments may be needed to achieve local control.

A. Cryotherapy. Intraoperative cryoablation is regarded as an effective form of palliative therapy and may cure some patients with small tumors. Intraoperative ultrasonography is used to monitor hepatic cryosurgery for nonresectable disease. Hepatic cryotherapy involves the freezing and thawing of liver tumors by means of a cryoprobe inserted into the tumors. During freeze/thaw cycles, ice forms within the intracellular and extracellular spaces, leading to tumor destruction. Tumors are then left in situ to be absorbed. Postoperative complications include hemorrhage, biliary fistula, myoglobinuria, and acute renal failure. Hepatic cryoablation is also associated with a rare syndrome of multiorgan failure, coagulopathy, and disseminated intravascular coagulation. Overall morbidity rates range from 6% to 50%. Mortality rates range from 0% to 8%. Hepatic cryosurgery is an option for patients with isolated liver metastases from colorectal cancer that are not surgically resectable but are limited enough to allow cryoablation of all lesions. However, owing to the rare systemic complications, other ablation techniques are favored in patients who are not candidates for formal resection of their solid tumors.

B. **Radiofrequency ablation.** The radiofrequency ablation (RFA) technique involves percutaneous or intraoperative insertion of a radiofrequency (RF) probe into the center of a hepatic tumor under ultrasonography or CT guidance. RF energy is then emitted from the electrode and absorbed by the surrounding tissue. This process generates heat, leading to coagulation necrosis of the treated tissue. It relies on the ability of the tissue to conduct current, so it is less reliable for desiccated tissue or tissue with high impedance, such as lung or bone. Also, large blood vessels adjacent to the tumor can result in a "heat sink" effect, preferentially conducting current away from the lesion. The initial limitation of this therapy was the small (1.5 cm) diameter of necrosis achievable with a single RF probe. Newer probes allow treatment of larger volumes. The primary advantage of RF ablation over cryosurgery lies in the low incidence of complications and the ease of performance under CT or ultrasonography guidance. RF ablation can be performed percutaneously in many cases, thereby avoiding laparotomy or laparoscopy. It has been best studied in the treatment of cancers localized to the liver, particularly metastatic colorectal cancer and primary hepatocellular carcinomas. Radiofrequency ablation is currently the most widely used ablative therapy, and it has been the most extensively studied.

C. **Microwave ablation.** Microwave ablation is similar to RFA in that it generates an electromagnetic field, resulting in the production of heat within the target tissue. An antenna probe is placed into the tumor to deliver the energy, which can heat tissue up to 2 cm from the antenna. Multiple antennas can also be used simultaneously, allowing the treatment of large or multifocal lesions. Unlike RFA, microwave ablation is not as influenced by the ability of the tissue to conduct electricity, making it a better choice for tissues with higher impedance. It is also less vulnerable to "heat sink" effect and can treat large tumor volumes more reliably than RFA. A disadvantage of microwave ablation is the tendency of the antenna to overheat and potentially damage other tissues along the track of the probe.

D. **Irreversible electroporation.** The irreversible electroporation (IRE) technique differs from the others in that it does not induce a thermal injury to the treated tissues. IRE uses a pulsed direct current that causes irreversible cell damage, leading to apoptosis. It is thought to do so by disrupting the cell membrane and inducing the formation of pores within the lipid bilayer. Because of this, it is not subject to "heat sink" effect and does not exhibit thermal spread to nearby tissues. It is theorized that this will make IRE safer and more reliable to use for lesions close to critical anatomic structures or large blood vessels. Irreversible electroporation is a new technology, and it is still under active investigation for the treatment of multiple cancer types.

VIII. **SURGICAL INTERVENTION FOR ONCOLOGIC EMERGENCIES.** Although true oncologic emergencies are rare, surgeons are often consulted regarding the management of complications that are a result of tumor progression or cytotoxic therapy. In cases of widespread metastasis or unresectable disease, it is essential that part of the discussion about prognosis should include the patient's wishes for surgical intervention in the event that such a complication occurs. Ideally, this would occur when the patient is relatively well and able to express their wishes and ask appropriate questions. Frequently, these discussions take place only in the context of the emergency itself, when the patient and family are unable to have a well-considered discussion about goals of care. Emergent surgery carries a higher risk of complications than elective surgery, and generally delays palliative chemotherapy during the recovery.

A. **Bowel perforation.** Perforation of the gastrointestinal (GI) tract in patients with cancer carries a high morbidity and mortality. Although most perforations are from benign causes (diverticulitis, appendicitis, and peptic ulcer disease), they can also occur as a result of chemotherapy or radiation therapy or as a primary presentation of a malignancy. Undiagnosed colorectal cancers can present with perforation as a result of full-thickness colonic involvement or proximal perforation from a distal obstructing mass. The response of some malignancies, such as GI lymphomas, is so great to chemotherapy that full-thickness necrosis of the bowel wall occurs. Patients undergoing cancer therapy are often immunosuppressed and malnourished, which masks the traditional signs of a perforation (peritonitis, leukocytosis, fever, and tachycardia). Immunosuppression and poor nutrition are associated with an increase in the operative mortality and morbidity of these patients. Mortality rates as high as 80% have been reported in patients who undergo an emergency laparotomy and in those who have metastatic disease and are undergoing chemotherapy. Comfort care and nonsurgical treatments should be discussed in patients with an overall poor prognosis. In patients who undergo abdominal exploration, ostomies, gastrostomy, and feeding jejunostomy tubes should be considered.

B. **Bowel obstruction.** Intestinal obstruction is commonly found in cancer patients presenting with nausea, vomiting, abdominal distention, and obstipation. Benign sources of obstruction such as adhesions from previous surgery and radiation enteritis account for approximately one-third of cases in these patients. Primary (ovarian, colonic, and stomach) malignancies or metastatic disease (lung, breast, and melanoma) are the cause of intestinal obstruction in two-thirds of cases. In a small percentage of cancer patients, functional obstruction can also occur without a mechanical cause from electrolyte abnormalities, radiation therapy, malnutrition, narcotic analgesics, and prolonged immobility. In these patients, correction of the underlying cause and bowel decompression are the cornerstones of treatment.

The approach to the diagnosis and treatment of obstruction in patients with cancer should be similar to that for patients with benign disease. Diagnosis is most frequently made by CT scan, though additional studies using oral or rectal contrast may be diagnostic and/or therapeutic in some cases. CT scans of the abdomen with oral and rectal contrast can be helpful for determining the presence of a transition point, bowel wall thickening, or the presence of recurrent disease.

All patients should be initially resuscitated with IV fluids, have electrolyte abnormalities corrected, be decompressed with a nasogastric tube, and have urine output monitored. Patients who have signs of compromised bowel viability or perforation (abdominal tenderness, leukocytosis, fever, persistent tachycardia, and free intra-abdominal air) should undergo immediate exploratory laparotomy. Patients with a complete bowel obstruction rarely respond to medical management and require surgical exploration. Between 25% and 50% of patients with a partial small bowel obstruction will resolve their obstruction with conservative measures. Those patients who do not demonstrate resolution after a finite period or progress to complete obstruction should undergo laparotomy. Cancer patients with benign obstructions from adhesions or internal herniation benefit from surgery. If malignant obstruction is present, resection or bypass of the obstructed segment may be performed; however, only 35% of patients will have durable relief of symptoms after surgical treatment. These patients should be strongly considered for gastrostomy tube placement at the time of surgery, which provides significant palliation by relieving emesis and obviating the need for nasogastric suction. Radiation-induced enteritis may be clinically indistinguishable from adhesive small bowel obstruction. In cases of radiation enteritis, short segments of narrowed bowel may be resected; however, long segments should be treated with bypass. Surgical intervention for a malignant bowel obstruction is associated with a significant morbidity (30%) and mortality (10%), and patients have a mean survival of approximately 6 months only following laparotomy for a malignant bowel obstruction.

C. **Neutropenic enterocolitis (typhlitis).** Neutropenic enterocolitis most often occurs in patients who are undergoing chemotherapy and are neutropenic for more than 7 days. Symptoms include febrile neutropenia, diarrhea, abdominal distention, and right lower quadrant pain. Initially, the presentation can be very similar to appendicitis. Radiologic findings are often nonspecific or may demonstrate thickening of the cecum. Serial abdominal examinations are critical for proper diagnosis and treatment. Most episodes will resolve with conservative management with bowel rest, IV fluid resuscitation, nasogastric decompression, and broad-spectrum antibiotics. However, if patients develop perforation, uncontrolled hemorrhage, become septic, or symptoms continue to worsen despite medical therapy, a laparotomy should be performed. A right hemicolectomy with ileostomy and mucous fistula is the surgery of choice and may be reversed after several months.

D. **Biliary obstruction.** In addition to pancreatic and bile duct carcinomas, lymphomas, melanomas, and breast, colon, stomach, lung, and ovarian cancers can cause biliary obstruction due to metastasis to the portal lymph nodes or hilum of the liver. The prognosis for patients with biliary obstruction from metastatic disease is poor. Two-month mortality rates approaching 70% have been reported. Treatment should be aimed at preventing cholangitis and palliating jaundice. Endoscopic retrograde cholangiopancreatography (ERCP) with stent placement or percutaneous transhepatic drainage should be the initial treatment strategy.

E. **Hemorrhage.** Patients with malignancies who develop GI bleeding should undergo the same workup as those without malignant disease. Resuscitation, correction of coagulopathies, and a workup to define the bleeding site should be initiated immediately. Bright blood per rectum or hematemesis can give clues to a lower or upper GI source. Malignant tumors are rarely the source of significant intra-abdominal hemorrhage. If the bleeding is not at a life-threatening rate, tagged red blood cell scan, angiography, embolization, and endoscopic interventions can all be used to diagnose and treat the hemorrhage. The timing of surgical intervention is based on the rate and volume of blood loss, the underlying pathology, and the overall prognosis of the patient.

F. **Pericardial tamponade.** Metastatic disease to the pericardium leading to malignant obstruction of the pericardial lymphatics is the most common cause of pericardial tamponade in cancer patients. Lung cancer, breast cancer, lymphoma, leukemia, melanoma, and primary neoplasms of the heart are most commonly implicated in tamponade. The development of symptoms in a patient depends on the rate of accumulation of the volume of the pericardial fluid and compliance of the sac. If the accumulation is gradual, more than 2 L can be found in the pericardial sac. Patients often present with vague symptoms of chest pain, dyspnea, and anxiety. On examination, decreased heart sounds, tachycardia, pulsus paradoxus, and jugular venous distention can be found. Echocardiography is the best test to determine whether there is excess pericardial fluid. Pericardiocentesis with placement of a drainage catheter can be life-saving in a patient in tamponade and shock. Additional options in more stable patients include tetracycline sclerosis, radiation therapy, subxiphoid pericardiotomy, window pericardectomy, and complete pericardectomy. A subxiphoid approach avoids the need for a thoracotomy.

G. **Superior vena cava syndrome.** Superior vena cava syndrome (SVCS) results from an impedance to outflow from the superior vena cava (SVC) due to external compression by malignancy, fibrosis, or thrombosis. In more than 95% of patients, SVCS results from a malignancy. The SVC is a thin-walled vessel in the middle mediastinum, and any enlargement of the perihilar or paratracheal lymph nodes or abnormalities of the aorta, pulmonary artery, or mainstem bronchus could lead to impingement on the SVC. The SVC is responsible for venous drainage of the head, neck, upper extremities, and upper thorax. Small cell lung cancer and other pulmonary malignancies are the most common etiology of SVCS, although lymphomas, germ cell tumors, and metastatic lesions to the supraclavicular nodal basins are also responsible. In most cases, SVCS develops gradually. The most common symptoms are dyspnea and facial fullness. Other symptoms associated with SVCS are venous engorgement of the neck and chest wall, cyanosis, and upper extremity edema. Symptoms are worse when the patient bends forward or reclines. Unless SVCS causes impedance of the airway from laryngeal edema (an emergency treated with intubation, tracheostomy, or emergent radiation therapy), a thorough workup can be conducted. Chest radiography, CT, and biopsy can be useful in determining the etiology of SVC obstruction. Treatment includes diuretics, elevation of the head, and steroids, and chemotherapy and/or radiation therapy directed at treating the underlying cause. SVCS can be secondary to indwelling central venous catheters causing thrombosis. This can often be successfully treated with thrombolytic agents followed by systemic anticoagulation. Balloon angioplasty and vascular stenting can be used if initial therapies fail. Surgical innominate vein–right atrial bypass is the last option.

H. **Spinal cord compression.** Spinal cord compression is an acute emergency. The severity of neurologic impairment at presentation dictates the potential reversibility of symptoms.

Early recognition is essential in preventing progressive or irreversible neurologic deterioration that can lead to paralysis and loss of sphincter control. Extradural metastatic lesions of the vertebral body or neural arch are the most common cause of spinal cord compression in patients with malignancies. As tumors expand, they often impinge on the anterior aspect of the spinal cord. Metastatic lesions from lung, breast, prostate cancers, and multiple myeloma are the most common lesions responsible for spinal cord compression. Of these, 10% occur in the cervical vertebrae, 70% in the thoracic vertebrae, and 20% in the lumbosacral vertebrae. 90% of patients will present with localized back pain. The pain usually precedes the onset of neurologic deterioration by weeks to months. Patients will develop motor loss and weakness followed by sensory loss. Patients often describe an ascending tingling sensation beginning in the distal extremities. The onset of urinary retention, constipation, and/or loss of bowel or bladder control is a late and ominous manifestation. In addition to plain radiographs, MRI is the study of choice for evaluating patients with suspected spinal cord compression. Gadolinium contrast provides optimal imaging of extramedullary and intramedullary lesions. In cases of rapid compression of the spinal cord, therapeutic intervention must be performed immediately to avoid irreversible neurologic deficits. The patient should be immediately started on steroids, and treatment options include radiation therapy, surgery, chemotherapy, or a combination of all three. Laminectomy is effective in managing patients with epidural masses, and in select cases, surgical resection of the mass may be possible. As mentioned earlier, the functional status at the time of presentation clearly correlates with the posttreatment outcome; early diagnosis and recognition is crucial.

IX. VASCULAR ACCESS

A. Central venous catheterization. Many cancer patients require frequent venous catheterization for phlebotomy, chemotherapy, or infusions. Peripheral venous sites for catheterization can become quickly exhausted because of the venotoxic effects of the cytotoxic agents, the trauma of repeated use, and the undesirability of performing access procedures in limbs with proximal lymphadenectomies. Central venous catheters are designed for repeated venous access. Although they are generally easily placed, complications of placement include pneumothorax, hemothorax, air embolism, cardiac arrhythmia, and arterial injury. Over the long term, these catheters can cause central vein thrombosis, embolism, infection, and scarring. Infection and symptomatic catheter-associated thrombosis are indications for catheter removal. Relative contraindications to placement include uncorrected thrombocytopenia or coagulopathy and previous irradiation to the head or neck, which can result in scarring. For these latter patients or patients with a known history of central vein thrombosis, an ultrasonography before the procedure may be useful to establish the patency of their veins. Patients who are hypercoagulable from their cancers may benefit from low-dose warfarin (1 to 2 mg/day) to prevent central venous thrombosis. Catheters are available in tunneled externalized types (Hickman, Broviac) or implantable types (Portacath, Infusaport). They may be placed under local anesthesia, with or without sedation, on an outpatient basis. The choice of catheter type and placement location will depend on a number of factors, including the expected duration of therapy requiring the catheter, the anticipated infection risk to the patient, any history of prior central lines or central vein thrombosis, and the number of lumens needed. It is important to discuss these factors beforehand with the surgeon or radiologist who will be performing the procedure.

B. Arterial catheters: hepatic artery infusion catheters. Hepatic artery infusion (HAI) catheters are an option for treating hepatic metastases in patients with unresectable disease. HAI chemotherapy targets liver metastases, which derive most of their blood supply from the hepatic arterial circulation, in contrast to normal liver, which derives most of its blood supply from the portal circulation. In addition, higher levels of local therapy can be achieved without concomitant systemic toxicity owing to the clearance of many chemotherapeutic agents from first pass through the liver. HAI chemotherapy is generally reserved for patients without evidence of extrahepatic disease. Traditionally, catheters have been placed surgically by laparotomy, though percutaneous placement under radiographic guidance by interventionalists is currently under study in clinical trials. Before placement, patients undergo an angiogram to define regional arterial anatomy because of the highly variant arterial anatomy in this area. The infusion port or continuous infusion pump is placed in the abdominal subcutaneous tissues over the rectus muscle fascia, and the catheter is tunneled into the abdomen. The tip of the catheter is placed in the gastroduodenal artery at its junction with the common hepatic artery. Cholecystectomy is required to prevent chemotherapy-induced chemical cholecystitis, and complete separation of the hepatic arterial circulation from the gastroduodenal blood supply must be achieved to prevent GI toxicity. Postoperatively, radiolabeled microaggregated albumin is injected into the infusion pump, and a scintillation scan is obtained to verify hepatic infusion and exclusion of extrahepatic perfusion. Chemotherapeutic agents are injected into the port reservoir, which is designed to ensure continuous infusion of a constant amount of agent. Studies have demonstrated higher response rates with HAI than with systemic chemotherapy; however, no survival advantage has been observed. Current strategies combine liver resection, residual tumor ablation, and HAI pump placement.

X. ENTERAL FEEDING TUBES. Malnutrition is common in the cancer patient and may be related to inadequate voluntary intake, altered metabolism, or the effects of therapy. Enteral alimentation can be useful before or after surgery or during therapy. Early concerns that hyperalimentation would lead to rapid tumor growth have not been borne out by experience, and in severely malnourished patients (less than 80% standard weight for height), there is a measurable improvement in operative morbidity if nutritional supplementation is provided 7 to 10 days before surgery. Postoperatively, enteral or parenteral alimentation can support the cancer patient who is unable to eat because of a healing anastomosis or a postoperative ileus. During chemotherapy or radiation therapy, inflammation, infection, or strictures may lead to inadequate oral intake requiring enteral alimentation. The route of administration of nutritional support is selected on the basis of length of anticipated need, intestinal tract function, degree of malnutrition, access for administration, and potential complications. In patients with adequate GI function, enteral alimentation is preferred over the parenteral route. Enteral alimentation is less expensive, leads to fewer metabolic imbalances, preserves the GI architecture, and is thought to prevent bacterial translocation. The most common morbidities associated with enteral alimentation are abdominal distention, nausea, or diarrhea, which can occur in 10% to 20% of patients. These symptoms usually abate with a decreased rate of infusion or strength of the formula.

A. Gastrostomy tubes. Gastrostomy tubes (G-tubes) may be placed percutaneously, laparoscopically, or via laparotomy. They can serve the dual functions of conduits for feeding or intestinal decompression. Other advantages of a G-tube are bolus feeding with high-osmolar formulas because of the reservoir capacity of the stomach, and the ability to replace dislodged tubes easily through the gastrocutaneous fistula. Disadvantages include risk of aspiration in patients with lower esophageal sphincter dysfunction or without an intact gag reflex. Enteral feeds can be administered by bolus (200 to 400 mL over a 5- to 10-minute period) and is the preferred feeding method in ambulatory patients because it is less confining. Crushed pills may be administered through G-tubes.

B. Jejunostomy tubes. Jejunostomy tubes (J-tubes) are small-caliber feeding tubes placed distal to the ligament of Treitz by laparotomy or laparoscopy. The advantages of J-tubes are the minimal risk of aspiration and the ability to feed distal to the obstruction or fistula. Because there is no reservoir capacity, enteral feeds are administered continuously over 12- to 24-hour periods, and there is limited tolerance to high-osmolar loads. Once dislodged, these tubes are not easily replaced. In addition, because of the small caliber, these tubes may become clogged with inspissated material and require vigorous flushing to reestablish patency. For this reason, crushed pills should not be administered via most standard J-tubes, although medications in liquid form may be given via this route.

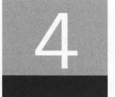

4 Principles and Practice of Radiation Oncology

Pawel Dyk • Clifford G. Robinson • Jeffrey D. Bradley • Joseph Roti Roti • Sasa Mutic

I. **INTRODUCTION.** Optimal care of patients with malignant tumors is a multidisciplinary effort that often combines two or more of the classic disciplines: surgery, radiation therapy, and chemotherapy. Pathologists, radiologists, clinical laboratory physicians, and immunologists are integral members of the team that renders the correct diagnosis. Many professionals, including physicists, laboratory scientists, nurses, social workers, and others, are intimately involved in the care of the patient with cancer.

Radiation oncology is a clinical and scientific discipline devoted to management of patients with cancer and other diseases through use of ionizing radiation, alone or in combination with other modalities, investigation of the biologic and physical basis of radiation therapy, and training of professionals in the field. The aim of radiation therapy is to deliver a precisely measured dose of radiation to a defined tumor volume with as minimal damage as possible to surrounding healthy tissue, resulting in eradication of the tumor, a high quality of life, and prolongation of survival at competitive cost. In addition to curative efforts, radiation therapy plays a major role in the effective palliation or prevention of symptoms of cancer including improving pain and restoring luminal patency, skeletal integrity, and organ function with minimal morbidity.

The radiation oncologist, like any other physician, must assess all conditions relative to the patient and the tumor under consideration for treatment, systematically review the need for diagnostic and staging procedures, and determine the best therapeutic strategy.

II. **TYPES OF RADIATION USED IN RADIATION THERAPY.** Many types of radiation are used for treatment of both benign and malignant diseases. The most common form of radiation is through the use of external beam photons or electrons. Photons are x-rays or γ-rays and may be considered as bundles of energy that deposit dose as they pass through matter. The term x-ray is used to describe radiation that is produced by machines, while γ-rays define radiation that is emitted from radioactive isotopes. Typical radiotherapy units used in modern-day x-ray therapy are linear accelerators with energies spanning 4 to 25 million volts or MV. The most common source of γ-rays for external beam radiotherapy has been ^{60}Co. Most radiotherapy facilities no longer use γ-rays because of their low energy profile, unfavorable dose distribution, and the need to replace and recalculate for decaying sources. An exception is the Gamma Knife unit used for intracranial stereotactic radiosurgery, which houses 192 or 201 (depending on the version) ^{60}Co sources to deliver high doses of radiation to relatively small target volumes within the brain. A recently developed radiotherapy unit, the ViewRay system, uses ^{60}Co sources to deliver radiotherapy simultaneously with real-time magnetic resonance imaging (MRI).

Electrons or β-particles can also be used to treat patients. Similar to the distinction between x-rays and γ-rays, the term *electron* is used to describe radiation produced by machines, while β-particles describe electrons emitted by radioactive isotopes. Electrons deposit their maximal energy slightly beyond the skin surface and have a sharp falloff beyond their range. Electrons are used mainly for treating skin or superficial tumors.

Other sources of external beam radiation are protons and neutrons. Protons are charged particles that have the advantage of depositing dose at a constant rate over most of the beam, but depositing most of the dose at the end of their range, creating a Bragg peak. The advantage of protons over photons is that beyond the Bragg peak, protons fall off rapidly and avoid dose deposition beyond the target. This vastly limits radiation dose to normal tissues beyond the target, as well as the total amount of radiation (integral dose) delivered to the patient. Proton dose-deposition characteristics are useful in situations where limiting dose to surrounding organs is critical, such as treating within a previously irradiated field where the structures surrounding the target have received the maximum tolerated radiation dose. Protons also have unique advantages in the treatment of pediatric malignancies by avoiding the irradiation of developing organs and skeletal structures, and potentially decreasing the risk of radiation-induced malignancies by lowering the delivered integral dose. The use of protons is also being investigated in other cancer sites, such as esophagus and lung, where improved reduction in dose to multiple uninvolved adjacent organs (lung, heart, esophagus, etc.) may be possible compared with other photon-based treatment techniques like 3D conformal radiation therapy (3D-CRT) or intensity modulated radiation therapy (IMRT). Because of the cost, few radiotherapy facilities in the United States currently have proton units available for patient treatment. The recent development of relatively cheaper proton delivery systems may substantially increase the availability of protons across the United States, potentially expanding their application and use to other clinical tumor sites.

Neutrons are uncharged heavy particles that are produced by a variety of mechanisms. They deposit large amounts of energy very close to their initial interaction sites with the nuclei of a treated medium. Experience with neutrons has been limited to a few centers because of the cost of producing and maintaining these radiotherapy units. An example of depth–dose characteristics for photons, electrons, protons, and neutrons is shown in Figure 4-1.

Brachytherapy is an alternative method of irradiating targeted tissues. *Brachy* is translated from Greek, meaning short distance. In brachytherapy, sealed or unsealed radioactive sources are placed very close to or in contact with the targeted tissue. The absorbed dose falls off rapidly with increasing distance from the source ($1/radius^2$ for a point source and $1/radius$ for a line source); thus, higher doses can be delivered safely to the targeted tissue over a short time. Prescribed brachytherapy doses are generally delivered in days for low-dose rate (LDR) or minutes for high-dose rate (HDR). Brachytherapy sources can be placed temporarily, as in the use of ^{192}Ir for HDR applications in cervix cancer, or permanently, as in the use of ^{125}I in the treatment of prostate cancer. Some common applications of sealed brachytherapy include the treatment of prostate (both HDR and permanent LDR), breast (mainly HDR), soft tissue sarcoma (HDR), and cervix (both HDR and LDR) cancers. In selective cases, sealed brachytherapy sources may also be used intraluminally in the palliative setting to relieve malignant obstruction in a previously irradiated field, such as obstructing esophageal and endobronchial tumors. Unsealed sources are radioactive substances in soluble form that are

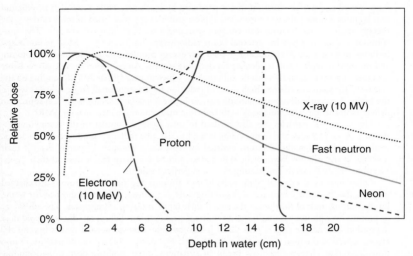

Figure 4-1. Depth–dose curves for photons (x-rays), electrons, protons, and neutrons at energies used in radiation therapy.

administered through ingestion or injection. Examples include ^{131}I ingested to treat thyroid cancer, ^{90}Y embedded resin or glass microspheres injected into the hepatic vasculature to treat metastatic or primary liver malignancies, and ^{223}Ra delivered intravenously to treat metastatic prostate cancer to the bone.

III. **GOALS OF RADIATION THERAPY.** The clinical use of radiation is a complex process that involves many professionals and a variety of interrelated functions. The aim of therapy should be defined at the beginning of the therapeutic intervention.

A. **Curative.** The patient has a probability of long-term survival after adequate therapy. Oncologists may be willing to risk both acute and chronic complications as a result of therapy in an attempt to eradicate the malignant disease.

B. **Palliative.** There is no hope that the patient will survive for extended periods; symptoms that produce discomfort or an impending condition that may impair the comfort or self-sufficiency of the patient require treatment.

In curative therapy, some side effects, even though undesirable, may be acceptable. However, in palliative treatment, no major side effects should be seen. In palliation of epithelial solid tumors causing complications due to mass effect or pain, relatively high doses of radiation (sometimes 75% to 80% of curative dose) are required to control the tumor for the survival period of the patient. There are some exceptions to high-dose palliative radiotherapy, including patients with lymphoma or multiple myeloma or for treatment of bleeding such as patients with cervical or endobronchial malignancies. Some disease conditions, such as low-grade lymphoma, are long-standing and incurable. These conditions also fall into the palliative category because one is generally willing to sacrifice some long-term tumor control to avoid the development of treatment-related complications.

IV. **BASIS FOR PRESCRIPTION OF RADIATION THERAPY**

A. Evaluation of tumor extent (staging), including radiographic, radioisotopic, and other studies

B. Knowledge of the pathologic characteristics of the disease

C. Definition of goal of therapy (cure vs. palliation)

D. Selection of appropriate treatment modalities (irradiation alone or combined with surgery, chemotherapy, or both)

E. Determination of the optimal dose of irradiation and the volume to be treated, according to the anatomic location, histologic type, stage, potential regional nodal involvement, and other characteristics of the tumor, and the normal structures present in the region

F. Evaluation of the patient's general condition, periodic assessment of tolerance to treatment, tumor response, and status of the normal tissues treated

In addition to coordinating the patient's care with the surgical and medical oncology teams, the radiation oncologist must work closely with the physics, treatment planning, and dosimetry staff within the radiotherapy facility to ensure the greatest possible accuracy, practicality, and cost benefit in the design of treatment plans. The ultimate responsibility for treatment decisions and the technical execution of the therapy will always rest with the physician.

V. **RADIOBIOLOGIC PRINCIPLES**

A. **Probability of tumor control.** It is axiomatic in radiation therapy that higher doses of radiation produce better tumor control. Numerous dose–response curves for cell killing of a variety of tumors by single dose and multiple repeated-dose radiation have been published. For every increment of radiation dose, a certain fraction of cells will be killed. Therefore, the total number of surviving cells will be proportional to the initial number of tumor cells present and the fraction killed with each. As such, various total doses will yield different probabilities of tumor control, depending on the extent of the lesion (number of clonogenic cells present) and the sensitivity to radiation. Additional factors that affect the efficacy of radiation therapy include repair of radiation damage (to DNA), the presence of hypoxic cells and their reoxygenation, cell cycle checkpoints, and tumor cell repopulation rates.

Subclinical disease has been referred to as deposits of tumor cells that are too small to be detected clinically and even microscopically but, if left untreated, may subsequently evolve into clinically apparent tumor. For subclinical disease in squamous cell carcinoma of the upper respiratory tract or for adenocarcinoma of the breast, doses of 45 to 50 Gy will result in disease control in more than 90% of patients. **Microscopic tumor,** as at the surgical margin, should not be regarded as subclinical disease; cell aggregates of 10^6/cc or greater are required for the pathologist to detect them. Therefore, these volumes must receive higher doses of radiation, in the range of 60 to 65 Gy in 6 to 7 weeks for epithelial tumors.

For **clinically palpable tumors,** doses of 60 (for T1) to 75 to 80 Gy or higher (for T4 tumors) are required (2 Gy/day, five fractions weekly). This dose range and tumor control probability (TCP) has been documented for squamous cell carcinoma and adenocarcinoma (Fletcher GH. *Textbook of Radiotherapy.* Philadelphia, PA: Lea & Febiger, 1980). Ideally, the radiation oncologist would have the ability to deliver doses in this range. However, these doses are often beyond the tolerance of normal tissues. Exceeding normal tissue tolerance may result in debilitating or life-threatening complications.

B. **Effects of radiation on tissues and the linear–quadratic equation.** Radiation causes cell death by inducing DNA double-strand breaks. The presence of DNA double-strand breaks in cells leads to lethal, sublethal, and potentially lethal damage. Lethal damage is a level of DNA damage that is too much for the cell to repair. *Sublethal damage* is defined as damage that can be repaired when a single dose of x-rays is divided into two or more fractions. Potentially lethal damage is defined as damage that can be repaired or fixed to lethal damage by modifying growth conditions (i.e., cell cycle progression) during or after a dose of x-rays. Sublethal damage repair (SLDR) and potentially lethal damage repair (PLDR) are important concepts in considering normal tissue repair. Normal tissues have a substantial capacity to recover from sublethal or potentially lethal damage induced by radiation (at tolerable dose levels). Injury to normal tissues may be caused by the radiation effect on the microvasculature or the support tissues (stromal or parenchymal cells).

A variety of changes in tissues are induced by ionizing radiation, depending on the total dose, fractionation schedule (daily dose and time), and volume treated. For many tissues, the necessary dose to produce a particular sequela increases as the irradiated fraction of volume of the organ decreases.

Chronologically, the effects of irradiation have been subdivided into **acute** (first 6 months), **subacute** (second 6 months), or **late,** depending on the time at which they are observed. The gross manifestations depend on the kinetic properties of the cells (slow or rapid renewal) and the dose of radiation given. No correlation has been established between the incidence and severity of acute reactions and the same parameters for late effects (Karcher KH, Kogelnik HD, Reinartz G, eds. *Progress in Radio-Oncology II.* New York, NY: Raven Press, 1982:287).

Formulations based on dose–survival models have been proposed to describe the dependence of cell killing on radiation dose and fractionation. These models are very useful in evaluating the biologic equivalence of various doses and fractionation schedules. These assumptions are based on a linear–quadratic survival curve represented by the equation

$$\ln S = \alpha D + \beta D^2 \text{ for a single dose or } \ln S = \alpha(nd) + \beta(nd)d \qquad (4.1)$$

for a fractionated dose, where n = number of fractions, d = dose/fraction, and nd = total dose. In this equation, α represents the linear (i.e., first-order dose-dependent) component of cell killing, and β represents the quadratic (i.e., second-order dose-dependent) component of cell killing. Thus, α represents the less reparable component of lethal radiation damage, that is, damage for which the lethality is not reduced by fractionating the radiation dose. Conversely, β represents damage that can be repaired (i.e., its lethality is reduced) when the radiation dose is fractionated. At low doses, the α (linear) component of cell killing predominates. At high doses, the β (quadratic) component of cell killing predominates. The dose at which the two components of cell killing are equal constitutes the α/β ratio.

In general, tissues reacting immediately to acute effects, like the skin and mucosa, have a high α/β ratio (between 8 and 15 Gy), whereas tissues involved in late effects, like the brain and spinal cord, have a low α/β ratio (1 to 5 Gy). Therefore, the severity of late effects changes more rapidly with a variation in the size of dose per fraction when a total dose is selected to yield equivalent acute effects. With a decreasing size of dose per fraction, the total dose required to achieve a certain isoeffect increases more for late-responding tissues than for immediately responding tissues. Therefore, in hyperfractionated regimens, the tolerable dose would be increased more for late effects than for early effects. Conversely, if large doses per fraction are used, the total dose required to achieve isoeffects in late-responding tissues would be reduced more for late effects than for early effects. A biologically equivalent dose (BED) can be obtained by using the following equations, derived from the equation for cell survival after a fractionated dose:

$$BED = -\ln S/\alpha = nd[1 + d/(\alpha/\beta)] = D[1 + d/(\alpha/\beta)] \qquad (4.2)$$

To compare two treatment regimens (with some reservations), the following formula can be used:

$$Dx = Dr[(\alpha/\beta + dx)/(\alpha/\beta + dr)] \qquad (4.3)$$

in which Dr is the known total dose (reference dose), Dx is the new total dose (with different fractionation schedule), dr is the known dose per fraction (reference), and dx is the new dose per fraction.

The following is an example of use of this formula (with some reservations!): suppose 50 Gy in 25 fractions is delivered to yield a given biologic effect. If one assumes that the subcutaneous tissue is the limiting parameter (late reaction), it is desirable to know what the total dose to be administered will be, using 4-Gy fractions. Assume $\alpha/\beta = 5$ Gy.

Using the earlier equation

$$Dx = 50 \text{ Gy}(5 + 2)/(5 + 4) = 38 \text{ Gy} \qquad (4.4)$$

Answer: A dose of 50 Gy in 25 fractions provides the same BED as 39 Gy in 4-Gy fractions.

As the total dose to a particular tumor and surrounding normal tissues increases, both TCP and normal tissue complication probability (NTCP) increase. Both TCP and NTCP are sigmoidal in shape. The farther these two curves diverge, the more favorable the **therapeutic ratio** (Fig. 4-2). When the curves are close together, increases in irradiation dose will lead to exponential increases in NTCP. The TCP and NTCP curves can be separated

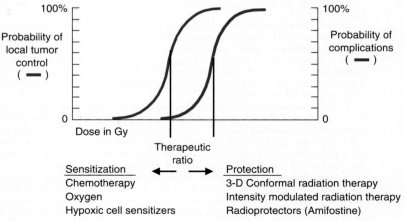

Figure 4-2. The therapeutic ratio represents the relationship between two sigmoidal curves; the TCP and the NTCP curves. The further the two curves are separated, the higher the TCP and the lower the NTCP.

by the use of biologic modifiers, radioprotectors, three-dimensional conformal irradiation, IMRT, or proton therapy. When the TCP and NTCP curves are well separated, higher doses of radiation therapy can be delivered more safely. Chemotherapy also modifies the TCP and NTCP curves, often by shifting both curves to the left. Therefore, with chemoradiation, lower doses of radiotherapy are required to produce a given TCP/NTCP. Biologic factors can also contribute to the TCP and NTCP. Defects in DNA repair will lower the dose for both curves unless the defect is unique to the tumor. In contrast, defective apoptotic pathways tend to increase radiation resistance.

An acceptable complication rate for severe injury is 5% to 10% in most curative clinical situations. Moderate sequelae are noted in varying proportions depending on the dose and fractionation of radiation given and the volume irradiated of the specific organ at risk. In 2010, a seminal series of articles was published that provides clinicians with evidence-based dosimetric tools to guide radiation treatment planning in order to minimize normal tissue complications. This **QU**antitative **A**nalysis of **N**ormal **T**issue **E**ffects in the **C**linic (QUANTEC) is an evaluable source that describes dose and volume parameters that have been shown in the literature to be associated with organ-specific radiation toxicity. Table 4-1 is a QUANTEC summary of dose, volume, and outcome data for organs at risk treated with conventional fractionation (1.8 to 2 Gy per fraction) (*Int J Radiat Oncol Biol Phys* 2010;76(3):S10).

Combining irradiation with surgery or cytotoxic agents frequently modifies the tolerance of normal tissues and/or tumor response to a given dose of radiation, which may necessitate adjustments in treatment planning and dose prescription. For example, in curative radiation therapy for cancer of the esophagus, concurrent chemotherapy consisting of 5-fluorouracil (5-FU) and cisplatin and radiation therapy to 50 Gy result in improved local tumor control and similar esophagitis rates when compared with irradiation alone to doses of 64 Gy.

C. **Dose–time factors.** Dose–time considerations constitute a complex function that expresses the interdependence of total dose, time, and number of fractions in the production of a biologic effect within a given tissue volume.

Short overall treatment times are required for tumors with rapid proliferation, and more slowly proliferating tumors can be treated with longer overall treatment times. With regard to fractionation, five fractions per week, for example, are preferable to three fractions because it has been shown that there is approximately 10-fold less cell killing per week with the latter schedule (Fowler JR. Fractionation and therapeutic gain. In: Steel GG, Adams GE, Peckham MJ, eds. *Biological Basis of Radiotherapy*. Amsterdam: Elsevier Science, 1983:181).

In general, fractionation of the radiation dose will spare acute tissue reactions, as in the skin and mucosa, because of compensatory accelerated proliferation in the epithelium. Therefore, a prolonged course of therapy with small daily fractions will decrease early acute reactions. However, such a strategy will not reduce serious late damage to normal tissue because such effects are not proliferation-dependent. Worse, extensively prolonging the treatment time will allow the growth of rapidly proliferating tumors. Therefore, prolonged treatment schedules are undesirable.

Radiation treatments may be delivered by conventional fractionation, hypofractionation, hyperfractionation, or accelerated fractionation schedules. In the United States, **conventional fractionation** is defined as a daily fraction size of 1.8 to 2.0 Gy, and in the nonpalliative setting it is typically delivered 5 days per week over 5 to 8 weeks to a total dose of 45 to 80 Gy. The other fractionation schedules are defined by overall treatment duration and total dose of radiation as compared with conventional fractionation.

Hypofractionation refers to fraction sizes that are larger than conventionally fractionated radiation therapy, and are delivered once daily. Typically, a lower total dose is delivered and designed to achieve the same tumor control probability (TCP) as conventional fractionation. Common examples of hypofractionation in the United States are palliative therapy regimens of 30 Gy in 10 fractions over a 2-week period or 8 Gy in a single fraction. The difficulty with hypofractionation is the effect of the larger dose per fraction on

TABLE 4-1 QUANTEC summary of dose, volume, and outcome data for OAR treated with conventional fractionation (1.8 – 2Gy per fraction). From Marks LB, et al. Use of NTCP Models in the Clinic.

Organ	Volume segmented	Irradiation type (partial organ unless otherwise stated)[†]	Endpoint	Dose (Gy), or dose/ volume parameters[†]	Rate (%)	Notes on dose/volume parameters
Brain	Whole organ	3D-CRT	Symptomatic necrosis	D_{max} <60	<3	Data at 72 and 90 Gy, extrapolated from BED models
	Whole organ	3D-CRT	Symptomatic necrosis	D_{max} = 72	5	
	Whole organ	3D-CRT	Symptomatic necrosis	D_{max} = 90	10	
	Whole organ	SRS (single fraction)	Symptomatic necrosis	V12 <5–10 cc	<20	Rapid rise when V12 >5–10 cc
Brain stem	Whole organ	Whole organ	Permanent cranial neuropathy or necrosis	D_{max} <54	<5	
	Whole organ	3D-CRT	Permanent cranial neuropathy or necrosis	D1–10 ccll ≤59	<5	Point dose <<1 cc
	Whole organ	3D-CRT	Permanent cranial neuropathy or necrosis	D_{max} <64	<5	
	Whole organ	SRS (single fraction)	Permanent cranial neuropathy or necrosis	D_{max} <12.5	<5	For patients with acoustic tumors
Optic nerve/ chiasm	Whole organ	3D-CRT	Optic neuropathy	D_{max} <55	<3	Given the small size, 3D CRT is often whole organ[‡‡]
	Whole organ	3D-CRT	Optic neuropathy	D_{max} 55–60	3–7	
	Whole organ	3D-CRT	Optic neuropathy	D_{max} >60	>7–20	
	Whole organ	SRS (single fraction)	Optic neuropathy	D_{max} <12	<10	
Spinal cord	Partial organ	3D-CRT	Myelopathy	D_{max} = 50	0.2	Including full cord cross-section
	Partial organ	3D-CRT	Myelopathy	D_{max} = 60	6	
	Partial organ	3D-CRT	Myelopathy	D_{max} = 69	50	
	Partial organ	SRS (single fraction)	Myelopathy	D_{max} = 13	1	Partial cord cross-section irradiated 3 fractions, partial cord cross-section irradiated

(continued)

TABLE 4-1 QUANTEC summary of dose, volume, and outcome data for OAR treated with conventional fractionation (1.8 - 2Gy per fraction). From Marks LB, et al. Use of NTCP Models in the Clinic. *(continued)*

Organ	Volume segmented	Irradiation type (partial organ unless otherwise stated)[†]	Endpoint	Dose (Gy), or dose/ volume parameters[†]	Rate (%)	Notes on dose/volume parameters
Cochlea	Partial organ	SRS (hypofraction)	Myelopathy	$D_{max} = 20$	1	Mean dose to cochlear, hearing at 4 kHz
	Whole organ	3D-CRT	Sensory neural hearing loss	Mean dose ≤45	<30	Serviceable hearing
	Whole organ	SRS (single fraction)	Sensory neural hearing loss	Prescription dose ≤14	<25	
Parotid	Bilateral whole parotid glands	3D-CRT	Long-term parotid salivary function reduced to <25% of pre-RT level	Mean dose <25	<20	For combined parotid glands[¶]
	Unilateral whole parotid gland	3D-CRT	Long-term parotid salivary function reduced to <25% of pre-RT level	Mean dose <20	<20	For single parotid gland. At least one parotid gland spared to <20 Gy[¶]
	Bilateral whole parotid glands	3D-CRT	Long-term parotid salivary function reduced to <25% of pre-RT level	Mean dose <39	<50	For combined parotid glands (per Fig. 3 in paper)[¶]
Pharynx	Pharyngeal constrictors	Whole organ	Symptomatic dysphagia and aspiration	Mean dose <50	<20	Based on Section B4 in paper
Larynx	Whole organ	3D-CRT	Vocal dysfunction	D_{max} <66	<20	With chemotherapy, based on single study (see Section A4.2 in paper)
	Whole organ	3D-CRT	Aspiration	Mean dose <50	<30	With chemotherapy, based on single study (see Fig. 1 in paper)
	Whole organ	3D-CRT	Edema	Mean dose <44	<20	Without chemotherapy, based on single study in patients without larynx cancer**
Lung	Whole organ	3D-CRT	Edema	V50 <27%	<20	
	Whole organ	3D-CRT	Symptomatic pneumonitis	V20 ≤30%	<20	For combined lung. Gradual dose response
	Whole organ	3D-CRT	Symptomatic pneumonitis	Mean dose = 7	5	Excludes purposeful whole lung irradiation

Organ	Anatomy	Technique	Endpoint	Dose (Gy)	Rate (%)	Notes
	Whole organ	3D-CRT	Symptomatic pneumonitis	Mean dose = 13	10	
	Whole organ	3D-CRT	Symptomatic pneumonitis	Mean dose = 20	20	
	Whole organ	3D-CRT	Symptomatic pneumonitis	Mean dose = 24	30	
	Whole organ	3D-CRT	Symptomatic pneumonitis	Mean dose = 27	40	
Esophagus	Whole organ	3D-CRT	Grade ≥3 acute esophagitis	Mean dose <34	5–20	Based on RTOG and several studies
	Whole organ	3D-CRT	Grade ≥2 acute esophagitis	V35 <50%	<30	A variety of alternate threshold doses have been implicated
	Whole organ	3D-CRT	Grade ≥2 acute esophagitis	V50 <40%	<30	Appears to be a dose/volume response
	Whole organ	3D-CRT	Grade ≥2 acute esophagitis	V70 <20%	<30	
Heart	Pericardium	3D-CRT	Pericarditis	Mean dose <26	<15	Based on single study
	Pericardium	3D-CRT	Pericarditis	V30 <46%	<15	
	Whole organ	3D-CRT	Long-term cardiac mortality	V25 <10%	<1	Overly safe risk estimate based on model predictions
Liver	Whole liver—GTV	3D-CRT or Whole organ	Classic RILD[††]	Mean dose <30-32	<5	Excluding patients with preexisting liver disease or hepatocellular carcinoma, as tolerance doses are lower in these patients
	Whole liver—GTV	3D-CRT	Classic RILD	Mean dose <42	<50	
	Whole liver—GTV	3D-CRT or Whole organ	Classic RILD	Mean dose <28	<5	In patients with Child-Pugh A preexisting liver disease or hepatocellular carcinoma, excluding hepatitis B reactivation as an endpoint
	Whole liver—GTV	3D-CRT	Classic RILD	Mean dose <36	<50	
	Whole liver—GTV	SBRT (hypofraction)	Classic RILD	Mean dose <13	<5	3 fractions, for primary liver cancer
				<18	<5	6 fractions, for primary liver cancer
	Whole liver—GTV	SBRT (hypofraction)	Classic RILD	Mean dose <15	<5	3 fractions, for liver metastases
				<20	<5	6 fractions, for liver metastases
	>700 cc of normal liver	SBRT (hypofraction)	Classic RILD	D_{max} <15	<5	Critical volume based, in 3–5 fractions

(continued)

TABLE 4-1 QUANTEC summary of dose, volume, and outcome data for OAR treated with conventional fractionation (1.8 - 2Gy per fraction). From Marks LB, et al. Use of NTCP Models in the Clinic. *(continued)*

Organ	Volume segmented	Irradiation type (partial organ unless otherwise stated)[†]	Endpoint	Dose (Gy), or dose/volume parameters[†]	Rate (%)	Notes on dose/volume parameters
Kidney	Bilateral whole kidney[‡]	Bilateral whole organ or 3D-CRT	Clinically relevant renal dysfunction	Mean dose <15–18	<5	
	Bilateral whole kidney[‡]	Bilateral whole organ	Clinically relevant renal dysfunction	Mean dose <28	<50	
	Bilateral whole kidney[‡]	3D-CRT	Clinically relevant renal dysfunction	V12 <55%	<5	For combined kidney
				V20 <32%		
				V23 <30%		
				V28 <20%		
Stomach	Whole organ	Whole organ	Ulceration	D100[‖] <45	<7	
Small bowel	Individual small bowel loops	3D-CRT	Grade ≥3 acute toxicity[§]	V15 <120 cc	<10	Volume based on segmentation of the individual loops of bowel, not the entire potential peritoneal space
	Entire potential space within peritoneal cavity	3D-CRT	Grade ≥3 acute toxicity[§]	V45 <195 cc	<10	Volume based on the entire potential space within the peritoneal cavity
Rectum	Whole organ	3D-CRT	Grade ≥2 late rectal toxicity, Grade ≥3 late rectal toxicity	V50 <50%	<15 <10	Prostate cancer treatment
	Whole organ	3D-CRT	Grade ≥2 late rectal toxicity, Grade ≥3 late rectal toxicity	V60 <35%	<15 <10	
	Whole organ	3D-CRT	Grade ≥2 late rectal toxicity, Grade ≥3 late rectal toxicity	V65 <25%	<15 <10	
	Whole organ	3D-CRT	Grade ≥2 late rectal toxicity, Grade ≥3 late rectal toxicity	V70 <20%	<15 <10	

Organ	Volume	Irradiation type	Endpoint	Dose/volume parameters	Rate (%)	Notes
	Whole organ	3D-CRT	Grade ≥2 late rectal toxicity	V75 <15%	<15	
	Whole organ	3D-CRT	Grade ≥3 late rectal toxicity		<10	
Bladder	Whole organ	3D-CRT	Grade ≥3 late RTOG	D_{max} <65	<6	Bladder cancer treatment. Variations in bladder size/shape/location during RT hamper ability to generate accurate data
	Whole organ	3D-CRT	Grade ≥3 late RTOG	V65 ≤50 % V70 ≤35 % V75 ≤25 % V80$^{\|}$ ≤15 %		Prostate cancer treatment Based on current RTOG 0415 recommendation
Penile bulb	Whole organ	3D-CRT	Severe erectile dysfunction	Mean dose to 95% of gland <50	<35	
	Whole organ	3D-CRT	Severe erectile dysfunction	D90$^{\|}$ <50	<35	
	Whole organ	3D-CRT	Severe erectile dysfunction	D60–70 <70	<55	

From Marks LB, Yorke ED, Jackson A, et al. Use of NTCP Models in the Clinic. Int J Radiat Oncol Biol Phys 2010;76(3):S10.

3D-CRT, 3-dimensional conformal radiotherapy; SRS, stereotactic radiosurgery; BED, biologically effective dose; SBRT, stereotactic body radiotherapy; RILD, radiation-induced liver disease; RTOG, radiation therapy oncology group.

*All data are estimated from the literature summarized in the QUANTEC reviews unless otherwise noted. Clinically, these data should be applied with caution. Clinicians are strongly advised to use the individual QUANTEC articles to check the applicability of these limits to the clinical situation at hand. They largely do not reflect modern IMRT.

†All at standard fractionation (i.e., 1.8–2.0 Gy per daily fraction) unless otherwise noted. V_x is the volume of the organ receiving ≥x Gy. D_{max} = Maximum radiation dose.

‡Non-TBI.

§With combined chemotherapy.

$^{\|}D_x$ = minimum dose received by the "hottest" x% (or x cc's) of the organ.

¶Severe xerostomia is related to additional factors including the doses to the submandibular glands.

**Estimated by Dr. Eisbruch.

††Classic radiation-induced liver disease (RILD) involves anicteric hepatomegaly and ascites, typically occurring between 2 weeks and 3 months after therapy. Classic RILD also involves elevated alkaline phosphatase (more than twice the upper limit of normal or baseline value).

‡‡For optic nerve, the cases of neuropathy in the 55–60 Gy range received ≈59 Gy (see optic nerve paper for details). Excludes patients with pituitary tumors where the tolerance may be reduced.

normal tissues, specifically negating the normal tissue-sparing effects of fractionation. As a consequence, this leads to lower total dose threshold tolerances for toxicity in normal tissues compared with conventional fractionation, and thus, historically, the reluctance to increase the total dose delivered to a tumor that may be adjacent to sensitive structures (e.g., the spinal cord). Recent technological advancements in patient immobilization and image-guided radiation therapy (IGRT) have allowed for the safe delivery of large cumulative doses of highly hypofractionated radiation (e.g., 10 to 18 Gy per fraction) with subcentimeter accuracy and excellent clinical outcomes. Reported results of hypofractionated stereotactic body radiation therapy (SBRT) in the treatment of early stage non–small cell lung cancer have shown local–regional control rates, metastatic disease control rates, and cancer-specific survival similar to surgical management, with minimal normal tissue toxicity (*JAMA* 2010;303(11):1070).

The basic rationale of **hyperfractionation** is that the use of small doses per fraction of 1.1 to 1.2 Gy allows higher total doses to be delivered over the same treatment duration as compared with conventional fractionation, but within the tolerance of late-responding tissues—late-responding tissues such as bowel, spinal cord, kidney, lung, and bladder have the same probability of complications with hyperfractionation. However, the patient will experience more acute reactions as a result of the larger total dose. The typical period between daily fractions is 6 hours to allow late tissue repair. An example of hyperfractionation is 69.6 Gy total dose delivered over a 6-week period in twice-daily fractions of 1.2 Gy for non–small cell lung cancer.

The basic rationale for **accelerated fractionation** is that a reduction in overall treatment time decreases the opportunity for tumor cell regeneration during treatment and therefore increases the TCP for a given total dose. Therefore, the fraction size is decreased, and the treatment duration is decreased as compared with conventional fractionation. An example of accelerated fractionation is the delivery of 45 Gy in 30 twice-daily fractions of 1.5 Gy separated by a minimum of 6 hours over a 3-week period in the treatment of small cell lung cancer.

D. **Prolongation of overall treatment time, tumor control, and morbidity.** Treatment interruptions result in a lower TCP for the same total dose received. The total dose of irradiation to produce a given TCP must be increased when fractionation is prolonged beyond 4 weeks because of repopulation of surviving cells, which may result in improved nutrition of those cells after early shrinkage of the tumor due to the initial radiation fractions. Taylor et al. (*Radiother Oncol* 1990;17:95) estimated a >1 Gy increment in isoeffect dose per day in 473 patients with squamous cell carcinoma of the head and neck treated with irradiation.

VI. RADIATION TREATMENT PLANNING

A. **Introduction to treatment planning.** The International Commission on Radiation Units and Measurements (ICRU) Report No. 50, and more recently No. 62, define the volumes of interest in treatment planning (*ICRU 50, Prescribing, Recording, Reporting, Photon Beam Therapy.* Washington, DC: International Commission on Radiation Units and Measurements, 1994; *ICRU 62, Prescribing, Recording, Reporting, Photon Beam Therapy (Supplement to ICRU Report 50).* Bethesda, MD: International Commission on Radiation Units and Measurements, 1999). The delineation of tumor and target volumes is a crucial step in radiation therapy planning. Gross tumor volume (GTV) is defined as all known gross disease, including involved regional lymph nodes, and is determined using physical examination findings and imaging tools, like computed tomography (CT) imaging, MRI, and/or positron emission tomography (PET). Clinical target volume (CTV) encompasses the GTV plus regions considered to harbor potential microscopic disease. The internal margin (IM) is a margin that accounts for variations in size, shape, and position of the CTV due to physiological processes, such as bladder filling/emptying and tumor movement during respiration, and is added to the CTV to constitute the internal target volume (ITV). The setup margin (SM) is a margin that accounts for day-to-day uncertainties in patient positioning and alignment of beams during treatment planning. The final volume, that is, the actual treated target, is called the planning target volume (PTV), and consists of the SM added to the ITV. In shorthand, PTV = (CTV + IM) + SM = ITV + SM. Additionally, organs and normal structures that surround the PTV are defined as organs at risk (OAR), and play a critical role in the planning phase and evaluation of a treatment plan. The planning organ at risk volume (PRV) is analogous to the PTV volume, and is defined as PRV = OAR + IM + SM.

Simulation is the process used to accurately identify the tumor volume(s) and OAR in order to determine the optimal configuration of radiation beam portals necessary to treat the tumor and avoid sensitive structures. Modern radiation therapy planning systems use CT scanning for simulation in which patients are placed in their planned treatment positions using various immobilization devices. Individual CT slices can be imaged several times during CT simulation to capture the movement of the GTV and OARs due to respiratory excursion and other physiological processes (also known as 4D-simulation). CT scan images are obtained of the area(s) of interest, and contours are delineated (GTV, CTV, ITV, PTV, OAR, and PRV) from the CT images at a computer workstation. The conventional simulator had been the workhorse of simulation in the past, consisting of a table and gantry with 360 degrees of rotation as well as fluoroscopy and diagnostic x-ray capability, but it has been replaced by CT simulation in the vast majority of treatment centers.

The goal of treatment planning is to adequately irradiate the PTV(s) while at the same time attempting to avoid surrounding OAR, thus minimizing acute and late toxicity. Various steps can be taken to decrease toxicity in normal tissues, including precise treatment planning and irradiation techniques, selectively decreasing the volume receiving higher doses, and maneuvers to exclude sensitive organs from the irradiated volume. With the emphasis on organ preservation (which is being applied to patients with tumors in the head and neck, breast, and rectosigmoid, and soft tissue sarcomas), treatment planning is critical to achieve a maximum therapeutic ratio.

B. Three-dimensional treatment planning and intensity modulated radiation therapy. The CT simulator allows more accurate definition of tumor volume and anatomy of critical normal structures, three-dimensional (3D) treatment planning to optimize dose distribution, and radiographic verification of volume treated, as is done with conventional simulators (*Int J Radiat Oncol Biol Phys* 1994;30:887). Advances in computer technology have augmented accurate and timely computation, display of 3D radiation dose distributions, and dose–volume histograms (DVHs). These developments have stimulated sophisticated 3D treatment-planning systems, which yield relevant information in evaluation of tumor extent, definition of target volume, delineation of normal tissues, virtual simulation of therapy, generation of digitally reconstructed radiographs, design of treatment portals and aids (e.g., compensators, blocks), calculation of 3D dose distributions and dose optimization, and critical evaluation of the treatment plan.

In addition, DVHs are extremely useful as a means of dose display, particularly in assessing several treatment plan dose distributions. They provide a graphic summary of the entire 3D dose matrix, showing the amount of target volume or critical structure receiving more than a specified dose level. Because they do not provide spatial dose information, they cannot replace the other methods of dose display such as room-view displays, but can only complement them. For example, the DVH may show the percentage PTV receiving the prescribed dose, but cannot locate the portion of the PTV receiving less than the prescribed dose. Treatment verification is another area in which 3D treatment-planning systems play an important role. Digitally reconstructed radiographs of sequential CT slice data are used to generate a simulation film that can be used to aid in portal localization and comparison with the treatment portal film for verifying treatment geometry.

Intensity modulated radiation therapy is an advanced form of 3D treatment planning and conformal therapy that optimizes the delivery of radiation to irregularly shaped volumes through a process of complex inverse treatment planning and dynamic delivery of radiation that results in modulated fluence (intensity) of photon beams. By varying the fluence across multiple treatment fields, the radiation dose can be modulated to conform to irregular shapes (i.e., concave) and to design a heterogeneous dose distribution. Several

IMRT hardware and software packages are commercially available including rotational slice-by-slice, dynamic multileaf, static (step and shoot) multileaf, milled compensator, and helical tomotherapy and arc delivery systems. Central to intensity modulation is the development of multileaf collimators (MLCs) and the concept of inverse treatment planning. MLCs are a set of shielding vanes measuring 0.5 to 1 cm wide that are located in the head of the linear accelerator and shape the radiation portal. Each vane is controlled independently and can remain static (static MLC) or move across the treatment field during "beam on" time (dynamic MLC). To understand inverse treatment planning, one must first understand traditional forward treatment planning. Under forward treatment planning, the radiation oncologist draws the radiation portals, considers the dose distribution generated by those portals, and adjusts the portals according to the desired dose distribution. Forward planning is cumbersome. Inverse planning reverses that order. The radiation oncologist contours the desired target volumes and critical structures to be avoided and prescribes an ideal dose distribution. Inverse planning starts with the ideal dose distribution and finds, through mathematical optimization algorithms, the beam characteristics (fluence profiles) that produce the best approximation of the ideal dose. IMRT is in widespread clinical use, and has clear advantages for treatment of many cancer sites.

C. **Image-guided radiation therapy and stereotactic radiation therapy.** The increased sophistication in treatment planning and radiation delivery requires parallel precision in patient immobilization, as well as patient and tumor position verification. This requirement has led to the development and implementation of IGRT. IGRT consists of the ability to image the patient, or optimally the tumor or a tumor surrogate, on a daily basis before or even during treatment. The daily images taken before or during treatment are used for patient and tumor positioning, greatly reducing random and systematic errors in daily localization between and during fractions of delivered radiation. Examples of common imaging modalities used before treatment include ultrasonography, optical (light-based) devices, on-board kV fluoroscopy, x-ray, and cone-beam CT, and megavoltage computed tomographic (MVCT) imaging. Image guidance systems that have the ability to image during radiation treatment include the Cyberknife kV-x-ray tracking system, the Calypso beacon localization system, and, most recently, the ViewRay radiation delivery system with on-board real-time MRI.

Because IGRT leads to improvements in daily patient and tumor localization, it allows the radiation oncologist to decrease the size of the setup margin when creating a PTV. In consequence, the PTV that is being irradiated to a particular dose can be significantly reduced without sacrificing local tumor control, and also can minimize normal tissue toxicity by reducing the irradiated volume of the surrounding OAR (*Int J Radiat Oncol Biol Phys* 2012;84(1):125). Additionally, there is evidence that the combination of IGRT and IMRT can further reduce complications compared with more conventional, non-IGRT, 3D treatment techniques (*Radiat Oncol* 2014;9:44). IGRT also allows for treatment gating, where the radiation beam can be turned on and off during treatment as the radiation therapist and radiation oncologist visualize the tumor, or tumor surrogate, on a computer screen as it moves in and out of the target volume because of normal physiologic processes like respiratory motion or bladder and rectal filling and emptying. The benefit of gating is the possibility of further reductions in margin size and PTV volume(s).

Continued improvements in the geometric accuracy of radiation delivery, as well as the development of advanced treatment techniques that allow for excellent coverage of irregularly shaped targets with surrounding steep dose gradients, has led to the development of effective treatment strategies that safely deliver very large doses of radiation to targets in very close proximity to sensitive structures or previously irradiated fields.

An excellent example is the ever-expanding use of hypofractionated SBRT in the definitive and palliative treatment of many different cancers. SBRT was initially developed to treat intracranial lesions with large single doses of radiation and is known as stereotactic radiosurgery (SRS) in this setting. The SRS system with the longest experience involves a frame that is rigidly attached to the patient's head using surgical screws and defines a three-dimensional coordinate system. The location of the lesion is defined within this coordinate system using different diagnostic imaging tools, like CT or MRI, with the frame in place. The patient is aligned on the treatment machine according to the location of the lesion within the coordinate system relative to the rigid frame rather than to anatomic surrogates. Using MRI-based localization techniques, the immobilization provided by the rigid stereotactic frame allows for the delivered radiation therapy to be accurate within 1 to 2 mm (*Neurosurgery* 2001;48(5):1092). The accuracy of the system allows for the safe delivery of large doses of radiation therapy near critical and sensitive structures, like the optic chiasm and optic nerves. It has been used mostly for the treatment of brain metastases, but also pituitary adenomas/carcinomas, meningiomas, and benign intracranial pathologies, such as arteriovenous malformations and trigeminal neuralgia. Examples of SRS delivery systems included linear accelerator–based cone or micro multileaf collimators systems, as well as the ^{60}Co Gamma-Knife radiosurgery system. Although very accurate, the invasiveness of the stereotactic frame has significantly limited its application to other tumor sites. Modern immobilization devices, such as the thermoplastic S-frame mask and the semi-rigid vacuum body fixation system, have achieved geographic accuracies similar to SRS rigid frames, both for intra- and extracranial targets (*Int J Radiat Oncol Biol Phys* 2012;84(2):520). The addition of image guidance allows for further refinement in patient positioning, and may also provide inter- and intra-fraction localization of targets and OAR that may move day-to-day because of normal physiologic processes. Failing to account for this movement can potentially lead to a geographic miss during high-dose radiation delivery, and unexpected irradiation of an adjacent sensitive structure to unacceptable dose levels.

SBRT is the application of SRS techniques to tumors or tumor surrogates in the body, but with the treatment machine being aligned to the tumor or tumor surrogate itself using image guidance. Spine SBRT is an excellent example of a growing treatment modality that uses the aforementioned technological advancements to deliver very high doses of radiation to lesions only a few millimeters from the spinal cord—a relatively radiosensitive structure with consequences of neurologic toxicity that can be devastating. Institutional studies have shown excellent pain and local control rates approaching 90% at 1 to 2 years, with <5% incidence of any severe toxicity, and no incidence of severe spinal cord toxicity (*J Neurosurg Spine* 2007;7(2):151–160; *Int J Radiat Oncol Biol Phys* 2011;81(2):S131). In addition to the treatment of early stage lung cancers, brain lesions, and spinal metastases, SBRT has also been used to treat liver malignancies, with promising results (*J Clin Oncol* 2013;31(13):1631). Recent interest has focused on the use of SBRT and its excellent local control rates in the treatment of patients with limited metastatic burden, or oligometastatic disease, typically defined as the presence of 1 to 5 metastatic lesions. It is believed that these patients do not have widespread subclinical metastases, but disease confined to 1 to 5 areas, with possibility of cure, and thus deserving of aggressive local treatment (*J Clin Oncol* 1995;13(1):8–10). This is an active area of research, and clinical trials are forthcoming.

It is imperative to understand that SBRT is a highly sophisticated and complex treatment technique that requires advanced equipment, and a dedicated staff of highly trained, competent, and experienced radiation therapists, dosimetrists, physicists, and radiation oncologists to deliver the treatment effectively and safely.

VII. COMBINATION OF THERAPEUTIC MODALITIES

A. **Irradiation and surgery.** The rationale for *preoperative radiation therapy* relates to its potential ability to eradicate subclinical or microscopic disease beyond the margins of the surgical resection, to diminish tumor implantation by decreasing the number of viable cells within the operative field, to sterilize lymph node metastases outside the operative field, to decrease the potential for dissemination of clonogenic tumor cells that might produce distant metastases, and to increase the possibility of resectability. The main disadvantage of preoperative irradiation is that it may interfere with normal healing of the tissues affected by the radiation. Such interference, however, is minimal when radiation doses are less than 45 to 50 Gy in 5 weeks.

The rationale for *postoperative irradiation* is based on the fact that it is possible to eliminate any residual tumor in the operative field by destroying subclinical or microscopic foci of tumor cells after the surgical procedure by eradicating adjacent subclinical foci of cancer (including lymph node metastases) and by delivering higher doses than can be achieved with preoperative irradiation, the greater dose being directed to the volume of high-risk or known residual disease.

The potential disadvantages of postoperative irradiation are related to the delay in initiation of radiation therapy until wound healing is completed. Theoretical and experimental evidence suggests that the radiation effect may be impaired by vascular changes produced in the tumor bed by surgery.

B. Irradiation and chemotherapy. Chemotherapy and radiation therapy are combined to obtain an additive or supra-additive effect (Halperin EC, Perez CA, Brady LW, eds. *Radiation Oncology: Technology and Biology.* Philadelphia, PA: WB Saunders, 1994:113). Enhancement describes any increase in effect greater than that observed with either chemotherapy or irradiation alone on the tumor or normal tissues. Calculation of the presence of additivity, supra-additivity, or sub-additivity is simple when dose–response curves for irradiation and chemotherapy are linear. When chemotherapeutic agents are used, the agents should not be cross-resistant, and each agent should be quantitatively equivalent to the other.

Chemotherapy alone or combined with irradiation may be used in several settings. **Primary chemotherapy** is used as part of the primary lesion treatment (even if later followed by other local therapy) and when the primary tumor response to the initial treatment is the key identifier of systemic effects. **Adjuvant chemotherapy** is used as an adjunct to other local modalities as part of the initial curative treatment. Frei (*J Natl Cancer Inst* 1989;80:1088) proposed the term **neoadjuvant chemotherapy** when this modality is used in the initial treatment of patients with localized tumors, before surgery or irradiation.

Administration of chemotherapy **before** irradiation produces some cell killing and reduces the number of cells to be eliminated by the irradiation. Use of chemotherapy **during** radiation therapy has a strong rationale because it could interact with the local treatment (additive and even supra-additive action) and could also affect subclinical disease early in treatment. Nevertheless, the combination of modalities may enhance normal tissue toxicity.

C. Integrated multimodality cancer management. Combinations of two or all three of the classic modalities are frequently used to improve tumor control and patient survival. Steel and Peckham (Steel GC, Adams GE, Peckham MJ, eds. *The Biological Basis of Radiotherapy.* Amsterdam, The Netherlands: Elsevier Science, 1983:239) postulated the biologic basis of cancer therapy as spatial cooperation, in which an agent is active against tumor cells spatially missed by another agent; addition of antitumor effects by two or more agents; and nonoverlapping toxicity and protection of normal tissues. Large primary tumors or metastatic lymph nodes must be removed surgically or treated with definitive radiation therapy. Regional microextensions are eliminated effectively by irradiation without the anatomic and at times physiologic deficit produced by equivalent medical surgery. Chemotherapy is applied mainly to control disseminated subclinical disease, although it also has an effect on some larger tumors.

Organ preservation is being vigorously promoted, as it enhances the quality of life and psychoemotional feelings of our patients with excellent tumor control and survival, as has been demonstrated in many tumors.

VIII. FOLLOW-UP. Continued support of the patient during therapy is mandatory, with at least one weekly evaluation by the radiation oncologist to assess the effects of treatment on the tumor and the side effects of therapy. Psychological and emotional reinforcement, medications, dietetic counseling, oral cavity care, and skin care instructions are integral parts of the management of these patients and should result in better therapeutic outcome.

IX. QUALITY ASSURANCE. A comprehensive quality assurance program is critical in any radiation oncology center to ensure the best possible treatment for the individual patient and to establish and document all operating policies and procedures.

Quality assurance procedures in radiation therapy will vary, depending on whether standard treatment or a clinical trial is carried out at single or multiple institutions. Particularly in multi-institutional studies, clear instructions and standardized parameters are needed in dosimetry procedures, treatment techniques, and treatment planning to be carried out by all participants. Many reports of the Patterns of Care Study demonstrate a definite correlation between the quality of the radiation therapy delivered at various types of institutions and the outcome of therapy.

The director of the department appoints the **Quality Assurance Committee**, which meets regularly to review the following: results of review and audit process, physics quality assurance program report, outcome studies, mortality and morbidity conference, any case of "misadministration" or error in delivery of more than 10% of the intended dose, and any chart in which an incident report is filed. Additional details can be obtained from the American College of Radiology.

SUGGESTED READINGS

Halperin EC, Bardy LW, Perez CA, et al. *Perez & Brady's Principles and Practice of Radiation Oncology*, 6th ed. Philadelphia, PA: Lippincott Williams & Wilkins, 2013.

ICRU 50, Prescribing, Recording, Reporting, Photon Beam Therapy. Washington, DC: International Commission on Radiation Units and Measurements, 1994.

ICRU 62, Prescribing, Recording, Reporting, Photon Beam Therapy (Supplement to ICRU Report 50). Bethesda, MD: International Commission on Radiation Units and Measurements, 1999.

Timmerman R, Paulus R, Galvin J, et al. Stereotactic body radiation therapy for inoperable early stage lung cancer. *JAMA* 2010;303(11):1070–1076.

5

Principles of Systemic Cancer Therapy: Cytotoxic Chemotherapy

Leigh M. Boehmer • Sara K. Butler • Janelle Mann

I. INTRODUCTION

A. **General.** Antineoplastic agents have a narrow therapeutic index and, as such, small changes in dose may result in unacceptable toxicity. Pretreatment characteristics including age, performance status, concurrent medications, renal and hepatic function, interpatient pharmacokinetic and pharmacodynamic variability, cachexia, obesity, and other comorbidities impact the efficacy and toxicity profile of many agents administered. In addition, many antineoplastic agents are extensively metabolized by cytochrome P-450 enzymes, resulting in the potential for drug–drug interactions and subsequent alterations in antineoplastic drug concentrations. The sequence of drug administration may also increase or decrease the antitumor effect or impact the severity of toxicities seen with these agents. Finally, calculation and manipulation of the actual dose to be administered is based on a variety of factors, including the patient's body size and commercially available antineoplastic vial size, as well as previous response and treatment intent. With that in mind, many factors should be considered when determining a patient's antineoplastic dose.

II. CALCULATION OF DOSE

A. **General.** The dose of antineoplastic agents may be based on a flat dose (e.g., imatinib), on body weight (e.g., conditioning regimens for hematopoietic stem cell transplantation), or, more commonly, a standardized reference body surface area (BSA) in order to provide consistent exposure of drug across various body types. Utilization of BSA is thought to be ideal because of its known relationship between body size and physiologic functions, including blood volume, cardiac output, glomerular filtration rate (GFR), and liver blood flow. The motivation for calculating the dose on the basis of BSA is to reduce interpatient variability of systemic antineoplastic exposure and to limit the toxicity exerted by the drug.

B. **Formulas**
1. **Dubois and Dubois.** This formula is the most widely utilized, originally derived in 1916 by making molds of nine nonobese individuals who varied in age, size, and shape. By trial and error, this formula was created by using height and weight alone to approximate BSA. However, caution should be used when applying this formula to infants and young adults. It is considered the gold standard for BSA calculations and the basis for many other nomograms.

$$BSA \ (m^2) = W^{0.425} \times H^{0.725} \times 0.007184$$
$$W = weight \ (kg) \ H = height \ (cm)$$

2. **Gehan and George.** In 1970, the DuBois and DuBois formula was validated by Gehan and George by directly measuring the skin surface area of 401 individuals, including a large number of children. However, it was found that the BSA was over-estimated by 15% in approximately 15% of the cases. In an effort to simplify the task of calculating the surface area, the authors provided tables and charts to estimate BSA from height and weight.

3. **Mosteller.** By modifying the equation proposed by Gehan and George, Mosteller et al. provided an equation that is easy to remember with a slight loss of accuracy of only 2%. Although the initial validation was only based on evaluations of adolescent and adult subjects, a subsequent study utilizing infants and children found it to be equally applicable.

$$BSA \ (m^2) \ \sqrt{\frac{Ht \ (cm) \times Wt \ (kg)}{3,600}} \qquad BSA \ (m^2) \ \sqrt{\frac{Ht \ (in) \times Wt \ (lbs)}{3,131}}$$

4. **Calvert.** Early studies of carboplatin noted that a patient's pretreatment renal function impacts the severity of thrombocytopenia observed. Approximately 70% of the drug is excreted unchanged via the urine within 24 hours, and pharmacokinetics suggests that the toxicity and efficacy of carboplatin is dictated primarily by pretreatment GFR. On the basis of these observations, Calvert et al. validated a simplified formula utilizing a targeted area under the curve (AUC) for carboplatin dose calculation and accounting for GFR in an effort to minimize the toxicity.

$$Carboplatin \ dose \ (mg) = target \ AUC \ (GFR + 25)$$

C. **Manipulation of Doses.** The dose of an antineoplastic agent administered to a patient depends not only upon patient factors and mathematical calculations, but also upon the treating physician's practice of rounding or capping of the dose. It is not uncommon for a dose to be rounded if it is within 5% to 10% of the nearest commercially available vial size. The practice of rounding, in fact, is supported by a sizeable literature base and does confer a potential cost savings to the health care system. Overall, modification of the antineoplastic dose must be done cautiously to prevent a clinically significant change from the intended dose.

D. **Amputees.** None of the above equations included amputees in the patient sample leading to their validation. Furthermore, some of the formulas found a loss in accuracy in children, short and/or obese patients, thereby questioning the accuracy of applying these same equations to amputees. Although the formulas have not been validated, it is recommended to evaluate the data provided by Colangelo et al., proposing two alternative equations for this patient population.

E. **Obesity.** It was once believed that dosing obese patients on their actual body weight would result in increased toxicities secondary to the distribution of lipid soluble drugs into adipose tissue. Therefore, ideal body weight, an adjusted body weight, or a capped BSA have historically been used to calculate the dose to be administered. Several reports have been published; however, assessing this practice and their results concluded that there was no increase in toxicity observed in obese patients with breast, colon, or small cell lung cancer who received antineoplastic doses based on actual body weight. Furthermore, manipulation of the dose downward in obese breast cancer patients who received cyclophosphamide, doxorubicin, and 5-fluorouracil negatively impacted overall survival. The American Society of Clinical Oncology released clinical practice guidelines on appropriate dosing for obese cancer patients in 2012. The expert panel recommended that full weight-based antineoplastic doses be used to treat obese patients, particularly when the treatment goal is cure.

F. **Elderly.** As a person ages, many physiologic changes may take place that influence the effects of antineoplastic agents. However, these changes do not take place at the same stage of life for each individual. There are no set guidelines addressing how to handle dose calculations in the elderly, but hypoalbuminemia, reduced hepatic and renal blood flow, cardiac dysfunction, and other comorbidities need to be considered when determining a treatment plan. In addition, this patient population is frequently taking medications that may interact with the efficacy and safety profile of any agent(s) administered.

G. **Hepatic dysfunction.** Several antineoplastic agents undergo hepatic metabolism and any alteration in their clearance or the metabolic capacity of the liver may result in potential complications. Data are limited in this situation, and many take the simple approach of assessing liver function by evaluating the total bilirubin. Other laboratory values such as the transaminases, serum alkaline phosphatase, and albumin may also impact systemic exposure and the ability of the liver to metabolize these medications. Therefore, all hepatic function tests may need to be taken into consideration prior to deciding the final dosage of an antineoplastic regimen. Although there is little data for combination regimens, there are some individual agents such as the taxanes, vinca alkaloids, anthracyclines, and irinotecan, which are known to necessitate a dose adjustment based on hepatic function. To further complicate the situation, one may find that the liver dysfunction is a result of the tumor and may need to determine whether dose alteration should be considered at all. Currently, there are no consensus recommendations for dosing antineoplastic drugs for tumor-related liver dysfunction.

H. **Renal dysfunction.** Several antineoplastic agents are eliminated through the kidneys, and even minor alterations in renal function may impact their safety. Furthermore, the literature is limited to case reports and small case series with regard to end-stage renal disease and the dosing of antineoplastics in patients with cancer. The choice and dose of the agent need to be considered carefully, as well as the method and optimal timing of dialysis in patients with renal dysfunction to assure maximal drug exposure while minimizing toxicity.

SUGGESTED READINGS

Arriagada R, Le Chevalier T, Pignon JP, et al. Initial chemotherapeutic doses and survival in patients with limited small-cell lung cancer. *N Engl J Med* 1993;329:1848–1852.

Calvert AH, Newell DR, Gumbrell LA, et al. Carboplatin dosage: prospective evaluation of a simple formula based on renal function. *J Clin Oncol* 1989;7:1748–1756.

Colangelo PM, Welch DW, Rich DS, et al. Two methods for estimating body surface area in adult amputees. *Am J Hosp Pharm* 1984;41:2650–2655.

DuBois D, DuBois EF. A formula to estimate the approximate surface area if height and weight be known. *Arch Intern Med* 1916;17:863–871.

Eklund JW, Trifilio S, Mulcahy MF. Chemotherapy dosing in the setting of liver dysfunction. *Oncology* 2005;19:1057–1063.

Eneman JD, Philips GK. Cancer management in patients with end-stage renal disease. *Oncology* 2005;19:1199–1212.

Gehan EA, George SL. Estimation of human body surface area from height and weight. *Cancer Chemother Rep* 1970;54:225–235.

Griggs JJ, Mangu PB, Anderson H, et al. Appropriate chemotherapy dosing for obese adult patients with cancer: American Society of Clinical Oncology Clinical Practice Guidelines. *J Clin Oncol* 2012;30:1553–1561.

Meyerhardt JA, Catalano PJ, Haller DG, et al. Influence of body mass index on outcomes and treatment-related toxicity in patients with colon carcinoma. *Cancer* 2003;98:484–495.

Mosteller RD. More on simplified calculation of body surface area. *N Engl J Med* 1988;318:1130.

Mosteller RD. Simplified calculation of body surface area. *N Engl J Med* 1987;317:1098.

Rosner GL, Hargis JB, Hollis DR, et al. Relationship between toxicity and obesity in women receiving adjuvant chemotherapy for breast cancer: results from cancer and leukemia group B study 8541. *J Clin Oncol* 1996;14:3000–3008.

6 Principles of Systemic Cancer Therapy: Molecularly Targeted Therapy

Leigh M. Boehmer • Sara K. Butler • Janelle Mann

I. **BACKGROUND.** Traditional cytotoxic chemotherapy generally affects rapidly dividing normal and malignant cells. Recent advances in cancer biology, however, have led to the identification of numerous specific molecular targets for drug therapy. These molecular targets often play a key role in the signal transduction pathways that regulate tumor cell growth, proliferation, migration, angiogenesis, and apoptosis. *Molecularly targeted therapy* is a broad term encompassing several classes of agents, including tyrosine kinase inhibitors and monoclonal antibodies (MAb).

II. **TYROSINE KINASE INHIBITORS**

A. **Tyrosine kinases.** Tyrosine kinases catalyze the transfer of γ-phosphate from adenosine triphosphate (ATP) to tyrosine residues in protein targets. They play a key role in the transduction of signals within cellular signaling cascades that are ultimately responsible for the regulation of gene transcription within the nucleus. Tyrosine kinases are further classified into receptor or nonreceptor tyrosine kinases.

1. **Receptor tyrosine kinases.** Receptor tyrosine kinases assist in the transmission of signals from extracellular ligands to the cell nucleus. They are composed of a ligand-binding extracellular domain, a lipophilic transmembrane domain, and an intracellular domain containing a catalytic site. Receptor tyrosine kinases are unphosphorylated, monomeric, and inactive without the presence of a ligand.

Ligand binding to the extracellular domain induces dimerization of the tyrosine kinase. This, in turn, leads to autophosphorylation of the intracellular domain, converting the tyrosine kinase to an active state. More specifically, when the intracellular domain undergoes autophosphorylation, binding sites for signaling proteins are formed. These signaling proteins are recruited to the membrane, and subsequently, multiple downstream signaling cascades are activated. Signals are conveyed from the cell membrane to the nucleus, resulting in alterations of DNA synthesis and cell growth, proliferation, migration, angiogenesis, and apoptosis. Examples of receptor tyrosine kinases include epidermal growth factor receptor (EGFR) (ErbB/HER) family members, vascular endothelial growth factor receptors (VEGFR), and platelet-derived growth factor receptors α and β (PDGFR α and β).

2. **Nonreceptor tyrosine kinases.** Nonreceptor tyrosine kinases play a role in the conveyance of intracellular signals. They lack the transmembrane domain and are primarily located intracellularly. More specifically, they are found on the inner surface of the plasma membrane, cytosol, and nucleus. Inhibitory proteins and lipids and intramolecular autoinhibitory mechanisms maintain the nonreceptor tyrosine kinases in an inactive state. Activation may occur by intracellular signals causing a dissociation of the inhibitory proteins and lipids, by other kinases causing phosphorylation, or by the recruitment of the tyrosine kinase to transmembrane receptors causing subsequent oligomerization and autophosphorylation of the tyrosine kinase. Similar to receptor tyrosine kinases, the nonreceptor tyrosine kinases activate multiple signaling pathways. Examples of nonreceptor tyrosine kinases include BCR-ABL, c-KIT, and c-Src.

B. **Functional alterations of tyrosine kinases in cancer.** Within tumor cells, there is a loss of tyrosine kinase regulation. The dysregulation of tyrosine kinases within cancer cells may occur through numerous mechanisms. Proteins may be fused to tyrosine kinases resulting in constant oligomerization, autophosphorylation, and activation. This typically occurs as the result of chromosomal translocations, with one of the most common examples being the formation of the BCR-ABL oncogene as a result of t(9;22) in chronic myeloid leukemia (CML). Other mechanisms described in the literature include mutations causing interruptions in the autoregulation of tyrosine kinases; abnormal expression of receptor tyrosine kinases, their associated ligands, or both; or a decrease in the processes that regulate tyrosine kinase activity, thereby causing an increase in tyrosine kinase activity. Through the action of tyrosine kinase inhibitors, unregulated tyrosine kinases and often multiple signaling pathways are inactivated, leading to a decrease in tumor cell growth, proliferation, migration, angiogenesis, and/or apoptosis.

III. MONOCLONAL ANTIBODIES

A. Background. MAbs are targeting agents that recognize cell surface proteins/receptors as antigens, particularly on the surface of tumor cells. There are three main classes of MAbs: unconjugated, conjugated, and radioimmunoconjugates.

Unconjugated MAbs directly affect signaling pathways by inhibiting ligand–receptor interactions. These are MAbs against either the receptor or its ligand. They may also indirectly stimulate host defense mechanisms, such as antibody-dependent cellular cytotoxicity (ADCC) or complement-mediated lysis, causing antitumor activity. Examples of unconjugated MAbs include rituximab, obinutuzumab, trastuzumab, cetuximab, panitumumab, and bevacizumab. Conjugated MAbs are MAbs combined with protein toxins or cytotoxic agents. These directly disrupt protein synthesis and cause tumor cell death. Examples of conjugated MAbs include brentuximab vedotin and ado-trastuzumab emtansine. Radioimmunoconjugates are MAbs in combination with radioisotopes intended to deliver a sterilizing dose of radiation to the tumor, such as ibritumomab tiuxetan.

Antibodies, or immunoglobulins, are Y-shaped molecules containing four chains—two identical light chains and two identical heavy chains. There is a fragment antigen binding (Fab) and a fragment crystalline (Fc) portion of the antibody. The Fab portion contains variable regions, including complementarity determining regions (CDR), that enable the antibody to bind to a specific antigen. The Fc portion contains constant regions that are identical in all immunoglobulins of the same isotype (i.e., IgA, IgG, and IgM) and function as binding sites for leukocytes and complement.

MAbs may be manufactured from multiple sources of B lymphocytes (i.e., murine, human, and primate). Murine MAbs are derived entirely from mice. Chimeric MAbs are composed of a murine variable region of the antibody with a constant region derived from humans, making approximately 65% to 90% of the agent of human origin. Humanized MAbs consist of variable and constant regions derived from humans with CDR derived from mice, making approximately 95% of the agent of human origin. Primatized MAbs contain variable regions from monkeys and constant regions from humans. Human MAbs are derived entirely from humans. MAbs are often manufactured by genetic manipulation to produce a humanized agent. Humanization of the agent decreases the immunogenicity of the MAb, thereby decreasing the production of human antimouse antibodies (HAMAs). HAMAs have the potential to inactivate and eliminate pure murine MAbs after repeated administration, decreasing the half-life of the agent. But HAMAs may also contribute to allergic reactions after the formation of antibody–HAMAs complexes. Pure murine MAbs also ineffectively stimulate host defense mechanisms, such as ADCC and complement-mediated lysis, because of differences between murine and human immune systems.

The United States Adopted Names (USAN) Council has developed guidelines for the nomenclature of MAbs for standardization purposes and to enable identification of the MAb composition for patient safety intent because of the potential for the development of source-specific antibodies. In general, the product source identifiers precede the suffix–*mab*. Also incorporated into the product name is a code syllable for the target disease state of the agent. Refer to Tables 6-1 and 6-2 for a list of product source identifiers and code syllables for the target disease states. Specific guidelines also exist for the nomenclature of radiolabeled and other conjugated MAbs.

TABLE 6-1	Product Source Identifiers
Source	**Identifier**
Human	-u-
Mouse	-o-
Rat	-a-
Humanized	-zu-
Hamster	-e-
Primate	-i-
Chimera	-xi-

TABLE 6-2	Code Syllables for the Targeted Disease State of the Agent		
Disease		**Tumor**	
Viral	-vir-	Colon	-col-
Bacterial	-bac-	Melanoma	-mel-
Immune	-lim-	Mammary	-mar-
Infectious Lesions	-les-	Testis	-got-
Cardiovascular	-cir-	Ovary	-gov-
		Prostate	-pr(o)-
		Miscellaneous	-tum-

IV. MOLECULAR TARGETS IN ONCOLOGY

A. BCR-ABL tyrosine kinase inhibition. The BCR-ABL tyrosine kinase is formed by the fusion of the BCR gene on chromosome 22 and the c-ABL tyrosine kinase gene on chromosome 9. This fusion protein forms as a result of the chromosomal t(9;22), or the Philadelphia chromosome, which has been implicated in approximately 95% of adult patients with CML, 15% to 20% of adult patients with acute lymphocytic leukemia (ALL), and 5% of adult patients with acute myeloid leukemia (AML). Subsequently, there is constitutive activation of the tyrosine kinase, leading to the activation of several transduction pathways, resulting in dysregulated cell proliferation and an inhibition of apoptosis. Imatinib inhibits the BCR-ABL tyrosine kinase, but also has inhibitory effects on other tyrosine kinases including c-KIT and PDGFR α and β. As a result of this non–BCR-ABL kinase inhibition, imatinib has shown efficacy in the treatment of other malignancies, including gastrointestinal stromal tumors (GISTs), which have mutations in c-KIT or PDGFRα. Dasatinib also has inhibitory effects on BCR-ABL as well as several other tyrosine kinases. This agent displays approximately 325-fold more potency than imatinib against ABL and has activity against imatinib-resistant BCR-ABL mutations.

1. Imatinib (Gleevec)
   a. FDA-approved indications. Philadelphia chromosome–positive CML, Philadelphia chromosome–positive ALL; *c-KIT* (CD117) –positive unresectable and/or metastatic malignant GISTs.
   b. Pharmacology. Tyrosine kinase inhibitor.
      i. Mechanism. Inhibits BCR-ABL tyrosine kinase, which blocks proliferation and causes apoptosis in BCR-ABL positive cell lines; inhibits stem cell factor (SCF; *c-KIT*) receptor tyrosine kinases, which inhibit proliferation and cause apoptosis in GIST cells that express *c-KIT* mutations; inhibits PDGFRα and β tyrosine kinases.

   ii. **Metabolism.** Hepatic metabolism through CYP 3A4 to active metabolite (N-demethylated piperazine derivative). Eliminated primarily in the feces (68%) with some urinary excretion (13%) as metabolite and unchanged drug.
  c. **Toxicity**
   i. **Common.** Nausea, vomiting, diarrhea, erythema multiforme rash, fluid retention/edema, fatigue, pyrexia, headache, hepatotoxicity, hemorrhage, myelosuppression, arthralgia, myalgia, cough, and dyspnea.
   ii. **Occasional.** Alopecia, gastrointestinal (GI) hemorrhage, ascites, increased transaminases and/or bilirubin, blurred vision, conjunctivitis, pruritus, chest pain, and upper respiratory tract infection.
   iii. **Rare.** Central nervous system (CNS) hemorrhage, angioedema, aplastic anemia, migraine, pulmonary fibrosis, Stevens–Johnson syndrome, syncope, electrolyte disturbances, and peripheral neuropathy.
  d. **Administration**
   i. **FDA-approved dose.** Chronic phase CML dose is 400 mg orally daily, may be increased to 600 mg daily. Accelerated phase or blast crisis dose is 600 mg once daily, may be increased to 800 mg daily (400 mg twice daily). Dosing for Ph+ ALL is 600 mg orally daily. Dosing for GIST is 400 to 800 mg daily.
   ii. **Dose modification.** Dose adjustment for severe hepatic impairment, hematologic and hepatotoxic adverse events, and inadequate hematologic or cytogenetic response.
   iii. **Supplied** as 100- and 400-mg tablets.
 2. **Bosutinib (Bosulif)**
  a. **FDA-approved indications.** Philadelphia chromosome–positive CML.
  b. **Pharmacology.** Tyrosine kinase inhibitor.
   i. **Mechanism.** Inhibits BCR-ABL tyrosine kinase, which blocks proliferation and causes apoptosis in BCR-ABL positive cell lines; inhibits SRC family (including SRC, LYN, and HCK); has activity in many imatinib-resistant BCR-ABL mutations (exceptions T315I and V299L).
   ii. **Metabolism.** Hepatic metabolism through CYP 3A4 to primarily inactive metabolites. Eliminated primarily in the feces (91%) with minimal urinary excretion (3%).
  c. **Toxicity**
   i. **Common.** Edema, fever, fatigue, headache, rash, decreased bicarbonate, hypermagnesemia, hypomagnesemia, diarrhea, nausea, vomiting, abdominal pain, decreased appetite, thrombocytopenia, anemia, neutropenia, increased transaminases, arthralgia, back pain, weakness, cough, and dyspnea.
   ii. **Occasional.** Chest pain, pericardial effusion, dizziness, pain, pruritis, acne, urticarial, dehydration, hypophosphatemia, uric acid elevation, hypocalcemia, gastritis, hepatotoxicity, tinnitus, renal failure, pleural effusion, and hypersensitivity reaction.
   iii. **Rare.** Anaphylactic shock, fixed drug eruption, GI hemorrhage, pancreatitis, QTc prolongation, and pulmonary hypertension.
  d. **Administration**
   i. **FDA-approved dose.** Chronic phase CML dose is 500 mg orally once daily. May be increased to 600 mg once daily if complete response not achieved.
   ii. **Dose modification.** Dose adjustment for hepatic impairment, hematologic and hepatotoxic adverse events, inadequate hematologic or cytogenetic response.
   iii. **Supplied** as 100- and 500-mg tablets.
 3. **Dasatinib (Sprycel)**
  a. **FDA-approved indications.** CML in chronic, accelerated, or blast phase in patients resistant or intolerant to prior therapy including imatinib; CML in patients newly diagnosed in chronic phase; Philadelphia chromosome–positive ALL with resistance or intolerance to prior therapy.

b. **Pharmacology.** Tyrosine kinase inhibitor.
  i. **Mechanism.** Multitargeted tyrosine kinase inhibitor affecting BCR-ABL, the SRC family, c-KIT, EPHA2, and PDGFRβ kinases; binds to both active and inactive ABL kinase domains.
  ii. **Metabolism.** Extensive hepatic metabolism through CYP 3A4. Primarily fecal elimination. 0.1% and 19% of the dose eliminated unchanged in the urine and feces, respectively.
c. **Toxicity**
  i. **Common.** Myelosuppression, fluid retention/edema, nausea, vomiting, diarrhea, abdominal pain, headache, hemorrhage, chest pain, arrhythmia, fatigue, pyrexia, rash, pruritus, mucositis, constipation, myalgia, arthralgia, dyspnea, cough, infection, and neuropathy.
  ii. **Occasional.** Congestive heart failure, pericardial effusion, pulmonary edema, ascites, febrile neutropenia, electrolyte abnormalities, and elevated transaminases.
  iii. **Rare.** QTc prolongation, elevated bilirubin.
d. **Administration**
  i. **FDA-approved dose.** Chronic phase CML: 100 mg orally once daily with optional dose escalation to 140 mg once daily. Accelerated or blast phase CML: 140 mg orally once daily. ALL, Ph+: 140 mg orally once daily.
  ii. **Dose modification.** Dose adjustment for hematologic toxicity or other non-hematologic adverse events. Consider when administered with strong CYP 3A4 enzyme inducers or inhibitors, or if inadequate hematologic or cytogenetic response.
  iii. **Supplied** as 20-, 50-, 70-, 80-, 100-, and 140-mg tablets.
4. **Nilotinib (Tasigna)**
  a. **FDA-approved indications.** Newly diagnosed chronic phase CML, CML in chronic or accelerated phase in patients resistant or intolerant to prior therapy including imatinib.
  b. **Pharmacology.** Tyrosine kinase inhibitor.
    i. **Mechanism.** Inhibits BCR-ABL tyrosine kinase, which blocks proliferation and causes apoptosis in BCR-ABL positive cell lines; inhibits *c-KIT* and PDGFR.
    ii. **Metabolism.** Hepatic metabolism through CYP 3A4 to inactive metabolites. Eliminated primarily in the feces (93%) with 69% being parent drug.
  c. **Toxicity**
    i. **Common.** Peripheral edema, hypertension, headache, fatigue, fever, insomnia, rash, pruritus, alopecia, hypophosphatemia, hyperglycemia, nausea, vomiting, diarrhea, constipation, neutropenia, thrombocytopenia, anemia, hyperbilirubinemia, elevated transaminases, arthralgia, and cough.
    ii. **Occasional.** Arterial stenosis, cerebrovascular accident, arrhythmia, atrial fibrillation, QTc prolongation, dizziness, depression, dry skin, acne, erythema, hypokalemia, hyponatremia, hyperkalemia, and dyspepsia.
    iii. **Rare.** Arteriosclerosis, cardiac failure, coronary artery disease, diplopia, dysuria, gastric ulcer, and hepatitis.
  d. **Administration**
    i. **FDA-approved dose.** Chronic phase CML: 300 mg orally twice daily. Chronic or accelerated phase in resistant or intolerant patients: 400 mg po twice daily.
    ii. **Dose modification.** Dose adjustment for hepatic impairment, hematologic and hepatotoxic adverse events, inadequate hematologic or cytogenetic response.
    iii. **Supplied** as 150- and 200-mg capsules.
5. **Ponatinib (Iclusig)**
  a. **FDA-approved indications.** CML or ALL, Ph+ for whom no other TKI therapy is indicated or who are T315I-positive.

   b. Pharmacology. Tyrosine kinase inhibitor.
      i. Mechanism. Pan-inhibitor of BCR-ABL tyrosine kinase including T315I, which blocks proliferation and causes apoptosis in BCR-ABL positive cell lines; inhibits VEGFR, FGFR, PDGFR, EPH, and SRC kinases and KIT, RET, TIE2, and FLT3.
      ii. Metabolism. Hepatic metabolism through CYP 3A4, 2C8, 2D6, and 3A5. Eliminated primarily in the feces (87%) with some urinary excretion (5%).
   c. Toxicity
      i. Common. Hypertension, peripheral edema, heart failure, arterial ischemia, fatigue, headache, fever, pain, dizziness, rash, dry skin, hyperglycemia, hypophosphatemia, hypocalcemia, abdominal pain, constipation, nausea, diarrhea, vomiting, mucositis, weight loss, neutropenia, thrombocytopenia, anemia, elevated transaminases, elevated bilirubin, arthralgia, myalgia, and peripheral neuropathy.
      ii. Occasional. Myocardial infarction, SVT, atrial fibrillation, venous thromboembolism, pericardial effusion, stroke, and TIA.
      iii. Rare. Ascites, atrial flutter, cerebral edema, heart block, and hepatic failure.
   d. Administration
      i. FDA-approved dose. 45 mg orally once daily.
      ii. Dose modification. Dose adjustment for moderate-to-severe hepatic impairment, hematologic and hepatotoxic adverse events, inadequate hematologic or cytogenetic response.
      iii. Supplied as 15- and 45-mg tablets.
B. ALK fusion targeting. Anaplastic lymphoma kinase (ALK) is a membrane-associated tyrosine kinase receptor of the insulin receptor superfamily. ALK was first identified as a fusion protein in anaplastic large cell lymphoma cell lines. ALK chromosomal rearrangements have been discovered in anaplastic large cell lymphoma (50% to 60%), inflammatory myofibroblastic tumors (27%), and non–small cell lung cancers (NSCLC; 4% to 7%).
   In NSCLC, the EML4-ALK fusion oncogene is the most commonly reported ALK mutation. This inversion on chromosome 2 leads to a fusion of the kinase domain of ALK and EML-4 echinoderm microtubule-associated protein-like 4 region, inv(2)(p21p23). The EML4-ALK fusion mediates ligand-independent dimerization of the kinase, leading to the continuous downstream signaling of the PI3K-AKT, STAT3, and Ras-Raf-ERK pathways causing cell survival and proliferation.
   Crizotinib has a classical ATP-competitive mechanism of action with dose-dependent inhibition on the phosphorylation of ALK as well as c-MET, preventing cellular proliferation and inducing apoptosis.
   1. Crizotinib (Xalkori)
      a. FDA-approved indications. Frontline therapy for metastatic anaplastic lymphoma kinase positive NSCLC.
      b. Pharmacology. Tyrosine kinase inhibitor.
         i. Mechanism. Binds to the ATP intracellular domain of activated ALK, which inhibits phosphorylation and subsequent downstream signaling.
         ii. Metabolism. Extensive hepatic metabolism primarily through CYP 3A4. Eliminated primarily by feces (63%) with a small amount in the urine (22%).
      c. Toxicity
         i. Common. Vision disorder (visual impairment, photopsia, blurred vision, vitreous floaters, photophobia, and diplopia), dizziness, neuropathy, fatigue, decreased appetite, nausea, diarrhea, vomiting, edema, and constipation.
         ii. Rare. Pneumonitis, pneumonia, QTc prolongation, liver function test elevations (AST/ALT, bilirubin), and hepatotoxicity.
      d. Administration
         i. FDA-approved dose. 250 mg orally twice daily.
         ii. Dose modification. Recommendations regarding dose adjustment for corrected QTc >500 ms without serious signs or symptoms of arrhythmia are to hold therapy until QTc <480 ms and then resume at 200 mg orally twice

daily. Dose adjustment for AST/ALT elevations of $\geq 5 \times$ ULN with grade ≤ 1 total bilirubin is to hold until toxicity improves and then resume at 200 mg orally twice daily. Evaluate for drug interaction with strong inducers or inhibitors of CYP3A and concomitant use of QTc prolonging medications.

   iii. Supplied as 200-, 250-mg capsules.

C. EGFR targeting. The EGFR is one of the four tyrosine kinase receptors within the ErbB receptor family—ErbB1 (EGFR/HER1), ErbB2 (HER2/neu), ErbB3 (HER3), and ErbB4 (HER4). Several malignancies have been associated with an overexpression or alteration of EGFR and include head and neck, esophageal, gastric, pancreatic, colorectal, renal cell, prostate, breast, bladder, ovarian, and cervical cancers, as well as NSCLC and glioblastoma.

Activation of these receptor tyrosine kinases result in multiple downstream signaling pathways being activated, including the Ras/Raf mitogen-activated protein kinase (MAPK) pathway, the phosphatidylinositol 3′-kinase (PI3K)/Akt pathway, the protein kinase C pathway, and the Janus kinase (JAK)/signal transducer and activator of transcription (STAT) pathway. These pathways affect cell proliferation, migration, differentiation, and inhibit apoptosis. The activation of EGFR also causes an upregulation of vascular endothelial growth factor (VEGF) expression, leading to an increase in angiogenesis.

EGFR tyrosine kinase inhibitors are small molecules that bind to the ATP-binding site on the tyrosine kinase domain of the receptor and inhibit the catalytic activity of the kinase or they may inhibit fusion tyrosine kinases by blocking dimerization. The available EGFR tyrosine kinase inhibitors include erlotinib and afatinib. The EGFR-targeting MAbs available, cetuximab and panitumumab, inhibit ligand binding to the receptor.

   1. Erlotinib (Tarceva)
   a. FDA-approved indications. Frontline therapy for metastatic NSCLC expressing an EGFR exon 19 deletion or exon 21 substitution. Additionally, for refractory, locally advanced, or metastatic NSCLC, in combination with gemcitabine for locally advanced, unresectable, or metastatic pancreatic cancer.
   b. Pharmacology. Tyrosine kinase inhibitor.
      i. Mechanism. Inhibits intracellular phosphorylation of the EGFR tyrosine kinase.
      ii. Metabolism. Extensive hepatic metabolism primarily through CYP 3A4. Eliminated primarily by feces (83%) with a small amount in the urine (8%).
   c. Toxicity
      i. Common. GI upset (diarrhea, nausea, vomiting, and anorexia), mucositis, dermatologic toxicity (acneiform rash, erythematous rash, maculopapular dermatitis, dry skin, and pruritus), fatigue, headache, depression, dizziness, insomnia, dyspnea, cough, infection, edema, eye irritation/conjunctivitis, elevated hepatic transaminases, and/or bilirubin.
      ii. Occasional. Deep vein thrombosis, myocardial infarction/ischemia, cerebrovascular events, ileus, and pancreatitis.
      iii. Rare. Corneal ulcerations, epistaxis, GI bleeding, interstitial lung disease–like events, and hemolytic anemia.
   d. Administration
      i. FDA-approved dose. Dose for NSCLC is 150 mg orally once daily. Dose for pancreatic cancer is 100 mg orally once daily in combination with gemcitabine. Administer at least 1 hour before or 2 hours after food.
      ii. Dose modification. No adjustment for renal impairment. May need dose adjustment if severe liver impairment exists. Dose modifications may be made for intolerance or concomitant CYP 3A4 inhibitor or inducer administration.
      iii. Supplied as 25-, 100-, 150-mg tablets.
   2. Afatinib (Gilotrif)
   a. FDA-approved indications. Frontline therapy for metastatic NSCLC expressing the EGFR exon 19 deletion or exon 21 substitution.

    b. Pharmacology. Tyrosine kinase inhibitor.

        i. Mechanism. Irreversibly inhibits intracellular phosphorylation of the EGFR tyrosine kinase.

        ii. Metabolism. Metabolism is negligible, inhibitor/substrate of P-glycoprotein. Eliminated primarily by feces (85%) with a small amount in the urine (4%).

    c. Toxicity

        i. Common. GI upset (diarrhea, anorexia), stomatitis, dermatologic toxicity (acneiform rash, erythematous rash, maculopapular dermatitis, dry skin, and pruritus), paronychia, fatigue, dyspnea, cough, and eye irritation/conjunctivitis.

        ii. Occasional. Elevated hepatic transaminases, hypokalemia, and cystitis.

        iii. Rare. Interstitial lung disease–like events, pneumonia, sepsis, diastolic dysfunction, bullous skin eruption, and hepatotoxicity.

    d. Administration

        i. FDA-approved dose. Dose for NSCLC is 40 mg orally once daily. Administer at least 1 hour before or 2 hours after food.

        ii. Dose modification. Dose adjustment for renal impairment should be considered if CrCl <59 mL/min and patient is showing intolerance to therapy. Reduce afatinib daily dose by 10 mg if patient is using concurrent P-glycoprotein inhibitor(s) and not tolerating treatment. If taking P-glycoprotein inducers, it is recommended to increase afatinib daily dose by 10 mg.

        iii. Supplied as 20-, 30-, 40-mg tablets.

3. Cetuximab (Erbitux)

    a. FDA-approved indications. Metastatic colorectal cancer; squamous cell carcinoma of the head and neck.

    b. Pharmacology. Chimeric MAb.

        i. Mechanism. Binds to the extracellular domain of the EGFR inhibiting the binding of epidermal growth factor (EGF) to the receptor; inhibits cell growth and metastasis, induces apoptosis, inhibits VEGF production, causes ADCC, and downregulates EGFR.

        ii. Metabolism. Elimination through EGFR binding/internalization.

    c. Toxicity

        i. Common. Dermatologic toxicities (acneiform rash, skin drying and fissuring, inflammatory/infectious reactions), malaise, fever, hypomagnesemia, nausea, constipation, abdominal pain, diarrhea, headache, weakness, cough, peripheral edema, alopecia, and anemia.

        ii. Occasional. Sepsis, pulmonary embolism, kidney failure, dehydration, conjunctivitis, infusion-related reactions, and cardiopulmonary arrest.

        iii. Rare. Interstitial lung disease, leukopenia.

    d. Administration

        i. FDA-approved dose. Initial loading dose: 400 mg/m^2 intravenously on day 1. Maintenance dose: 250 mg/m^2 intravenously once a week starting on day 8.

        ii. Dose modification. Dose adjustment for toxicities. No adjustment needed for renal or hepatic impairment.

        iii. Supplied as 100-mg vials.

4. Panitumumab (Vectibix)

    a. FDA-approved indications. Metastatic colorectal cancer (*KRAS* mutation negative).

    b. Pharmacology. Human MAb.

        i. Mechanism. Binds to the extracellular domain of the EGFR inhibiting the binding of EGF and other ligands to the receptor; inhibits cell growth, survival, proliferation, and transformation.

        ii. Metabolism. Elimination through EGFR binding/internalization.

   c. **Toxicity**

      i. **Common.** Dermatologic toxicities (acneiform rash, skin drying and fissuring, inflammatory/infectious reactions), peripheral edema, fatigue, hypomagnesemia, abdominal pain, nausea, diarrhea, constipation, vomiting, ocular toxicity, and cough.

      ii. **Occasional.** Infusion-related reactions, stomatitis, mucositis, conjunctivitis, eyelash growth, and antibody formation.

      iii. **Rare.** Sepsis, pulmonary fibrosis, and skin necrosis.

   d. **Administration**

      i. **FDA-approved dose.** 6 mg/kg intravenously every 14 days.

      ii. **Dose modification.** Dose adjustment for toxicities. No adjustment needed for renal or hepatic impairment.

      iii. **Supplied** as 100- and 400-mg vials.

D. HER2 targeting. The human epidermal growth factor receptor 2 (HER2) is a member of the ErbB receptor family, which includes ErbB1/EGFR/HER1, ErbB3/HER3, and ErbB4/HER4. HER2 is the only one out of the four ErbB receptors that does not have a known ligand. Interactions between the other HER family members and the extracellular domain of HER2 result in the formation of heterodimer complexes after ligand binding. Therefore, the primary role of HER2 is as a coreceptor, facilitating signal transduction after ligand binding to other HER family members. Activation of HER2 may also occur by homodimerization. The HER2 intracellular domain displays tyrosine kinase activity upon activation and regulates cell growth, differentiation, and migration. Amplification of the *HER2/neu* oncogene results in overexpression of HER2, which occurs in approximately 20% to 30% of breast cancer tumors. HER2-overexpressing breast cancers generally have a worse prognosis than non-overexpressing breast tumors. Trastuzumab and pertuzumab are humanized MAbs against HER2, while lapatinib is a tyrosine kinase inhibitor against EGFR and HER2.

   1. Lapatinib (Tykerb)

      a. **FDA-approved indications.** Metastatic breast cancer whose tumors overexpress the HER2/*neu* protein in combination with chemotherapy, hormonal therapy, or trastuzumab.

      b. **Pharmacology.** Tyrosine kinase inhibitor.

         i. **Mechanism.** Dual tyrosine kinase inhibitor against EGFR and HER2 blocking phosphorylation and activation of downstream second messengers.

         ii. **Metabolism.** Hepatic via extensively CYP3A4/5 and to a lesser extent via CYP2C19 and 2C8 to oxidized metabolites.

      c. **Toxicity**

         i. **Common.** Fatigue, headache, hand–foot syndrome, rash, dry skin, alopecia, nail disorder, diarrhea, nausea, vomiting, abdominal pain, stomatitis, dyspepsia, anemia, neutropenia, thrombocytopenia, increased transaminases, increased bilirubin, limb pain, and weakness.

         ii. **Occasional.** Left ventricular dysfunction, insomnia.

         iii. **Rare.** Anaphylaxis, hepatotoxicity, interstitial lung disease, pneumonitis, and QTc prolongation.

      d. **Administration**

         i. **FDA-approved dose.** In combination with capecitabine: 1,250 mg orally daily; in combination with letrozole: 1,500 mg orally daily; in combination with trastuzumab: 1,000 mg orally daily.

         ii. **Dose modification.** Recommend decreased dose for severe hepatic impairment.

         iii. **Supplied** as 250-mg tablets.

   2. Trastuzumab (Herceptin)

      a. **FDA-approved indications.** Breast cancer whose tumors overexpress the HER2/*neu* protein in the adjuvant or metastatic setting; metastatic gastric cancer whose tumors overexpress the HER2/*neu* protein.

    b. Pharmacology. Humanized MAb.

        i. Mechanism. Binds to the extracellular domain of the HER2/*neu* protein. It mediates several intracellular effects including internalization of the HER2 receptor and downregulation of surface HER2 expression; alters downstream signaling pathways and leads to a decrease in cell proliferation and VEGF production, induces apoptosis, and potentiates chemotherapy. It also causes several extracellular effects including interference with homodimer and heterodimer formation between HER-family receptors and induces antibody-dependent cellular toxicity against cells that overproduce HER2.

        ii. Metabolism. Elimination through internalization after receptor binding.

    c. Toxicity

        i. Common. Infusion-related reactions (fever, chills), rash, headache, diarrhea, myelosuppression, and infections.

        ii. Occasional. Left ventricular dysfunction, cardiomyopathy, congestive heart failure, and arthralgia.

        iii. Rare. Severe hypersensitivity reactions (anaphylaxis, urticaria, bronchospasm, angioedema, and/or hypotension), severe infusion-related reactions (fever, chills, nausea, vomiting, pain at the tumor site, headache, dizziness, dyspnea, hypotension, rash, and asthenia), pulmonary events (dyspnea, pulmonary infiltrates, pleural effusions, noncardiogenic pulmonary edema, pulmonary insufficiency and hypoxia, acute respiratory distress syndrome [ARDS], pneumonitis, and pulmonary fibrosis).

    d. Administration

        i. FDA-approved dose. Weekly dosing: initial loading dose is 4 mg/kg intravenously on day 1. Maintenance dose is 2 mg/kg intravenously once weekly starting on day 8. Every 3-week dosing: initial loading dose is 8 mg/kg intravenously on day 1. Maintenance dose is 6 mg/kg intravenously every 3 weeks starting on day 22.

        ii. Dose modification. Recommended to hold for at least 4 weeks for LVEF ≥16% decrease from baseline or LVEF below normal limits and ≥10% decrease from baseline.

        iii. Supplied as a 440-mg vial.

  3. Pertuzumab (Perjeta)

    a. FDA-approved indications. Treatment of HER-2/neu positive breast cancer in the metastatic or neoadjuvant setting.

    b. Pharmacology. Humanized MAb.

        i. Mechanism. Targets the extracellular HER2/*neu* dimerization domain and inhibits HER2 dimerization blocking downstream signaling. Binds to a different HER2 epitope than trastuzumab, resulting in a more complete inhibition of HER2 signaling when combined with trastuzumab.

        ii. Metabolism. Elimination through internalization after receptor binding.

    c. Toxicity

        i. Common. Fatigue, headache, fever, dizziness, rash, diarrhea, mucosal inflammation, nausea, stomatitis, vomiting, neutropenia, anemia, and infusion reactions.

        ii. Occasional. Paronychia, anorexia.

        iii. Rare. Heart failure, insomnia, left ventricular ejection fraction decreased, peripheral edema, and pleural effusion.

    d. Administration

        i. FDA-approved dose. In combination with docetaxel and trastuzumab: 840 mg intravenously on day 1 followed by 420 mg intravenously every 3 weeks.

        ii. Dose modification. No dose adjustments recommended.

        iii. Supplied as a 420-mg vial.

E. VEGF targeting. VEGF is a member of the PDGF family. Several ligands for VEGFRs exist including VEGF-A through -E and placenta growth factor. These ligands are capable of binding to various VEGFRs that are expressed on vascular endothelial cells. Binding to VEGFR-1 (Flt-1; Fms-like tyrosine kinase-1) induces endothelial cell migration. Binding to VEGFR-2 (KDR) stimulates endothelial cell proliferation, antiapoptotic effects, and vascular permeability. This receptor is primarily responsible for the activation of the tyrosine kinase domains once ligands are bound.

Binding to VEGFR-3 (Flt-4) induces lymphangiogenesis. VEGF also plays a key role in the induction of angiogenesis, or the growth of new blood vessels from existing vasculature, which helps sustain tumor growth and survival by supplying nutrients and oxygen. The overexpression of VEGF occurs in various tumor types including colorectal, breast, cervical, endometrial, gastric, renal, pancreatic, and hepatic cancers, and NSCLC, melanoma, glioblastoma, and AML. Several factors may upregulate VEGF expression including hypoxia, acidosis, embryogenesis, endometriosis, wound healing and various growth factors (PDGF, fibroblast growth factor [FGF], epidermal growth factor [EGF], tumor necrosis factor [TNF], transforming growth factor beta, interleukin 1 [IL-1]). Within tumor cells, hypoxia is the key mediator of VEGF overexpression. Agents with effects on VEGF/VEGFRs include axitinib, pazopanib, sunitinib, bevacizumab, and ziv-aflibercept.

1. **Axitinib (Inlyta)**
   a. **FDA-approved indications.** Advanced renal cell cancer.
   b. **Pharmacology.** Tyrosine kinase inhibitor, second generation.
      i. **Mechanism.** Blocks angiogenesis and tumor growth by inhibiting VEGFR 1, 2, and 3.
      ii. **Metabolism.** Hepatic, primarily through CYP 3A4/5 and to a lesser extent via CYP 1A2, CYP 2C19, and UGT 1A1. Primarily excreted in the feces (41%) with a smaller amount excreted renally (23%).
   c. **Toxicity**
      i. **Common.** Hypertension, fatigue, dysphonia, headache, hand–foot syndrome, rash, hypocalcemia, hyperglycemia, hypernatremia, hypoalbuminemia, decreased bicarbonate, diarrhea, nausea, increased lipase/amylase, weight loss, vomiting, constipation, myelosuppression, increased liver function tests (LFTs), weakness, arthralgias, increased creatinine, proteinuria, and cough.
      ii. **Occasional.** Venous/arterial thrombotic events, transient ischemic attack, dizziness, dry skin, pruritus, alopecia, erythema, hyperthyroidism, dyspepsia, hemorrhoids, myalgias, tinnitus, hematuria, and epistaxis.
      iii. **Rare.** Cerebral bleeding, cerebrovascular crisis, reversible posterior leukoencephalopathy syndrome, and heart failure.
   d. **Administration**
      i. **FDA-approved dose.** 5 mg orally twice daily with or without food with a glass of water. If dose is tolerated for at least 2 consecutive weeks, may increase the dose to 7 mg orally twice daily, and then further increase (using the same criteria) to 10 mg orally twice daily.
      ii. **Dose modification.** For adverse events, reduce dose from 5 mg orally twice daily to 3 mg orally twice daily; further reduction to 2 mg orally twice daily can be performed. Avoid concomitant administration with strong CYP 3A4 inhibitors. If strong CYP 3A4 inhibitors are used, a 50% dosage reduction is recommended. No dose adjustment necessary for mild to severe renal dysfunction. No dose adjustment necessary for Child–Pugh class A; 50% dose reduction for Child-Pugh class B; and has not been studied in Child–Pugh class C.
      iii. **Supplied** as 1- and 5-mg tablets.
2. **Pazopanib (Votrient)**
   a. **FDA-approved indications.** Advanced renal cell cancer, advanced or refractory soft tissue sarcoma.
   b. **Pharmacology.** Tyrosine kinase (multikinase) inhibitor.
      i. **Mechanism.** Blocks angiogenesis and tumor growth by inhibiting VEGFR 1, 2, and 3, PDGFR, FGFR-1 and 3, cKIT, interleukin-2 receptor inducible T-cell kinase, leukocyte-specific protein tyrosine kinase (LcK), and c-Fms.

    ii. **Metabolism.** Hepatic, primarily through CYP 3A4 and to a lesser extent via CYP1A2, CYP2C8, and UGT 1A1. Primarily excreted in the feces with a smaller amount excreted renally (<4%).

  c. Toxicity

    i. **Common.** Hypertension, edema, fatigue, headache, dizziness, hair discoloration, hand–foot syndrome, rash, hyperglycemia, hypophosphatemia, hyponatremia, increased TSH, diarrhea, nausea, weight loss, vomiting, constipation, myelosuppression, increased LFTs, weakness, and cough.

    ii. **Occasional.** Venous/arterial thrombotic events, transient ischemic attack, chest pain, QTc prolongation, insomnia, chills, dyspepsia, and blurred vision.

    iii. **Rare.** Cerebral bleeding, cerebrovascular crisis, reversible posterior leukoencephalopathy syndrome, and heart failure.

  d. Administration

    i. **FDA-approved dose.** 800 mg orally once daily on an empty stomach.

    ii. **Dose modification.** Modify doses for moderate-to-severe hepatic impairment.

    iii. **Supplied** as 200-mg tablets.

3. Sunitinib (Sutent)

  a. FDA-approved indications. GIST after disease progression on or intolerance to imatinib; advanced renal cell cancer (RCC); locally advanced or metastatic pancreatic neuroendocrine tumors (PNET).

  b. Pharmacology. Tyrosine kinase inhibitor.

    i. **Mechanism.** Inhibits multiple tyrosine kinases including VEGFR 1, 2, and 3; SCF receptor (*c-KIT*); PDGFR α and β; and Fms-like tyrosine kinase-3 (Flt-3).

    ii. **Metabolism.** Hepatic through CYP 3A4 to the active *N*-desethyl metabolite SU12662. Primarily excreted in the feces (61%) with a small amount excreted renally (16%).

  c. Toxicity

    i. **Common.** Hypertension, rash, hand–foot syndrome, alopecia, skin discoloration (yellow–orange), hair pigmentation changes, dry skin, diarrhea, nausea, vomiting, mucositis/stomatitis, constipation, dyspepsia, dyspnea, cough, edema, fever, fatigue, hyperuricemia, increased LFTs, increased amylase/lipase, myelosuppression, arthralgia, myalgia, increased serum creatinine, decreased left ventricular ejection fraction (LVEF), and hemorrhage.

    ii. **Occasional.** Electrolyte disturbances, hypothyroidism, oral pain, thromboembolism, myocardial ischemia/infarction, anorexia, and peripheral neuropathy.

    iii. **Rare.** Febrile neutropenia, pancreatitis, reversible posterior leukoencephalopathy syndrome, and seizure.

  d. Administration

    i. **FDA-approved dose.** 50 mg orally once daily with or without food for 4 weeks in a 6-week treatment cycle (4 weeks on, 2 weeks off) for GIST and advanced RCC. Dosing for PNET is 37.5 mg orally once daily with or without food; maximum daily dose used in clinical trials: 50 mg.

    ii. **Dose modification.** Dose reductions to 37.5 mg daily (GIST/RCC) or 25 mg daily (PNET) should be considered with concomitant use of strong CYP 3A4 inhibitors. Dosage increment to 87.5 mg daily (GIST/RCC) or 62.5 mg daily (PNET) should be considered with concomitant use of strong CYP 3A4 inducers.

    iii. **Supplied** as 12.5-, 25-, and 50-mg capsules.

4. Bevacizumab (Avastin)

  a. FDA-approved indications. Treatment of metastatic colorectal cancer (first- or second-line treatment and second line after progression on a firstline treatment containing bevacizumab); metastatic nonsquamous NSCLC (firstline treatment in combination with paclitaxel and carboplatin); metastatic renal cell carcinoma (RCC).

b. Pharmacology. Humanized MAb.

   i. Mechanism. Recombinant, humanized MAb that binds to and neutralizes VEGF.

c. Toxicity

   i. Common. Hypertension, headache, abdominal pain, nausea, vomiting, diarrhea, anorexia, constipation, proteinuria, leukopenia, weakness, exfoliative dermatitis, stomatitis, epistaxis, dyspnea, upper respiratory infection, and wound healing.

   ii. Occasional. Venous thromboembolic events, hemorrhagic events, GI perforation, arterial thromboembolic events, left ventricular dysfunction, and infusion-related reactions.

   iii. Rare. CNS hemorrhage, nephrotic syndrome, fistula development, severe or fatal hemorrhage, necrotizing fasciitis, and wound dehiscence.

d. Administration

   i. FDA-approved dose. For metastatic colorectal cancer: 5 mg/kg intravenously every 2 weeks (in combination with bolus-IFL); 10 mg/kg intravenously every 2 weeks (in combination with FOLFOX4). 5 mg/kg intravenously every 2 weeks or 7.5 mg/kg intravenously every 3 weeks (in combination with fluoropyrimidine-irinotecan or fluoropyrimidine-oxaliplatin–based regimen). For metastatic nonsquamous NSCLC: 15 mg/kg intravenously every 3 weeks (in combination with paclitaxel and carboplatin). For metastatic RCC: 10 mg/kg intravenously every 2 weeks (in combination with interferon alfa).

   ii. Dose modification. Temporary suspension of therapy is warranted in patients with moderate or severe proteinuria or severe, uncontrolled hypertension. Permanent discontinuation is recommended for wound dehiscence requiring intervention, GI perforation, hypertensive crisis, serious bleeding, severe arterial thromboembolic events, or nephrotic syndrome.

   iii. Supplied as 100- and 400-mg vials.

5. Ziv-aflibercept (Zaltrap)

a. FDA-approved indications. Treatment of metastatic colorectal cancer (in combination with fluorouracil, leucovorin, and irinotecan [FOLFIRI]) in patients who are resistant to or have progressed on an oxaliplatin-based regimen.

b. Pharmacology. Recombinant fusion protein.

   i. Mechanism. Recombinant fusion protein, comprised of portions of binding domains for VEGFR 1 and 2 attached to the Fc portion of human IgG1, which acts as a decoy receptor for VEGF-A, -B, and placental growth factor that prevent VEGFR binding/activation to their receptors, leading to angiogenesis and tumor regression.

c. Toxicity (reported in combination with FOLFIRI)

   i. Common. Hypertension, fatigue, dysphonia, hand–foot syndrome, diarrhea, stomatitis, decreased appetite, weight loss, abdominal pain, myelosuppression, increase AST/ALT, weakness, proteinuria, increased creatinine, epistaxis, and dyspnea.

   ii. Occasional. Venous/arterial thromboembolic events, reversible posterior encephalopathy syndrome (RPLS), hyperpigmentation, dehydration, hemorrhoids, neutropenic fever, oropharyngeal pain, pulmonary embolism, and fistula formation.

   iii. Rare. Hypersensitivity resections, thrombotic microangiopathy, and impaired wound healing.

d. Administration

   i. FDA-approved dose. 4 mg/kg intravenously every 2 weeks (in combination with FOLFIRI).

      ii. **Dose modification.** Temporary suspension of therapy is warranted in patients with uncontrolled hypertension, neutropenia, or moderate-to-severe proteinuria. Permanent discontinuation is recommended for arterial thrombotic events, fistula formation, GI perforation, serious bleeding, hypertensive crisis, nephrotic syndrome or thrombotic microangiopathy, RPLS, or wound dehiscence requiring intervention.

      iii. **Supplied** as 100- and 200-mg vials.

F. Raf tyrosine kinase inhibition. The Raf/mitogen extracellular kinase (MEK)/extracellular signal-related kinase (ERK) signal transduction pathway is overactivated in different cancers including thyroid, hepatocellular, pancreatic, colorectal, ovarian, prostate, breast, and kidney tumors, as well as in NSCLC, AML, and melanoma. Once extracellular ligands such as transforming growth factor alpha (TGF-α), EGF, VEGF, and PDGFβ bind to their respective receptors, the Raf/MEK/ERK pathway is activated. The pathway transmits signals from the cell surface through autophosphorylation to the nucleus. The Raf/MEK/ERK pathway is involved in the regulation of proliferation, differentiation, survival, angiogenesis, metastasis, and adhesion. Various Raf isoforms exist and sorafenib has shown inhibitory effects on several of the Raf kinases.

1. **Sorafenib (Nexavar)**
   a. **FDA-approved indications.** Advanced renal cell carcinoma; hepatocellular cancer; and differentiated thyroid cancer.
   b. **Pharmacology.** Multitargeted tyrosine kinase inhibitor.
      i. **Mechanism.** Inhibits several intracellular Raf kinases including C-Raf, wild-type B-Raf, and mutant B-Raf. Also inhibits several cell surface kinases including VEGFR1-3, PDGFRβ, c-KIT, RET, and Flt-3. These inhibitory effects decrease tumor cell proliferation and angiogenesis.
      ii. **Metabolism.** Hepatic metabolism primarily through CYP 3A4 and glucuronidation by UGT1A9. Elimination occurs primarily by the fecal route (77%; 51% as unchanged drug); 19% of the dose undergoes urinary excretion.
   c. **Toxicity**
      i. **Common.** Rash, hand–foot syndrome, diarrhea, hypertension, elevations in amylase/lipase, bleeding events, fatigue, hypophosphatemia, alopecia, pruritus, dry skin, diarrhea, nausea, vomiting, constipation, dyspnea, cough, myelosuppression, and neuropathy.
      ii. **Occasional.** Cardiac ischemia/infarction, mucositis/stomatitis, headache, hypokalemia, and dyspepsia.
      iii. **Rare.** GI perforation, thromboembolism, interstitial lung disease, and RPLS.

2. **Regorafenib (Stivarga)**
   a. **FDA-approved indications.** GIST, locally advanced, unresectable, or metastatic; metastatic colorectal cancer previously treated with fluoropyrimidine-, oxaliplatin-, and irinotecan-based chemotherapy, an anti-VEGF therapy, and, if *KRAS* wild-type, an anti-EGFR therapy.
   b. **Pharmacology.** Multitargeted tyrosine kinase inhibitor.
      1. **Mechanism.** Inhibits intracellular Raf-1, wild-type B-Raf, and mutant B-Raf. Also inhibits several cell surface kinases including VEGFR 1-3, PDGFRα, PDGFRβ, RET, and Abl. These inhibitory effects decrease tumor cell proliferation and angiogenesis.
      2. **Metabolism.** Hepatic metabolism primarily through CYP 3A4 and glucuronidation by UGT1A9. Elimination occurs primarily by the fecal route (71%; 47% as unchanged drug); 19% of the dose undergoes urinary excretion.
   c. **Toxicity**
      i. **Common.** Hypertension, fatigue, dysphonia, pain, headache, fever, hand–foot syndrome, rash, alopecia, hypocalcemia, hypophosphatemia, hyponatremia, hypothyroidism, increased lipase, diarrhea, nausea, vomiting, elevations in AST/ALT, and proteinuria.

    ii. Occasional. Taste disturbance, xerostomia, gastroesophageal reflux, tremor, and myocardial ischemia.

    iii. Rare. GI fistula, hypertensive crisis, RPLS, and skin cancer (squamous cell carcinoma or keratoacanthoma).

  d. Administration

    i. FDA-approved dose. 160 mg orally once daily for the first 21 days of each 28-day cycle with a low-fat (<30% fat) breakfast.

    ii. Dose modification. Modifications recommended for skin toxicities. No adjustments in mild or moderate preexisting renal impairment; not studied in severe renal dysfunction. No adjustments necessary for Child–Pugh Class A or B hepatic dysfunction; not studied in Child–Pugh Class C.

    iii. Supplied as 40-mg tablets.

3. Vemurafenib (Zelboraf)

  a. FDA-approved indications. Unresectable or metastatic melanoma with a V600E mutation on the BRAF gene.

  b. Pharmacology. BRAF inhibitor.

    i. Mechanism. Inhibits BRAF V600E and blocks downstream phosphorylation in BRAF-mutated cells

    ii. Metabolism. Hepatic metabolism occurs via CYP3A4. Elimination occurs primarily by the fecal route (94%); 1% of the dose undergoes urinary excretion.

  c. Toxicity

    i. Common. Alopecia, papilloma, photosensitivity, pruritus, rash, nausea, arthralgia, and fatigue.

    ii. Occasional. Prolonged QT interval, squamous cell carcinoma of the skin, Stevens–Johnson syndrome, toxic epidermal necrolysis, and hand–foot syndrome.

    iii. Rare. Immune hypersensitivity reaction, malignant melanoma.

  d. Administration

    i. FDA-approved dose. 960 mg orally twice daily

    ii. Dose modification. Modifications recommended for QT prolongation. No adjustments in mild or moderate preexisting renal impairment; not studied in severe renal dysfunction. No adjustments necessary for Child–Pugh Class A or B hepatic dysfunction; not studied in Child–Pugh Class C.

    iii. Supplied as 240-mg tablets.

4. Dabrafenib (Tafinlar)

  a. FDA-approved indications. Treatment of unresectable or metastatic melanoma with BRAF V600E mutation.

  b. Pharmacology. BRAF inhibitor.

    i. Mechanism. Inhibits BRAF V600E kinase, as well as BRAF V600K, BRAF V600D, and wild-type BRAF and CRAF kinases and competitively blocks phosphorylation at the ATP-binding site of these kinases.

    ii. Metabolism. Hepatic metabolism primarily through CYP 2C8 and CYP3A4. Elimination occurs primarily by the fecal route (71%); 23% of the dose undergoes urinary excretion.

  c. Toxicity

    i. Common. Peripheral edema, alopecia, hand–foot syndrome, hyperkeratosis, night sweats, papilloma, rash, hyperglycemia, hypoalbuminemia, hypokalemia, hypophosphatemia, abdominal pain, constipation, decreased appetite, diarrhea, nausea, vomiting, anemia, leukopenia, neutropenia, elevated liver enzymes, lymphocytopenia, arthralgia, myalgias, headache, cough, fatigue, pyrexia, and shivering.

    ii. Occasional. Cardiomyopathy, deep venous thrombosis, pancreatitis, interstitial nephritis, and renal failure.

    iii. Rare. New primary cutaneous malignancies, febrile drug reaction, hemolytic anemia in G6PD-deficient patients, uveitis, and iritis.

    d. Administration

        i. FDA-approved dose. 150 mg orally twice daily taken 1 hour before or 2 hours after a meal.

        ii. Dose modification. May be considered based on side effects. No data exist to guide dose adjustments in patients with renal or hepatic insufficiencies; however, dose adjustments are not recommended for mild-to-moderate renal dysfunction or mild hepatic dysfunction. It is recommended to avoid strong inhibitors and inducers of CYP3A4, CYP2C8, and p-glycoprotein.

        iii. Supplied as 50- and 75-mg capsules.

5. Trametinib (Mekinist)

    a. FDA-approved indications. Treatment of unresectable or metastatic melanoma with BRAF V600E or V600K mutations.

    b. Pharmacology. MEK inhibitor.

        i. Mechanism. Inhibitor that reversibly inhibits mitogen-activated extracellular regulated kinase 1 (MEK1) and MEK2 activation and of MEK1 and MEK2 activity. It also inhibits BRAF V600 mutation-positive cells when used in combination with dabrafenib.

        ii. Metabolism. Predominantly metabolized via deacetylation alone or with mono-oxygenation in combination with glucuronidation. Elimination occurs primarily by the fecal route (80%); 20% of the dose undergoes urinary excretion.

    c. Toxicity

        i. Common. Peripheral edema, night sweats, rash, hyperglycemia, hypoalbuminemia, hypokalemia, hypophosphatemia, abdominal pain, constipation, decreased appetite, diarrhea, nausea, vomiting, anemia, leukopenia, neutropenia, thrombocytopenia, elevated liver enzymes, lymphedema, arthralgia, myalgias, cough, fatigue, pyrexia, and shivering.

        ii. Occasional. Cardiomyopathy, prolonged QT interval, interstitial nephritis, and renal failure.

        iii. Rare. New primary cutaneous malignancies, febrile drug reaction, retinal pigment epithelial detachment, thrombosis of retinal vein, pulmonary embolism, and interstitial lung disease.

    d. Administration

        i. FDA-approved dose. 2 mg orally once daily taken 1 hour before or 2 hours after a meal.

        ii. Dose modification. May be considered based on side effects. Reduce, hold, or discontinue doses based on organ-specific toxicities, specifically cutaneous, cardiac, ocular, and pulmonary toxicities.

        iii. Supplied as 0.5- and 2-mg tablets.

G. mTOR targeting. The mammalian target of rapamycin (mTOR) is a serine/threonine kinase that integrates signals from several molecular pathways that regulate cell functions including translation, transcription, and cell growth, differentiation, and survival. Dysregulation of the mTOR pathway has been associated with several human cancers, and thus mTOR inhibitors hold therapeutic promise as anticancer agents. Agents with effects on mTOR include everolimus and temsirolimus.

1. Everolimus (Afinitor)

    a. FDA-approved indications. Advanced renal cell carcinoma (RCC) after failure of sorafenib or sunitinib; advanced, metastatic, or unresectable PNET.

    b. Pharmacology. mTOR inhibitor.

        i. Mechanism. Binds to the FK binding protein-12 to form a complex that inhibits activation of mTOR serine-threonine kinase activity, which leads to reduced protein synthesis and cell proliferation. Also inhibits VEGF and hypoxia-inducible factor, thereby reducing angiogenesis.

        ii. Metabolism. Extensively metabolized in the liver via CYP 3A4; forms six weak metabolites. Elimination occurs via feces (80%) and urine (~5%).

 c. Toxicity

  i. Common. Peripheral edema, hypertension, fatigue, headache, fever, seizure, behavioral changes, insomnia, dizziness, rash, acneiform eruption, pruritus, xeroderma, contact dermatitis, excoriation, hypercholesterolemia, hyperglycemia, hypertriglyceridemia, hypophosphatemia, hypocalcemia, diabetes mellitus, hypomagnesemia, stomatitis, constipation, nausea, diarrhea, gastroenteritis, myelosuppression, abnormal liver function tests, weakness, arthralgias, limb pain, otitis, increased serum creatinine, epistaxis, cough, dyspnea, and rhinitis.

  ii. Occasional. Chest pain, depression, migraine, paresthesia, chills, eczema, alopecia, hand–foot syndrome, hypermenorrhea, menstrual disease, gastritis, vaginal hemorrhage, increased serum bilirubin, muscle spasm, tremor, jaw pain, pleural effusion, pneumonia, and rhinitis.

  iii. Rare. Cardiac arrest, azoospermia, fluid retention, intrahepatic cholestasis, pulmonary embolism, thrombotic microangiopathy, and thrombotic thrombocytopenic purpura.

 d. Administration

  i. FDA-approved dose. 10 mg orally once daily with or without food with a glass of water. To reduce variability, take consistently with regard to food.

  ii. Dose modification. No dosage adjustment necessary for renal dysfunction. For Child–Pugh class A, reduce dose to 7.5 mg orally once daily; if not tolerated, may further reduce to 5 mg orally once daily. For Child–Pugh class B, reduce dose to 5 mg orally once daily; if not tolerated, may further reduce to 2.5 mg orally once daily. For Child–Pugh class C, if potential benefit outweighs risks, a maximum dose of 2.5 mg orally once daily may be considered.

  iii. Supplied as 2.5-, 5-, 7.5-, and 10-mg tablets.

2. Temsirolimus (Torisel)

 a. FDA-approved indications. Advanced RCC.

 b. Pharmacology. mTOR inhibitor.

  i. Mechanism. Binds to the FK binding protein-12 to form a complex that inhibits activation of mTOR serine-threonine kinase activity, which leads to reduced protein synthesis and cell proliferation. Also inhibits VEGF and hypoxia-inducible factors, thereby reducing angiogenesis.

  ii. Metabolism. Primarily hepatic metabolism via CYP 3A4 to sirolimus (active metabolite) and four minor metabolites. Excretion occurs via feces (78%) and the urine (<5%).

 c. Toxicity

  i. Common. Edema, chest pain, fever, pain, headache, insomnia, rash, pruritus, nail thinning, dry skin, hyperglycemia, hypercholesterolemia, hypophosphatemia, hyperlipidemia, hypokalemia, mucositis, nausea, anorexia, stomatitis, constipation, weight loss, vomiting, myelosuppression, abnormal liver function tests, weakness, back pain, arthralgia, increased creatinine, dyspnea, cough, epistaxis, and infections.

  ii. Occasional. Hypertension, venous thromboembolism, acne, impaired wound healing, hyperbilirubinemia, bowel perforation, myalgias, conjunctivitis, interstitial lung disease, and hypotension.

  iii. Rare. Acute renal failure, glucose intolerance, angioneurotic edema, pericardial effusion, pleural effusion, pneumonitis, and seizure.

 d. Administration

  i. FDA-approved dose. 25 mg intravenously once weekly until disease progression or unacceptable toxicity. Avoid concomitant administration with CYP 3A4 inhibitors. If a strong CYP 3A4 inhibitor cannot be avoided, consider dose reduction to 12.5 mg intravenously once weekly. If a strong CYP 3A4 inducer is concomitantly used, consider dose adjustment up to 50 mg intravenously once weekly.

      ii. Dose modification. No renal dose adjustments are necessary; has not been studied in dialysis. For mild hepatic dysfunction (bilirubin >1–1.5 times upper limit of normal (ULN) or AST >ULN with bilirubin ≤ULN), reduce dose to 15 mg intravenously once weekly. Use is contraindicated in moderate-to-severe hepatic dysfunction.

      iii. Supplied as 25-mg vials.

H. Bruton's tyrosine kinase inhibition. Bruton's tyrosine kinase is an integral component of the B-cell receptor and cytokine receptor pathways. This tyrosine kinase is important for the survival of malignant B cells. Ibrutinib has been approved as an irreversible inhibitor of Bruton's tyrosine kinase.

  1. Ibrutinib (Imbruvica)

    a. FDA-approved indications. Chronic lymphocytic leukemia (CLL), mantle cell lymphoma.

    b. Pharmacology. Bruton's tyrosine kinase inhibitor.

      i. Mechanism. Potent and irreversible binding of Bruton's tyrosine kinase, resulting in decreased malignant B-cell proliferation and survival.

      ii. Metabolism. Metabolized in the liver via CYP 3A (major) and CYP2D6 (minor) to an active metabolite. Elimination occurs via feces (80%) and urine (<10%).

    c. Toxicity

      i. Common. Peripheral edema, fatigue, skin rash, diarrhea, nausea, constipation, thrombocytopenia, neutropenia, anemia, musculoskeletal pain, and dyspnea.

      ii. Occasional. Dehydration, stomatitis, dyspepsia, arthralgias, increased serum creatinine, sinusitis, and epistaxis.

      iii. Rare. Malignant neoplasm of skin, renal failure.

    d. Administration

      i. FDA-approved dose. CLL: 420 mg orally once daily; Mantle cell lymphoma: 560 mg orally once daily. Administer with water at approximately the same time each day.

      ii. Dose modification. Avoid concurrent use with moderate or strong inhibitors of CYP3A. If concomitant use is necessary, reduce dose to 140 mg orally once daily.

      iii. Supplied as 140-mg capsules.

V. OTHER TARGETS

A. Unconjugated monoclonal antibodies

  1. Alemtuzumab (Campath)

    a. FDA-approved indication. B-cell CLL.

    b. Pharmacology. Humanized MAb.

      i. Mechanism. Binds to CD52, resulting in complement-mediated and/or antibody-dependent cellular cytotoxicity.

      ii. Metabolism. Initial half-life is 11 hours but increases to 6 days after repeated dosing (due to depletion of CD52-positive cells).

    c. Toxicity

      i. Common. Hypotension, fever, chills, headache, rash, nausea, vomiting, diarrhea, rigors, chest pain, dyspnea, pharyngitis, infection, neutropenia, thrombocytopenia, and anemia.

      ii. Occasional. Pancytopenia, autoimmune idiopathic thrombocytopenia, and hemolytic anemia.

      iii. Rare. Pulmonary fibrosis, bone fracture, tumor lysis syndrome, and electrolyte disturbances.

    d. Administration

      i. FDA-approved dose. Initial dose is 3 mg intravenously once daily, which is then increased to 10 mg intravenously once daily as tolerated. Once the 10-mg dose is tolerated, the dose is increased to 30 mg intravenously once daily. Most patients can tolerate dose escalation in 4 to 7 days. The maintenance dose is 30 mg intravenously once daily, three times per week, on alternate days for 12 weeks. If therapy is interrupted for more than 7 days, dose escalation should gradually be reinitiated.

    ii. Dose modification. Hematologic toxicities.

    iii. Supplied as 30-mg vials.

2. Obinutuzumab (Gazyva)

  a. FDA-approved indications. CLL

  b. Pharmacology. Humanized MAb.

    i. Mechanism. Binds to CD20, which regulates cell cycle initiation. Obinutuzumab induces complement-dependent cytotoxicity and antibody-dependent cell-mediated cytotoxicity.

    ii. Metabolism. Not appreciably metabolized. Elimination is uncertain, but it may undergo phagocytosis by the reticuloendothelial system.

  c. Toxicity

    i. Common. Cytokine release syndrome (fever, chills, dyspnea, bronchospasm, hypoxia, hypotension, urticaria, and angioedema), hypocalcemia, hyperkalemia, hyponatremia, hypoalbuminemia, hypokalemia, leukopenia, lymphocytopenia, neutropenia, thrombocytopenia, increased transaminases, antibody development, infection, and increased serum creatinine.

    ii. Occasional. Tumor lysis syndrome, cough, fever

    iii. Rare. Progressive multifocal leukoencephalopathy, reactivation of HBV.

  d. Administration

    i. FDA-approved dose. Cycle 1: 100 mg intravenously on day 1, followed by 900 mg intravenously on day 2, followed by 1,000 mg intravenously weekly for 2 doses (days 8 and 15). Cycles 2 to 6: 1,000 mg intravenously on day 1 every 28 days for 5 doses.

    ii. Dose modification. No specific recommendations.

    iii. Supplied as 1,000-mg vials.

3. Ofatumumab (Arzerra)

  a. FDA-approved indications. CLL.

  b. Pharmacology. Human MAb.

    i. Mechanism. Binds to extracellular (large and small) loops of CD20, which regulates cell cycle initiation. Ofatumumab induces complement-dependent cytotoxicity and antibody-dependent cell-mediated cytotoxicity.

    ii. Metabolism. Not appreciably metabolized. Elimination is uncertain, but it may undergo phagocytosis by the reticuloendothelial system.

  c. Toxicity

    i. Common. Cytokine release syndrome (fever, chills, dyspnea, bronchospasm, hypoxia, hypotension, urticaria, and angioedema), fatigue, rash, diarrhea, nausea, neutropenia, anemia, infection, cough, and dyspnea.

    ii. Occasional. Peripheral edema, hypertension, hypotension, tachycardia, chills, insomnia, headache, back pain, and sinusitis.

    iii. Rare. Abdominal pain, hemolytic anemia, hepatitis B, hypoxia, progressive multifocal leukoencephalopathy, and thrombocytopenia.

  d. Administration

    i. FDA-approved dose. Initial dose: 300 mg intravenously on week 1, followed 1 week later by 2,000 mg intravenously once weekly for 7 doses (doses 2 to 8), followed 4 weeks later by 2,000 mg intravenously once every 4 weeks for 4 doses (doses 9 to 12).

    ii. Dose modification. No specific recommendations.

    iii. Supplied as 100- and 1,000-mg vials.

4. Rituximab (Rituxan)

  a. FDA-approved indications. Relapsed or refractory low-grade or follicular CD20-positive, B-cell non-Hodgkin's lymphoma (NHL); diffuse large B-cell CD20-positive NHL.

    b. Pharmacology. Chimeric murine/human MAb.

        i. Mechanism. Binds to CD20, which regulates cell cycle initiation. Rituximab induces complement-dependent cytotoxicity and antibody-dependent cell-mediated cytotoxicity.

        ii. Metabolism. Not appreciably metabolized. Elimination is uncertain, but it may undergo phagocytosis by the reticuloendothelial system.

    c. Toxicity

        i. Common. Cytokine release syndrome (fever, chills, dyspnea, bronchospasm, hypoxia, hypotension, urticaria, and angioedema), headache, GI upset (nausea, vomiting, and diarrhea), myelosuppression, weakness, cough, rhinitis, infusion-related reactions (hypotension, angioedema, hypoxia, and bronchospasm), infections, rash, arthralgia, myalgia, and hypersensitivity reactions (hypotension, angioedema, bronchospasm).

        ii. Occasional. Edema, hypertension, dyspnea, sinusitis, and tumor lysis syndrome.

        iii. Rare. Severe infusion-related reactions (pulmonary infiltrates, ARDS, myocardial infarct, ventricular fibrillation, and cardiogenic shock), optic neuritis, serum sickness, severe mucocutaneous reactions (paraneoplastic pemphigus, Stevens–Johnson syndrome, lichenoid dermatitis, vesiculobullous dermatitis, and toxic epidermal necrolysis), and acute renal failure.

    d. Administration

        i. FDA-approved dose. Refer to individual protocols. Usual dose is 375 mg/m^2 intravenously once weekly for 4 to 8 doses.

        ii. Dose modification. No specific recommendations.

        iii. Supplied as 100- and 500-mg vials.

B. Conjugated monoclonal antibodies

  1. Ado-trastuzumab emtansine (Kadcyla)

    a. FDA-approved indication. Metastatic breast cancer, HER2-positive.

    b. Pharmacology. Humanized MAb.

        i. Mechanism. MAb drug conjugate directed at HER2, which incorporates the HER2-targeted actions of trastuzumab with the microtubule inhibitor DM1 (a maytansine derivative) resulting in cell cycle arrest and apoptosis.

        ii. Metabolism. DM1 undergoes hepatic metabolism via CYP 3A4/5.

    c. Toxicity

        i. Common. Fatigue, headache, fever, insomnia, rash, nausea, constipation, diarrhea, abdominal pain, vomiting, xerostomia, stomatitis, thrombocytopenia, anemia, increased transaminases, increased bilirubin, pain, peripheral neuropathy, arthralgia, weakness, myalgia, and cough.

        ii. Occasional. Peripheral edema, hypertension, left ventricular systolic dysfunction, dizziness, chills, pruritus, dysgeusia, neutropenia, and blurred vision.

        iii. Rare. Anaphylaxis, hepatic encephalopathy, hepatotoxicity, and portal hypertension.

    d. Administration

        i. FDA-approved dose. 3.6 mg/kg intravenously every 3 weeks until disease progression or toxicity.

        ii. Dose modification. No recommendation for renal and/or hepatic impairment.

        iii. Supplied as 100- and 160-mg vials.

  2. Brentuximab vedotin (Adcetris)

    a. FDA-approved indication. Hodgkin lymphoma (HL) after failure of at least two prior chemotherapy regimens or after stem cell transplant failure; systemic anaplastic large cell lymphoma (sALCL) after failure of at least one prior chemotherapy regimen.

    b. Pharmacology. Chimeric murine/human MAb.

        i. Mechanism. MAb drug conjugate directed at CD30, made up of three components: (1) a CD30-specific IgG1 antibody; (2) a microtubule-disrupting agent, monomethylauristatin E (MMAE); and (3) a protease cleavable dipeptide linker. After binding to cells that express CD30, the complex is internalized and releases MMAE, which binds to tubules and causes cell cycle arrest and apoptosis.

      ii. **Metabolism.** MMAE: minimal, primarily via CYP 3A4/5-mediated oxidation.

  c. **Toxicity**

      i. **Common.** Peripheral edema, fatigue, pain, headache, insomnia, dizziness, anxiety, rash, pruritus, alopecia, nausea, diarrhea, abdominal pain, constipation, weight loss, myelosuppression, peripheral sensory neuropathy, myalgias, arthralgias, dyspnea, oropharyngeal pain, and infusion reactions (fever, chills, rigors, and sweats).

      ii. **Occasional.** Supraventricular arrhythmia, dry skin, limb pain, muscle spasms, pyelonephritis, pneumonitis, pulmonary embolism, and septic shock.

      iii. **Rare.** Anaphylaxis, progressive multifocal leukoencephalopathy, tachycardia, and tumor lysis syndrome.

  d. **Administration**

      i. **FDA-approved dose.** 1.8 mg/kg intravenously (maximum dose: 180 mg) every 3 weeks for a maximum of 16 cycles. For patients weighing >100 kg, doses should be calculated using a weight of 100 kg.

      ii. **Dose modification.** No recommendation for renal and/or hepatic impairment.

      iii. **Supplied** as 50-mg vials.

C. Radioimmunoconjugates

  1. Ibritumomab Tiuxetan (Zevalin)

    a. **FDA-approved indications.** Relapsed or refractory low-grade, follicular, or transformed B-cell NHL.

    b. **Pharmacology.** Radioimmunoconjugated MAb.

      i. **Mechanism.** Ibritumomab is joined through covalent bonds to tiuxetan, a chelating agent. The chelator tightly binds to the radioisotopes indium 111 (^{111}In) or yttrium 90 (^{90}Y). Ibritumomab binds to the CD20 antigen found on normal and malignant B cells while allowing the emission of radiation against the target and neighboring cells. The agent causes antibody-dependent and complement-mediated cytotoxicity and induces apoptosis.

      ii. **Metabolism.** Primarily eliminated from circulation by binding to the tumor and metabolized through radioactive decay. The product of the radioactive decay of ^{90}Y is ^{90}Zr (nonradioactive); ^{111}In decays to ^{111}Cd (nonradioactive). Approximately 7% of the radiolabeled activity undergoes urinary excretion over 7 days.

    c. **Toxicity**

      i. **Common.** Chills, fever, GI upset (nausea, vomiting, abdominal pain), myelosuppression, weakness, infection, headache, dizziness, dyspnea, and cough.

      ii. **Occasional.** Hypotension, diarrhea, constipation, insomnia, anxiety, arthralgia, myalgia, epistaxis, allergic reactions, pruritus, rash, peripheral edema, and secondary malignancies.

      iii. **Rare.** Arthritis, encephalopathy, pulmonary edema, hemorrhagic stroke, angioedema, and pulmonary embolus.

    d. **Administration**

      i. **FDA-approved dose.** Step 1: inject ^{111}In ibritumomab tiuxetan 5 mCi (1.6-mg total antibody dose) over 10 minutes after rituximab infusion of 250 mg/m^2. Biodistribution is then assessed with a first image taken 2 to 24 hours after ^{111}In ibritumomab tiuxetan, a second image 48 to 72 hours after the infusion, and an optional third image 90 to 120 hours after the infusion. If biodistribution is considered acceptable, proceed to step 2. Step 2 (initiated 7 to 9 days after step 1): rituximab infusion 250 mg/m^2 followed by ^{90}Y ibritumomab tiuxetan 0.4 mCi/kg over 10 minutes (if platelet count >150,000) or 0.3 mCi/kg (if platelet count between 100,000 and 149,000). Ibritumomab should not be administered if platelet count is less than 100,000 cells/mm^3, and the maximum allowable whole-body dose should not exceed 32 mCi regardless of patient's weight.

    ii. Dose modification. No dosage modifications recommended for renal and/or hepatic impairment.

    iii. Supplied as 3.2-mg vials.

D. Proteasome inhibition. The 26S proteasome is a protein complex that degrades ubiquitinated proteins. The role of the ubiquitin–proteasome pathway is to regulate intracellular concentrations of specific proteins and maintain cellular homeostasis as it relates to cell cycle and transcriptional regulation, cell signaling, and apoptosis. Bortezomib reversibly inhibits the activity of the 26S proteasome, preventing proteolysis and affecting multiple signaling cascades within cells, which leads to cell cycle arrest and apoptosis. Carfilzomib, a novel epoxyketone proteasome inhibitor, irreversibly binds to active sites of 20S proteasome, within the 26S proteasome. It is more selective for chymotrypsin-like active sites of the proteasome and has activity against bortezomib-resistant cell lines.

1. Bortezomib (Velcade)

    a. FDA-approved indications. Multiple myeloma refractory to other treatments; relapsed or refractory mantle cell lymphoma.

    b. Pharmacology. Proteasome inhibitor.

        i. Mechanism. Selective, reversible inhibitor of the 26S proteasome.

        ii. Metabolism. Primarily hepatic through CYP 1A2, 2C19, and 3A4 with minor metabolism through CYP 2D6 and 2C9 to inactive metabolites. Elimination pathways in humans are unknown.

    c. Toxicity

        i. Common. Peripheral neuropathy, hypotension, thrombocytopenia, anemia, neutropenia, nausea, vomiting, diarrhea, constipation, pyrexia, psychiatric disorders, decreased appetite, asthenia, paresthesia, dysesthesia, anemia, headache, cough, dyspnea, rash, pain, insomnia, lower respiratory tract infections, arthralgia, myalgia, dizziness, herpes zoster, lower limb edema, blurred vision, and pneumonia.

        ii. Occasional. Heart failure events (acute pulmonary edema, cardiac failure, congestive cardiac failure, cardiogenic shock, and pulmonary edema).

        iii. Rare. QT-interval prolongation, pneumonitis, interstitial pneumonia, lung infiltration, ARDS, cardiac tamponade, ischemic colitis, encephalopathy, disseminated intravascular coagulation, hepatitis, pancreatitis, and toxic epidermal necrolysis.

    d. Administration

        i. FDA-approved dose. 1.3 mg/m^2 intravenously twice weekly for 2 weeks on days 1, 4, 8, and 11 in a 21-day cycle. Therapy extending beyond 8 cycles may be administered by the standard schedule or may be given once weekly for 4 weeks on days 1, 8, 15, and 22 followed by a 13-day rest (days 23 to 35). Doses given consecutively should be separated by at least 72 hours.

        ii. Dose modification. No dosage adjustment for mild hepatic dysfunction; reduce initial dose to 0.7 mg/m^2 in the first cycle for moderate hepatic dysfunction (bilirubin >1.5 to 3 times upper limit of normal). No dosage adjustment necessary for renal dysfunction. Recommend administration post-dialysis, given that dialysis may decrease bortezomib concentrations. Monitor closely for toxicity.

        iii. Supplied as 3.5-mg vials.

2. Carfilzomib (Kyprolis)

    a. FDA-approved indications. Multiple myeloma refractory to other treatments, including bortezomib.

    b. Pharmacology. Proteasome inhibitor.

        i. Mechanism. Selective, irreversible inhibitor of the 20S proteasome.

        ii. Metabolism. Primarily metabolized via peptidase and epoxide hydrolase activity. Elimination pathways in humans are unknown, but most likely extrahepatic clearance.

    c. Toxicity

        i. Common. Peripheral neuropathy, thrombocytopenia, anemia, neutropenia, nausea, vomiting, diarrhea, constipation, headache, backache, cough, dyspnea, rash, pain, insomnia, upper respiratory tract infections, elevated serum creatinine, fatigue, and pyrexia.

        ii. Occasional. Congestive heart failure, acute renal failure, pneumonia, pulmonary hypertension, pulmonary complications, and infusion reactions.

        iii. Rare. Dyspnea, cardiac arrest, myocardial ischemia, liver failure, tumor lysis syndrome, and febrile neutropenia.

    d. Administration

        i. FDA-approved dose. 20 mg/m^2/day intravenously on days 1, 2, 8, 9, and 16 to be given every 28 days for cycle 1. If cycle 1 is well tolerated, may increase dose to 27 mg/m^2/day on the same schedule. Utilize actual body weight and cap BSA at 2.2 m^2.

        ii. Dose modification. Recommendations on modifying or holding therapy based on the following toxicities, hematologic, cardiac, pulmonary, hepatic, renal, and peripheral neuropathy.

        iii. Supplied as 3.5-mg vials.

E. Histone Deacetylase inhibition. Histones are a family of proteins that interact with DNA, resulting in DNA being wound around a histone core within a nucleosome. Histone acetylation and deacetylation enzymes play key roles in modifying chromatin structure and, as such, contribute to the regulation of gene expression. The formation of histone deacetylation nuclear complexes is crucial for transcriptional repression and epigenetic regulation of cellular processes including cellular proliferation, self-renewal, and differentiation. Epigenetic alteration has been linked to the development of several cancers, including T-cell lymphomas, via silencing of tumor suppressor genes. Histone deacetylase inhibitors can induce cellular differentiation and/or cause apoptosis by allowing transcription of a variety of target genes to occur. Agents that can inhibit histone deacetylase enzymes include romidepsin and vorinostat.

    1. Romidepsin (Istodax)

        a. FDA-approved indications. Refractory cutaneous T-cell lymphoma (CTCL) and refractory peripheral T-cell lymphoma (PTCL).

        b. Pharmacology. Histone deacetylase inhibitor.

            i. Mechanism. Inhibition of histone deacetylase results in accumulation of acetyl groups, leading to changes in chromatin structure and transcription factor activation causing termination of cell growth and apoptosis.

            ii. Metabolism. Primarily hepatic via CYP 3A4, and to a lesser degree CYP 3A5, 1A1, 2B6, and 2C19.

        c. Toxicity

            i. Common. ST-T wave changes, hypotension, fatigue, fever, headache, chills, pruritus, dermatitis, hypocalcemia, hyperglycemia, hypoalbuminemia, hypermagnesemia, hyperuricemia, hypokalemia, hypophosphatemia, hyponatremia, nausea, diarrhea, constipation, taste alteration, weight loss, abdominal pain, myelosuppression, AST/ALT increase, cough, and dyspnea.

            ii. Occasional. Peripheral edema, tachycardia, dehydration, stomatitis, hyperbilirubinemia, hypoxia, and pulmonary embolism.

            iii. Rare. Acute renal failure, atrial fibrillation, cardiopulmonary failure, cardiogenic shock, and septic shock.

   d. Administration
   - **i. FDA-approved dose.** 14 mg/m² intravenously on days 1, 8, and 15 of a 28-day cycle.
   - **ii. Dose modification.** No dosage adjustments necessary for renal impairment. Use has not been studied, however, in patients with end stage renal disease. For mild hepatic dysfunction, no dosage adjustments are provided. Use with caution in patients with moderate-to-severe hepatic impairment.
   - **iii. Supplied** as 10-mg vials.

2. Vorinostat (Zolinza)
   - **a. FDA-approved indications.** Progressive, persistent, or recurrent CTCL on or following two systemic treatments.
   - **b. Pharmacology.** Histone deacetylase inhibitor.
     - **i. Mechanism.** Inhibition of histone deacetylase results in accumulation of acetyl groups, leading to changes in chromatin structure and transcription factor activation causing termination of cell growth and apoptosis.
     - **ii. Metabolism.** Glucuronidated and hydrolyzed (followed by beta-oxidation) to inactive metabolites. Excretion occurs via the urine (52%) as both inactive metabolites (~52%) and unchanged drug (<1%).
   - **c. Toxicity**
     - **i. Common.** Peripheral edema, fatigue, chills, dizziness, headache, fever, alopecia, pruritus, hyperglycemia, diarrhea, nausea, taste alteration, anorexia, vomiting, decreased appetite, muscle spasm, myelosuppression, proteinuria, increased creatinine, and cough.
     - **ii. Occasional.** QTc prolongation, squamous cell carcinoma, and pulmonary embolism.
     - **iii. Rare.** Angioneurotic edema, cholecystitis, deafness, diverticulitis, exfoliative dermatitis, GI bleeding, hemoptysis, MI, neutropenia, renal failure, sepsis, and ischemic stroke.
   - **d. Administration**
     - **i. FDA-approved dose.** 400 mg orally once daily until disease progression or unacceptable toxicity.
     - **ii. Dose modification.** Dosing was not studied in renal dysfunction; based on the minimal renal clearance, however, the need for adjustment is not expected. For patients with mild-to-moderate hepatic dysfunction, reduce dose to 300 mg orally once daily. For patients with severe hepatic dysfunction (bilirubin >3 times upper limit of normal), doses of 100 to 200 mg orally daily have been studied in a limited number of cases.
     - **iii. Supplied** as 100-mg capsules.

F. CTLA-4 target. Targeting tumor immunobiology and the complexity of the interactions between the host T cells and cancer has led to new approaches in cancer treatment. Tumors are able to avoid detection and destruction by the host immune system; thus, activating the immune system in the host may result in cancer cell death. Enhancing the patient's natural antitumor response consists of blocking the immunoregulatory mechanisms that break host responses. Cytotoxic T lymphocyte antigen-4 (CTLA-4) is a molecule that downregulates T-cell activation.

Ipilimumab is a first-in-class human monoclonal antibody against CTLA-4. Ipilimumab inhibits CD80 and CD 86 on antigen-presenting cell forms binding to CTLA-4 on T cells. The blockade of CTLA-4 signaling results in prolonged T-cell activation, proliferation and amplifies immunity.

1. Ipilimumab (Yervoy)
   - **a. FDA-approved indications.** Unresectable or metastatic malignant melanoma.
   - **b. Pharmacology.** Human monoclonal antibody directed against CTLA-4.
     - **i. Mechanism.** Binds to CTLA-4, which blocks the interaction of CTLA-4 with its ligands. This leads to T-cell activation and proliferation.

    c. Toxicity

       i. Common. Pruritus, rash, colitis, diarrhea, nausea, vomiting, injection site reaction, pyrexia, and fatigue.

       ii. Occasional. Hypothyroidism, enterocolitis, hepatotoxicity.

       iii. Rare. Pericarditis, dermatitis, adrenal insufficiency, disorder of endocrine system, hypogonadism, hypopituitarism, perforation of intestine, eosinophilia, hemolytic anemia, myositis, polymyositis, encephalitis, Guillain–Barré syndrome, meningitis, neuropathy, peripheral motor neuropathy, iritis, orbital myositis, uveitis, nephritis, renal failure, and pneumonitis.

    d. Administration

       i. FDA-approved dose. 3 mg/kg intravenously every 21 days for a total of 4 doses. Discontinue treatment if therapy cannot be completed in 16 weeks.

       ii. Dose modification. Moderate immune-mediated reactions require holding therapy until resolution and dosing with prednisone therapy. No dose adjustments required for renal impairment. Dose adjustments are not required for mild hepatic impairment. No data for moderate or severe hepatic impairment.

       iii. Supplied as 5 mg/mL solution.

SUGGESTED READINGS

Arora A, Scholar EM. Role of tyrosine kinase inhibitors in cancer therapy. *J Pharmacol Exp Ther* 2005;315(3):971–979.

Balmer CM, Valley AW, Iannucci A. Cancer treatment and chemotherapy. In: DiPiro JT, Talbert RL, Yee GC, et al, eds. *Pharmacotherapy: A Pathophysiologic Approach*, 6th ed. New York, NY: McGraw-Hill, 2005:2279–2328.

Carmeliet P. VEGF as a key mediator of angiogenesis in cancer. *Oncology* 2005;69 (Suppl 3):4–10.

Ferrara N. VEGF as a therapeutic target in cancer. *Oncology* 2005;69(Suppl 3):11–16.

Finley RS. Overview of targeted therapies for cancer. *Am J Health Syst Pharm* 2003;60(9): S4–S10.

Gollob JA, Wilhelm S, Carter C, et al. Role of Raf kinase in cancer: therapeutic potential of targeting the Raf/MEK/ERK signal transduction pathway. *Semin Oncol* 2006;33:392–406.

Harari PM. Epidermal growth factor receptor inhibition strategies in oncology. *Endocr Relat Cancer* 2004;11:689–708.

Harris M. Monoclonal antibodies as therapeutic agents for cancer. *Lancet Oncol* 2004;5:292–302.

Krause DS, Van Etten RA. Tyrosine kinases as targets for cancer therapy. *N Engl J Med* 2005;353: 172–187.

Mendelsohn J, Baselga J. Epidermal growth factor receptor targeting in cancer. *Semin Oncol* 2006;33(4):369–385.

O'Brien S, Albitar M, Giles FJ. Monoclonal antibodies in the treatment of leukemia. *Curr Mol Med* 2005;5:663–675.

Rotea W, Saad E. Targeted drugs in oncology: new names, new mechanisms, new paradigm. *Am J Health Syst Pharm* 2003;60:1233–1243.

Stern M, Herrmann R. Overview of monoclonal antibodies in cancer therapy: present and promise. *Crit Rev Oncol Hematol* 2005;54:11–29.

The United States Adopted Names (USAN) Council. *Monoclonal Antibodies*. http://www.ama-assn.org/ama/pub/physician-resources/medical-science. Accessed December 12, 2013.

Vlahovic G, Crawford J. Activation of tyrosine kinases in cancer. *Oncologist* 2003;8:531–538.

7 Cancer Immunotherapy

Gerald P. Linette • Beatriz M. Carreno

I. **DEFINITION.** Cancer immunotherapy is based on the principle that a patient's own immune system can be harnessed to reject a malignant tumor. The decade of the 1980s was arguably the beginning of modern human cancer immunotherapy. Prior to the 1980s, astute clinicians reported sporadic cases of cancer regression in patients exposed to infectious pathogens (either deliberately or by natural infection); however, mechanistic insights were minimal and skepticism prevailed. Fundamental discoveries on how the immune system recognizes and eliminates pathogens, a deeper understanding on how the innate and adaptive immune system can be modulated to eliminate neoplastic cells, and the development of humanized monoclonal antibodies provided the necessary foundation to develop rational approaches for cancer immunotherapy.

Multiple modalities of cancer immunotherapy are currently in the clinic or under development, including cytokines (systemic therapy); antibody-based (targeting cell surface molecules in cancer and immune cells), cellular therapies (DC vaccines and T/NK cell therapies), and gene transfer viral vectors (virus-mediated tumor-directed immunity). Collectively, these therapeutic modalities represent a paradigm shift in cancer treatment by targeting the immune system instead of the cancer cell and have coalesced into a burgeoning and credible discipline that offers tremendous potential to solidify its position as the fourth major modality of cancer treatment.

Importantly, the complexity of tumors cannot be overlooked, from the heterogeneity of the cancer genome to its dynamic relationship with the tumor microenvironment. It is now apparent that cancer immunotherapy will require the addition of other modalities (such as targeted agents or cytotoxic drugs) to promote optimal benefit in patients with advanced or metastatic disease. This chapter will focus on human cancer immunotherapy, emphasizing the agents and modalities that will likely be incorporated into the practice of oncology—some are FDA-approved drugs, and others are investigational therapies that have shown considerable activity in clinical trials.

II. **THE IMMUNE SYSTEM**

A. **The innate system.** Innate immunity is the first line of host defense that is activated upon initial encounter with infectious pathogens such as bacteria, fungi, parasites, and viruses. Innate immunity is defined by host pattern recognition receptors (PRR) that bind conserved pathogen-associated molecular pattern (PAMP) domains encoded by infectious pathogens. A variety of PAMP domains have been characterized including lipopolysaccharide, double/single stranded viral nucleic acid as well as β-1,3–linked glucan. Several PRR families have been identified including toll-like receptors (TLRs), NOD-like receptors (NLRs), retinoic acid-inducible gene-1 (RIG-1) receptors, and C-type lectin receptors. The key attribute of the various PRR families is signal transduction to activate the production of proinflammatory cytokines such as IL-1β, IL-12, TNF-α, and type-1 interferon. There are also dedicated "innate" receptors that serve to promote the process of phagocytosis such as the mannose receptors expressed on macrophages. Major cell types of the innate immune system include granulocytes, mast cells, macrophages, dendritic cells (DC), and natural killer (NK) cells. NK cells mediate immediate/short-lived (cytotoxicity or cytokine release) responses and play a critical role in tumor surveillance. DCs play a crucial role as professional antigen-presenting cells (APC) that capture and process antigen to initiate T cell immunity.

B. **The adaptive system.** Three features define adaptive immunity: diversity, specificity, and memory. Major cell types of the adaptive immune system are B lymphocytes that carry out humoral immunity and T lymphocytes that carry out cell-mediated immunity. B and T lymphocytes utilize a process of somatic recombination to generate the highly diverse repertoire of antigen receptors required for recognition of foreign pathogens and neoplastic cells (i.e., antigens). A central tenet of adaptive immunity is the clonal selection theory as proposed by Burnet and Talmage in 1957, which suggested that antigen stimulates specific lymphocyte clones through their antigen receptors, surface immunoglobulin for B lymphocytes, and T cell receptors (TCR) for T lymphocytes, to undergo mitosis, expand, and differentiate into effector cells. After the antigen (pathogen) is cleared, the lymphocytes die by apoptosis and a pool of "memory" lymphocytes survive to protect the host upon antigen re-exposure. Immunologic memory—both humoral and cellular—can last for decades. Antigen specificity is dictated principally by defined regions (CDR3 loops) contained within antibodies and TCRs. Two lineages ($\alpha\beta$ TCR and $\gamma\delta$ TCR) of T cell lymphocytes mediate cellular immunity. $\alpha\beta$ T lymphocytes are further subdivided into two major subsets, the CD4+ (helper) T cells and CD8+ (cytotoxic) T cells. Regulatory T cells often defined by the CD4+CD25+FoxP3+ phenotype infiltrate most tumor sites and are regarded as a significant barrier to effective tumor immunity. Newly characterized cell types that bear rearranged TCRs include invariant type 1 NKT cells, type 2 NKT cells, and mucosal invariant T cells that appear to play a role in the recognition of infectious pathogens; as such, their role in the tumor immune response is less well defined.

III. THERAPEUTIC MODALITIES

A. **Cytokines.** Cytokines are small proteins (5 to 20 kDa) that play an important role in cell-to-cell communication. They stimulate immunity by targeting cells that express the appropriate receptors and are important modulators of innate and adaptive immune responses.

1. **Interferon alpha.** The first biologic cancer therapy produced by recombinant DNA technology in the early 1980s. Interferon Alpha is a member of a family of related proteins made by white blood cells that regulate immune responses and inflammation; in addition, interferon Alpha can also interfere with virus replication and, accordingly, are used to treat certain chronic viral infections. There are two closely related types of interferon Alpha that are approved for use in cancer patients. Interferon Alpha 2a (Roferon-A) is approved for CML, hairy cell leukemia, AIDS-related Kaposi's sarcoma as well as chronic hepatitis C. Interferon Alpha 2b (Intron A) is used as adjuvant treatment of high-risk resected melanoma as well as condylomata acuminata, AIDS-related Kaposi's sarcoma, chronic hepatitis C, and chronic hepatitis B. Both cytokines are available as pegylated versions. Interferon Alpha n3 (Alferon-N, Hemispherx Biopharma) is approved for the treatment of genital and perianal warts caused by human papillomavirus (HPV). Other interferons (such as Interferon Beta and Interferon Gamma) are used for nononcology indications.

2. **Interleukin-2.** An important growth factor/activator of T cells and NK cells, developed in the 1980s, it is indicated for the treatment of renal cell carcinoma and metastatic melanoma. In view of the side effects and potential toxicities, high-dose IL-2 (600,000 to 720,000 IU/Kg/dose intravenously) (Proleukin) should be restricted to use in selected patients and administered in the hospital setting by an experienced oncologist.

3. **Investigational cytokines.** IL-7, IL-12, IL-15, and IL-21 are currently in early to midstage development in oncology primarily as mediators of T lymphocytes activation and homeostasis. Many clinical trials are focused on the use of cytokines in conjunction with cancer vaccines and adoptive T cell/NK cell therapies to enhance antitumor immunity.

B. **Antibody-based therapies.** The landmark development of monoclonal antibodies (mAbs) by Kohler and Milstein in 1975 laid the foundation for the use of antibodies in oncology; however, the full therapeutic potential of these agents remained unfulfilled until the process of antibody humanization was described in the 1980s.

1. **Immune checkpoint blockade.** T cell activation is dependent upon signals delivered through the antigen-specific TCR and accessory receptors. These accessory receptors do not function independently, but serve to enhance or inhibit TCR-mediated signals.

CTLA-4 (cytotoxic T lymphocyte antigen-4) and PD-1 (program death-1) are accessory receptors expressed on activated T cells that act as negative regulators to dampen T cell responses. "Immune Checkpoint Blockade," in general, refers to a therapeutic approach that uses antagonistic CTLA-4- or PD-1/PD-L1-targeted antibodies to increase T cell immunity.

a. **Anti-CTLA-4 (CD152) antibodies**

   i. Ipilimumab (Yervoy) is a humanized mAb (IgG1) that blocks the interaction of CTLA-4 with its ligands, CD80 and CD86 (expressed on immune cells, primarily antigen-presenting cells). This blockade overcomes the T cell inhibitory pathways elicited by CTLA-4 signaling, effectively enhancing T cell proliferation. Ipilimumab is indicated for the treatment of patients with unresectable or metastatic melanoma and was granted regulatory approval in March 2011. Ipilimumab has been shown to prolong overall survival in patients with metastatic melanoma (*N Engl J Med* 2010;363:711).

   A major issue related to the use of ipilimumab is the risk of immune-related adverse events. Treating physicians must be able to recognize, diagnose, and treat potential autoimmune-related toxicities, which are unique and distinct from the common toxicities seen with conventional cytotoxic agents and targeted kinase inhibitors. Immune-related adverse events such as rash, diarrhea, colitis, autoimmune hepatitis, endocrinopathy (hypophysitis), and peripheral neuropathy are frequently observed (*J Clin Oncol* 2012;30:2691). A Risk Evaluation and Mitigation Strategy is an important component of educating both physicians and patients on the immune-mediated adverse reactions unique to ipilimumab (Yervoy) administration in patients.

   ii. Tremelimumab (AstraZeneca) is a humanized mAb (IgG2) directed against CTLA-4 with a mechanism of action similar to ipilimumab. It was tested in a phase 3 randomized clinical trial in metastatic melanoma but failed to demonstrate superior clinical activity compared with dacarbazine (*J Clin Oncol* 2013;31:616). The safety profile of tremelimumab appears to be similar to that of ipilimumab. Clinical trials with this agent for various oncology indications are ongoing.

b. **Anti-PD-1 (CD279)/PD-L1 (CD274) antibodies.** PD-1 is expressed on the surface of activated T cells and when bound by its ligands (PD-L1 and PD-L2) acts to transduce a negative signal to modulate T cell activation after TCR engagement. Among PD-1 ligands, PD-L1 is of particular interest given that it is expressed on the cell surface of various neoplasms, including melanoma, non–small cell lung carcinoma, and renal cell carcinoma. Thus, the PD-1: PD-L1 interaction appears to downregulate T cell function and effectively impairs tumor recognition by activated T cells within the tumor microenvironment. Antagonistic antibodies directed at either PD-1 or PD-L1 are being tested in clinical trials in a wide variety of malignancies and the data from phase 1 and phase 2 clinical trials is very encouraging with response rates ranging from 10-40% in solid tumors (*N Engl J Med 2012; 366: 244, N Engl J Med 2012; 366: 2455, N Engl J Med 2013*; 369: 134). FDA approval for anti-PD-1 mAb (Pembrolizumab) was granted in September 2014 for treatment of patients with advanced or unresectable melanoma after BRAF inhibitor and ipilimumab. Regulatory approval of additional anti-PD-1 (Nivolumab) and anti-PD-L1 (MPDL3280A) mAbs is anticipated in 2015 and beyond. Although immune-related adverse events are seen with anti-PD-1 and anti-PD-L1 mAbs, the rate and severity appear to be lower when compared with that reported for ipilimumab. The combination of ipilimumab with nivolumab is under investigation in patients with metastatic melanoma (*N Engl J Med* 2013;369:122).

   Given the clinical benefit demonstrated by targeting CTLA-4 and PD-1/PD-L1, mAbs directed at other checkpoint molecules (OX-40, GITR, CD137, LAG-3, and TIM-3) are under development for the treatment of multiple malignancies.

2. **Dual-targeting agents.** Dual-targeting agents act, in most instances, as a bridge between distinct cell types promoting immune cell-mediated tumor destruction.

    a. Bispecific antibodies are agents that combine the antigen-recognition sites of two antibodies within a single antibody molecule (150 kDa).

       Catumaxomab (Removab) is a bispecific rat–mouse hybrid mAb directed against CD3, the signaling complex on T lymphocytes, and EpCAM, an epithelial cell surface antigen present on several malignancies. Catumaxomab is indicated for treatment of malignant ascites. Catumaxomab is approved only for use in the EU as of April 2014.

    b. Bispecific T cell Engagers (BiTES) and dual affinity retargeting proteins (DARTS) are ~50 kDa molecular entities that combine the antigen-recognition sites of two antibodies. Most frequently, one of the antigen-recognition sites is directed against CD3, while the other targets a tumor-specific molecule. In BiTES, both recognition sites are presented on a single polypeptide. In DARTS, separate polypeptides linked via disulfide bridges combine to make two antigen-recognition sites.

       i. Blinatumomab (Amgen) is an anti-CD19 × anti-CD3 BiTE in development for Acute Lymphoblastic Leukemia (ALL) and Non-Hodgkin's Lymphoma (NHL)..

       ii. MGD006 (Macrogenics) is an anti-CD123 × anti-CD3 DART in development for AML.

    c. Immune mobilizing mTCR Against Cancer (ImmTACs) are of similar molecular weight to BiTES and DARTS, but these entities combine an antigen-recognition site directed at CD3 and a soluble, high-affinity TCR specific for a tumor (peptide) antigen/MHC complex.

       IMCgp100 (Immunocore) is an anti-CD3 × YLEPGPVTA /HLA-A*02:01-specific TCR in development for melanoma.

C. Cancer vaccines. Broadly speaking, there are two categories of cancer vaccines. Prophylactic cancer vaccines are intended to prevent cancer in high-risk populations, while therapeutic vaccines are designed to treat existing malignancies.

    1. Prophylactic cancer vaccines. There are two indications for which vaccines have been shown to reduce the incidence of viral infections that are associated with cancer: Hepatitis B virus (HBV) and Human Papilloma Virus (HPV). On the basis of a 20-year follow-up, the HBV vaccine has been proven to lower the incidence of hepatocellular carcinoma in children and young adults in Taiwan. Since the HPV vaccine was approved in 2006, additional follow-up is needed before a definitive assessment can be made regarding its impact on the incidence of cervical cancer.

    a. HBV. Hepatitis B is a DNA virus that infects the liver and can cause both acute and chronic disease. It can be transmitted through blood, bodily fluids (intimate contact), and the maternal–fetal route. Most individuals can clear the virus within 6 months; however, approximately 3% of immunocompetent adults become chronic carriers and are at substantial (15% to 25% chance) risk of developing cirrhosis and/or hepatocellular carcinoma. High-risk groups that are more prone to develop chronic HBV infection include newborn infants, children infected before the age of six, and HIV-infected individuals. According to the World Health Organization, there are more than 240 million people worldwide with chronic liver infections. It is estimated that 600,000 people die each year due to HBV. Prevalence rates for HBV infection are highest in sub-Saharan Africa and East Asia (5% to 10% adults chronically infected), moderate in the Amazon, Eastern/Central Europe, Middle East, and lowest in Western Europe and North America (<1%). Mother-to-child transmission at birth is common in highly endemic areas.

       i. HBV vaccine. The HBV subunit vaccine was approved in 1981. The initial formulation used HBV surface antigen (HBsAg) purified and inactivated from the plasma of infected individuals. A recombinant HBsAg derived vaccine was approved in 1986 and remains in current use as the standard formulation. Universal infant vaccination in the United States began in 1991, while adolescent vaccinations began in 1996. Three vaccine doses are typically administered over a 6-month period. In most vaccinated healthy individuals, immunity is lifelong, and booster vaccine doses are not normally suggested.

The current vaccine induces protective antibody levels in >95% of infants, children, and young adults. The rate of protective immunity declines with age (>40 years), concurrent HIV infection, and certain comorbid illnesses such as diabetes and renal failure.

b. HPV. Human Papilloma virus is a DNA sexually transmitted virus that causes genital warts. It is estimated that HPV causes approximately 5% of all cancers in men and 10% in women—most notably anogenital cancers and oropharyngeal carcinoma. Of the more than 100 HPV genotypes, 15 are considered high-risk mucosatropic types associated with cancer. HPV 16 and 18 are considered the most prevalent high-risk types that are associated with cancer, while HPV 6 and 11 are low-risk types often associated with genital warts. HPV 16 and 18 are detected in approximately 70% of all cervical cancer cases worldwide, with the rest associated with the remaining high-risk HPV genotypes.

    i. HPV vaccine. The first HPV subunit vaccine was approved in 2006. There are two formulations in use in the United States. Gardasil quadrivalent formulation contains the yeast-derived major capsid L1 protein of HPV types 6, 11, 16, and 18 emulsified in aluminum hydroxyphosphate sulfate as adjuvant. Cervarix bivalent formulation contains the yeast-derived major capsid L1 protein of HPV types 16 and 18 emulsified in aluminum hydroxide and monophosphoryl lipid A. According to current CDC guidelines, HPV vaccines are recommended for preteen girls and boys starting at age 11 to 12 years. HPV vaccination is highly efficacious in preventing the development of persistent vaccine-type HPV infections and associated intraepithelial neoplasia in both females and males (Nature Reviews. Clin. Oncology 2013;10:400). Interestingly, the quadrivalent HPV vaccine protects against nonvaccine HPV type 31, while the cross-protective efficacy of the bivalent vaccine extends to HPV types 31, 33, 45, and 51.

2. Therapeutic cancer vaccines. Sipuleucel-T (Provenge, Dendreon) is an autologous cellular product indicated for the treatment of asymptomatic or minimally symptomatic metastatic castrate resistant (hormone refractory) prostate cancer and was FDA-approved in 2010. The active components of sipuleucel-T are autologous APCs and the polyprotein PAP-GM-CSF (Prostate acid phosphatase/granulocyte macrophage colony-stimulating agent). Other cell types (T cells, B cells, NK cells) are included in the cell product, which is administered in 250 ml of Lactated Ringer's solution. Sipuleucel-T is administered intravenously in a three-dose schedule at approximately 2-week intervals. Each dose given as a 60-minute infusion contains a minimum of 50 million CD54+ APCs loaded with PAP-GM-CSF protein. Sipuleucel-T increases overall survival by 4 months compared with placebo infusions (25.8 m vs. 21.4 m, p=0.032, HR0.775) (*N Engl J Med* 2010;363:411).

D. Adoptive cell therapies

1. T cell therapies. T cell therapy is currently the focus of intense scientific interest in early stage clinical development. Donor lymphocyte infusions (DLI) are considered in this section despite the fact that most DLI products are not manipulated prior to infusion. Virtually all other T cell products are manipulated by in vitro culture and in many instances genetically modified using viral vectors. T cell retargeting with antigen-receptor gene therapy via viral vectors is the current focus of much of the research.

    a. Donor lymphocyte infusion (DLI). Patients that relapse after an allogeneic bone marrow transplant can be given an infusion of bulk or purified lymphocytes from the donor in order to induce a remission. In relapsed CML after allogeneic transplant, DLI induces long-term remissions in >50% of patients. The potential risks include graft-versus-host disease and bone marrow aplasia.

    b. Tumor infiltrating lymphocytes (TIL). Metastatic deposits of melanoma are infiltrated by a variety of immune-related cells, including T cells that are specific for the tumor. Surgical resection of tumor metastases allows the isolation and subsequent propagation of the T cells in culture for ex vivo expansion in the presence of IL-2. TIL consists of a mixture of CD4+ and CD8+ T lymphocytes; however, in most instances, the fine antigen specificity of TIL remains unknown. A course of high doses of IL-2 (720,000 IU/kg q 8h) is given with infused T cells. Response rates range from 40% to 70%, and 10% to 20% responses can be durable (*Clin Cancer Res* 2011;17:4550).

   c. Chimeric antigen receptor (CAR). Engineered antigen-targeting receptors that are genetically inserted into patient effector T lymphocytes for adoptive transfer. The most common form of antigen-targeting receptors is single-chain variable fragments (scFv) derived from monoclonal antibodies specific for cell surface tumor antigens such as CD19, a molecule expressed on a variety of hematologic malignancies. The scFv is fused to a transmembrane/signaling module that typically encodes either the co-stimulatory CD28 or CD137 domain coupled to the TCR signaling (CD3ζ) domain. CAR T cell adoptive therapy directed against CD19 is especially promising with early phase 1 results from multiple centers documenting response rates >50% in adult Chronic Lymphoblastic Leukemia (CLL)/ALL and pediatric ALL. Durable complete remissions beyond 3 years have been reported in adult CLL patients given a single T cell infusion.

   d. TCR gene therapy. Engineered TCR are genetically inserted into patient effector T lymphocytes for adoptive cell transfer. In principle, the TCR are modified to create higher affinity receptors to recognize the antigenic peptide-MHC complex present on tumor cells. Pilot human trials with the NY-ESO-1 specific TCR show activity with regression of synovial sarcoma and multiple myeloma.

   e. Polyclonal T cell lines. Antigen-specific T cells (either CD4+ or CD8+) clones or polyclonal cell lines expanded ex vivo have been adoptively transferred to patients with cancer, typically melanoma. Response rates have been <20%, and poor T cell persistence has been the biggest obstacle to date.

      Current protocols for T cell therapy, particularly those described in Sections III.D.1.b to III.D.1.d, involve a conditioning regimen for the patient prior to adoptive T cell transfer. This conditioning consists of nonmyeloablative chemotherapy (i.e., cyclophosphamide ± fludarabine and in certain instances, total body irradiation with stem cell support) several days prior to the T cell infusion. The current thinking is that ablation of lymphocytes and myeloid cells results in increased availability of "space" and homeostatic cytokines (IL-7, IL-15) to support expansion of the infused T cells.

  2. NK cell therapy. NK cells are large granular lymphocytes, phenotypically characterized as CD3 (TCR)- CD56+. NK cells exhibit natural cytotoxicity to tumors, and low cytotoxicity has been associated with increased cancer risk. NK cell recognition of tumors is complex and involves activating and inhibitory invariant receptors. Clinical studies using autologous and allogeneic NK cells have aimed to promote NK activity by modulating inhibitory and activating signals. The most promising disease indications for NK cell therapies are the hematological malignancies, especially in high-risk/relapsed AML after allogeneic transplantation. In this indication, adoptive transfer of allogeneic (mismatched inhibitory receptors) NK cells enhances cytotoxicity directed at tumors and the ability to control AML relapse.

E. Oncolytic viral therapies. These therapies are based on the use of viruses that either have tropism or can selectively replicate in tumors. Several viral platforms (herpes simplex type-1, vaccinia, and reovirus) are under development, and these viruses can be modified to promote tumor cell death, improve susceptibility to radiation and chemotherapy, or generate host antitumor immune responses. None of these therapies are FDA-approved at this time, and only those agents with the most promising clinical results are mentioned here.

  1. Pexa-Vec (JX-594) consists of a vaccinia-virus backbone expressing GM-CSF and is designed to induce virus-replication–dependent tumor death as well as promote tumor immunity. The therapy has been delivered intratumorally and intravenously, and it is currently undergoing phase II trials in advanced hepatocellular carcinoma.

2. Talimogene laherparepvec (T-VEC) consists of a modified herpes simplex virus type-1 vector backbone expressing GM-CSF and is designed to induce virus-replication–dependent tumor death as well as elicit antitumor immunity. In a randomized phase III trial in melanoma, intratumoral delivery of T-VEC has shown a durable response rate of 16.3% versus 2.1% with the control GM-CSF.

IV. **IMMUNE-RELATED RESPONSE CRITERIA.** Until recently, most oncology protocols required treatment discontinuation if there was any evidence of disease progression. During clinical development of ipilimumab, four distinct response patterns were noted: (a) shrinkage in baseline lesions without new lesions; (b) durable stable disease followed by a slow, steady decline in total tumor burden; (c) response after an increase in total tumor burden; and (d) response in the presence of new lesions. Each pattern of response was associated with a prolonged survival. It was found that 9.7% of treated patients (n=227) with ipilimumab had disease progression at the week 12 assessments; however, at later time points they were found to have a radiographic response associated with patterns (c) and (d) (*Clin Cancer Res* 2009;15:7412). Given this type of "unconventional" responses observed, a new set of "Immune-related Response Criteria" incorporating the appearance of new measurable (and nonmeasurable) lesions with increased tumor burden has been proposed as more reliable response assessment criteria for use with immunotherapy clinical development programs. Investigators postulate that the apparent increased tumor burden reflects a brisk immune cell infiltration with edema into the tumor site as well as a transient increase in tumor volume prior to the development of a sufficient immune response that can lag temporally and take weeks to months after completion of ipilimumab treatment. For patients with modest disease progression and stable (ECOG 0-1) performance status after a course of ipilimumab, it is our practice to observe (no further therapy) and repeat imaging in 6 to 8 weeks to determine whether response pattern (c) or (d) is evident.

SUGGESTED READINGS

Barrett DM, Singh N, Porter DL, et al. Chimeric antigen receptor therapy for cancer. *Ann Rev Med* 2014;65:333–347.

Brahmer JR, Tykodi SS, Chow LQ, et al. Safety and activity of anti-PD-L1 antibody in patients with advanced cancer. *N Engl J Med* 2012;366:2455–2465.

Hamid O, Robert C, Daud A, et al. Safety and tumor responses with lambrolizumab (anti-PD-1) in melanoma. *N Engl J Med* 2013;369:134–144.

Hodi FS, O'Day SJ, McDermott DF. Improved survival with ipilimumab in patients with metastatic melanoma. *N Engl J Med* 2010;363:711–723.

Kantoff PW, Higano CS, Shore ND, et al. Sipuleucel-T immunotherapy for castration-resistant prostate cancer. *N Engl J Med* 2010;363:411–422.

Mellman I, Coukos G, Dranoff G. Cancer immunotherapy comes of age. *Nature* 2011;480:480–489.

Page DB, Postow MA, Callahan MK, Allison JP, Wolchok JD. Immune modulation in cancer with antibodies. *Ann Rev Med* 2014;65:185–202.

Ribas A, Kefford R, Marshall MA, et al. Phase III randomized clinical trial comparing tremelimumab with standard-of-care chemotherapy in patients with advanced melanoma. *J Clin Oncol* 2013;31:616–622.

Robert C, Thomas L, Bondarenko I, et al. Ipilimumab plus dacarbazine for previously untreated metastatic melanoma. *N Engl J Med* 2011;364:2517–2526.

Rosenberg SA, Yang JC, Sherry RM, et al. Durable complete responses in heavily pretreated patients with metastatic melanoma using T-cell transfer immunotherapy. *Clin Cancer Res* 2011;17:4550–4557.

Topalian SL, Hodi FS, Brahmer JR, et al. Safety, activity, and immune correlates of anti-PD-1 antibody in cancer. *N Engl J Med* 2012;366:2443–2454.

Weber JS, Kahler KC, Hauschild A. Management of immune-related adverse events and kinetics of response with ipilimumab. *J Clin Oncol* 2012;30:2691–2697.

Wolchok JD, Hoos A, O'Day S, et al. Guidelines for the evaluation of immune therapy activity in solid tumors: immune-related response criteria. *Clin Cancer Res* 2009;15:7412–7420.

Principles of Hematopoietic Cell Transplantation

Jesse Keller • Rizwan Romee

I. **INTRODUCTION.** Hematopoietic cell transplantation (HCT) involves the administration of dose-intense chemotherapy and/or radiation followed by the infusion of either autologous or allogeneic (donor-derived) hematopoietic cells. The number of hematopoietic cell transplants performed each year has been steadily increasing for both benign and malignant hematologic conditions. This chapter summarizes the underlying principles and clinical aspects of both autologous and allogeneic HCT.

II. **TYPES OF TRANSPLANTS.** Hematopoietic cell transplants are classified by the source of donor cells as (a) autologous, (b) syngeneic, and (c) allogeneic.

  A. **Autologous transplantation.** In an autologous transplant, a patient's hematopoietic cells are harvested and cryopreserved. Autologous hematopoietic cells, including hematopoietic stem cells (HSCs), are then reinfused after administration of high-dose chemotherapy and/or radiation therapy. Autologous transplantation (auto-HCT) allows the delivery of high doses of drugs to maximize efficacy in situations where myelosuppression would otherwise be dose-limiting.

  B. **Syngeneic transplantation.** Transplantation from an identical twin is similar to an autologous transplant with the benefit of providing a "clean" graft of hematopoietic cells that are free of contaminating malignant cells. The advantage of using syngeneic over auto-HCT, however, has never been demonstrated in a large clinical trial. Syngeneic HCT is not associated with either the graft-versus-host or graft-versus-tumor (GvT) effect of an allogeneic transplant and does not require posttransplant immunosuppression. Even when available, syngeneic transplant is rarely done owing to the lack of GvT effect, a key component in preventing disease relapse.

  C. **Allogeneic transplantation.** Allogeneic hematopoietic cell transplantation (allo-HCT) involves the infusion of hematopoietic cells including HSCs from a human leukocyte antigens (HLA) matched or mismatched donor. Allo-HCT can be performed either from a related family member or an unrelated donor. In addition to permitting myeloablative doses of chemotherapy and/or radiation therapy to be administered, an allo-HCT allows for potent immunologic effects mediated by donor lymphocytes (predominantly by T cells and NK cells). This effect is known as the GvT or the graft-versus-leukemia (GvL) effect. Allo-HCT has efficacy in the treatment of malignant and nonmalignant disorders, including congenital immune deficiencies, sickle-cell anemia, thalassemia, and some inborn errors of metabolism. The possible donor choices in allo-HCT are HLA-matched sibling donors, HLA-matched or HLA-mismatched unrelated donors, related HLA-haploidentical donors, and cord blood.

    1. **Matched sibling donors.** For those requiring allo-HCT, use of a matched sibling is still considered an ideal graft source when available. An allo-HCT from an HLA-matching sibling donor is associated with the best survival rates and with less morbidity, including lower rates of acute and chronic GVHD. However, the availability of an appropriate donor is a concern, as roughly 70% of patients do not have a suitable HLA-matched sibling.

    2. **Matched unrelated donors (MUD).** The majority of patients who do not have access to a matched sibling are eligible for an MUD. Donor searches, however, are costly and time-consuming. Notably, availability of appropriate donors for minority populations is limited. Currently, less than 25% of African American patients are able to find an appropriate HLA-matched donor.

3. **Mismatched related donors.** In some cases, transplantation may be performed with related donors mismatched at one or two HLA loci. Drawbacks to this approach include increased risks of GVHD and graft failure.

4. **Related haploidentical donors.** Related HLA-haploidentical donors are mismatched at three of the six possible loci (HLA-A, HLA-B, and HLA-DR) for which HLA typing is performed (in reality, they are mismatched for an entire maternal- or paternal-derived HLA haplotype, but the related family donors are typically tested only for the above-mentioned HLA loci). This is an expanding area of transplantation with emerging data supporting that outcomes may be equivalent to patients receiving an HLA-matched unrelated donor and possibly even HLA-matched sibling donor transplantation. Donor availability is simplified and expedited as usually multiple eligible donors can be found within a family.

III. PATIENT SELECTION

A. **Indications for transplantation.** HCT has been successfully used in the treatment of a number of malignant and nonmalignant conditions (Table 8-1). The choice of autologous-versus-allogeneic transplantation largely depends on the disease being treated and the availability of a compatible donor. Currently, multiple myeloma and lymphomas are the most frequent indications for autologous transplants, whereas acute leukemia and myelodysplastic syndromes are the most frequent indications for allo-HCT. Guidelines for transplant referrals in adult patients have been published by the American Society for Blood and Marrow Transplantation (ASBMT) (Table 8-2).

B. **Pretransplant evaluation of candidates for hematopoietic cell transplantation.** Pretransplant evaluation of patients considered for HCT is required to identify candidates with comorbid conditions that may preclude the administration of high-dose therapy with their associated toxicity. Although the risk of transplant-related complications increases with advancing age, age alone is no longer considered an absolute contraindication, but rather one of many factors affecting the overall suitability of a patient for HCT. Guidelines for pretransplant evaluations are listed in Table 8-3.

IV. DONOR SELECTION

A. **HLA typing.** For allo-HCT, donors are selected on the basis of their histocompatibility with the recipient. The major histocompatibility complex (MHC) locus, also called HLA locus, on chromosome 6 encodes class I and class II HLA antigens that allow for the immune recognition of foreign antigens. In hematopoietic and solid organ

---

TABLE 8-1	Diseases Treatable with HCT

Autologous transplantation
Multiple myeloma
Hodgkin's and non-Hodgkin's lymphoma
Acute promyelocytic leukemia
Neuroblastoma
Germ cell tumors

Allogeneic transplantation
Acute and chronic myeloid leukemia
Acute and chronic lymphocytic leukemia
Myelodysplastic and myeloproliferative syndromes
Hodgkin's and non-Hodgkin's lymphoma
Multiple myeloma
Aplastic anemia and other bone marrow failure disorders
Hemoglobinopathies: thalassemia major and sickle-cell anemia
Immunodeficiency syndromes: severe combined immunodeficiency, Wiskott–Aldrich
Inborn errors of metabolism: Hurler's syndrome, adrenoleukodystrophy

TABLE 8-2	Recommended Timing for Transplant Consultation

AML

High-risk AML

Antecedent hematologic disease
(e.g., myelodysplasia)

Treatment-related leukemia

Induction failure

Presence of minimal residual disease after
initial or subsequent therapy

CR1 (except favorable risk cytogenetics)

CR2 and beyond

ALL

CR1 with high-risk features

Primary induction failure or relapse

Presence of minimal residual disease after
initial or subsequent therapy

CR2 and beyond, if not previously evaluated

MDS

Any intermediate or high IPSS score

Any MDS with poor prognostic features,
including:

Treatment-related MDS

Refractory cytopenias

Adverse cytogenetics

Transfusion dependence

CML

Inadequate hematologic or cytogenetic
response after tyrosine kinase inhibitor
(TKI) treatment including the second
generation TKIs

Disease progression

Accelerated phase

Intolerance and or resistance to the currently
available TKI

Blast crisis (myeloid or lymphoid)

Chronic Lymphocytic Leukemia (CLL)

High-risk cytogenetics or molecular features

Short initial remission

Poor initial response

Resistant/refractory

Richter's transformation

Non-Hodgkin's lymphomas

Follicular

Poor response to initial treatment

Initial remission duration <12 mo

First relapse

Transformation to diffuse large B cell lymphoma

Diffuse large B cell

At first or subsequent relapse

CR1 for patients with high or high-
intermediate IPI risk

No CR with initial treatment

Second or subsequent remission

Mantle cell

Following initial therapy

Hodgkin's lymphoma

No initial CR

First or subsequent relapse

Multiple myeloma

After initiation of therapy

At first progression

AML, acute myelogenous leukemia; ALL, acute lymphoblastic leukemia; WBC, white blood corpuscles; CNS, central nervous system; CR, complete remission; MDS, myelodysplastic syndromes; IPSS, International Prognostic Scoring System; CML, chronic myelogenous leukemia; IPI, International Prognostic Index.

transplantation, HLA molecules function as alloantigens that can trigger immune recognition and graft rejection in mismatched recipients.

1. **HLA alleles.** HLA antigens are defined serologically by testing for reactivity against a panel of monoclonal antibodies. DNA-based testing has largely replaced serologic testing and utilizes sequence-specific DNA primers and probes to define HLA alleles. High-resolution molecular typing of 10 HLA genes (HLA-A, HLA-B, HLA-C, HLA-DRB1, and HLA-DQB1) is the current standard. High-resolution molecular typing permits precise HLA matching between donors and transplant patients, which has resulted in improved patient outcomes. Because the MHC complex is tightly clustered on chromosome 6, HLA alleles are inherited as a set also referred to as the patient's *haplotype*. The chance of any individual sibling being HLA-matched is 25%, whereas the probability of having a fully HLA-matched sibling donor is $1-(3/4)^n$, where n is the number of full siblings.

2. **HLA matching of unrelated donor transplants.** In individuals who do not have an HLA-identical sibling, selection of an unrelated donor is required. Typing of HLA-A,

TABLE 8-3	Pretransplant Evaluation

Test	Comment
History and physical examination	Assess: performance status, active infection, significant organ system dysfunction
Review of tissue samples	Confirmation of diagnosis
Review of initial staging and restaging tests	Assess responsiveness to therapy and current disease status
Bone marrow biopsy/aspirate	
Confirmatory donor and recipient HLA and ABO and Rh blood typing (allogeneic HSCT candidates)	
Serum chemistry panel (electrolytes, creatinine, bilirubin, AST, ALT, alkaline phosphatase, LDH)	Creatinine >2 may result in altered metabolism of drugs commonly used in HSCT (certain antibiotics, methotrexate); AST, ALT, bilirubin >2 times normal increases the risk of veno-occlusive disease
Radioventriculogram or echocardiogram	LVEF >40%–45% desirable
ECG	Evaluate for underlying cardiovascular disease
Chest radiograph	Evaluate for underlying pulmonary disease or infection
Pulmonary function tests	FEV_1, FVC, DLCO >50% predicted
Viral serologies (CMV, HSV, HIV, HTLV-I, hepatitis A, hepatitis B core antigen and surface antibody, and hepatitis C)	HSV seropositivity requires antiviral prophylaxis; hepatitis seropositivity without evidence of active disease increases the risk of veno-occlusive disease, but is not a contraindication to HSCT
Radiation oncology evaluation	TBI conditioning regimen candidates
Nutrition evaluation	
Pregnancy test (premenopausal women)	
Sperm/oocyte banking	

HLA, human leukocyte antigen; HSCT, hematopoietic stem cell transplant; AST, aspartate aminotransferase; ALT, alanine aminotransferase; LDH, lactate dehydrogenase; LVEF, left ventricular ejection fraction; ECG, electrocardiogram; FEV_1, forced expiratory volume in the first second; FVC, forced vital capacity; DLCO, carbon dioxide diffusion in the lung; CMV, cytomegalovirus; HSV, herpes simplex virus; HIV, human immunodeficiency virus; HTLV-I, human T-cell lymphoma virus type 1; TBI, total body irradiation.

-B, -C, -DR (DRB1), and DQB1 is routinely used to select unrelated donors. In addition, other class II loci HLA-DPB1 and -DRB3/4/5 are often tested although there is no definite association with the patient outcomes. In the United States, unrelated donor transplant searches are coordinated by the National Marrow Donor Program (NMDP). The likelihood of finding an unrelated donor for a given patient depends upon the frequency of the patient's HLA haplotype in the general population. For all patients, the likelihood of finding a potential unrelated marrow or peripheral blood stem cells (PBSC) donor in the donor registries is largely tied to race. In the United States, Caucasians are much more likely to find a match than African Americans or Asian Americans.

3. **HLA matching of haploidentical donor transplants.** Haploidentical donors are matched at 3 of 6 loci (HLA-A, HLA-B, and HLA-DR). The likelihood of finding a successful haploidentical relative is significantly higher than that of finding a successful MUD match. Additionally, the time and expense of a donor search may be spared when seeking a haploidentical donor.

B. **Non-HLA factors.** Other factors are often considered when donors are selected, including cytomegalovirus (CMV)—negative serology (for patients with CMV-negative serology), male sex, younger age, ABO compatibility, larger body weight, and matched race. Multiparous female donors are associated with a higher risk of chronic graft-versus-host disease (cGVHD), but with no effect on overall survival.

V. SOURCES OF HEMATOPOIETIC STEM CELLS

A. **Bone marrow.** Historically, bone marrow was used as the sole graft source in transplantation. Bone marrow is collected from the posterior iliac crest by performing repeated aspirations while the donor is under general or regional anesthesia. The volume collected varies, but generally ranges from 10 to 15 mL/kg of donor weight. Improved survival has been correlated with higher transplanted HSC dose with more robust engraftment and fewer infectious complications. A total nucleated cell (TNC) dose of approximately 2×10^8 cells/kg in the harvested bone marrow product is considered adequate for HCT. Side effects of marrow collection include fatigue and pain at the collection site and effects related to general anesthesia such as nausea and vomiting.

B. **Peripheral blood as a graft source.** HSCs normally circulate in low levels in the peripheral circulation, but can be recruited into the peripheral blood from the marrow in response to stressors such as inflammation or infection. In addition, the exogenous administration of hematopoietic growth factors can increase the numbers of peripheral blood stem cells by 40- to 80-fold in a process termed *stem cell mobilization*. These mobilized HSCs along with other mononuclear cells can then be harvested and used for HCT. Currently, the majority of autologous and allogeneic transplants are performed using peripheral blood as a graft source.

1. **Stem cell mobilization.** Although a number of cytokines and cytokine combinations can mobilize HSCs, the FDA-approved medications for stem cell mobilization include granulocyte-stimulating factor (G-CSF) (filgrastim, 10 to 16 µg/kg), granulocyte-macrophage colony-stimulating factor (GM-CSF) (sargramostim), and plerixafor. Donors may experience myalgia, bone pain, headache, nausea, and low-grade fevers with G-CSF. Splenic rupture due to extramedullary hematopoiesis has been reported as a rare complication.

   HSCs also increase in the peripheral circulation during neutrophil recovery after the administration of chemotherapy. For autologous stem cell collection, high-dose cyclophosphamide or other forms of chemotherapy may be used to mobilize HSCs, and this can be augmented with the administration of G-CSF or GM-CSF to increase the stem cell yield.

   Plerixafor is a CXCR4 antagonist used for the mobilization of stem cells. CXCR4 is a receptor for the chemokine CXCL12 (stromal-derived factor-1 [SDF-1]) produced by marrow stromal cells and is critical for the homing and retention of HSCs in the marrow. By disrupting the CXCR4/CXCL12 axis, plerixafor has been shown to be effective for the mobilization of stem cells either alone or in combination with G-CSF. Plerixafor is FDA-approved for use in combination with G-CSF for HSC mobilization for patients with a diagnosis of non-Hodgkin's lymphoma (NHL) or multiple myeloma (MM) undergoing autologous transplantation.

2. **HSC harvesting from peripheral blood.** Following mobilization, HSCs are collected by large volume apheresis (up to 20 liters) through the antecubital veins or a central venous catheter. The mononuclear fraction containing the HSCs along with other mononuclear cells like lymphocytes and monocytes is retained, and the remainder is reinfused into the patient. Hypocalcemia from the anticoagulation with acid-citrate-dextrose solution used during apheresis may cause perioral numbness, paresthesias, and carpopedal spasm and is treated with calcium supplementation. A minimum of 2×10^6 CD34$^+$/kg recipient weight is required for an autologous transplant, whereas a goal of 5×10^6 CD34$^+$/kg increases the probability of early platelet recovery. Similarly ideal dose of CD34$^+$ collected for allo-HCT is around 5×10^6/kg recipient weight but doses $\geq 3 \times 10^6$/kg are considered sufficient, especially in the absence of donor–recipient

HLA mismatch. Most normal donors require only a single apheresis session to collect adequate numbers of stem cells, while autologous donors may require multiple (five or more) sessions, depending on their degree of exposure to previous chemotherapy.

Compared with marrow, PBSC contain higher numbers of CD34$^+$ cells than bone marrow and are associated with faster neutrophil and platelet recovery. In addition, PBSC grafts have approximately 10 times as many T lymphocytes, which are associated with higher rates of cGVHD but without an effect on overall survival. Aplastic anemia is an exception to the expanding use of peripheral blood as a graft source, as for these patients, bone marrow is the preferred graft source and has been associated with better outcomes.

C. **Umbilical cord blood.** Blood present in the umbilical cord and placenta following childbirth is a rich source of HSCs. After delivery of the placenta, the umbilical cord is clamped, and approximately 50 to 100 mL remaining in the placenta and umbilical cord is drained and cryopreserved. Cord blood typically contains about a 10- to 20-fold smaller dose of nucleated and CD34$^+$ cells than an adult bone marrow. Because of the limitations in stem cell dose, cord blood transplants have been primarily performed in pediatric populations with a minimum of 2.0×10^7 mononuclear cells/kg typically required for successful transplantation and greater than 3.0×10^7 mononuclear cells/kg for optimal results. In the adult population, typically two cord blood units (double cord allo-HCT) are pooled for a single recipient, which can result in a more rapid hematopoietic recovery. Of interest, in double cord allo-HCT, only one of the two cord blood units dominates hematopoiesis over the long term.

Cord blood transplants are associated with lower of risks of GVHD and can be performed successfully with a greater degree of HLA mismatch than adult stem cell sources. In addition, cord blood units are more readily available than stem cells from adult donors and are associated with lower rates of viral transmission. Cord blood registries, unlike adult donor registries, do not suffer from loss to the donor pool due to advancing age or difficulties in locating potential donors. Major problems with cord blood transplantation include delayed engraftment, higher risk of posttransplant infections, mildly increased rates of graft failure, and the inability to collect additional donor cells for patients with graft failure and/or relapse.

VI. CONDITIONING REGIMENS

A. **Myeloablative conditioning.** Traditional conditioning regimens used in HCT use myeloablative doses of alkylating agents (cyclophosphamide, busulfan, melphalan) with or without total body irradiation (TBI) before transplant to (a) eliminate residual disease and to (b) suppress immune function to allow engraftment of donor stem cells. Standard conditioning regimens vary by disease with commonly used regimens listed in Table 8-4. In addition to severe myelosuppression, agents used in HCT are typically associated with side effects such as mucositis, alopecia, nausea, and may cause significant organ damage including hepatic or pulmonary dysfunction.

B. **Reduced intensity conditioning.** In the allogeneic setting, nonmyeloablative or reduced intensity conditioning (RIC) regimens were designed to reduce the toxicity associated with high-dose therapy. These regimens do not attempt to completely eliminate malignant cells before transplant, but instead provide enough immunosuppression to allow donor engraftment and rely predominantly upon a GvT effect mediated by the donor-derived T cells to achieve their therapeutic goal. Some of the commonly used RIC regimens are listed in Table 8-5.

RIC regimens allow the elderly and patients with significant comorbid conditions to be eligible for allo-HCT. In retrospective analyses conducted in myeloid malignancies, RIC regimens are associated with lower treatment-related mortality but with higher relapse rates and no change in overall survival. Rates of acute and cGVHD after RIC are comparable to those observed in standard high-dose transplants, but the onset of acute GVHD (aGVHD) is often delayed by weeks to months. In view of the increased risk of relapse, these regimens are best suited to patients who are otherwise in complete remission at the time of transplant.

TABLE 8-4	Common Myeloablative Conditioning Regimens

Regimen	Total dose	Daily dose
		Allogeneic regimens
Cy/TBI		
TBI	1,225 cGy	175 cGy b.i.d. d−6/−5/−4, 175 cGy d−3
Cyclophosphamide	120 mg/kg	60 mg/kg/d i.v. × 2, d−3/−2
MESNA	120 mg/kg	60 mg/kg CIVI over 24 h × 2, d−3/−2
Bu/Cy		
Busulfan	16 mg/kg	1 mg/kg p.o. q6h, d−7/−6/−5/−4
Cyclophosphamide	120 mg/kg	60 mg/kg/d i.v. × 2, d−3/−2
MESNA	120 mg/kg	60 mg/kg CIVI over 24 h × 2, d−3/−2
		Autologous regimens
Multiple myeloma		
Mel-200		
Melphalan	200 mg/m^2	100 mg/m^2 i.v. × 2, d−3/−2
Lymphoma		
BEAM		
BCNU	450 mg/m^2	450 mg/m^2, d, d−8
Etoposide	800 mg/m^2	100 mg/m^2 i.v. b.i.d. × 4, d−7/−6/−5/−4
Ara-C	800 mg/m^2	100 mg/m^2 i.v. b.i.d. × 4, d−7/−6/−5/−4
Melphalan	140 mg/m^2	140 mg/m^2, d−3
Solid tumors		
MEC		
Etoposide	1,200 mg/m^2	300 mg/m^2 × 4, d−6/−5/−4/−3
Carboplatinum	1,400 mg/m^2	700 mg/m^2 × 2, d−4/−3
Melphalan	140 mg/m^2	140 mg/m^2, d−2

TBI, total body irradiation; MESNA, [sodium-2]-mercaptoethane sulfonate; VP, vincristine/prednisone; CIVI, continuous intravenous infusion; BCNU, 1,3- bis-(2-chloroethyl)- 1-nitrosourea; Ara-C, acytosine arabinose.

TABLE 8-5	Common Reduced Intensity and Nonmyeloablative Conditioning Regimens

Regimen	Total dose	Daily dose
Cyclophosphamide	120 mg/kg	60 mg/kg/d × 2, d−7/−6
Fludarabine	125 mg/m^2	25 mg/m^2 × 5, d−5/−4/−3/−2/−1
MESNA	120 mg/kg	60 mg/kg CIVI over 24 h × 2, d−4/−3
Cyclophosphamide	200 mg/kg	50 mg/kg/d × 4, d−6/−5/−4/−3
Thymic RT	700 cGy	d−1
ATG	45–90 mg/kg	15–30 mg/kg × 3, d−2/−1/ + 1
MESNA	200 mg/kg	50 mg/kg CIVI over 24 h × 4, d−6/−5/−4/−3
Flu/Bu ± ATG		
Busulfan (oral)	8 mg/kg	4 mg/kg/d × 2, d−6/−5
Fludarabine	150 mg/m^2	30 mg/m^2/d × 5, d−10/−9/−8/−7/−6/−5
ATG	40 mg/kg	10 mg/kg/d × 4, d−4/−3/−2/−1

RT, reverse transcription; ATG, antithymocyte globulin.

VII. HEMATOPOIETIC CELL GRAFT INFUSIONS. Cells collected for autologous transplant are cryopreserved in the liquid or vapor phase of liquid nitrogen with 10% dimethyl sulfoxide (DMSO) used as a cryoprotectant. Before reinfusion of the cells, a bicarbonate infusion is used to alkalinize the urine to protect against renal injury caused by the hemolysis of contaminating red cells. Stem cells products are rapidly thawed at 37-degree water bath and typically infused over a 15-minute period as longer infusion times potentially subject the HSCs to DMSO toxicity. Side effects associated with DMSO include flushing, unpleasant taste, nausea, and vomiting with rare hypotension, atrial arrhythmias, and anaphylactic reactions. Allogeneic grafts are usually infused fresh, with patients monitored for any hypersensitivity reactions. Large volume bone marrow products should be infused over the period of 3 to 4 hours and the patient monitored for fluid overload. Also, the grafts for allo-HCT typically undergo RBC reduction in case of major ABO donor–recipient blood group mismatch prior to the cell infusion.

VIII. POSTTRANSPLANT CARE AND COMPLICATIONS

A. Hematopoietic

1. **Engraftment.** Following stem cell infusion, progenitor cells home to the marrow microenvironment, guided by interactions between adhesion molecules and their receptors expressed on hematopoietic cells and the marrow stroma. These cells must then proliferate and differentiate to repopulate the peripheral blood with mature blood cells in a process termed engraftment. Neutrophil engraftment (ANC greater than 500/mm^3) typically occurs between 10 and 15 days' posttransplant with PBSC transplants and slightly later in bone marrow transplants. The administration of colony-stimulating factors, either G-CSF or GM-CSF, posttransplant has been demonstrated to lessen the duration of neutropenia, though without improving survival. Platelet recovery tends to be much more variable posttransplant.

   Donor/recipient chimerism is evaluated post-HCT by analyzing either peripheral blood or bone marrow for differences in donor- and recipient-specific Short Tandem Repeats (STRs) using polymerase chain reaction (PCR)-based assays. In the case of sex-mismatched transplantation, chimerism can also be analyzed by the ratio of sex chromosome–specific fluorescence in situ hybridization (FISH) probes.

2. **Transfusion support.** Transfusions of red blood cells and platelets are common in HCT. Although transfusion parameters are somewhat arbitrary, it is reasonable to maintain hemoglobin levels greater than 8 g/dL and platelet counts greater than 10,000/mm^3. To reduce the risk of transfusion-associated GVHD, all blood products should be irradiated with 2,500 cGy before administration.

3. **ABO incompatibility.** Because stem cell products are matched on the basis of HLA compatibility, ABO-incompatible HSCTs frequently occur. Red cell incompatibility is classified according to whether donor isoagglutinins, isoantigens, or both are incompatible with those of the recipient. Major incompatibility occurs when the recipient has antibodies directed against donor red blood cell antigens (e.g., A donor, O recipient); minor incompatibility occurs when donor plasma contains antibodies directed against patient red cells (e.g., O donor, A recipient). Mixed or bidirectional incompatibility occurs when there is both major and minor ABO incompatibility (e.g., A donor, B recipient, or vice versa). Red cells are typically reduced from the harvested grafts in major incompatible allo-HCT, especially when using bone marrow as the graft source to reduce the risk of clinically significant hemolysis of large quantities of red cells contained in the cell product. Immune-mediated hemolysis is indicated by a positive direct antiglobulin test (direct Coombs) in the setting of other markers of hemolysis such as an elevated lactate dehydrogenase (LDH) or indirect bilirubin. In cases of mild hemolysis, RBC transfusion support is adequate. In more severe cases, plasma exchange may be used. In contrast, patients receiving minor incompatible transplants have a risk of immediate hemolysis from the infusion of incompatible plasma. Immediate hemolysis can be prevented by removal of plasma from the bone marrow grafts by centrifugation. In transplants using peripheral blood mononuclear cells, apheresis used to collect the cells product effectively removes most of the donor plasma, and there is significantly less contamination with RBCs.

4. **Graft failure.** Rejection of the donor hematopoietic cells by the immune system of the recipient is termed *graft failure* and may be classified as primary (ANC $<500/mm^3$ after 28 days posttransplant, although various definitions exist) or secondary (transient donor hematopoiesis). Causes of graft failure include HLA disparity at major and minor loci, inadequate conditioning of the host, inadequate number of donor stem cells, T cell depletion of the donor graft, inadequate immunosuppression, and presence of high titers of donor-specific antibodies (DSAs) caused by allo-sensitization to donor HLA antigens by blood transfusions, especially platelet products and multiple pregnancies before transplantation. Therapeutic options include more intensive immunosuppression, the administration of hematopoietic growth factors, donor lymphocyte infusions (DLIs), and even a second HCT.

B. **Acute graft-versus-host disease (aGVHD)**

1. **Pathogenesis.** aGVHD is caused by allo-reactive donor T cells that recognize recipient antigens as foreign, resulting in inflammatory disease affecting multiple organs. Cytokine storm in the early posttransplant period caused by either the conditioning regimen and/or infection is thought to further activate donor-derived lymphocytes, exacerbating the aGVHD-associated inflammation. Further, recipient antigen presenting cells (APCs), especially the dendritic cells, are thought to play an important role in initiating acute inflammatory cascade associated with aGVHD. aGVHD can be particularly severe in the setting of a major MHC class mismatch, but also occurs because of disparities in minor histocompatibility antigens.

2. **Clinical manifestations.** aGVHD typically manifests itself after the first 25 to 28 days after transplantation, and most commonly involves skin, liver, and gut, the three largest organs in our body. The skin manifestation of aGVHD varies from a mild maculopapular rash to overt sloughing. Liver involvement is commonly seen with a conjugated hyperbilirubinemia and elevation of the alkaline phosphatase as the biliary ductules are the first targeted components in the liver. Lower gastrointestinal (GI) involvement typically presents as diarrhea and abdominal cramping, while upper GI involvement usually presents as nausea and vomiting.

Although several scoring systems are used to grade GVHD, most are based on the original Glucksberg criteria, with those having stage III and IV disease having a significantly poorer outcome (Table 8-6). Rates of grade III–IV aGVHD vary by study and donor source. Large studies have shown cumulative rates of aGVHD through 40 months of 39% and 49% respectively for sibling-allogeneic and unrelated donor transplants. For haploidentical transplantation using posttransplant cyclophosphamide, rates of grade III–IV aGVHD have ranged from 5% to 11%.

3. **GVHD prophylaxis**

a. **Pharmacologic prophylaxis.** Because of the high morbidity and mortality associated with the development of aGVHD, routine prophylaxis against GVHD is required in all patients undergoing allo-HCT. Although a number of different pharmacologic agents can be used, a typical regimen uses an antimetabolite agent like methotrexate (at a dose of 10 mg/m^2 on days 1, 3, 6 $\pm$ 9) or mycophenolate mofetil (MMF) continued until day 30 after allo-HCT combined with a calcineurin inhibitor, either cyclosporine or tacrolimus. Immunosuppression with a calcineurin inhibitor is generally continued until day 100 posttransplant and gradually tapered in the absence of GVHD or disease relapse. Recently, other novel regimens have included sirolimus plus tacrolimus, as well as vorinostat- and bortezomib-based regimens. Further GVHD prophylaxis using high-dose cyclophosphamide (50 mg/kg given on days 3 and 4 after allo-HCT) has revolutionized haploidentical transplantation as its use has dramatically reduced both aGVHD and cGVHD rates after haploidentical transplantation. This has also been successfully been used in HLA-matched sibling and unrelated donor transplants with very favorable GVHD rates.

b. **T cell depletion.** T cell depletion may be used as either an alternative or adjuvant to pharmacologic prophylaxis for GVHD. As donor-derived T cells are central to

TABLE 8-6	Glucksberg aGVHD Grading

Clinical grading of aGVHD

Stage	Skin	Liver	Gut	Functional impairment
0	0	0	0	0
I	1+–2+	0	0	0
II	1+–3+	1+	1+	1+
III	2+–3+	2+–3+	2+	2+
IV	2+–4+	2+–4+	3+	3+

Clinical staging of aGVHD

Stage	Skin	Liver	Gut
1+	Maculopapular rash <25% body surface	Bilirubin 2–3 mg/dL	Diarrhea 500–1,000 mL/d; persistent nausea
2+	Maculopapular rash 25%–50% body surface	Bilirubin 3–6 mg/dL	Diarrhea 1,000–1,500 mL/d
3+	Generalized erythroderma	Bilirubin 3–6 mg/dL	Diarrhea >1,500 mL/d
4+	Desquamation and bullae	Bilirubin >15 mg/dL	Pain ± ileus

the pathogenesis of aGVHD, T cell depletion of the donor graft can effectively reduce the incidence of GVHD. A number of methods for T cell depletion have been used and include physical adsorption of T cells to proteins such as lectins, elutriation, or depletion with T cell or lymphocyte-specific antibodies. A loss of donor T cells is associated "however, with higher rates of graft rejection mediated by residual host T cells and a disease relapse due to partial loss of the GvT effect." In addition, T cell depletion results in delayed immune reconstitution in recipients, leading to higher rates of viral infections and, in particular, cytomegalovirus (CMV) and Epstein–Barr virus (EBV).

4. **Treatment.** Corticosteroids are the primary treatment for aGVHD. For mild (grade I) GVHD of the skin, topical steroids may be sufficient. For grade II or higher disease, prednisone or methylprednisolone 1 to 2 mg/kg/day is usually initiated. Steroid doses are then generally tapered gradually after clinical improvement. For patients with steroid refractory disease, a number of agents have been used with modest success. These include agents such as mycophenolate mofetil, cyclosporine, tacrolimus, sirolimus, pentostatin, thalidomide, and monoclonal antibodies including daclizumab and infliximab. Recently, use of extracorporeal photopheresis (ECP) has also been tested for the treatment of aGVHD with variable results.

C. **Infections**
1. **Timing of infectious complications.** HCT recipients are at increased risk for opportunistic infections. The risk of developing specific types of infections seen in stem cell transplant recipients varies by the type of transplant (autologous or allogeneic) and the length of time since undergoing the transplant. Before neutrophil engraftment, patients are at increased risk for infection due to neutropenia caused by the conditioning regimen and breaks in mucosal barriers from chemotherapy or indwelling vascular access devices. During this period, febrile neutropenia caused from both gram-positive and gram-negative organisms are common. In addition, Candida infections and herpes

simplex virus (HSV) reactivation may occur. The postengraftment period (days 30 to 100) is characterized by impaired cell-mediated immunity. After engraftment, the herpes viruses, particularly CMV, are major pathogens. Other dominant pathogens during this phase include *Pneumocystis carinii* and *Aspergillus* species.

2. **Prophylaxis and management of specific infections**

   a. **CMV.** CMV infections in HSCT recipients most commonly present as fever or interstitial pneumonitis. Other clinical manifestations include bone marrow suppression, retinitis, or diarrhea. Patients at risk for developing CMV infection include those undergoing allogeneic HSCT where either the donor or recipient is CMV positive. Prevention of CMV disease in allogeneic transplant can be accomplished using either a prophylactic or a preemptive strategy. A prophylactic strategy of ganciclovir through day +100 posttransplant is effective at preventing CMV disease but may result in drug-induced marrow suppression and prevent reconstitution of CMV-specific T cell immunity, resulting in late occurrences of CMV disease. A preemptive strategy uses sensitive PCR techniques to detect viremia and initiates therapy with ganciclovir before the development of overt disease. For patients with resistant disease, foscarnet or cidofovir may be used.

   To reduce the risk of transfusion-acquired CMV infection, all donors and recipients are screened for their CMV serostatus. CMV antibody–negative blood products should be given to CMV-negative recipients. Alternatively, leukofiltration to reduce the white cell fraction in the transfused produce may be used as an alternative if no CMV-negative products are available.

   b. **HSV and VZV.** Routine prophylaxis with either acyclovir 400 mg t.i.d. or valacyclovir 500 mg qd. to prevent reactivation of HSV and varicella zoster virus (VZV) is given to patients until neutrophil engraftment in autologous transplant patients and immunosuppression are discontinued in allogeneic transplant patients.

   c. **PCP prophylaxis.** Prophylaxis with TMP-SMX one DS tablet b.i.d. 2× a week, dapsone 100 mg daily or aerosolized pentamidine should be given to all patients undergoing allogeneic transplant and selected patients undergoing autologous transplant. PCP prophylaxis is continued while patients remain on immunosuppressive medications.

D. **Veno-occlusive disease of the liver.** Veno-occlusive disease (VOD) of the liver is a clinical diagnosis based on the presence of hyperbilirubinemia associated with fluid retention and painful hepatomegaly. Histologically, VOD is associated with central vein occlusion, centrilobular hepatocyte necrosis, and sinusoidal fibrosis. Ultrasonography may reveal reversal of flow in the portal and hepatic veins. The etiology of VOD is believed to arise from damage to the hepatic endothelium secondary to high-dose chemotherapy and/or radiation.

Risk factors for VOD include preexisting hepatic disease (e.g., viral hepatitis, cirrhosis), high-dose radiation as part of the conditioning, mismatched or unrelated donor HSCT, and the use of cyclosporine and methotrexate for GVHD prophylaxis. Spontaneous resolution of VOD is observed in approximately 70% of cases, but can frequently evolve into fatal multisystem organ failure. Low-dose heparin or ursodeoxycholic acid may provide some protection when used in a prophylactic manner. Supportive care measures are the mainstay of treatment for VOD with attention to fluid and electrolyte management. Other agents used for the treatment of VOD include defibrotide, alteplase and high-dose methylprednisolone, although the evidence supporting their use is mixed.

E. **Management of relapsed disease.** For relapsed disease following allogeneic transplant, maneuvers that attempt to maximize the GvL effect of the allograft may be useful. Withdrawal of immunosuppression is usually attempted first. If no effect is seen, a DLI can augment the immunologic effect of the allograft. DLI can result in significant toxicity including acute and cGVHD and severe pancytopenia. Responses are seen more frequently in diseases thought to be most sensitive to a graft-versus-disease effect such as chronic myeloid leukemia (CML) and in those patients who develop GVHD. Currently, the outcomes of patients who relapse after allo-HCT and are unable to achieve remission with salvage therapies remain extremely poor.

IX. LATE COMPLICATIONS OF ALLOGENEIC TRANSPLANTATION
A. cGVHD
1. **Clinical manifestations.** The clinical manifestations of cGVHD are heterogeneous in terms of the organ systems involved, the disease severity, and the clinical course. Historically, GVHD was classified as chronic when it occurred after day +100 post-HSCT. However, currently if patients have features of aGVHD even after day +100 in the absence of features diagnostic of cGVHD, it is still classified as persistent, recurrent, or late-onset aGVHD. Based on NIH consensus guidelines, cGVHD includes classic cGVHD when patients have manifestations that are only present in cGVHD and overlap syndrome, which has diagnostic or distinctive features of cGVHD along with features typical of aGVHD (skin, GI tract, liver).

    Based on the NIH scoring system, cGVHD is classified into mild, moderate, or severe disease, depending on the number of affected organs and organ-specific severity (scored from 0 to 3). Mild cGVHD involves two or fewer organs/sites with no clinically significant organ impairment. Moderate cGVHD involves three or more organs/sites with no clinically significant impairment or at least one organ/site with clinically significant functional impairment, but no major disability. Severe cGVHD involves major disability caused by cGVHD.

    The most frequently affected organs in cGVHD include the skin, liver, GI tract (predominantly esophagus), and lungs. Epidermal involvement is characterized as an erythematous rash that may appear papular, lichen planus–like, papulosquamous, or poikiloderma. Dermal and subcutaneous involvement is characterized by sclerosis, fasciitis, and ulcerations. Oral manifestations of cGVHD include erythema, lichenoid hyperkeratosis, ulcerations, or mucoceles. Lacrimal gland dysfunction frequently results in keratoconjunctivitis sicca, also known as the dry eye syndrome, and can manifest as burning irritation, pain, blurred vision, and photophobia. GI symptoms include nausea, vomiting, anorexia, and unexplained weight loss. Liver involvement is characterized by rising bilirubin and transaminases. Pulmonary cGVHD can result in a debilitating bronchiolitis obliterans syndrome with pulmonary function testing often demonstrating decreases in the forced expiratory volume in the first second (FEV_1) and the diffusing capacity of the lung for carbon monoxide (DLCO).

2. **Diagnosis and treatment.** The diagnosis of cGVHD can often be made on the basis of classical features of skin involvement, manifestations of gastrointestinal involvement, and a rising serum bilirubin concentration. Often the diagnosis is less clear, in which case histologic confirmation may be desirable.

    Systemic immunosuppression with corticosteroids and other agents are often required to treat cGVHD. In addition, ancillary and supportive care measures tailored to the organ system involved are critical for the management of cGVHD, and in many circumstances reduce or eliminate the need for systemic immunosuppression.

B. Late infections.
Autologous HCT patients have a more rapid recovery of immune function and a lower risk of opportunistic infections than allogeneic HSCT patients. Because of cell-mediated and humoral immunity defects and impaired functioning of the reticuloendothelial system, allogeneic HSCT patients with cGVHD are at risk for various infections during this phase. Late infections include EBV-related posttransplant lymphoproliferative disease, community-acquired respiratory virus infection, and infections with encapsulated bacteria. In addition, fungal infections with Aspergillus species and zygomycosis can be seen in the late period, particularly in patients with cGVHD.

C. Secondary malignancies.
Patients undergoing both autologous and allogeneic transplantation are at risk for the development of either treatment-related myelodysplastic syndromes (MDS) or acute myelogenous leukemia (AML) due to the high-dose alkylators and irradiation typically used as part of the conditioning regimens. Exposure to radiation and the photosensitizing effects of many commonly used transplantation-related medications increase the risk of skin cancers among recipients. Posttransplant lymphoproliferative disorders due to EBV can be observed particularly in patients receiving T cell–depleted grafts.

D. Other complications. Although stem cell transplantation can result in long-term survival with an excellent quality of life, late sequelae of the transplantation can result in significant morbidity. For example, TBI is associated with hypothyroidism and development of cataracts. Patients receiving prolonged corticosteroids can develop muscle weakness and bone loss. Recommendations for screening and preventative practices for long-term survivors of HSCT have been published.

SUGGESTED READINGS

Bray RA, Hurley CK, Kamani CK, et al. National marrow donor program HLA matching guidelines for unrelated adult donor hematopoietic cell transplants. *Biol Blood Marrow Transplant* 2008;14:45–53.

Bashey A, Solomon SR. T-cell replete haploidentical donor transplantation using post-transplant CY: an emerging standard-of-care option for patients who lack and HLA-identical sibling donor. *Blood and Marrow Transplant* 2014;49(8):999–1008.

Bashey A, Zhang X, Sizemore CA, et al. T-cell replete HLA-haploidentical hematopoietic transplantation for hematologic malignancies using post-transplantation cyclophosphamide results in outcomes equivalent to those of contemporaneous HLA-matched related and unrelated donor transplantation. *J Clin Oncol* 2013; 31:1310–1316.

Gragert L, Eapen M, Williams E, et al. HLA match likelihoods for hematopoietic stem-cell grafts in the U.S. registry. *New Engl J Med* 2014;371:339–348.

Jagasia M, Arora M, Flowers ME, et al. Risk factors for acute GVHD and survival after hematopoietic cell transplantation. *Blood* 2012;119:296–307.

Copelan E. Hematopoietic stem-cell transplantation. *New Engl J Med* 2006;354:1813–1826.

Holtan SG, Pasquini M, Weisdorf DJ. Acute graft-versus-host disease: a bench-to-bedside update. *Blood* 2014;124:363–373.

Gerard S, Jerome R. Current issues in chronic graft-versus host disease. *Blood* 2014;124:374–384.

Dignan FL, Amrolia P, Clark A, et al. Diagnosis and management of chronic graft-versus-host disease. *Br J Haematol* 2012;158:46–61.

Majhail NS, Rizzo JD, Lee SJ, et al. Recommended screening and preventive practices for long-term survivors after hematopoietic cell transplantation. *Bone Marrow Transplant* 2012;47:337–341.

Filipovich AH, Weisdorf D, Pavletic S, et al. National Institutes of Health consensus development project on criteria for clinical trials in chronic graft-versus-host-disease: I Diagnosis and staging working group report. *Biol Blood Marrow Transplant* 2005;11:945–956.

Biostatistics as Applied to Oncology

Kathryn M. Trinkaus • Feng Gao • J.Philip Miller

I. **INTRODUCTION.** Statistics is the mathematical science of estimation in the presence of uncertainty. Its strengths are identifying patterns and teasing out relations in complex data, comparing information from multiple sources, quantifying similarities or differences, and estimating the degree of uncertainty or level of confidence with which to regard the results. Statistics includes an extensive toolbox of solutions for practical problems, with a well-established mathematical foundation. Statistics is more than just tricks, tests, and theorems, however. In a broader sense, it is an efficient, systematic, and reproducible means of investigating patterns and relations in complex data. It is a framework for organized thinking about the issues that generate these data.

A. **A few words about data.** The **hypotheses** of a study state the scientific ideas being tested, the **objectives** state the tasks required to test those hypotheses, and the **end points** are the quantities that will be measured while carrying out the tests. A good end point is clearly related to the biological or behavioral process that it measures, ascertainable with minimal error, and readily reproducible.

If an end point cannot be directly observed, a related quantity may be substituted as a **surrogate**. Surrogates are ethically preferable if the true end point requires invasive procedures or otherwise puts the patient at additional risk. They may be more efficient if the true end point takes a long time to observe or is costly to obtain. To be valid, a surrogate must provide the same conclusion as a test of the true end point, so it must respond to disease and treatment in the same manner as the true end point. Association alone is not sufficient, nor is availability of a more precise measurement. A surrogate end point will produce useless or misleading results if it is precise at the expense of accurately capturing the quantity of interest.

A useful end point is consistently observable and easy to record accurately as **missing data** put a study at risk of failure. **Primary end points** are used to achieve the primary objectives, so every missing value of a primary end point is the loss of a participant. **Systematic data loss** is the absence of most end points from individuals or from most individuals for a single end point. Dropping variables or individuals with missing data may substantially influence, or **bias**, results by narrowing the scope of the study or reducing the power of the study to identify patterns and differences accurately. Numerous methods of substituting values for those that are missing are available. The most effective is multiple **imputation**, which uses a probability model to impute values based on known characteristics of the subject. Values are imputed several times and the results are combined to provide estimates of the missing value and of the precision of the imputation. Missing data may be important indicators that a study is encountering logistic, administrative, or procedural difficulties. The best solution is to monitor data loss and address the underlying problems as promptly as possible. A study is only as successful as its data are accurate, precise, and consistently recorded. Good experimental design and data analysis strategies can help with the complex realities of biomedical and clinical research, but they are no substitute for good data.

II. A SHORT INTRODUCTION TO PROBABILITY.
Probabilities are used to describe discrete events, such as "response to therapy," as well as the likelihood that a continuous measurement, such as serum creatinine or blood pressure, will take on a specific value. For brevity, both are referred to as events. The individuals to whom results of a clinical study will be generalized make up the **target population**. The probability that an event will occur can be defined as the frequency with which the event or value occurs in the target population; this definition is referred to as "**frequentist**." A clinical study usually estimates frequencies in a **sample** from the target population. The **sample size** should be large enough to include all relevant features of the target population. The selection process is designed so that all members of the target population have the same (or a predefined) probability of being chosen for the sample; that is, the sample is **randomly chosen**. Randomness helps ensure that no characteristic of the target population is over- or underrepresented, so the selection process does not bias the conclusions of the study.

The frequency of all possible states of an event (e.g., all possible levels of response) in the target population is the event's **probability distribution**. Hypotheses are tested, inferences drawn, and conclusions reached by comparing frequencies observed in the sample with those expected from the probability distribution in the target population. Clearly defining the target population can be difficult but is necessary for sound frequentist statistical analysis.

An alternative is to use existing knowledge, beliefs, or assumptions to define a **prior (probability)** distribution and the **likelihood** of each possible outcome. The prior distribution, **likelihood function**, and observed data are combined to generate a revised, **posterior probability distribution** for the measure of interest. This reasoning is based on a theorem about conditional probabilities first stated by Thomas Bayes; hence the term "**Bayesian**" **statistics**. Bayesian approaches are well-suited to predictive modeling and iterative decision making, as in dose-finding studies or sequential toxicity monitoring, because the posterior distribution provides a new prior for the next stage of data collection. Even so-called "vague" or "noninformative" priors can have a substantial effect on conclusions and must be chosen with care.

Defining a likelihood function also can be challenging. Frequentist and Bayesian approaches have a common mathematical foundation, and most standard analyses can be carried out using either way.

Generally speaking, two events are **independent** if the occurrence of one provides no information about the probability of occurrence of the second. In most cases, observations taken on separate and unrelated biological organisms are considered independent, whereas repeated observations taken from the same biological organism are dependent. Common sources of dependence are association in space (e.g., expression levels of two proteins from a single individual), time (e.g., measures at time of treatment and subsequent weekly intervals), function (e.g., blood pressure and heart rate of the same individual), or inheritance (e.g., genetic studies of family members). Dependence is a matter of degree and can be modeled.

Repeated observations may be incorporated into experimental design and methods of analysis. **Replication** of a measure within an individual helps to better estimate within-subject differences, whereas taking measurements on additional individuals helps to better estimate differences between subjects. Repeating an experiment with the same samples already analyzed (**technical replication**) is primarily useful for quality control and adds little to any conclusion drawn about the study sample or target population.

In general, the **effective sample size** is the number of independent observations, not the number of events or measurements. The more complex or variable a quantity is, the larger the number of independent measurements needed to adequately describe it.

III. **MEASUREMENT WITH ERROR. Random error** occurs by chance alone and is a part of most measurements in a clinical study. Over a large series of measurements, random error has an average value of zero, so it can be reduced by replication. Systematic error is a more serious problem as it is due to some aspect of the biological phenomenon of interest, the sample being studied, or the measurement process. **Systematic error** has an average value greater or less than zero in the long run, so it shifts (biases) estimates away from the true value of the quantities being observed. It may be amplified by replication rather than reduced. A study can be designed to minimize identified sources of error to improve its estimates of the quantities of interest. **Biological variability** also contributes to the overall variability of observations. Variability in quantities of interest to the study are considered "signal"; those not of interest to the study contribute "noise." A good experimental or clinical study design maximizes the capture of signal and minimizes the capture of noise.

Most clinical measurements are **random variables (RV)**, measurements that take on a different value for each experimental subject with each value having a specific probability distribution. **Discrete RVs** fall into unordered (nominal) or ordered (ordinal) categories. The probability distributions of discrete RVs are often known, such as the binomial or multinomial probabilities of falling into two or more categories, respectively. Counts, especially of events per unit time or space, may approximate a Poisson distribution. **Continuous RVs** are measured on a real or complex number scale with or without upper or lower boundaries. The values that completely describe a continuous distribution are its **parameters**. The parameters of a distribution are usually related to its mean (location of the center) or variance (the spread). Common **parametric** distributions are generalizations from observation of natural processes, not merely mathematical abstractions, and many are related to one another. For a large number of observations of a relatively rare event, the binomial is a good approximation of the Poisson. For a large number of observations, both the binomial and the Poisson approach the normal/Gaussian distribution.

If the parameters of a distribution can be estimated, so can the probability that the random variable will take on any given value. If it is very improbable that two sets of observations could have been drawn from a distribution with a single set of parameters, then there is evidence that the groups differ in that respect. This reasoning is the basis of most frequentist **hypothesis tests**. It also explains the large role of estimating means and variances in statistical analysis.

If the observations do not seem to fit any known distribution, some eccentricities of shape can be adjusted by analyzing the data on an alternative scale, transforming the data to a shape with known properties. **Transformation** alters the intervals between observations, not their order, so it does not alter conclusions drawn from hypothesis tests. A log transform, for example, makes a multiplicative relationship additive, a useful feature if additive models such as regression are to be used. Taking **ratios** is a way of adjusting each measurement with respect to a baseline or denominator. Mild eccentricity, such as skewness without a large number of duplicate measurements, can also be analyzed with **robust, nonparametric,** or **semiparametric** methods. These methods are less strongly influenced by a few unusual values (**outliers**) and have fewer, weaker assumptions about the distribution from which observed values are drawn.

Observations with multiple peaks, abrupt descents, and reascents ("singularities"), large numbers of single values (e.g., a "floor" at zero or a "ceiling" at the detection limit of the measuring instrument), or a combination of discrete and continuous elements are not adequately characterized by a few parameters. With some loss of information, the values can be **categorized** and discrete methods used. Another alternative is **resampling,** a form of simulation using probability ("**Monte Carlo**") methods to draw repeated samples from observed data. The repeated samples define an empirical probability distribution for a quantity of interest, such as a mean, and can be used to find confidence intervals or estimate bias, figuratively using the data to pull itself up by its **bootstraps.** The same strategy can be used to test hypotheses by randomly permuting sample subgroup labels, testing the hypothesis of interest in the many such subgroups with permuted labels. The **permutation test** *p-value* is the proportion of permuted sample *p-values* that are smaller than the *p-value* from the same hypothesis test in the correctly labeled subgroups.

If the data are too complex to be dealt with as a whole, piecewise methods, such as **locally weighted regression** and **splines,** including **multivariable adaptive regression splines (MARS),** may be preferable. These methods analyze the data in segments, estimating the regression curve over a small region rather than trying to find the curve appropriate for the observations as a whole.

IV. VIEWING THE DATA.

Given the complexity of biological phenomena, a preliminary overview is essential before diving into analysis. Plots, charts, lists, and frequency tables provide a comprehensive, visual representation of pattern, distribution, and difference. They highlight unusual data points, help with error checking, summarize the shape of individual variables, and illustrate relations between sets of variables. Visual summaries are so important for understanding data that it is essential to have a software program with good graphics capability.

For continuous, interval, or ordinal variables, **dot plots** and **stem-and-leaf plots** contain a symbol for each data point, stacking the occurrences of each value. The location of most common values, symmetry or skewness, and presence of unusual values (**outliers**) are readily seen. **Histograms** summarize counts or proportions in a solid column rather than representing each data value separately. Relative numbers or proportions in nominal or ordinal categories are easily identified. Histograms are most informative when the height of the column represents the amount being displayed. The magnitude of a single value, such as a mean, may not be well-represented by its height above zero, and as such is better illustrated by a point with error bars. **Bivariate scatter plots** are useful for examining relations between two or more continuous variables, as well as finding the center(s) of the distribution and the location and distance to outlying values. **Box plots** represent the distribution of a continuous variable in each of one or more categories. The "box" represents the middle of the distribution, usually the 25th to 75th percentiles. Lines extending outward from the ends of the box and plot symbols represent the spread of the data. A **lattice plot** is a matrix of scatter plots, one for each pair of a set of variables. Lattice plots make it easy to assess a number of variables at a glance; for example, for a first look at variables to be used in a multivariable analysis. **Robust smoothing methods** draw a curve through the bulk of data points, giving more weight to nearby observations than to distant ones.

A useful plot highlights patterns by suppressing detail, so it is often more useful to compare several kinds of plots than to add information to a single plot. The human eye is extraordinarily good at finding patterns in random scatters, especially when few data points are available. Plots are a starting point, but they do not replace a more rigorous statistical examination.

V. MAKING INFERENCES ABOUT DATA.

The goal of most clinical studies is to improve clinical decision making and patient outcomes, so the data that are gathered will be used for making inferences and testing hypotheses. Hypothesis testing, whether frequentist or Bayesian, is a well-defined, repeatable methodology for answering questions about observed data using probability models. Frequentist hypothesis tests require a **null hypothesis**, which describes the background against which research results will be interpreted, and an **alternative hypothesis**, stating the expected result or difference. The probabilities of all possible results are calculated assuming the null hypothesis is true. Results compatible with the null hypothesis, the **critical region**, are identified, as are those too extreme to be probable when the null hypothesis is true.

Samples are drawn from a well-defined target population, with randomization to reduce selection bias, and the measure of interest is observed. If the measure falls within the critical region, there is no evidence that the null hypothesis is false. If the measure falls outside the critical area, the result is not compatible with the null hypothesis, and the alternative is chosen instead. There are two correct decisions: to accept the alternative when the null hypothesis is false and to fail to reject a true null hypothesis. The corresponding errors are to reject the null hypothesis when it is true (a **false-positive or type I error**) or to fail to reject the null hypothesis when it is false (a **false-negative or type II error**).

In practice, a **p-value** is usually calculated, expressing the probability of results that are as extreme as or more extreme than the observed results, assuming that the observations are drawn from the probability distribution specified by the null hypothesis. "More extreme than" refers to values far from the center of the distribution, or in the "tails" of the distribution. If the alternative hypothesis is concerned with any difference from the null hypothesis, then the p-value measures the probability of falling into either tail of the distribution, a **two-tailed test**. If the alternative is concerned only with values greater than, or only values less than, the null value, then the p-value measures the probability of falling into a single tail, a **one-tailed test**. Two-tailed tests are more demanding as the area in each tail is smaller, and are generally preferred unless there is a strong reason for a one-tailed test.

Studies are designed to minimize the probability of a false-positive (the **significance level,** or α), while maximizing the probability of a correct positive (the **study power**). Conventional significance levels are 0.01 and 0.05, whereas power is usually no less than 0.8. Calculating study power is a routine part of designing any clinical trial using inferential procedures. Calculating power requires information about the expected values of end points under standard conditions (the null hypothesis) and the study treatment (the alternative hypothesis) as well as the expected variability and precision of measurement. If some of this information is not available, the maximum detectable difference can be calculated for a given null hypothesis and a specified study power. In the absence of any preliminary evidence, no inferential procedures can be planned, and only an observational trial is possible. If the preliminary information is weak or of uncertain relevance, study power can be reviewed at one or more **interim analyses** to ensure that the entire study does not rest on a shaky foundation. There is no useful information to be had from a *post hoc* **power calculation** carried out after the data have been gathered.

Estimates of study power generally refer to single tests. If many tests are to be carried out, then some positive results may be observed purely by chance. A significance level of 0.05 implies that any result that is expected to occur less frequently than 5 in 100 times, or 1 in 20 times, is considered "unlikely." If a large number of tests are carried out, the probability of at least one false-positive result can be large, making it necessary to adjust for the effect of **multiple testing**. Most such adjustments were developed for moderate numbers of tests in a single analysis or model. Their usefulness for combining results from several types of analyses on related data or from multiple studies (**meta-analyses**) is unclear. Genomic and proteomic studies, which may involve tens of thousands of tests, are also not well-served by traditional multiple testing correction methods. Multiple testing corrections are more useful in confirmatory studies, where the goal is to avoid a false-positive result, than in discovery studies, where overcorrection may prevent recognition of interesting results. Results from discovery studies usually require validation in fully independent studies.

If the conditions of a hypothesis test are too difficult to meet or if a more information-rich result is needed, then a Bayesian procedure may be preferable. These make more efficient and comprehensive use of prior information. The *caveat* is that prior data must be substantially accurate if a reliable prior distribution and likelihood function are to be found.

VI. MODELING RELATIONS. Modeling provides a richer, more nuanced approach to data analysis than simple hypothesis testing. Traditional single or multiple linear models describe the relation between independent variables and Gaussian-distributed dependent variables. The effect of each independent variable is adjusted for the effect of the others, so the model describes the joint effect of several covariates on the outcome. Models may be stratified, allowing different curves to be fit to subsets of the data and their distinctness tested. **Generalized linear, nonlinear**, and **time-to-event** models allow the same strategies to be applied to non-Gaussian or nonlinear dependent variables, as well as to events for which some patients' times are unknown (censored). **Mixed models** have extended the linear framework to random effect, independent variables that represent a sample of the values to which conclusions will be generalized. **Hierarchical models** allow inclusion of multiple levels of dependence, such as multiple observations taken from each individual and at several points in time or space. **Robust methods** can accommodate some forms of eccentrically distributed data by modeling a curve or surface in segments, estimating the value of the dependent variable based on nearby observations. Splines take a similar piecewise approach in a more formal way, fitting a model to each segment.

The complexity of relations being modeled is both a strength and a weakness of the modeling process. **Confounding** occurs when two or more independent variables are related to one another as well as to the outcome. Confounding can exaggerate or mask the effect of one or more covariates on the outcome, and it is best dealt with in the study design. A related problem is **collinearity**, in which two or more covariates provide redundant information about the outcome. One or more will appear less strongly related to the outcome than is actually the case. If it is important to estimate the effect of each covariate, several models can be created.

The joint effect of several covariates may be quite different than their individual effects, or main effects. When the effect of a covariate differs depending on the presence or level of another covariate, an **interaction** is present. In this case, there is no way to interpret the effect of a single covariate; only their joint effects can be interpreted.

If there are few observations to work with, then only large effects are likely to be identified even if the sample is a good representation of the target population. Some real effects may not be measurable with a given sample, and a difficult **choice of covariates** is usually necessary. The *p-values* indicate whether a covariate contributes to a model, but they are not sensitive measures of how much information is provided. **Measures of information** or tests, such as **likelihood ratio tests**, are better indicators of how much information is gained or lost with each independent variable. If a model is based on most of the variation in the input data, with few anomalies and little ignored information, then it is said to fit well. Any change in the model can alter its fit, so the fit must be reexamined after each change. Diagnostic tools, such as **residuals**, measure unexplained variability, while tests for **goodness-of-fit** estimate how closely the model fits the input data. **Outliers** occur where the model's estimation of the outcome value differs from the observed value for a specific set of covariates. **Influential points** are closely approximated by the model, although at the expense of a substantial number of the remaining observations. Any of these may distort the model and render its conclusions inaccurate or misleading. To fit a sound model and interpret it correctly, the analyst must know the input data well, understand the model being used, test the fit with care, and examine the output results in detail.

VII. PREDICTION. Well-fitting descriptive models often fail to produce accurate predictions when given new data. A model may be **overfitted** to a specific data set, so it does not accommodate systematic differences between the data on which it was built and new data about which predictions are made. Predictive modeling can be improved by splitting the data into parts, a **training set** on which the model is built and an independent **validation set** on which its performance is assessed. **K-fold cross-validation** divides the data into K equal-sized parts and creates K-1 models, each leaving out one part to be used as a validation set. Training sets also may be **randomly sampled**, leaving the remainder of observations as a validation set and repeating the process many times. Model performance is summarized over the results from each validation set. Performance criteria include overall deviation from predicted values, such as the root mean square error (**RMSE**), and data visualization such as **residual plots**, which show where deviations from prediction are largest or most common. At each training and test step, it is essential that data used to assess performance come only from the validation set and are not used in training the model.

VIII. STATISTICAL LEARNING. Statistical learning is a rapidly expanding set of methods for analyzing and interpreting complex or very large data sets. **Classification** methods are used to predict a qualitative outcome or response, **regression** methods to predict a quantitative outcome or response. If the outcome or response of interest is known at the outset, the analysis is a **supervised learning** process. In some cases, the goal is to illuminate structure in the data, treating all input alike, a process referred to as **unsupervised learning**. **Bootstrap** and **cross-validation** are used to estimate precision and predictive accuracy, select the best among alternative methods, and avoid overfitting a specific model or set of classes. Classification analyses split the observations into subsets, clusters, or nodes, aiming to maximize homogeneity within and heterogeneity between nodes. Some common classification procedures include **K-nearest neighbor analysis**, **logistic regression, discriminant analysis**, and many forms of **cluster analysis**. More complex underlying structure can be identified using **latent class analysis**. Tree-based classification methods repeatedly split a data set, as in **recursive partitioning**, or create a forest of many bootstrap-based trees, as in **random forest**. Classification accuracy may be increased by bootstrap aggregating ("**bagging**") the results of repeated classifications. In a supervised analysis, classification accuracy can be assessed by developing classifiers with a proportion of observations and assessing their accuracy using the remaining, out-of-bag observations. The **Gini index** is a measure of homogeneity within and heterogeneity between classes. Tree-based methods, such as **random forest**, also find distances ("proximities") between observations that can be used to visualize their structure using **multidimensional scaling**. Regression analyses attempt to predict the value of a continuous quantity by such methods as **linear regression, partial least squares, principal components**, and **factor analysis**. More complex, partly prespecified structures can be represented with **structural equation modeling** and **latent profile analysis**. **Random forest** also can be used to build regression trees.

IX. CONCLUSION. A basic knowledge of statistics allows one to investigate data at first hand in a systematic and organized manner as well as to collaborate more effectively with a statistician when more extensive analyses are needed.

    A. How to learn more. JMP (www.jmp.com), SPSS (www.spss.com), and Stata (www.stata.com) provide immediate access with good graphics and user-friendly, menu-driven interfaces. JMP includes extensive genomic data analysis methods, and all four have power and sample size calculators. For more complex or customized analyses, SAS (www.sas.com), R (www.r-project.org), MATLAB (www.mathworks.com), and Python (www.python.org/psf, www.learnpython.org) are powerful programming and scripting languages that require some study to be used effectively. R and Python are open source and can be used without charge. SAS and MATLAB require a license.

SUGGESTED READINGS

General Interest

Hacking I. *The Taming of Chance*. Cambridge, England: Cambridge University Press, 1990.

Huff D, Geis I. *How to Lie with Statistics*. New York, NY: W.W. Norton & Co, 1993.

McGrayne SB. *The Theory That Would Not Die: How Bayes' Rule Cracked the Enigma Code, Hunted Down Russian Submarines, and Emerged Triumphant from Two Centuries of Controversy*. Yale University Press, 2012.

Salsburg D. *The Lady Tasting Tea: How Statistics Revolutionized Science in the Twentieth Century*. New York, NY: Henry Holt, 2002.

Silver N. *The Signal and the Noise: Why So Many Predictions Fail – But Some Don't*. Penguin Press HC, 2012.

Stigler S. *Statistics on the Table: A History of Statistical Concepts and Methods*. Cambridge, England: Harvard University Press, 2002.

Basics

James G, Witten D, Hastie T, et al. *An Introduction to Statistical Learning*. Springer, 2013.

Klein G, Dabney A. *The Cartoon Introduction to Statistics*. New York, NY: Hill and Wang, 2013.

Kuhn M. *Applied Predictive Modeling*. New York, NY: Springer, 2013.

Motulsky H. *Intuitive Biostatistics: A Nonmathematical Guide to Statistical Thinking*, 3rd ed. London, England: Oxford University Press, 2013.

Rosner B. *Fundamentals of Biostatistics*, 7th ed. Boston, USA: Cengage Learning, 2010.
Salkind N. *Statistics for People Who (Think They) Hate Statistics*, 5th ed. Thousand Oaks, CA: Sage Publications, 2013.

Software-Guided Learning
Cody R. *SAS Statistics by Example*. Cary, NC: SAS Institute, 2011.
Delwiche L, Slaughter S. *The Little SAS Book: A Primer*, 5th ed. Cary, NC: SAS Institute, 2012.
Field A. *Discovering Statistics Using IBM SPSS Statistics*. Thousand Oaks, CA: Sage Publications, 2013.
Hahn B, Valentine D. *Essential MATLAB for Engineers and Scientists*, 5th ed. New York, NY: Academic Press, 2013.
Kohler U, Kreuter F. *Data Analysis Using Stata*, 3rd ed. College Station: Stata Press, 2012.
Kruschke JK. *Doing Bayesian Data Analysis: A Tutorial with R and BUGS*, 1st ed. New York, NY: Academic Press, 2010.
Lutz M. *Learning Python*, 5th ed. O'Reilly Media, 2013.
Maindonald J, Braun J. *Data Analysis and Graphics Using R: An Example-Based Approach*, 3rd ed. Cambridge, England: Cambridge University Press, 2010.
Sall J, Lehman A, Stephens M, et al. *JMP Start Statistics: A Guide to Statistics and Data Analysis Using JMP*, 5th ed. Cary, NC: SAS Institute, 2012.

Neuro-oncology

Andrew Lin • Jian Campian • Michael R. Chicoine • Jiayi Huang • David D. Tran

I. GENERAL APPROACH TO EVALUATING AN INTRACRANIAL MASS LESION

A. **Presentation.** Intracranial mass lesions can be found during an evaluation for headache, seizure, or a focal neurological deficit; occasionally, they are also found incidentally. Brain tumors may cause an obstructive hydrocephalus or increased intracranial pressure through mass effect, resulting in headache, nausea, and vomiting. If they cause hydrocephalus, depending on the severity, brain tumors can cause global neurologic dysfunction. More typically, brain tumors give rise to focal deficits or changes in behavior that are slowly evolving or occasional, sudden in onset, particularly in the setting of a seizure.

B. **Evaluation.** Intracranial mass lesions have a wide spectrum of differential diagnoses, and it can be difficult to distinguish among the possible etiologies by imaging characteristics. Lesions due to a primary or secondary brain tumor can be difficult to differentiate from one another and from lesions of other etiologies such as infection (e.g., an abscess), areas of demyelination, and even subacute stroke. Therefore, definitive management of an intracranial mass lesion often requires a tissue diagnosis.

   Common primary brain tumors and their relative frequencies can be found in Table 10-1.

C. **Treatment.** Prior to tissue diagnosis, two important management considerations are the treatment of seizures and increased intracranial pressure.

   1. **Seizures.** Seizures are a common complication of supratentorial tumors, and treatment should be initiated after the first seizure. In patients with a tumor who have never had a seizure, there is data supporting the use of short-term perioperative seizure prophylaxis, but no definitive data supporting the use of long-term seizure prophylaxis. Levetiracetam and lacosamide are the antiepileptic drugs of choice as they do not have significant drug–drug interactions and are unlikely to interfere with chemotherapy unlike older antiepileptic drugs.

TABLE 10-1 Primary Brain Tumors and Their Frequency

Primary brain tumors	% Primary brain tumors	Tumor type		% Gliomas	WHO grade
Gliomas	28%	*Astrocytic tumors*	Pilocytic astrocytoma	2%–5.1%	I
			Diffuse astrocytoma	9.1%	II
			Anaplastic astrocytoma	6.0%–13%	III
			Glioblastoma multiforme	54.4%–57%	IV
		Oligoastrocytoma	Low-grade oligoastrocytoma	3.3%–5%	II
			Anaplastic oligoastrocytoma		III
			GBM with oligodendroglial component		IV
		Oligodendroglioma	Low-grade oligodendroglioma	6.1%–10%	II
			Anaplastic oligodendroglioma		III
			GBM with oligodendroglial component		IV
		Ependymal tumors	Subependymoma	1%–6.8%	I
			Myxopapillary ependymoma		I
			Ependymoma		II
			Anaplastic ependymoma		III
Embryonal tumors	1.2%	Medulloblastoma			IV
		Supratentorial PNET			IV
		Atypical teratoid/rhabdoid tumor			IV
Meningioma	35.8%	Atypical			I
		Anaplastic			II
Germ cell tumors	0.4%				III
Pituitary tumors	14.7%				
Craniopharyngioma	0.8%				
Schwannomas and neurofibromas	8.1%				
PCNS lymphoma	2.1%				

Rare tumor types: choroid plexus tumors, neuronal tumors, pineal parenchymal tumors. *Neuro Oncol* 2013;15:ii1–ii56; *Neuro Oncol* 2006;8(1):12–26.

2. **Increased intracranial pressure.** Another common neurologic complication of brain tumors is mass effect and vasogenic edema. Tumor-induced edema is commonly treated with corticosteroids such as dexamethasone. However, if there is clinical or radiological suspicion for CNS lymphoma, corticosteroid treatment should be withheld if possible until after the tissue biopsy, as corticosteroids may severely hamper diagnostic yield. Once symptoms improve, attempts should be made to wean patients off or to a lower dose of dexamethasone as soon as clinically safe to avoid the potentially debilitating, long-term side effects of chronic corticosteroid treatment. In recent years, bevacizumab, an anti-VEGFA monoclonal antibody, has increasingly been used to decrease symptoms from mass effect, that is, as a steroid-sparing agent.

II. GLIOMAS

A. **Introduction.** Gliomas account for 30% of all primary CNS tumors, but cause a disproportionate amount of morbidity and mortality as they comprise 80% of all malignant primary brain tumors.

   The World Health Organization (WHO) grades gliomas on a scale of I to IV and then subclassifies gliomas by histology (Table 10-1). In this classification scheme, gliomas are classified by the cell type(s) that the predominant tumor cell population resembles. Historically, gliomas were thought to arise following the transformation of fully differentiated glia: that is, astrocytomas arise from astrocytes and oligodendrogliomas arise from oligodendrocytes. It is now hypothesized that these tumors result from the transformation of neural stem cells (*N Engl J Med* 2005;353:811) and that the phenotype is a function of their molecular makeup. An early mutation that gives rise to slow-growing, indolent gliomas is the *IDH1* mutation. Greater than 90% of *IDH1* mutations occur at R132H; this mutation can be identified by immunohistochemistry and is an important pathologic finding as it has prognostic, and likely predictive, significance.

B. **WHO grade IV (Glioblastoma Multiforme)**

   1. **Epidemiology.** Glioblastoma multiforme (GBM) is the most common subtype of gliomas, accounting for approximately 50% with an incidence of 2 to 3 per 100,000 people. These tumors can arise de novo as grade IV astrocytomas (primary GBM) or less frequently, following transformation of lower grade gliomas (secondary GBM). Primary GBMs occur most commonly in older patients with a median age of 55 years, whereas secondary GBMs typically occur in younger patients with a median age of 39 years. Despite maximal medical management and an improved understanding of their genetic compositions, prognosis remains poor.

   2. **Imaging.** On magnetic resonance imaging (MRI), GBMs typically demonstrate a prominent enhancement pattern that can be peripheral or solid. The tumor is T2 hyperintense with surrounding vasogenic edema, T1 hypointense, and frequently crosses to the contralateral hemisphere. Because these tumors are highly cellular, they often restrict diffusion weakly in comparison with bacterial brain abscesses, which typically have prominent area of restricted diffusion.

   3. **Pathology.** When GBMs arise de novo, GBMs are almost exclusively *IDH1* mutation–negative. In these tumors, the methylation status of the *MGMT* promoter is the marker of prognostic and predictive significance. *MGMT* encodes a DNA repair enzyme. When the expression of the *MGMT* gene is silenced via methylation of CpG islands in the promoter, GBMs are less aggressive and more sensitive to alkylating agents like temozolomide (*N Engl J Med* 352:997). The median survival of patients with GBM possessing a methylated *MGMT* promoter and treated with concurrent chemoradiotherapy is 21.7 months—in contrast to a median survival of 12.7 months in similarly treated tumors with an unmethylated promoter.

   4. **Treatment.** When a lesion suspicious for GBM is in an eloquent location within the brain and is unresectable, a biopsy is indicated. When the lesion is amenable to surgery, a gross total resection or maximal debulking is preferred. In fact, there is limited class I evidence that demonstrates a survival advantage when the grossly abnormal brain tissue is completely resected. Unfortunately, GBMs are diffusely infiltrative, and therefore surgery is not curative. To further reduce the tumor burden regardless

of the extent of resection, standard of care in the treatment of newly diagnosed GBM includes concurrent conformal fractionated radiation and temozolomide chemotherapy, as protocoled by EORTC 22981 (*N Engl J Med* 2005;352:987). In this trial, 18- to 70-year-old patients with newly diagnosed, resected GBM were randomized to radiotherapy alone or concurrent radiotherapy and temozolomide chemotherapy. The median survival was extended by 2.5 months with the addition of temozolomide to radiation—12.1 to 14.6 months, and the 2-year survival rate increased from 10.4% to 26.5% in the combined modality arm. Notably, survival in GBM favors young persons with a better performance status.

3-D conformal radiotherapy to the volume of the tumor and a surrounding margin is administered in daily fractions of 2 Gy given 5 days per week for 6 weeks for a total dose of 60 Gy. Temozolomide is administered concurrently with radiation at 75 mg/m^2 orally daily during the entire 6-week period of radiation. After a 4- to 6-week break, maintenance temozolomide is given at 150 to 200 mg/m^2 orally daily for five consecutive days every 28 days for a minimum of six cycles. Throughout the treatment course, frequent laboratory testing, in particular complete blood counts and complete metabolic panel, is recommended. Thrombocytopenia, neutropenia, and severe lymphopenia are common reasons for the discontinuation and/or dose modifications of temozolomide. In patients who become severely immunosuppressed with CD4 counts less than 200 cells/mm^3, trimethoprim-sulfamethoxazole is often used as prophylaxis against Pneumocystis jirovecii (PCP) pneumonia.

In 2009, bevacizumab, a humanized monoclonal antibody that targets VEGF, was granted accelerated approval by the U.S. Food and Drug Administration (FDA) as a single agent in recurrent GBM. The approval was based on demonstration of durable objective response rates observed in two prospective single-arm phase II studies (*J Clin Oncol* 2009;27:4733; *J Clin Oncol* 2009;27:740). However, two recent Phase III randomized, placebo-controlled, double-blinded trials using bevacizumab in combination with standard conformal radiation and concurrent temozolomide in newly diagnosed GBM have shown an improvement in progression-free survival of 3 to 4 months, but failed to show an improvement in overall survival. The AVAglio trial conducted in Europe reported an improvement in patients' quality of life with the addition of bevacizumab. In contrast, the RTOG 0825 study in North America registered a negative impact on neurocognitive function in the bevacizumab arm. As a result, the ultimate utility of antiangiogenic therapy in the management of newly diagnosed GBM remains unclear.

5. **Monitoring.** Radiologic surveillance by MRI is routine practice. During the first 3 months after chemoradiotherapy, patients can develop worsening contrast enhancement that is indistinguishable from true tumor progression. This is due to breakdown of the blood–brain barrier from robust peritumoral inflammation induced by therapy. This phenomenon is known as *pseudoprogression*. Late pseudoprogression, often referred to as radiation necrosis, can also occur months, and rarely years, after radiotherapy has been completed and is thought to be related to delayed ischemic changes caused by radiation damage. Pseudoprogression and radiation necrosis are not only a radiologic phenomenon, but also can precipitate significant neurologic complications when they are associated with significant vasogenic edema and mass effect. Distinguishing between pseudoprogression/radiation necrosis and true tumor progression is difficult. Radiologic techniques such as 18-Fluoro-deoxyglucose positron emission tomography (FDG-PET) and MRI perfusion may be helpful in distinguishing between the two processes, but their use has not been validated prospectively. The only definitive way to differentiate the two is by obtaining additional tissue or by serially imaging the lesion in question and monitoring for regression or stability—which is evidence of pseudoprogression—or enlargement of the contrast enhancement, which is evidence of progression.

C. **WHO grade III**
1. **Epidemiology.** Approximately 10% of gliomas that are diagnosed each year are anaplastic (WHO grade III) astrocytomas, and another 5% to 10% are anaplastic oligodendrogliomas and mixed oligoastrocytomas.

2. **Imaging.** Anaplastic astrocytomas have poorly defined borders with heterogeneous signal intensity on T1 and T2, and these tumors frequently contrast enhance, although not as intensely as GBM. Anaplastic oligodendrogliomas are frequently T2 hyperintense and T1 hypointense, and are frequently calcified, which can be seen on susceptibility-weighted imaging. Contrast enhancement occurs less frequently in oligodendrogliomas, and when it occurs, the enhancement is typically faint.

3. **Pathology.** WHO grade III gliomas can be histologically classified as astrocytomas, oligodendrogliomas, or mixed oligoastrocytomas. These tumors are frequently *IDH1* mutated and are predicted to follow a more indolent growth pattern. In oligodendrogliomas and rarely mixed oligoastrocytomas, a recurrent cytogenetic abnormality of prognostic and predictive importance is loss of heterozygosity at chromosomes 1p and 19q. In one large series, 89% of oligodendrogliomas, 19% of mixed oligoastrocytomas, and 0% of pure astrocytomas harbor the 1p and 19q codeletions (*J Clin Oncol* 2006;24:5419). Therefore, oligodendrogliomas typically carry the best prognosis, followed by mixed oligoastrocytomas and then astrocytomas.

4. **Treatment.** Like GBM, WHO grade III gliomas are considered high-grade, malignant gliomas and are often managed similarly to GBM, with maximal resection followed by radiotherapy and temozolomide. The exception is anaplastic oligodendrogliomas and mixed oligoastrocytomas with 1p and 19q codeletions, in which activity of an older chemotherapy regimen, PCV (procarbazine, CCNU, and vincristine), and not temozolomide, has been clearly demonstrated in the randomized, controlled RTOG 9402 trial. Overall survival was extended with the addition of PCV to radiation in patients with 1p and 19q codeletions from a median of 7.3 years to a median of 14.7 years. Patients without 1p, 19q codeletions derived no appreciable survival benefit with the addition of PCV. Randomized studies are currently ongoing to prospectively examine the benefit of temozolomide for grade III gliomas and to compare it with PCV chemotherapy.

5. **Monitoring.** The natural history of these tumors is that they tend to progress to grade IV. Therefore, routine MRI surveillance is required. Like GBM, pseudoprogression and radiation necrosis are frequent imitators of true progression following chemoradiotherapy.

D. **WHO grade II**
   1. **Epidemiology.** Low-grade gliomas (WHO grade II) are also astrocytomas, oligodendrogliomas, or mixed oligoastrocytomas and account for about 20% of all gliomas.
   2. **Imaging.** Typically, these tumors do not contrast enhance and are more homogeneously T1 hypointense and T2 hyperintense.
   3. **Pathology.** Again, these tumors are frequently *IDH1* mutated. In low-grade gliomas with an oligodendroglial component, the presence or absence of 1p and 19q codeletions is again of prognostic, and perhaps predictive, significance.
   4. **Treatment.** Patients with low-grade gliomas also undergo resection if the tumor is surgically amenable. Once the diagnosis is made, they are often watched expectantly, unless the patient and tumor carry markers of poor prognosis (such as age >40 years, a high proliferative index, a substantial amount of residual disease, and significant neurological symptoms), as upfront radiation therapy has been shown to improve progression-free survival, but failed to enhance overall survival compared with patients who were followed expectantly and treated at the time of disease recurrence of progression (*Lancet* 2005;366(9490):985). The rationale behind postponing radiotherapy is to delay the neurocognitive side effects of treatment, especially in younger patients.
   5. **Monitoring.** Again routine surveillance with MRI is required as the natural history of these low-grade tumors is their tendency to transform into higher grade tumors. When treatment is deferred, it is important that the patient is closely monitored for radiographic evidence of transformation to a higher grade tumor.

E. **Pilocytic astrocytomas (WHO grade I)**
   1. **Epidemiology.** Pilocytic astrocytomas are the most common WHO grade I gliomas. These tumors are slow-growing, circumscribed, often cystic lesions that occur more frequently in children and young adults.

2. **Presentation.** They often occur in the cerebellum, anterior optic pathways, and brain stem, and present with chronic signs of neurologic dysfunction related to location, such as obstruction of cerebrospinal fluid (CSF) pathways causing hydrocephalus, focal neurologic deficits, and, rarely, seizures.

3. **Imaging.** These tumors are circumscribed and often have a cystic component and a nodule that is intensely contrast enhancing.

4. **Pathology.** A significant proportion of pilocytic astrocytomas occur in the setting of the neurofibromatosis type 1 (NF1) tumor predisposition syndrome, caused by a germline mutation in the tumor suppressor, *NF1*. Owing to a less aggressive phenotype, NF1-associated pilocytic astrocytomas are managed more conservatively than the sporadic variety. Sporadic pilocytic astrocytomas do not harbor mutations in *NF1*, but are frequently associated with molecular changes in the *BRAF* serine/threonine kinase gene (in 50% to 65% of tumors of all locations and 80% of cerebellar tumors) and are associated with a less aggressive clinical phenotype.

5. **Treatment.** In sporadic (non-NF1–associated) pilocytic astrocytomas, complete surgical excision is the preferred treatment when the tumor is surgically amenable as this approach is potentially curative (10-year survival rate is >80%). For unresectable tumors, radiation was for many years the primary treatment modality. However, in recent years, chemotherapy and debulking surgeries have been used as the primary treatment to delay radiation and the cognitive side effects that occur with radiation.

6. **Monitoring.** Long-term follow-up with serial imaging is warranted even when total resection has been performed, as these tumors may recur after resection.

F. **Ependymoma (WHO grade II and III)**

1. **Epidemiology.** This subset of tumors comprises 5% to 8% of gliomas and occurs in all age groups but is more common in children.

2. **Presentation.** These tumors typically occur along the ventricular system at the 4th ventricle, the lateral ventricles, the cerebral aqueduct, or within the spinal cord. Presenting symptoms are variable and depend on the location of the tumor.

3. **Imaging/Diagnostic testing.** On MRI, these tumors are hyperintense on T2, hypo- to isointense on T1, and the majority of tumors are contrast enhancing.

   In children, ependymomas typically develop in the posterior fossa. In adults, and patients with NF2, the majority of ependymomas occur along the spinal cord. Ependymomas infrequently develop supratentorially—when this occurs they can be intraparenchymal or intraventricular.

   Ependymomas often track along CSF pathways into the cisterns; hence, at the time of diagnosis, 10% to 30% have disseminated disease and have seeded the spinal column with "drop metastases." Because of the high incidence of CSF dissemination, all patients with ependymomas should have imaging of the entire neuroaxis. Of note, the role of CSF cytology is not completely defined, as it is unclear whether CSF cytology can detect microscopic dissemination that cannot be appreciated on imaging.

4. **Treatment.** In all patients with ependymoma, extent of surgical resection is an important prognostic factor in that complete surgical removal will cure a small percentage of cases. As these tumors frequently recur even in patients with a complete resection, focal radiation to the tumor bed is recommended and has been shown to result in a survival advantage. In the case of CSF dissemination, radiation to the entire neuroaxis may provide some benefit.

   Overall, children have a poorer prognosis than adults, possibly related to the infratentorial predominance. Subtotal resection, age younger than 3 years, and anaplastic features are all associated with a poorer prognosis.

   Tumor recurrence often occurs at the original tumor site, and the recurrent tumor usually remains a similar grade, although progression can occur. Overall, 5-year survival ranges are 30% to 40% in children and 40% to 50% in adults.

III. METASTASES TO THE CNS

A. Brain metastases

1. **Epidemiology.** Secondary brain tumors that arise from a primary tumor outside the CNS are overwhelmingly the most common malignant intracranial masses found in adults. Autopsy studies have revealed the presence of intracranial metastasis in ~25% of cancer patients. The majority of brain metastases in adults result from primary malignancies arising from lung, breast, and melanoma.

2. **Presentation.** The presenting signs and symptoms of intracranial metastases are similar to those of most primary brain neoplasms (i.e., focal neurologic deficit, headaches, and seizures). Close to 10% of brain metastases present as foci of intraparenchymal hemorrhage. The intraparenchymal hemorrhage can conceal the tumor at the time of initial presentation, resulting in a delay in diagnosis. In particular, melanoma, choriocarcinoma, thyroid carcinoma, and renal cell carcinoma are commonly associated with symptomatic hemorrhage. Other cancers, such as lung cancer, hemorrhage less frequently, but owing to the sheer numbers of metastatic cases, account for a significant proportion of hemorrhages associated with brain metastases.

3. **Imaging.** Brain metastases may be single or multiple, and tend to be located at the gray–white junction. They are usually well circumscribed, demonstrate peripheral enhancement on computed tomography (CT) or MRI, and often cause significant vasogenic edema. The finding of multiple synchronous lesions in an immunocompetent individual strongly supports the diagnosis of brain metastasis and is helpful in differentiating them from primary brain tumors or other mass lesions. In a patient who is found to have a brain mass that looks like it could be a metastasis but no primary is known, the evaluation should focus on the lungs, as 66% of these patients will have a lesion on chest radiography that represents primary lung cancer or pulmonary metastasis from other sites.

4. **Treatment.** The mainstays of treatment for metastatic disease are corticosteroids and, where appropriate, surgery and/or radiotherapy. Prognosis with treatment is related to age, Karnofsky performance score (KPS), number of metastases, response to therapy, and status of systemic disease.

   After the diagnosis of brain metastasis, corticosteroids are typically started, then either tapered off or down to the lowest tolerated dose following cytoreduction of the tumor. Antiepileptic drugs are indicated in patients that have had a seizure and may be used prophylactically in patients following surgery, but again, there is no data supporting the use of long-term seizure prophylaxis in patients who have not had a seizure.

   a. **Whole brain radiation.** Without treatment, patients with metastases to the brain have a life expectancy of about 1 month, though there is wide variability. With the addition of corticosteroids, median survival is extended to approximately 2 months. The first major advance in the treatment of brain metastases was whole brain radiation, which provides symptomatic improvement in most patients and extends survival to approximately 4 months. It is still widely used in patients with brain metastases that are too numerous to be treated with surgery or stereotactic radiosurgery. It is also used in patients in whom the primary goal is palliation due to their poor prognosis.

   In patients that have received surgery or stereotactic radiosurgery, whole brain radiation has not been shown to improve overall survival, though it may improve control of intracranial tumor burden over a period of months. Since whole brain radiotherapy has significant potential neurocognitive effects, it may be reasonable to withhold in this setting until the time of recurrence. A recent randomized study has shown that memantine (an NMDA receptor antagonist) when given concurrently with (and for at least 6 months after) whole brain radiotherapy appears to reduce the decline in delayed recall and cognitive function (*Neuro-Oncology* 2013;15:1429).

b. **Surgery versus stereotactic radiosurgery.** Surgery is the current treatment of choice for solitary brain metastases in patients with fair control of systemic disease, and in whom the lesion is in a surgically amenable location. Surgical excision not only appears to improve survival, it provides a tissue diagnosis and results in rapid decompression in patients with a large tumor with significant mass effect and vasogenic edema, and provides relief in patients with hydrocephalus from a posterior fossa tumor.

Alternatively, patients may be treated with stereotactic radiosurgery if the lesion is 3 to 4 cm or smaller. Several retrospective studies of radiosurgery have demonstrated a survival benefit that is comparable to surgery. The downside of radiosurgery is that it does not provide a tissue diagnosis. Nevertheless, it is a viable treatment option, especially for metastases that are surgically inaccessible and occur in the setting of poorly controlled systemic disease. It is often used when there are multiple but limited lesions, such as less than 4 to 5.

In patients that undergo surgery in whom whole brain radiation is withheld, adjuvant radiosurgery to the resection site is an alternative to reduce the risk of local recurrence.

Chemotherapy has an increasing, although still emerging, role in the treatment of brain metastases. The blood–brain barrier is a limiting factor in the use of chemotherapy for brain metastases in that it prevents the efficient passage of many therapeutic agents. For the vast majority of brain metastases, chemotherapy has an ancillary role. That said, early successes have been reported with antibody-based therapies and small molecule targeted therapies that may have better blood–brain barrier penetration, such as sorafenib in renal cell carcinoma that is metastatic to the brain or BRAF inhibitors in melanomatous brain metastases. The only tumors where chemotherapy is used as first-line treatment is in exquisitely chemosensitive tumors such as metastatic germ cell tumors, choriocarcinoma, and lymphoma.

B. **Leptomeningeal metastasis**
   1. **Overview.** Leptomeningeal metastasis is also known as carcinomatous meningitis or leptomeningeal carcinomatosis and is the metastatic spread of a malignancy to the leptomeninges (pia and arachnoid mater, which make up the subarachnoid space).
   2. **Epidemiology.** Autopsy studies have shown that leptomeningeal metastasis is present in 1% to 8% of cancer patients. The same solid tumors that frequently metastasize to the brain parenchyma, such as lung, breast, and melanoma, also metastasize to the leptomeninges. Additionally, in leptomeningeal carcinomatosis, leukemia and systemic lymphoma are also frequent perpetrators.
   3. **Presentation.** The presenting signs and symptoms of leptomeningeal metastasis are widely variable and include diffuse neurologic dysfunction. These patients may have signs of hydrocephalus and increased intracranial pressure, headache, nausea and vomiting, focal neurologic deficits, seizures, cranial neuropathies, meningismus, cerebellar symptoms, or myelopathy.
   4. **Imaging/Diagnostic tests.** Patients with suspected leptomeningeal metastasis should receive an MRI of the brain and entire spinal cord. MRI is fairly sensitive in evaluating for leptomeningeal involvement of solid tumors, but is significantly less sensitive in detecting leptomeningeal spread in hematopoietic malignancies.

      CSF cytology may provide a definitive diagnosis. The sensitivity of CSF cytology increases with repeated sampling from 71% after the first lumbar puncture to 86% after two and 90% after three lumbar punctures. The diagnostic yield of CSF sampling can also be increased by performing flow cytometry for hematopoietic malignancies and by testing for tumor markers for solid tumors.
   5. **Treatment.** Treatment options include radiation and systemic or intrathecal chemotherapy. The main role of surgery is palliation of hydrocephalus via shunting.
      a. **Symptomatic therapy.** In patients with headache, intracranial pressure should be evaluated by lumbar puncture. In the setting of increased intracranial pressure, corticosteroids can be used to treat edema, and even in the absence of hydrocephalus, shunting can be considered.

b. **Radiation.** With the exception of hematologic malignancies, in which radiation to the brain and the entire spinal cord is fairly common, radiation is primarily used for directed palliation of symptoms and bulky disease seen on imaging, as radiation of the entire neuroaxis is often poorly tolerated. With radiation, noncommunicating hydrocephalus from leptomeningeal carcinomatosis can frequently be treated without shunting.

c. **Chemotherapy.** For leptomeningeal carcinomatosis, chemotherapy can be delivered intrathecally or systemically. Intrathecal chemotherapy is the delivery of chemotherapy through an Ommaya reservoir or a lumbar puncture catheter. The typical agents used for intrathecal treatment are methotrexate, thiotepa, and cytarabine. Intrathecal administration of chemotherapy bypasses the blood–brain barrier—the main barrier in treating patients with systemic chemotherapy. Because of the blood–brain barrier, only certain drugs can achieve therapeutic levels in the CNS when administered systemically. The benefit of systemic chemotherapy compared with intrathecal chemotherapy is that it treats both CNS and non-CNS disease.

6. **Prognosis.** The prognosis of leptomeningeal metastasis is poor with the median survival between 2 and 3 months for solid tumors and closer to 5 months for hematological malignancies.

IV. MENINGIOMAS

A. **Epidemiology.** Meningiomas are benign, slow-growing, extra-axial tumors that are attached to the dura mater and arise from arachnoidal cap cells. They represent 30% of primary intracranial tumors and are a common incidental finding at autopsy. Advances in cranial imaging have increased the number of incidentally discovered asymptomatic lesions.

The peak age for meningiomas is 45 years of age, and there is a female predominance of almost 3:1, which increases to almost 10:1 for spinal meningiomas. These tumors are rare in children, except in association with neurofibromatosis type 2 in whom multiple meningiomas can develop at a younger age.

B. **Presentation.** Most meningiomas are present for many years prior to diagnosis, but are asymptomatic until they slowly reach a size where they begin to compress adjacent structures. Neurologic deficits that can occur include vision loss, cranial nerve palsies, hearing loss, mental status changes, motor weakness, and deficits arising from obstructive hydrocephalus. These tumors may also come to attention during the evaluation of seizures or headaches.

C. **Imaging.** These tumors may occur in almost any location but favor the falx cerebri, the cerebral convexity, the skull base (at the sphenoid bone, olfactory groove, parasellar region, the posterior fossa), the tentorium cerebelli, the ventricles, and the spinal canal.

Meningiomas frequently demonstrate calcifications and typically have an extra-axial location. On MRI, these tumors are typically isointense on T1 sequences without contrast, and homogeneously enhancing on T1 sequences with intravenous gadolinium administration. An attachment to adjacent dura may be visualized on the MRI (a "dural tail"), and significant edema in the surrounding brain parenchyma may be seen.

Imaging is problematic in differentiating atypical (grade II) and malignant (grade III) meningiomas from benign (grade I) meningiomas. Nevertheless, peritumoral vasogenic edema, intratumoral cystic change, boney destruction, arterial encasement, hyperostosis of adjacent bone, and extension through the skull base might suggest a higher grade, but not reliably.

D. **Pathology.** Many histologic variants have been described and are not useful for predicting clinical behavior, except in determining grade. The majority of meningiomas are WHO grade I, although up to 35% of meningiomas are grade II. Only a small minority of the tumors are malignant, WHO grade III tumors.

The grade of the meningioma is of prognostic significance. Grade I tumors often remain stable in size or grow very slowly and are frequently observed. In contrast, grade II tumors recur locally after treatment in 30% to 40% of cases, and the median survival in one reported series was around 12 years. Malignant grade III tumors have a higher recurrence rate of ~80% and have a reduced median survival of about 3 years.

Meningiomas occur in 45% to 60% of persons with neurofibromatosis type 2, which is caused by a germline mutation in the *NF2* tumor suppressor. As it turns out, 50% of sporadic meningiomas also harbor *NF2* mutations; however, in these sporadic meningiomas, mutations in oncogenes like Smoothened (*SMO*) and PI3K/AKT and in tumor suppressors, other than *NF2*, have also been identified.

E. **Treatment.** The decision about whether to treat an asymptomatic meningioma is often difficult and requires consideration of multiple factors including patient age, general medical condition, operative morbidity, as well as tumor size, grade, and location.

Expectant management with serial imaging is often reasonable for incidentally discovered asymptomatic lesions that do not appear to be expanding, infiltrating, or causing significant edema. Surgical removal offers the greatest chance of cure and is usually feasible, depending on the location.

Recent advances in radiotherapy techniques including stereotactic radiosurgery make it an option for treatment including the use of fractionated and stereotactic radiosurgical modalities. Radiotherapy is used in nonoperative cases, as it can result in regression of the tumor after 2 or 3 years; it is also used as adjuvant therapy, when a meningioma is incompletely resected and in grade II and III tumors—even when the tumor is completely resected—since these meningiomas have a high rate of recurrence without additional therapy. Prospective trials are underway that will clarify the indications for radiotherapy in grade II and III meningiomas.

V. PRIMARY CENTRAL NERVOUS SYSTEM LYMPHOMA

A. **Overview.** Primary central nervous system lymphoma (PCNSL) is an uncommon, typically aggressive form of non-Hodgkin's lymphoma that does not represent spread from systemic disease. PCNSL can occur in immunocompetent individuals but occurs most commonly in people who are immunosuppressed from HIV infection, immunosuppressive medications, or an inherited immunodeficiency.

B. **Epidemiology.** The median age at diagnosis is 52 years in an immunocompetent individual and 34 years in an immunosuppressed person, and accounts for 4% of primary CNS tumors.

C. **Presentation.** Patients with PCNSL come to medical attention because of a focal neurologic deficit, a personality change, or symptoms related to increased intracranial pressure, such as headache, nausea, and vomiting. Seizures and vision changes are less common presentations.

D. **Imaging/Diagnostic tests.** PCNSL typically causes parenchymal lesion(s) that can be found anywhere, though the most common sites are periventricular and superficial regions of the brain that are adjacent to the ventricle or the meninges. On MRI, noncontrast T1-weighted images are generally hypo/isointense, whereas T2 weighted images are generally iso/hyperintense. Lesions due to PCNSL have moderate-to-marked contrast enhancement and tend to show restricted diffusion due to their high cellularity, even more so than high-grade gliomas and metastases.

For the most part, PCNSL starts intraparenchymally, and the leptomeninges are involved secondarily (in approximately 10% to 25% of patients). In contrast, systemic lymphoma that involves the CNS favors the leptomeninges, and a parenchymal lesion is found only in a third of these patients.

A CT chest/abdomen/pelvis, lumbar puncture if safe, bone marrow biopsy, and at times, testicular ultrasound (especially for men >60 years old) is indicated to evaluate for systemic disease. Many tumors have a rapid lytic response to corticosteroid treatment, so corticosteroids should be withheld until a diagnostic biopsy has been performed, unless there is severe mass effect. In the case when the biopsy is nondiagnostic in the setting of corticosteroid administration, the biopsy should be repeated after stopping the corticosteroid for 10 to 14 days. If CSF cytology is positive, spine MRI should also be acquired.

Patients with suspected PCNSL should be checked for HIV infection and should undergo a detailed ophthalmological evaluation for intraocular involvement, as ocular involvement is present in as many as 20% of all cases and is a more accessible site for biopsy. The diagnosis can be made minimally invasively by lumbar puncture, though the sensitivity of cytology and flow cytometry is low. Brain biopsy is often needed to make the diagnosis.

E. Treatment. 90% of immunocompetent individuals with PCNSL have an aggressive diffuse large B-cell lymphoma. There is no benefit to surgical resection, and so the only surgical indication is stereotactic biopsy for diagnosis.

Although PCNSL is quite radiosensitive, whole brain radiation for this indication is falling out of favor. Radiotherapy can cause progressive memory loss and ataxia, especially in older patients when given concurrently with high-dose methotrexate chemotherapy. Hence, most experts do not recommend its use as an initial treatment unless there is a contraindication to chemotherapy. Radiation can be given as consolidation therapy after induction chemotherapy, or (more commonly) it is reserved for progressive PCNSL that is refractory to treatment with chemotherapy.

In PCNSL, high-dose methotrexate is considered the most active single agent and is frequently used in combination with other chemotherapeutics. In addition to traditional cytotoxic agents, rituximab is used by some experts in CD20-positive non-Hodgkin's lymphomas, though its use has not been validated by a randomized clinical trial.

F. AIDS-associated PCNSL

1. **Epidemiology.** PCNSL that occurs in the setting of AIDS has a particularly poor prognosis. PCNSL occurs in HIV-positive patients with a CD4 count less than 50 cells/microL and is an AIDS-defining illness.

2. **Imaging/Diagnostic tests.** In AIDS patients, the two most common causes of brain lesions are toxoplasmosis and PCNSL. SPECT and PET may be useful in differentiating these two entities.

   The pathogenesis of PCNSL in an immunosuppressed person is strongly tied to EBV infection, as the virus immortalizes B cells and drives their proliferation. In AIDS-associated PCNSL, the rate of EBV infection is 80% to 100%, in contrast to immunocompetent patient populations, where the EBV virus is detected in only 0 to 20% of individuals.

   CSF EBV PCR is thus highly sensitive and specific for HIV-associated PCNSL in an AIDS patient with an intracranial mass. Like PCNSL in immunocompetent individuals, CSF cytology is minimally invasive and can make a definitive diagnosis, but has a low sensitivity of around 25%. Again, the sensitivity of CSF analysis can be increased by concurrently performing flow cytometry.

3. **Treatment.** Many of the same principles of treatment described above apply to PCNSL in immunocompromised patients. The only difference is that in AIDS-associated PCNSL, the initiation of highly active antiretroviral therapy (HAART) is a cornerstone of treatment since spontaneous remission has been seen with initiation of HAART.

VI. EMBRYONAL TUMORS (WHO Grade IV)

A. Overview. Embryonal tumors encompass a wide variety of clinically important, mainly pediatric tumors that do not have a universally accepted classification scheme based on histopathologic criteria. They may demonstrate many different patterns of histologic differentiation. Some tumors included in this class are medulloblastoma, ependymoblastoma, medulloepithelioma, atypical teratoid/rhabdoid tumors, and all other tumors known as *supratentorial primitive neuroectodermal tumors* (PNETs). As a group, they represent aggressive, malignant tumors that are all rather rare with the exception of medulloblastoma. All are WHO grade IV tumors. Medulloblastoma, in particular, accounts for almost a fourth of all pediatric brain tumors and is the most common malignant brain tumor of childhood and in young adults, and as a result, will be reviewed in detail here. Of note, supratentorial PNETs occur most frequently in young adults in their second and third decades of life, and treatment options follow a similar approach as for medulloblastoma.

B. Medulloblastoma

1. **Epidemiology.** Medulloblastoma occurs primarily in children: 70% of these tumors are found in children younger than age 16 with a peak incidence between ages 5 and 7 years. Less commonly, medulloblastomas develop in adults; when it does, it occurs primarily in the third or fourth decade of life.

2. **Presentation.** These tumors are typically found in the cerebellum and frequently compress the fourth ventricle. Hence, most patients present with signs and symptoms of hydrocephalus such as papilledema, lethargy, headache, nausea/vomiting, and diplopia; or cerebellar signs and symptoms like nystagmus, clumsiness, and incoordination.

3. **Imaging/Diagnostic tests.** Radiographic features are of a midline, well-demarcated, densely enhancing cerebellar mass that is often hyperdense on noncontrast CT scan. Obstructive hydrocephalus is a common feature. On MRI, medulloblastomas are iso/hypointense on T1 and heterogeneous on T2 with heterogeneous contrast enhancement.

   In one-third of patients, there is dissemination through the CSF pathways, and rarely the tumor spreads systemically, usually to bone or lung. Hence, neuroimaging of the entire neuroaxis and CSF cytology (preoperatively if it can be performed safely or 10 to 14 days following surgical decompression if the patient is at risk of herniation) are mainstays of the initial evaluation.

4. **Pathology.** Medulloblastomas have been subclassified by gene expression profiling. It has been found that tumors with activation of *WNT* have the best prognosis, and tumors with amplification of *MYC* have the worst prognosis.

5. **Treatment.** A combined-modality approach is necessary for optimal treatment of these tumors. The goal of surgery in these tumors is always gross total resection, as this improves survival; unfortunately, invasion of the brainstem often limits the surgeon's ability to completely resect this tumor. Additionally, CSF diversion (temporary ventricular drainage, ventricular shunt, or third ventriculostomy) is often a necessary step in the surgical management of these patients.

   Since medulloblastomas are fairly radiosensitive, craniospinal radiation is often needed to achieve the best possible outcome. As CSF dissemination is common, patients with medulloblastoma are typically treated with radiation to the entire neuroaxis with a boost to the primary site. A notable exception is in children younger than 3 years old, in whom radiation is often withheld or minimized since the toxicity of radiation is significantly greater in this population. In these patients, chemotherapy is used to delay, avoid, or reduce the need for radiotherapy and is widely used. It is also frequently used as adjuvant therapy to reduce the risk of relapse. Chemosensitivity is variable, and a variety of protocols are used. At the time of disease recurrence or progression or in patients with high-risk genetic features and high disease burden, high-dose chemotherapy with hematopoietic stem cell rescue has demonstrated evidence of survival benefit, especially in pediatric and young adult patients.

   Unfavorable prognostic factors for these tumors include an age of presentation of less than 3 years, subtotal resection, dissemination at the time of diagnosis, MYC amplification, and large cell variance. In the last 30 years, outcomes have improved with the current 5-year survival ranging from 50% to 70%.

VII. NEURONAL TUMORS (WHO Grade I and II)

A. **Overview.** These tumors are varied in location and histology but share some degree of differentiation into neuronal cell types. All of these tumors are unusual and relatively benign. All are WHO grade I or II and are almost always controlled with surgical excision.

B. **Gangliogliomas and gangliocytomas** are benign tumors of either ganglionic and glial cells, or ganglionic cells alone. Gangliogliomas may occur anywhere in the CNS, but have a tendency to occur in the temporal lobe, where they are a frequent cause of medically intractable epilepsy. Rarely, the glial component may demonstrate anaplastic or malignant features and designate the tumor as high grade. Surgery is usually curative.

C. **Dysembryoplastic infantile astrocytomas/gangliogliomas** are large, cystic tumors of the cerebral cortex, often involving the leptomeninges, which are composed of poorly differentiated cells mixed with either neoplastic astrocytes or a neuronal component. They are often large, and typically cause macrocephaly in the affected infant.

D. **Dysembryoplastic neuroepithelial tumors** are hamartomata-like lesions that have been described in children and young adults, and are found predominantly in males. These tumors are frequently found during resection of lesions for treatment of refractory epilepsy. They are usually supratentorial, retain a cortical topography, and may deform the overlying skull. They may also be associated with areas of cortical dysplasia.

E. **Central neurocytoma** is a tumor of young adults that characteristically occurs in the lateral and third ventricles in the region of the foramen of Monro. They histologically resemble ependymomas or oligodendrogliomas and are designated WHO grade II. Typically, they cause obstructive hydrocephalus and result in headache, visual changes, or lethargy. In cases in which total resection cannot be performed, postoperative radiotherapy may be considered, although experience is limited.

VIII. TUMORS OF SPECIAL LOCATION

A. **Vestibular schwannomas (also known by the older term, acoustic neuroma)**

1. **Epidemiology.** These tumors represent 5% to 7% of intracranial tumors, but 80% of tumors in the cerebellopontine angle (CPA). They are slightly more common in women and are another important tumor type in neurofibromatosis type 2 (NF2). In NF2, they are present in 95% of patients; when vestibular schwannomas occur bilaterally, it is pathognomonic for this tumor predisposition syndrome since the development of bilateral sporadic vestibular schwannomas is exceedingly unlikely.

2. **Presentation.** Initial symptoms include hearing loss, tinnitus, and disequilibrium, which can progress to further neurologic deficits due to brainstem compression if not treated.

3. **Imaging/Diagnostic tests.** MRI evaluation demonstrates a rounded, enhancing mass extending into the internal auditory canal. CT imaging of the temporal bone often shows expansion of the internal auditory meatus. Evaluation of individuals must also include audiometric testing to assess hearing quantitatively.

4. **Pathology.** In sporadic vestibular schwannoma, like NF2-associated cases, these tumors harbor *NF2* mutations. Although they are histologically benign, they may cause significant morbidity because of its proximity to the brainstem and adherence to the cranial nerves.

5. **Treatment.** The decision regarding whether to proceed with treatment using either surgery and/or radiosurgery, considers the age and general medical condition of the patient, hearing status, patient symptoms, and the size of the tumor. Many vestibular schwannomas can be safely monitored with serial imaging studies and assessments of hearing and other neurological functions. Several surgical techniques exist, including middle fossa approaches, translabyrinthine approaches, and retro-sigmoid suboccipital approaches, each with inherent advantages and disadvantages. The goal of surgery is complete resection when safely possible, but may be limited because of close proximity to other cranial nerves and occasionally the brainstem. Some patients, particularly with larger vestibular schwannomas, develop hydrocephalus, which may require a diversionary CSF shunt. Radiosurgery is often an excellent and well-tolerated option, particularly for patients with smaller tumors, but can carry some risk of delayed hearing loss and cranial nerve dysfunction. Subtotal resection followed by stereotactic radiation is a reasonable treatment option as well in some situations, particularly for larger tumors in an effort to improve preservation of the function of the facial nerve and other structures.

   Management decisions are probably best made by a collaborative team including neurosurgeons, radiation oncologists, neuro-oncologists, neuro-otologists, and neuroradiologists.

Until recently, there were no promising medical therapies for vestibular schwannomas, and so the management of these tumors entailed balancing the risks of surgery or radiosurgery with the natural history of continued observation. It has recently been found that bevacizumab (which carries its own risks) has activity in controlling this tumor and preserving hearing. Currently, a phase II clinical trial (NCT01767792) is underway, to further evaluate bevacizumab's efficacy and safety in treating vestibular schwannoma, although it is currently being used off-label based on retrospective data.

The decision-making process is even more difficult in the patient with NF2 and bilateral vestibular schwannomas since these patients tend to be first seen at a younger age, have a higher morbidity associated with resection, and hearing is often compromised in both ears—increasing the stakes of any further hearing loss.

B. Pineal region tumors

1. **Overview.** Several tumor types occur in the pineal region and are therefore considered as a group under this heading, but in general are relatively uncommon tumors.

2. **Germ cell tumors**

   a. **Epidemiology.** Intracranial germ cell tumors generally occur in the midline, more often in the pineal region in men or the suprasellar region in women. Over half of the tumors that occur in the pineal region are germ cell tumors, and most of these are germinomas. These tumors are predominantly pediatric tumors, are unusual after young adulthood, and are predominately found in boys. They have an increased incidence in individuals with Klinefelter (XXY) syndrome and are more common in Asia, where it makes up greater than 10% of pediatric CNS tumors in case series from Japan.

   b. **Presentation.** These tumors, when they present as a pineal region tumor, commonly cause obstructive hydrocephalus because of their location and can cause Parinaud's syndrome including paresis of upgaze and convergence-retraction nystagmus.

   c. **Imaging/Diagnostic tests.** Radiologic appearance is somewhat nonspecific, but generally these tumors are T1 iso- or hypointense, T2 hyperintense, and contrastenhancing.

   The evaluation of someone with a suspected germ cell tumor includes serum and CSF markers such as human chorionic gonadotropin (HCG), alpha-fetoprotein (AFP), and placental alkaline phosphatase (PLAP). These markers are suggestive of certain histologies and are useful in determining prognosis and response to treatment. As many as 35% of germ cell tumors may show metastasis throughout the CNS at the time of discovery; therefore, it is imperative that an MRI is obtained of the entire spinal cord.

   d. **Pathology.** Germinomas are the most common type of germ cell tumor, and 30% will consist of a mixture of cell types. Germinomas make up 60% to 70% of germ cell tumors. They typically demonstrate positivity for PLAP, although HCG may also be present, as they are known to contain elements of syncytiotrophoblastic cells. These tumors are distinct from choriocarcinoma tumors that are positive for HCG, and histologically have evidence of both cytotrophoblastic and syncytiotrophoblastic elements.

   The remainder of germ cell tumors consist of teratomas (mature and immature), embryonal carcinomas, and yolk sac tumors. Positivity for AFP helps distinguish yolk sac tumors. Embryonal carcinoma may express HCG, AFP, or PLAP, although this is inconsistent. With the exception of mature teratomas, most germ cell tumors are considered malignant neoplasms.

   e. **Treatment.** Patients frequently present with hydrocephalus that needs to be addressed with a procedure that diverts CSF. Subsequently, tissue confirmation is typically necessary, particularly in the case of pure germinomas or mature teratomas, in which the tumor markers (HCG and AFP) are not helpful, in order to distinguish them from other types of pineal region tumors. Diagnostic tissue may be obtained by a stereotactic needle biopsy, a transventricular endoscopic technique, or an open transcranial approach, depending upon the circumstances.

Germinomas are exceptionally radiosensitive, and radiotherapy results in high rates of long-term survival. Chemotherapy is often used to reduce the dose of radiation needed to treat patients with germinomas, and it is used in nongerminomatous germ cell tumors, which are relatively insensitive to radiation, to improve long-term overall survival.

C. **Pineal parenchymal tumors.** The cells that make up the pineal gland perform a diverse array of neuroendocrine functions, and when neoplasias occur, a spectrum of differentiation from primitive to relatively terminal pineocytes occurs. Tumors are classified as pineocytomas, pineoblastomas, or some intermediate forms, and make up 15% of tumors in the region of the pineal gland. They appear similar to other tumor types in this area, and no serum markers are available.

Pineocytomas tend to occur in adults, are slow growing, and may show a variety of phenotypes such as neuronal or glial lesions. Pineoblastomas are more aggressive tumors that often disseminate throughout the CNS and resemble PNETs histologically.

D. **Other.** The remainder of pineal region tumors consist of small numbers of miscellaneous tumor types such as meningiomas, craniopharyngiomas, and hemangiomas.

E. **Treatment.** Management of these lesions is multidisciplinary and somewhat controversial. The pineal region remains a difficult region to access surgically, although an aggressive approach has been advocated by centers with more experience in lesions of this region. Some tumors that are benign may be more amenable to aggressive surgical resection, such as meningioma, epidermoid, and mature teratoma. Stereotactic biopsy is generally safe, although it also carries risk for morbidity and the chance for sampling error because of the mixed nature of many lesions. Several series have demonstrated the usefulness and safety of stereotactic biopsy in initial management of pineal tumors and cysts. The role of radiotherapy including stereotactic radiosurgery and chemotherapy in these tumors is significant.

SUGGESTED READINGS

Batchelor T, Loeffler JS. Primary CNS lymphoma. *J Clin Oncol* 2006;24(8):1281–1288.

Brastianos PK, Horowitz PM, Santagata S, et al. Genomic sequencing of meningiomas identifies oncogenic SMO and AKT1 mutations. *Nat Genet* 2013;45(3):285–289.

Caincross G, Wang M, Shaw E, et al. Phase III trial of chemoradiotherapy for anaplastic oligodendroglioma: long-term results of RTOG 9402. *J Clin Oncol* 2013;31(3):337–343.

Friedman HS, Prados MD, Wen PY. Bevacizumab alone and in combination with irinotecan in recurrent glioblastoma. *J Clin Oncol* 2009;27:4733–4740.

Hegi ME, Diserens AC, Gorlia T, et al. MGMT gene silencing and benefit from temozolomide in glioblastoma. *N Engl J Med* 2005;352(10):997–1003.

Kreisl TN, Kim L, Moore K, et al. Phase II trial of single-agent bevacizumab followed by bevacizumab plus irinotecan at tumor progression in recurrent glioblastoma. *J Clin Oncol.* 2009;27:740–745.

Lin AL, Gutmann DH. Advances in the treatment of neurofibromatosis-associated tumours. *Nat Rev Clin Oncol* 2013;10:616–624.

Lu-Emerson C, Eichler AF. Brain Metastases. *Continuum* 2012;18(2):295–311.

Stupp R, Mason WP, van den Bent MJ, et al. Radiotherapy plus concomitant and adjuvant temozolomide for glioblastoma. *N Engl J Med* 2005;352(10):987–996.

van den Bent MJ, Afra D, de Witte O, et al; EORTC radiotherapy and brain tumor groups and the UK Medical Research Council. Long-term efficacy of early versus delayed radiotherapy for low-grade astrocytoma and oligodendroglioma in adults: the EORTC 22845 randomized trial. *Lancet* 2005;366(9490):985–990.

Weller M, Pfister SM, Wick W, et al. Molecular neuro-oncology in clinical practice: a new horizon. *Lancet Oncology* 14(9):e370–e379.

I. APPROACH TO THE HEAD AND NECK CANCER PATIENT. Although there are many similarities between head and neck cancers arising from different sites, there are important site-specific differences in anatomy, etiology, molecular biology, and natural history. Collectively, these differences produce functional consequence that must be considered when deciding the optimal treatment approach. In addition, patients with head and neck cancer often have comorbid illnesses related to the effects of tobacco and alcohol use that may further complicate therapy.

II. BACKGROUND

   A. Squamous cell cancer of the head and neck (SCCHN) is an example of the multistep process of carcinogenesis consisting of accumulated genetic mutations that result in histologic changes ranging from hyperplasia to dysplasia to carcinoma in situ to invasive cancer. A number of genetic aberrations have been identified. Loss of tumor suppressor gene function, including *p16*, *p53*, and *RB*, are frequent, and amplification of the proto-oncogene cyclin D1, overexpression of the epidermal growth factor receptor (EGFR), and mutations in NOTCH1, FBXW7, and FAT1 also occur.

   B. Risk factors. For most patients, tobacco, often augmented by alcohol, is the source of carcinogens that results in these genetic aberrations. The incidence of new cancers of the head and neck is estimated at 45,000 per year in the United States, most of which are smoking-related. These figures underscore the importance of educating patients about smoking cessation. The male-to-female ratio is approximately 3:1. Among nonsmokers (estimated 15% of patients with SCCHN), viruses, including human papilloma virus (HPV) and Epstein–Barr virus (EBV), are causal factors. While smoking may induce SCC across all oral mucosal sites, HPV and EBV are most strongly implicated in the development of SCC of the oropharynx and nasopharynx, respectively.

III. OVERVIEW OF THERAPY FOR CANCERS OF THE HEAD AND NECK

   A. General considerations. Care of patients with cancers of the head and neck requires a multidisciplinary team that includes specialists in surgery, radiation oncology, medical oncology, nursing, speech pathology, dentistry, and supportive care. Nutritional support often plays an essential role in the care of these patients because swallowing may be impaired by the disease or as a consequence of therapy. Placement of a gastrostomy tube is often needed to provide an avenue to administer nutrition, fluids, and medications. Narcotics (transdermal and oral) are necessary to control pain due to tumor or treatment-related effects. The functional status of the patient and location of the tumor play a key role in determining the management of the patient. The following overview addresses the approach to the patient with SCCHN. Variation in therapy does occur, depending on site, and these variations will be discussed in their appropriate sections.

   The staging system for all sites of head and neck cancer, except for nasopharyngeal cancer, follows the same principles. T stage is subdivided into T0 (no evidence of primary tumor), T1 (≤2 cm), T2 (>2 but ≤4 cm), T3 (>4 cm), T4a (moderately advanced), and T4b (very advanced). N stage is subdivided into N0 (no regional lymph node involvement), N1 (single ipsilateral lymph node ≤3 cm), N2a (single ipsilateral lymph node >3 cm but ≤6 cm), N2b (multiple ipsilateral lymph nodes, none >6 cm), N2c (bilateral or contralateral lymph nodes, none >6 cm), and N3 (lymph node >6 cm). M stage is divided into M0 (no distant metastases) and M1 (distant metastases present). Stages I and II are defined by the presence of T1N0M0 and T2N0M0, respectively. Stage III is defined by T3N0M0 or T1-3N1. Stage IV may be subdivided into IVA (T4aN0-1M0 or T1-3N2), IVB (T4bN0-3M0 or T0-4N3), and IVC (any T and N plus M1).

B. Management of early-stage cancers (stage I to II). Early-stage SCCHN is managed with either surgery or definitive radiation therapy. Both approaches have similar cure rates. Advantages of surgery include shorter treatment and recovery time and avoidance of radiation toxicity including mucositis, xerostomia, and dental caries. However, surgery can result in organ dysfunction including speech and/or swallowing problems, particularly with open techniques, and has limited applicability in patients with poor performance status and comorbidities. Radiation therapy is an alternative to a surgical procedure that would result in unacceptable cosmesis and/or organ function. However, radiation therapy is given over an extended interval, and resolution of acute toxicities often requires several months. Also, chronic radiation toxicity (particularly xerostomia) is common, but can be somewhat mitigated with advanced techniques. Regional differences in the general approach to early-stage cancers exist, often hinging on advanced surgical or radiation expertise among members of the treatment team. The ultimate goal is a high cure rate with minimum morbidity.

C. Management of locally advanced, nonmetastatic disease (III to IVB)

1. **Primary surgery.** Surgery to remove all visible tumors may be used as the initial therapy for locally advanced cancers of the head and neck. Current approaches to surgery increasingly involve procedures such as transoral endoscopic CO_2 laser or robotic resection and selective neck dissections. In contrast to open procedures and radical neck dissections, these more recent approaches to surgery lower the morbidity of the procedure and improve the likelihood of acceptable postoperative function. Following complete resection, adjuvant radiation-based therapy is usually recommended to most patients with locally advanced disease. In some patients, a biopsy of the primary tumor by the surgeon and fine needle aspiration biopsy of suspicious regional nodes is performed for diagnosis, after which the patient is referred for definitive radiation-based therapy. Critical information regarding the delineation of tumor can be obtained with operative-based and sometimes with office endoscopy prior to proceeding with definitive nonsurgical therapies.

2. **Adjuvant therapy.** Following complete tumor resection, adjuvant therapy with post-operative radiation (POART) or radiation and concurrent chemotherapy (POACRT) is usually given to patients with locally advanced disease. Adjuvant therapy is recommended when there is involvement of one or more cervical lymph nodes, perineural involvement, lymphovascular invasion, and/or a positive surgical margin at the site of primary tumor resection. The total radiation dose in the adjuvant setting is 60 to 66 Gy administered to the primary and involved lymph nodes, and 50 Gy to lower risk nodal stations in the neck. The duration of radiation therapy is 6 to 7 weeks, with treatment optimally starting 4 to 6 weeks postoperatively. The exact fractionation schema, portals, and use of boost-dose radiation are determined by site. POACRT is recommended for tumors with high-risk pathologic features: involved cervical lymph nodes with extra-nodal extension and/or positive surgical margins (*N Engl J Med* 2004;350:1937; *N Engl J Med* 2004;350:1945). Some also include the following as high-risk features: tumors with perineural and lymphovascular invasion, multiple positive cervical nodes, and/or large (T3 or T4) primary tumors.

3. **Definitive chemoradiation.** Concurrent chemotherapy and radiation (CRT) is the standard of care for the nonsurgical management of locally advanced cancers of the head and neck in patients who are able to tolerate such therapy (those with good performance status and few or no comorbidities). The MACH-NC meta-analysis of 93 randomized trials of 17,346 patients demonstrated a significant overall survival (OS) benefit with CRT compared with radiation therapy alone (*Radioth Oncol* 2009;92:4). The OS benefit is 6.5% at 5 years with CRT. However, the acute toxicity (particularly mucositis and renal dysfunction) of CRT is greater than that of radiation alone, which may partly explain why the OS benefit of CRT is greatest for patients under age 60 years and who have good performance status and few comorbidities.

    Several chemotherapy agents have been combined concurrently with radiation therapy; however, the most commonly used agent is cisplatin. Recently, the EGFR inhibitor cetuximab was also shown to improve OS when given concurrently with definitive radiation therapy. Other chemotherapy agents that may be given with radiation therapy include carboplatin or taxanes (paclitaxel or docetaxel).

Cisplatin is widely recognized as the gold standard that other agents are compared to when given concurrently with radiation therapy in SCCHN. Two common regimens include cisplatin 100 mg/m^2 administered on days 1, 22, and 43 of radiation or cisplatin 30 to 40 mg/m^2 administered weekly during radiation.

A randomized trial of cetuximab given concurrently with radiation therapy versus radiation alone for definitive treatment of locally advanced squamous cell carcinoma of the oropharynx, larynx, and hypopharynx demonstrated an OS benefit with cetuximab. In the cetuximab arm of the trial, cetuximab (400 mg/m^2) was given 1 week before initiation of radiation, followed by 250 mg/m^2 weekly for the duration of the radiation (total of eight doses). Median OS increased from 29.3 months in the radiation alone arm to 49 months in the cetuximab plus radiation arm ($p = 0.006$). Survival at 3 years favored the cetuximab and radiation arm over the radiation alone arm (55% vs. 45%, $p = 0.05$, respectively). The toxicities were similar between the two arms with the exception of a greater risk of skin toxicities (acneiform rash and radiation dermatitis) and infusion reactions in the cetuximab arm. Surprisingly, the risk of mucositis with cetuximab and radiation was similar to that with radiation alone. An update of this trial confirmed that the OS benefit of cetuximab added to radiation persisted through 5 years of follow-up (*Lancet Oncol* 2010;11:21). Also, a retrospective analysis of this study found an association of grade 2 or greater acneiform rash with better OS and disease control in the cetuximab and radiation arm. Interestingly, the patients who benefited the most from the addition of cetuximab to radiation had the phenotypic features of HPV-related SCCHN: oropharyngeal site, younger age, limited smoking history, small T classification, and better performance status.

Thus, level I evidence supports the use of single agent cisplatin or cetuximab in combination with radiation therapy. However, a recent randomized trial (RTOG 0522) demonstrated that the addition of cetuximab to cisplatin and radiation resulted in more toxicity and no benefit. Retrospective analysis of RTOG trials found poorer disease control rates and OS when delivered doses of cisplatin were lower than the target doses, supporting the importance of dose intensity. The benefit of adding 5-FU or taxanes to cisplatin with radiation is uncertain.

4. **Salvage surgery following definitive chemoradiation.** If a complete tumor response is not achieved following definitive CRT or if the cancer recurs locally or regionally after CRT, salvage surgical resection of the primary tumor site and/or the neck nodes may result in long-term survival in a fraction of patients. However, salvage surgery may be technically challenging following CRT, and the morbidity of the procedure may be significant.

5. **Induction chemotherapy before definitive chemoradiation.** Randomized trials of induction chemotherapy have shown mixed results. The MACH-NC meta-analysis of these trials found that a survival benefit was not consistently observed with induction chemotherapy except in the subset of patients given cisplatin and 5-FU (PF). The TAX 324 trial compared two different induction regimens consisting of PF or PF plus docetaxel (TPF) given before definitive CRT with weekly carboplatin (*N Engl J Med* 2007;357:1705). TPF (docetaxel 75 mg/m^2 on day 1, cisplatin 100 mg/m^2 on day 1, and 5-FU 1,000 mg/m^2 CIVI daily on days 1 to 4 every 3 weeks) was compared with PF (cisplatin 100 mg/m^2 on day 1 and 5-FU 1,000 mg/m^2 CIVI daily on days 1 to 5 every 3 weeks) given for three cycles before definitive CRT. The median OS was significantly longer in the TPF arm compared with that in the PF arm (70.6 months vs. 30.1 months; $p = 0.0058$). The OS benefit of TPF over PF persisted at 6 years in an updated analysis (*Lancet Oncol* 2011;12:153). The TAX 323 trial was a randomized trial of similar design that compared TPF versus PF except that all patients had unresectable disease and all were treated with definitive radiation therapy alone (*N Engl J Med* 2077;357:1695). This trial also showed an OS benefit in the TPF arm compared with the PF arm.

The PARADIGM trial compared induction chemotherapy followed by definitive CRT with CRT alone using TPF as the induction chemotherapy (*Lancet Oncol* 2013;14:257). There was no improvement in OS for induction chemotherapy, possibly related to the failure to accrue the target number of patients and unexpectedly high OS in both arms perhaps due in part to the rising incidence of HPV-related oropharynx squamous cell carcinoma (OPSCC), which carry a better prognosis. In a recently reported randomized trial by the Spanish Head and Neck Cancer Cooperative Group (TTCC), induction chemotherapy failed to improve PFS or OS (*Ann Oncol* 2014;25:216). However, most patients in the induction chemotherapy arms did not receive the full dose of radiation therapy owing to excessive toxicity, which arguably may have been mitigated by more aggressive supportive care. The results of another randomized trial (GCTCC Italy) of induction chemotherapy followed by CRT compared with CRT alone are pending.

Induction chemotherapy may also be used as a method to predict tumor response to CRT. Early trials showed that a favorable response (partial or complete) at the primary tumor site to induction chemotherapy as assessed by clinical examination predicted for better long-term disease control after definitive CRT, whereas if the primary tumor site response to induction chemotherapy was unfavorable, it was less likely that the cancer would be cured by CRT alone. Such patients are usually treated by surgery followed by postoperative adjuvant therapy.

Current studies are investigating the use of induction chemotherapy as a method to select patients with favorable prognosis to be candidates for de-intensification CRT. ECOG 1308 is a phase II trial of patients with HPV-related OPSCC that uses the tumor response to induction chemotherapy to direct patients to standard dose (69.3 Gy) RT (if less than complete response [CR]) or to lower dose (54 Gy) RT (if CR). All patients receive cetuximab with RT. With early follow-up, the 1-year progression-free survivals were similar in both arms.

D. Management of locally and/or regionally recurrent disease. Patients with local or regional recurrence only should be evaluated for potential salvage surgery or radiation therapy. If salvage surgery is not possible, and radiation therapy has previously been administered, concurrent chemotherapy with repeat irradiation may be effective in some patients. However, tissue tolerance, the extent of earlier radiation, and significant toxicity limit routine recommendation for this approach. Patients who are not candidates for local therapies may be treated with palliative chemotherapy.

E. Management of metastatic disease. Median OS of patients with metastatic SCCHN is 6 to 8 months. Lung, bone, and liver are the most common sites of distant disease. HPV-related OPSCC may display unusual patterns of metastases delayed and multiorgan recurrences. Several standard chemotherapeutic agents have activity against SSCHN and can provide palliation of symptoms. These include cisplatin, carboplatin, 5-FU, paclitaxel, docetaxel, methotrexate, pemetrexed, ifosfamide, and gemcitabine. The most common first-line therapy is a platin combined with a second agent, usually a taxane or 5-FU. Combination chemotherapy results in a greater tumor response rate than single agent therapy, but median OS is similar with both treatment options (*J Clin Oncol* 1992;10.2:257). First-line chemotherapy has a tumor response rate of 20% to 40%. The ECOG 1395 study showed similar response rates, OS, and toxicity for the combinations of cisplatin and 5-FU or paclitaxel. (*J Clin Oncol* 2005;23:3562) (E1395). Furthermore, the ECOG 1393 showed no differences between high-dose (175 mg/m^2) and low-dose (135 mg/m^2) paclitaxel when combined with cisplatin (*J Clin Oncol* 2001;19:1088). In patients with platinum-refractory SCCHN, the tumor response rate of alternative standard chemotherapy is low.

Cetuximab has activity as first-line therapy and in platinum-refractory SCCHN. A randomized trial showed that the addition of cetuximab to platinum and 5-FU significantly improved median OS (10.1 vs. 7.4 months, respectively) and PFS (5.6 vs. 3.3 months, respectively) (*N Engl J Med* 2008;359:1116). This trial was the first to demonstrate an OS benefit with a targeted agent in incurable SCCHN. In platinum-refractory SCCHN, single agent cetuximab resulted in a tumor response rate of 13% and a disease control rate of 46% (*J Clin Oncol* 2007;25:2171). However, median time to progression (TTP) and OS were only 70 and 178 days, respectively. Erlotinib and gefitinib are EGFR tyrosine kinase inhibitors that have also been used to treat SCCHN. In a phase II trial, erlotinib resulted in a tumor response rate of 4%, a disease control rate of 38%, and a median OS of 6 months (*J Clin Oncol* 2004;22:77). Similar outcome data were seen with gefitinib. Both drugs are generally well tolerated, with the most common side effects being fatigue, rash, and diarrhea. The addition of gefitinib to docetaxel did not improve outcomes in poor prognosis patients with SCCHN (*J Clin Oncol* 2013;31:1405).

F. Complications of disease

1. **Aspiration** with risk of pneumonia should be considered in the patient with fever or cough. Weight loss or risk of aspiration may require placement of feeding gastrostomy tubes. Some patients will minimize aspiration with certain postures (chin tuck maneuver) or dietary modification, and consultation with a speech pathologist is often helpful in rehabilitation. Shortness of breath should prompt evaluation of the airway and the potential need for tracheostomy.

2. **Fungating tumors** may ulcerate, bleed, and cause airway obstruction. Invasion of the carotid artery by tumor may be a terminal event and may be heralded by an episode of sentinel bleeding.

3. **Pain control.** Inability to swallow may limit narcotic analgesic choices. Transdermal fentanyl patches allow longer pain relief, with concentrated opiate elixirs for breakthrough pain. Opiate doses should be titrated to achieve pain control. Tumors invading nerves at the skull base may produce neuropathic pain syndromes that are helped by coanalgesics such as amitriptyline or gabapentin.

4. **Paraneoplastic syndromes** may include hypercalcemia due to tumor secretion of PTHrP and syndrome of inappropriate secretion of antidiuretic hormone (SIADH).

G. Complications of treatment

1. **Complications of surgery** may affect cosmesis, speech, airway patency, and ability to swallow. Reconstructive flap techniques and prosthetics may minimize these problems. Neck dissection may result in shoulder weakness if resection or injury of the 11th cranial nerve occurs. After total laryngectomy, a tracheoesophageal puncture (TEP) may allow speech by diverting expired air into the esophagus to vibrate the remaining pharyngeal tissue or flap. An electrolarynx, a handheld device that serves as a vibratory source for phonation, may also be used to allow communication following laryngectomy.

2. **Acute radiation toxicity** may include severe painful mucositis, loss of taste sensation, and inability to swallow. Oral candidiasis complicating mucositis may be treated with topical agents (nystatin or clotrimazole) or systemic agents (fluconazole). A cocktail of equal volumes of diphenhydramine suspension, nystatin, viscous lidocaine, and aluminum hydroxide/magnesium hydroxide suspension may be used as a topical oral swish solution for mucositis. Some patients may prefer a solution of one teaspoon of baking soda and 1/2 teaspoon of salt in a quart of water for milder mucositis. Opiates are indicated for more severe pain. Skin toxicity in the radiation port should be treated with emollients such as Aquaphor or Biafine and wound dressings, as appropriate.

3. **Late radiation effects include xerostomia**, which may be addressed by frequent oral hydration, or pilocarpine. Pilocarpine may cause uncomfortable sweats, especially at higher doses. Artificial saliva is available but poorly accepted by most patients. Dental caries is a chronic toxicity that may lead to tooth loss. Good dental hygiene and use of fluoride preparations may minimize this complication. Osteoradionecrosis may be treated conservatively with antibiotics, surgical debridement, or hyperbaric oxygen therapy. Fibrosis of the neck tissues may result in trismus, lymphedema, and loss of range of motion. Exercises may be helpful in preventing trismus. Impaired swallowing due to weakness of pharyngeal constrictor muscles and aspiration may occur. Laryngeal edema may require tracheostomy for management and should prompt consideration of possible disease recurrence.

4. **Chemotherapy toxicities** vary according to the agents used. Chemotherapy given with radiation may increase the severity of mucositis. Cisplatin may cause nausea/

vomiting, nephrotoxicity, peripheral neuropathy, ototoxicity, and myelosuppression. 5-FU may cause myelosuppression and mucositis. Taxanes may result in alopecia, myelosuppression, myalgias, and allergic reactions. Cetuximab is associated with acneiform rash, dry skin or skin fissuring, paronychial inflammation, and hypersensitivity infusion reactions. Minocycline may be helpful in managing the rash.

IV. LIP AND ORAL CAVITY

A. **Anatomy.** Cancer of the lip and oral cavity is the most common site of malignancy in the head and neck representing 30% of total cancers. Sites contained within this group are cancers originating from the lip, floor of mouth, anterior two-thirds of the tongue, buccal mucosa, gingiva, hard palate, and retromolar trigone.

B. **Presentation.** Although this region is easily accessible, patients often present after a prolonged interval of symptoms and with advanced disease. Patients may present with symptoms such as nonhealing oral lesions, pain in the mouth or ear, trismus, and weight loss. A pertinent history should include assessment of tobacco use including chewing tobacco and alcohol consumption. Dental problems and a history of chronic mucosal irritation should also be noted. Determination of oral functional status (biting, chewing, swallowing, and speech) is essential.

On physical examination, complete evaluation of the nares, oral cavity, oropharynx, hypopharynx, and larynx should be performed by clinical exam and fiberoptic endoscopy or mirror exam. Evaluation for trismus and tongue movement is also important. Fixation of the tongue (ankyloglossia) and trismus suggest an advanced lesion. Palpation with a gloved finger should be used to inspect the lips, buccal mucosa, oral tongue, retromolar trigone, and floor of mouth. The state of the patient's dentition should also be noted. Cranial nerve evaluation should also be performed. The neck should be evaluated for lymphadenopathy. Level 1 neck nodes are located in the submandibular–submental region, level 2 nodes along the proximal third of the sternocleidomastoid muscle at the angle of the mandible, level 3 nodes along the middle third of the sternocleidomastoid muscle, level 4 nodes along the distal third of the sternocleidomastoid muscle, and level 5 nodes in the posterior triangle. Cancers of the lip and oral cavity tend to metastasize to level 1 and level 2 nodes first.

C. **Staging.** In addition to the history and physical examination, the staging evaluation should include an examination under anesthesia (EUA) and radiographic imaging. Computed tomography (CT) or magnetic resonance imaging (MRI) of the head and neck is necessary to obtain a better anatomical understanding of the extent of the cancer. A CT scan shows details of bone involvement, whereas MRI gives a better view of soft tissue involvement. Often these techniques are complementary. A panorex may also be helpful in examining for mandibular bony involvement. CT scan of the chest should be performed to rule out pulmonary metastasis. Fluorodeoxyglucose (FDG)-Positron Emission Tomography (PET)/CT is widely used in staging of patients with advanced disease and may aid in developing radiation ports.

D. **Pathology.** Squamous cell carcinoma is the leading histology of lip and oral cancers. Adverse pathologic features include depth of invasion, infiltrative borders, poorly differentiated tumors, and perineural and lymphovascular invasion. Sarcomatoid, spindle cell, and basaloid features may also portend a worse prognosis. Less common histologies include adenoid cystic carcinoma and mucoepidermoid cancer of the minor salivary glands. These will be discussed in more detail later in this chapter.

E. **Natural history of disease.** Squamous cell cancer of the lip and oral cavity presents most commonly as local or local–regional disease with relatively late spread to distant sites.

1. **Field cancerization** is an important concept in the natural history of head and neck cancer, especially oral cavity tumors. Because the exposure of the mucosa to carcinogens in tobacco is diffuse across the aerodigestive tract, invasive cancer may be surrounded by areas of dysplasia or carcinoma in situ. Patients with head and neck cancer are at an increased risk of development of second primary cancers in the head and neck, lung, and esophagus. The risk is approximately 3% to 4% per year and generally tapers at a lifelong risk of 20% to 25% in survivors of the first treated head and neck squamous cell carcinoma.

2. **Leukoplakia and erythroleukoplakia** are premalignant lesions of the oral mucosa, related to the epithelial injury due to tobacco and ethanol. Leukoplakia is a white patch of mucosa that cannot be scraped off. Erythroleukoplakia may appear red and velvety and more commonly demonstrates dysplasia or carcinoma in situ on biopsy. The risk of malignant transformation increases with duration of these lesions and is higher with erythroleukoplakia compared with leukoplakia.

Treatment may include close observation or surgical resection, particularly if high-grade dysplasia is present. Early studies of retinoids such as isotretinoin (13 *cis*-retinoic acid) showed promising results in the treatment of leukoplakia. Isotretinoin (1.5 mg/kg/day by mouth for 3 months followed by 0.5 mg/kg/day) produced a response rate of 55%, with most patients maintaining their response over the course of 1 year. However, a large randomized trial failed to show a reduction in the risk of second cancers or recurrence of the primary cancer with isotretinoin in patients who had been treated with definitive radiation therapy for stage I and II SCCHN (*J Natl Cancer Inst* 2006;98:441). This trial did show that smoking cessation after radiation treatment of the SCCHN was associated with a significantly lower risk of second cancers and improved OS compared with continued smoking.

F. **Treatment of lip and oral cavity SCC**
   1. **stages I and II.** Most patients are treated by surgery alone. Neck dissections are performed in patients with thick (>3 to 5 mm) or larger tumors. Radiation is an alternative to surgery in patients who decline surgery or are not surgical candidates.
   2. **stages III and IV.** Most patients are treated by surgery followed by adjuvant therapy based on pathologic features. CRT is an alternative to surgery in patients who decline surgery or are not surgical candidates.

V. OROPHARYNX

A. **Anatomy.** Cancer of the oropharynx includes sites in the soft palate, palatine tonsils, posterior and lateral oropharyngeal walls, and the base of tongue. Its borders include the junction of the hard and soft palate, the tonsillar arch, and the circumvallate papillae on the tongue.

B. **Presentation.** Many of the features described earlier for cancers of the oral cavity also apply to cancers of the oropharynx.
   1. **Pertinent history** should include an assessment of tobacco and alcohol use and comorbid diseases. Odynophagia, dysphagia, neck mass, otalgia, trismus, and weight loss should also be noted.
   2. **The physical examination** includes an assessment of performance status, complete evaluation of the nares, oral cavity, oropharynx, hypopharynx and larynx, and neck, and the cranial nerves. An evaluation for trismus, status of dentition, and tongue movement and atrophy should be performed along with palpation of the tongue, tonsils, and soft palate. Lymph nodes in the neck should be examined with measurements of palpable nodes, noting their size, level, and whether they are fixed to underlying tissue. Primary tumors of the oropharynx tend to first metastasize to level 2 and 3 nodes.

C. **Staging.** Along with history and physical examination, the staging evaluation of patients with oropharynx cancers includes diagnostic imaging, EUA with biopsy of the primary lesion, and evaluation for distant metastasis and synchronous primaries. CT or MRI of the primary site and neck and CT of the chest should be performed. FDG-PET/CT is often performed. The staging of oropharynx cancer is defined by the size and extent of the primary tumor, extent of nodal disease, and presence or absence of distant metastasis.

D. **Pathology.** Squamous cell carcinoma is the histology found in more than 90% of cancers of the oropharynx. Less common pathologies include lymphomas involving Waldeyer's ring (palatine and lingual tonsils, and adenoids), mucosal melanomas, and tumors arising in the minor salivary glands that lie in the mucosa, including adenocarcinomas, adenoid cystic carcinomas, and mucoepidermoid carcinomas. Distinction should be made between well-differentiated and poorly differentiated squamous cell carcinomas. Adverse pathologic features include increasing depth of invasion, infiltrative borders, poorly differentiated tumors, and perineural and lymphovascular invasion. Sarcomatoid differentiation or basaloid features may also portend a worse prognosis.

An increasing number of cancers of the oropharynx are found in younger patients who have little or no prior exposure to smoking (*J Clin Oncol* 2013;31:4550). Most of these patients are Caucasian males in their 40s or 50s who present with a level 2 or level 3 neck mass. These cancers are typically nonkeratinizing SCCs that are strongly positive for p16 expression (by immunohistochemical stain), a surrogate marker for HPV. HPV-related OPSCC often presents with small primary tumors, large necrotic neck nodes, and have an excellent prognosis with current multimodality therapy. However, smoking history as a continuous variable increases the risk for cancer recurrence (*J Clin Oncol* 2012;30:2102).

E. **Natural history of disease.** Squamous cell cancer of the oropharynx usually presents with locally advanced-stage disease. A significant proportion of patients who present with level two or three neck masses and unknown primary SCC are found on EUA with an operating room microscope and with directed biopsies to have HPV-related OPSCC. In smoking-related OPSCC, the effects of tobacco and alcohol on the mucosa increase the risk of second primary cancers due to field cancerization.

F. **Treatment of OPSCC**
   1. **Stages I and II.** Patients may be treated with surgery that includes resection of the primary tumor and possibly at-risk neck nodes. Radiation provides clinical equipoise with surgery, and is an alternative in patients who decline surgery or are not surgical candidates.
   2. **Stages III and IV.** Patients may be treated with surgery that includes resection of the primary tumor and grossly involved and at-risk neck nodes followed by adjuvant therapy based on pathologic features, CRT, or induction chemotherapy followed by CRT (*Cancer* 2013;119:766). It is not clear that there are any differences in overall disease control rates between these treatment approaches.

VI. LARYNX AND HYPOPHARYNX

A. **Anatomy.** Cancers of the larynx and hypopharynx represent challenges in treatment because of their key involvement with speech and swallowing. As such, these sites have been associated with the most research on organ preservation, attempts to avoid total laryngectomy, while maintaining the best chance for cure. The boundaries of the hypopharynx are the level of the hyoid bone superiorly and the lower border of the cricoid inferiorly. Tumors in this area may be divided into those arising from the pyriform sinuses, the posterior wall of the hypopharynx, and the postcricoid area. Tumors of the larynx may be divided into those located predominantly above the true vocal cords (supraglottic), those arising from the true vocal cords (glottic), or those below the true vocal cords (subglottic). Cancers of the larynx are far more common than cancers of the hypopharynx.

B. **Presentation.** The presentation of cancers of the larynx and hypopharynx varies greatly with their primary site. Tumors of the supraglottic larynx or the pyriform sinus are often diagnosed only after cervical metastasis appears because of their greater access to lymphatics and vague symptoms of dysphagia or odynophagia. Conversely, glottic cancers present with hoarseness, often despite a small tumor size, and the tumors may remain localized to the primary site until thyroid cartilage invasion occurs. Cancers of the larynx and hypopharynx may cause airway obstruction resulting in stridor and requirement for immediate tracheostomy. Weight loss is also frequent at presentation.
   1. **Pertinent history** should include tobacco and alcohol use, the existence of comorbid diseases, and symptoms of dysphagia, odynophagia, weight loss, dyspnea, and hoarseness. Unilateral paralysis of a vocal cord may result in speech that deteriorates with longer use of the voice and improves with rest. Patients may also become dyspneic with speech. Symptoms of aspiration should be sought. A history of gastroesophageal reflux should be noted.
   2. **Physical examination** includes assessment of performance status, complete evaluation of the oral cavity, oropharynx, hypopharynx, and larynx with indirect examination or fiberoptic laryngoscopy, testing of cranial nerves, and palpation of the neck. Palpation and visualization of the base of tongue should be done to note whether there is

superior extension of the tumor to this site. Pooling of saliva in the hypopharynx may interfere with the office examination and requires better visualization at the time of EUA and biopsy. Fixation of the true vocal cord should be noted, as this affects staging, and diagrams of the extent of the lesion are helpful.

C. **Staging.** The staging of cancers in the larynx and hypopharynx requires EUA with biopsy to determine the extent of the lesion and search for synchronous primary cancers. CT or MRI imaging is performed to define the extent of the primary disease and involved neck nodes. Chest CT and/or FDG-PET/CT are used to assess for distant metastases and second primary cancers. The tendency of the thyroid cartilage to display irregular calcification should be noted, as it may result in overestimating cartilage invasion on staging. In addition to size of the primary tumor, the staging criteria for the primary (T stage) include whether adjacent subsites of the hypopharynx (pyriform sinus, pharyngeal wall, and postcricoid region) or supraglottic larynx (suprahyoid epiglottis, infrahyoid epiglottis, aryepiglottic folds, arytenoids, and false vocal cords) are involved.

D. **Pathology.** Squamous cell carcinoma, or one of its variants, is the histologic description of more than 95% of tumors arising in the larynx and hypopharynx. Tumors of minor salivary gland histology (adenoid cystic, adenocarcinoma, and mucoepidermoid carcinoma) occur infrequently. The supraglottic larynx may be the site for neuroendocrine small cell carcinomas and should be recognized because of their tendency for distant spread and sensitivity to chemotherapy and radiation.

E. **Stage-directed approach to therapy**

1. **Stage I to II.** Early-stage disease is most likely to be encountered in glottic carcinomas owing to early symptoms of hoarseness. The primary approach may consist of surgical resection or radiation therapy with similar cure rates. In most cases, a larynx-conservation surgery approach is feasible, including a transoral endoscopic laser resection, open supraglottic, or open vertical hemilaryngectomy. These approaches permit preservation of speech but may be limited (particularly with the open approaches) by problems with aspiration, which can be problematic in patients with chronic pulmonary disease. Posttreatment voice quality is usually excellent with transoral surgery and radiation therapy, but may be less satisfactory with open approaches.

2. **Stage III to IV.** The traditional approach to locally advanced tumors of larynx and hypopharynx has been surgical resection with total laryngectomy or laryngopharyngectomy and adjuvant radiation therapy. However, CRT is also effective and allows preservation of speech and swallowing in the majority of patients.

   Interest in larynx preservation led to trials of chemotherapy and radiation in an attempt to avoid total laryngectomy and preserve anatomy and function. The Veterans Administration (VA) Larynx Trial compared laryngectomy and postoperative adjuvant radiation with induction chemotherapy followed by definitive radiation therapy for those patients whose tumors responded favorably to induction chemotherapy and total laryngectomy and adjuvant radiation for those patients whose tumors did not respond favorably to induction chemotherapy (*N Engl J Med* 1991;324:1685). Cisplatin and 5-FU were administered every 3 weeks, with primary tumor response assessment after the second cycle. Patients with tumors that responded favorably received an additional cycle of chemotherapy followed by definitive radiation, whereas patients whose tumors did not respond favorably underwent total laryngectomy followed by adjuvant radiation therapy. Salvage total laryngectomy was performed in patients with persistent or locally recurrent disease after radiation therapy. This treatment approach resulted in equivalent OS with induction chemotherapy and radiation therapy as compared with total laryngectomy and adjuvant radiation therapy and permitted 64% of the surviving patients in the nonsurgical treatment arm to retain their larynx.

   A European Organization for the Research and Treatment of Cancer (EORTC) trial in cancers of the pyriform sinus compared the results of surgical resection and adjuvant radiation therapy with a similar induction chemotherapy and radiation therapy strategy (*N Engl J Med* 2003;349:2091). Patients were randomized to surgery and adjuvant radiation therapy or induction chemotherapy with cisplatin and 5-FU followed by definitive radiation therapy. Patients with chemosensitive tumors as assessed after cycle 1 received a total of three cycles of chemotherapy followed by definitive radiation therapy with salvage surgery for nonresponders to chemotherapy or in those patients with persistent or recurrent disease following definitive radiation. As in the VA larynx trial, OS was equivalent between these two treatment approaches, and functional larynx preservation at 3 years was achieved in 42% (95% CI, 31% to 53%) of patients on the induction chemotherapy arm.

RTOG 91-11 was an intergroup, three-arm randomized trial that compared induction chemotherapy followed by definitive radiation therapy (as given in the VA trial) to CRT to radiation therapy alone. The CRT arm received three cycles of high dose (100 mg/m^2) bolus cisplatin given every 21 days concurrent with radiation therapy. Eligible patients included patients with stage III to IV laryngeal cancer who would require total laryngectomy as surgical management. Patients with T4 primaries were excluded if they had more than minimal thyroid cartilage invasion or more than 1-cm tumor extension onto the base of the tongue. The larynx preservation rate was significantly higher with CRT compared to induction chemotherapy followed by radiotherapy therapy and to radiation therapy only (83.6% vs. 70.5% vs. 65.7%, respectively). The 5-year OS were similar in the three arms (55%). Long-term (10-year) follow-up of the RTOG 91-11 trial showed that induction chemotherapy followed by radiation therapy and CRT had similar laryngeal-free survival, whereas deaths not due to larynx cancer or treatment were higher with CRT (30.8% vs. 20.8% with induction chemotherapy vs. 16.9% with radiation therapy alone) (*J Clin Oncol* 2013;31:845). Together, these trials demonstrate the feasibility of organ preservation in most cases of locally advanced cancers of the larynx and hypopharynx without adversely affecting survival.

The TREMPLIN trial was a phase II randomized trial comparing induction chemotherapy with TPF followed by CRT with cisplatin or with cetuximab in favorable responders (*J Clin Oncol* 2013;31:853). Poor responders underwent salvage surgery. No significant differences in early laryngeal preservation or OS occurred in the two arms. Long-term follow-up of this trial is required to determine whether these results are maintained.

F. **Natural history of disease.** Local–regional control is a major challenge in the treatment of patients with cancer of the larynx and hypopharynx. The lack of symptoms in early pyriform sinus cancers can be contrasted with the frequent development of symptoms (hoarseness) with early glottic cancer. The effect of anatomy with confinement of many laryngeal cancers to the primary site due to surrounding thyroid cartilage contrasts with the advanced disease typically seen in hypopharynx cancers, which typically have submucosal spread and local lymphovascular spread. Although most recurrences of laryngeal and hypopharyngeal cancers occur within the first 3 years after treatment, continued vigilance is warranted for the development of metachronous primary head and neck cancers. All patients should be repeatedly counseled about the benefits of smoking cessation. Also, patients with cancers of the larynx and hypopharynx are at significant risk for subsequent development of lung cancer.

VII. NASOPHARYNX CANCER

A. **Anatomy.** The borders of the nasopharynx include the choanae (anterior), the soft palate (inferior), and lateral walls, including the fossae of Rosenmuller and the eustachian tube orifices. Its sloping roof along the skull base (superior and posterior) lies in close proximity to the foramen lacerum and the carotid artery as it enters the cavernous sinus. Tumors may extend through the foramen ovale to access the middle cranial fossa and the cavernous sinus with access to the oculomotor (CN III), trochlear (CN IV), trigeminal (CN V), and abducens (CN VI) nerves. Optic nerve (CN II) and orbital invasion is possible in advanced cases. There is a rich lymphatic supply with retropharyngeal nodes, including the lateral retropharyngeal nodes (of Rouvière), representing an important route of spread.

B. **Presentation.** The presentation of nasopharyngeal cancer has many unique features. Symptoms at diagnosis may be related to the primary site, disease in the neck, or distant metastases. The epidemiology of this cancer is different from that of other head and neck sites. Causes of nasopharyngeal cancer include EBV infection, HPV infection, and smoking.

1. **Pertinent history** may include geographic, genetic, and environmental factors. The highest incidence of nasopharyngeal cancers is found in southern China and Southeast Asia. Genetic factors related to host response to EBV infection may explain the increased risk among people of Asian ancestry. Other risk factors have been implicated, including diet (consumption of salted fish and low intake of fresh fruits and vegetables) and smoking. Symptoms may include a painless neck mass, nasal obstruction, epistaxis, headache, persistent sinusitis symptoms, dysphagia, odynophagia, eustachian tube dysfunction with sterile middle ear effusion, or cranial neuropathies (particularly the abducens and trigeminal nerves). Trismus may indicate invasion of the pterygoid region.

2. **Physical examination** includes assessment of performance status, complete evaluation of the nares and oral cavity, and a thorough evaluation of the cranial nerves. Proptosis may indicate orbital invasion. Evaluation of the nasopharynx with fiberoptic endoscopy or examination under anesthesia with biopsy is appropriate. The status of dentition should be noted, as any needed restoration or extractions should precede the initiation of radiation therapy. Lymph nodes in the neck should be palpated and palpable nodes measured.

C. **Staging.** Along with history and physical examination, the staging evaluation of patients with nasopharynx cancers includes diagnostic imaging, including MRI and CT from the base of skull to clavicles, EUA, and Chest CT or FDG-PET/CT to look for distant metastases. MRI and CT are complementary and helpful for delineating disease extent due to early skull base involvement. The neck nodal staging system is different for nasopharyngeal carcinoma as compared with other mucosal sites of head and neck cancers. The staging for nasopharyngeal cancer is distinct from the other head and neck sites. T stage is subdivided into T0 (no evidence of primary tumor), T1 (no parapharyngeal extension), T2 (parapharyngeal extension), T3 (involvement of skull base or paranasal sinuses), and T4 (involvement of cranial nerves, hypopharynx, orbit, infratemporal fossa, or intracranial extension). The lymph node staging includes N0 (no regional lymph node metastasis), N1 (unilateral metastasis in cervical lymph nodes $\leq$6 cm above the supraclavicular fossa and/or unilateral or bilateral retropharyngeal lymph nodes $\leq$6 cm), N2 (bilateral cervical lymph nodes $\leq$6 cm), and N3 (lymph nodes >6 cm or extension to the supraclavicular fossa). Stage I is defined as T1N0M0, stage II as T1N1M0 or T2N0-1M0, and stage III as T1-2N2M0 or T3N0-2M0. Stage IV is subdivided into IVA (T4N0-2M0), IVB (T0-4, N3M0), and IVC (any T and N plus M1).

D. **Pathology.** Carcinomas represent 85% of nasopharynx tumors (less common are lymphoma, adenocarcinoma, melanoma, plasmacytoma, rhabdomyosarcoma, and others). Nasopharyngeal carcinoma is classified according to a World Health Organization (WHO) schema. WHO-Type 1 is keratinizing squamous cell carcinoma. WHO-Type 2 is nonkeratinizing squamous cell carcinoma, and WHO-Type 3 is undifferentiated carcinoma (lymphoepithelioma). EBV tumors are most closely associated with WHO Types 3 and 2 histologies. Nasopharyngeal carcinoma has recently been shown to also be more rarely associated with HPV infection.

E. **Stage-directed approach to therapy**
   1. **Early-stage disease** is infrequently diagnosed in the Western world because of lack of symptoms and no screening programs due to rarity of the disease. Radiation therapy alone is the usual treatment for early-stage disease. Surgical resection or repeat radiation therapy may be considered for the rare local recurrence.
   2. **Advanced-stage disease** is treated with CRT. The Intergroup 0099 trial demonstrated better OS with CRT compared with radiation therapy alone (*J Clin Oncol* 1998;16:1310). This randomized trial compared radiation therapy (70 Gy) alone with CRT (with cisplatin 100 mg/m^2 given every 21 days, total of three doses) and three cycles of adjuvant cisplatin and 5-FU given every 4 weeks after completion of CRT. The 3-year progression-free survival was 24% versus 69% (p <0.001), and 3-year OS was 47% versus 78% (p = 0.005) for radiation therapy alone versus CRT, respectively. This trial included all three WHO types. Other randomized trials confirmed the

benefit of CRT over radiation therapy alone in populations enriched in EBV-driven tumors and in stage II disease. Randomized trials have also established that adjuvant chemotherapy does not improve outcomes after CRT (*Lancet Oncol* 2012;13:163) and that carboplatin was noninferior to cisplatin when administered concurrently with radiation therapy (*Euro J Cancer* 2007;43:1399).

F. **Natural history of disease.** Nasopharyngeal carcinoma is a disease with unique features. A younger age at presentation compared with that for other sites of head and neck cancers and a higher incidence in endemic geographic areas are seen. Most patients present with locally advanced disease, and for many decades the most common pattern of recurrence was local–regional failure. However, with the advent of combined CRT and advanced radiation techniques, distant failure is now more common, and the risk of distant metastasis is higher than with other sites. The role of genetic factors and EBV are well recognized but poorly understood. Viral titers assessed by polymerase chain reaction (PCR) that remain elevated or rise after therapy may identify a group at risk for disease recurrence.

VIII. LESS COMMON TUMORS OF THE HEAD AND NECK

A. **Salivary gland cancers** most commonly arise in the parotid gland, but may arise in the submandibular, sublingual, or minor salivary glands that line the mucosa of the upper aerodigestive tract.

1. **Pathology.** The histology of salivary gland carcinoma is varied. Perineural invasion, high-grade tumors, and nodal metastases are adverse prognostic features.

    a. **Mucoepidermoid** carcinomas are the most common type arising in the parotid glands and are classified as low, intermediate, or high grade. Low-grade tumors respond well to surgical resection, whereas high-grade tumors are associated with more aggressive local invasion, and nodal and distant metastases.

    b. **Adenoid cystic carcinoma** is the most frequent histology seen in the submandibular and minor salivary glands. Perineural invasion may lead to facial nerve (CN VII) paralysis and involvement of the skull base. It is also classified by grade and has a significant incidence of distant metastatic disease. Patients with distant metastasis to the lung have a much longer survival as compared with the more uncommon patients that develop metastasis to the liver or bones.

    c. **Malignant mixed tumors** (carcinoma ex-pleomorphic adenoma) arise from a preexisting benign mixed tumor (pleomorphic adenoma).

    d. **Adenocarcinomas** commonly arise from the minor salivary glands but may also arise in the major salivary glands. They have an aggressive behavior and a significant risk of distant metastasis. Low-grade polymorphous adenocarcinomas arise in the oral cavity and have an excellent prognosis with complete resection.

    e. **Acinic cell carcinomas** usually arise in the parotid glands. They are typically low grade, slow growing tumors, but may invade adjacent structures. Unpredictably, a small number will behave very aggressively. These tumors can be bilateral. Late recurrences and distant metastases may occur.

    f. **Squamous cell carcinomas** arising from the excretory duct of the salivary glands have an aggressive course with a poor prognosis despite aggressive therapy.

    g. **Metastatic regional disease** to intraparotid nodes can occur from skin cancers arising from the face, scalp, or ears. These are primarily from squamous cell carcinoma, melanoma, and Merkel cell carcinoma.

2. **Treatment.** Management of salivary gland cancers is surgical resection. In the parotid gland, this may consist of total or superficial parotidectomy, depending on the location of the tumor and histology tumor type. When possible, the facial nerve may be preserved. High-grade tumors and low-grade tumors with a positive resection margin benefit from adjuvant radiation therapy. Recurrent or metastatic tumors may be treated with chemotherapy, including cisplatin, doxorubicin, 5-FU, and cyclophosphamide combinations. Recent reports have documented the expression of c-kit, her-2-neu, EGFR, and/or the androgen receptors in salivary gland cancers and case reports of tumor response to targeted therapy directed (*J Clin Oncol* 2006;24:2673).

B. **Tumors of the nasal cavity and paranasal sinuses** are rare tumors that include a variety of histologies. Risk factors may include occupational exposures to wood dust, shoe manufacture, nickel refining, and Thorotrast contrast media.

1. **Squamous cell carcinoma** is the most common type in the nasal cavity and paranasal sinuses, and the maxillary sinus is the most common primary site. Minor salivary gland tumors may also occur. Surgical resection and postoperative radiation therapy is the preferred treatment approach.

2. **Esthesioneuroblastoma** (olfactory neuroblastoma) arises from the olfactory neuroepithelium. Surgical resection and adjuvant radiation therapy is the preferred treatment approach. The benefit of the addition of chemotherapy to radiation therapy is unclear.

3. **Sinonasal undifferentiated carcinomas (SNUCs)** are high-grade epithelial malignancies that may occur with or without neuroendocrine differentiation. Ideal treatment is controversial and may include surgery and adjuvant radiation therapy, or CRT.

IX. UNKNOWN PRIMARY

A. **The patient with a neck mass** may not have a primary site identified on initial inspection of the oral cavity and pharynx. The location (level) of the neck mass should direct close evaluation of the head and neck mucosal sites that are drained by that nodal group.

1. **Fine needle aspiration for cytology** of the neck mass should be pursued as the primary diagnostic procedure. Open biopsy should be pursued if a lymphoma is suggested. Evaluation of the thyroid, parotid, and any suggestive skin lesions should be performed. A mass in the supraclavicular fossa should prompt evaluation of possible primary sites below the clavicles.

2. **If squamous cell carcinoma is suggested by the cytology,** EUA with operative endoscopy should be used to try to identify the primary tumor site. Use of an operating microscope or surgical robot during the endoscopy might assist with identification of the primary tumor, particularly when small. If no primary is found, then bilateral or ipsilateral palatine tonsillectomy and ipsilateral lingual tonsillectomy should be performed, as these would be the most common sites for an occult primary, and the pathologist should perform serial step sectioning on the specimens. True occult primaries without an easily identifiable mucosal site are usually p16-positive oropharyngeal cancers.

3. **If no primary site is found,** several approaches are considered. If the neck mass is unresectable, then radiation therapy or CRT with a nasopharyngeal port, which will include the likely potential primary sites, may be used. If a nasopharyngeal primary is suggested by the cytology, CRT may be considered. If the neck mass is resectable, neck dissection may be pursued as primary therapy. If the pathology shows extracapsular extension or if multiple nodes are involved, postoperative CRT may be given, with some controversy as to whether a nasopharyngeal port or involved neck-only port is most appropriate. If the neck mass is solitary, small (N1), and without extracapsular extension, adjuvant radiation therapy may be held and the patient closely observed.

X. MANAGEMENT OF THE NECK

A. **Patients with clinically negative** neck nodes that are at significant ($\geq$20%) risk for occult disease may be treated effectively with selective neck dissection or radiation therapy. Clinically involved nodes may require both modalities, especially if there are multiple nodes involved or extracapsular extension.

B. **Radical neck dissection** consists of removing all five lymph node groups on one side of the neck, as well as the sternocleidomastoid muscle, the internal jugular vein, and the spinal accessory nerve (CN XI). Modified radical neck dissections remove all five lymph node groups but may spare one or more of the latter structures. In a selective neck dissection, only lymph node groups at the highest risk are excised, and the sternocleidomastoid, jugular vein, and CN XI are preserved.

SUGGESTED READINGS

Adkins D, Ley J, Trinkaus K, et al. A phase 2 trial of induction *nab*-paclitaxel and cetuximab give with cisplatin and 5-fluorouracil followed by concurrent cisplatin and radiation for locally advanced squamous cell carcinoma of the head and neck. *Cancer* 2013;119:766–773.

Al-Sarraf M, LeBlanc M, Shanker Giri PG, et al. Chemoradiotherapy versus radiotherapy in patient with advanced nasopharyngeal cancer: phase III randomized intergroup study 0099. *J Clin Onol* 1998;16:1310–1317.

Argiris A, Ghebremichael M, Gilbert J, et al. Phase III randomized, placebo-controlled trial of docetaxel with or without gefitinib in recurrent or metastatic head and neck cancer: an eastern cooperative oncology group trial. *J Clin Oncol* 2013;31:1405–1414.

Chaturvedi AK, Anderson WF, Lortet-Tieulent J, et al. Worldwide trends in incidence rates for oral cavity and oropharyngeal cancers. *J Clin Oncol* 2013;31:4550–4559.

Gillison ML, Zhang Q, Jordan R, et al. Tobacco smoking and increased risk of death and progression for patients with p16-positive and p16-negative oropharyngeal cancer. *J Clin Oncol* 2012;30:2102–2111.

Haddad R, O'Neill A, Rabinowits G, et al. Induction chemotherapy followed by concurrent chemoradiotherapy (sequential chemoradiotherpy) versus concurrent chemoradiotherapy alone in locally advanced head and neck cancer (PARADIGM): a randomized phase 3 trial. *Lancet Oncol* 2013;14:257–264.

Hitt R, Grau JJ, Lopez-Pousa A, et al. A randomized phase III trial comparing induction chemotherapy followed by chemoradiotherapy versus chemoradiotherapy alone as treatment of unresectable head and neck cancer. *Ann Oncol* 2014; 25: 216–225.

Laura SA, Licitra L. Systemic therapy in the palliative management of advanced salivary gland cancers. *J Clin Oncol* 2006;24:2673–2678.

Vermorken JB, Remenar E, van Herpen C, et al. Cisplatin, fluorouracil, and docetaxel in unresectable head and neck cancer. *N Engl J Med* 2007;357:1695–1704.

Vermorken JB, Mesia R, Rivera F, et al. Platinum-based chemotherapy plus cetuximab in head and neck cancer. *N Engl J Med* 2008;359:1116–1127.

Posner MR, Hershock DM, Blajman CR, et al. Cisplatin and fluorouracil alone or with docetaxel in head and neck cancer. *N Engl J Med* 2007;357:1705–1715.

12 Lung Cancer

Ali Mohamed • Saiama N. Waqar

I. NON–SMALL CELL LUNG CANCER

A. Presentation

1. **Subjective.** Although patients with non–small cell lung cancer (NSCLC) can be asymptomatic at presentation and detected only by "routine" or screening radiographic examination, most patients present with symptoms related to local disease or distant metastasis. These symptoms may be secondary to a tumor in the lung, such as new or worsening cough, worsening or new dyspnea, and fever, secondary to postobstructive pneumonia. Hemoptysis, especially in the middle-aged or elderly smoker, should always raise the suspicion of lung cancer. Chest pain may signify chest wall involvement; dyspnea and hoarseness of the voice may indicate involvement of recurrent laryngeal nerve. Because of its long intrathoracic course, the left recurrent laryngeal nerve is more commonly affected than the right. Superior sulcus tumors can cause Pancoast syndrome; a triad of shoulder pain, lower brachial plexus palsy, and Horner syndrome. Swelling and engorgement of the face, upper trunk, and arms signal superior vena cava (SVC) syndrome, which is associated more with right-sided tumors. Patients with pleural effusions may have dyspnea and cough. Occasionally, dysphagia may be one of the dominant presenting symptoms secondary to mediastinal lymph node involvement. Symptoms suggesting distant metastasis are not specific and include weight loss, cachexia, and symptoms related to distant sites involved (e.g., bone pain or fractures from bone involvement, right upper quadrant abdominal pain with liver

metastases, and neurologic symptoms associated with central nervous system [CNS] involvement). Paraneoplastic syndromes associated with NSCLC include hypercalcemia (which can cause constipation, abdominal pain, and confusion) and hypertrophic pulmonary osteoarthropathy with marked clubbing, joint pains, and swelling.

2. **Objective.** Assessment of the performance status (PS) and signs of recent substantial weight loss carry a significant prognostic importance. The superficial lymph nodes, particularly the supraclavicular nodes, should be carefully examined, as enlargement of these nodes raises the high likelihood of metastatic involvement. Signs on examination of the chest can detect not only those signs related to pleural effusion, atelectasis, and postobstructive pneumonia, but can also help assess the severity of any underlying lung disease (e.g., chronic obstructive pulmonary disease [COPD]) that may influence subsequent management options. Careful abdominal examination may detect hepatomegaly suggesting metastatic disease. New focal neurologic signs may signify brain or spinal cord involvement.

B. Workup and staging

1. Laboratory data

Patients may present with laboratory abnormalities such as anemia due to chronic disease, hypercalcemia as part of a paraneoplastic syndrome, hyponatremia due to syndrome of inappropriate antidiuretic hormone syndrome, and elevated transaminases or hyperbilirubinemia due to liver metastasis. There are no reliable or clinically useful serum tumor markers for diagnosis or follow-up of lung cancer, though carcinoembryonic antigen (CEA) may be elevated in some patients.

2. Imaging

a. **Chest radiograph (CXR).** A perfectly normal CXR does not necessarily exclude lung cancer, as conventional CXR may not always identify hilar or mediastinal lesions. Lung cancer can present as a mass, peripheral nodule, hilar or mediastinal changes suggestive of lymphadenopathy, or pleural effusions. CXR may reveal areas of atelectasis suggesting endobronchial lesion, and pneumonic infiltrates may be seen in association with obstructing lesions.

b. **Computed tomography (CT)** scan of the chest is the most effective noninvasive study to evaluate suspected lung cancer. Although its sensitivity to detect mediastinal metastases is variable, it has a high negative predictive value. It can also help identify local invasion (e.g., chest wall, bones, and pleura). The upper abdomen is usually included in this study, and the liver and adrenal glands should be carefully inspected for evidence of metastases.

c. **Magnetic resonance imaging (MRI)** of the chest is not routinely used in the staging workup of patients with lung cancer. It is particularly helpful in the setting of suspected spinal cord, vascular, brachial plexus, or chest wall involvement. Brain MRI at presentation can help detect brain metastasis.

d. **Fluorodeoxyglucose (FDG) positron emission tomography (PET)** scan is a useful adjunct tool to complete the staging workup in patients with recently diagnosed NSCLC. The FDG PET scan has been demonstrated to be superior to CT scans in identifying mediastinal lymph node involvement and distant metastasis. FDG PET scan helps identify additional sites of disease in approximately 10% to 30% of patients that were not identified by the conventional workup.

3. Pathological diagnosis.
Flexible fiber optic bronchoscopy can help determine the extent of endobronchial lesions and obtain tissue for diagnosis (washings, brushings, bronchoalveolar lavage, transbronchial biopsy). Cytologic examination of sputum is sometimes helpful in diagnosing centrally located squamous cell cancer in patients who are not candidates for CT-guided needle biopsy or bronchoscopy.

Mediastinoscopy is very useful in determining the status of mediastinal lymph nodes in patients who are considered to be candidates for surgical resection. Evaluation of mediastinal lymph nodes by mediastinoscopy is critical before surgical resection. Normal-appearing mediastinal lymph nodes may contain metastatic disease, and sometimes enlarged lymph nodes in the mediastinum may represent only hyperplastic lymph nodes from postobstructive pneumonia or may represent old granulomatous infection. Cervical mediastinoscopy is more accurate for staging superior mediastinal lymph nodes, whereas extended or anterior (Chamberlain) approach is better for anterior mediastinal lymph nodes. Endoscopic and endobronchial ultrasonography are being increasingly utilized to biopsy the mediastinal lymph glands. Many thoracic surgeons do not perform preoperative mediastinoscopy if the CT chest and FDG PET reveal no abnormalities in the mediastinum.

Video-assisted thoracoscopic surgery (VATS) can be used to access peripheral nodules, suspected pleural disease, and effusions.

4. **Pathology.** Specific histopathological diagnosis is essential for the appropriate treatment of each patient. The vast majority of patients fall into two major subtypes: non–small cell lung cancer (NSCLC) and small cell lung cancer (SCLC). NSCLC accounts for 85% of lung cancers, with the most common histologies being adenocarcinoma, squamous cell carcinoma, and large cell carcinoma. The histological subtype and the molecular subtype influence treatment decisions. SCLC accounts for 13% of primary lung cancers, and the incidence has been declining.

5. **Staging.** The International Staging System (ISS) uses the TNM (tumor, node, metastasis) descriptive system. T stage is subdivided into T1 (≤3 cm), T2a (>3 to ≤5 cm), T2b (>5 to ≤7 cm), T3 (tumor >7 cm, separate nodules in the same lobe, atelectasis or obstructive pneumonitis of the entire lung, or direct involvement of adjacent organs), and T4 (invasion of the mediastinum, great vessels, trachea, recurrent laryngeal nerve, esophagus, vertebral body, carina, or separate nodules in an ipsilateral different lobe). N stage is subdivided into N1 (ipsilateral peribronchial or hilar lymph node), N2 (ipsilateral mediastinal lymph node), and N3 (contralateral mediastinal, contralateral hilar or any supraclavicular node involvement supraclavicular lymph node). M stage is subdivided into M1a (contralateral nodules, pleural nodules, malignant pleural or pericardial effusion) and M1b (distant metastases). Staging is subdivided into IA (T1N0M0), IB (T2aN0M0), IIA (T1a-2aN1M0 or T2bN0M0), IIB (T2bN1M0 or T3N0M0), IIIA (T1a-2bN2M0, T3N1-2M0, or T4N0-1M0), IIIB (TanyN3Mo), and IV (M1).

C. Therapy and prognosis

1. **Stages I and II.** Tl or T2 without extrapulmonary nodal disease (i.e., N2 or N3) is treated surgically whenever complete resection is possible. Preoperative assessment should determine the stage (for potential resection), cardiopulmonary reserve, and perioperative risk of intended procedure. Suitable surgical candidates are those with estimated forced expiratory volume in 1 second (FEV_1) or diffusing lung capacity for carbon monoxide (DLCO) after pneumonectomy of more than 40% and maximal O_2 consumption greater than 20 ml/kg/minute. Stage of disease, age of the patient, and extent of resection significantly affect mortality, which averages approximately 3% to 7%. Lobectomy is the most commonly used procedure and is preferred over pneumonectomy when complete resection is achieved. Segmentectomy and wedge resection are associated with two- to threefold increased risk of local recurrence (and should be reserved for situations in which the tumor is <3 cm and lobectomy cannot be done). If the chest wall is involved, then en bloc resection of the tumor with the involved chest mass and a minimum of 2 cm of normal chest wall in all directions beyond the tumor are recommended. Systemic mediastinal lymph node sampling during resection should be performed first. If nodes were not involved, complete lymph node dissection is not indicated. VATS is less invasive than open thoracotomy and associated with shorter recovery time as well as less surgical complications.

Definitive radiation therapy (RT) is an alternative for patients who are not candidates for surgery. Selection of patients for RT is based largely on the extent of the primary tumor and the prognostic factors. On the basis of retrospective data, the patterns of failure following surgery (lobectomy/pneumonectomy) or stereotactic body radiation therapy (SBRT) are comparable (*J Thorac Oncol* 2013;2:192). Survival after RT depends on the patient's overall health status, radiation dose, tumor size, and complete response by 6 months after completion of RT.

Preoperative RT is not considered appropriate in early-stage lung cancer. The role of postoperative radiotherapy (PORT) was evaluated in the PORT meta-analysis, which was a pooled analysis of 2,128 patients with lung cancer treated in nine randomized trials between 1966 and 1994, and demonstrated a 7% absolute reduction in 2-year overall survival, with the greatest detrimental effect in patients with stage I disease. In patients with Nl or N2 disease, two studies by the Lung Cancer Study Group (LCSG) and the British Medical Research Council (BMRC) concluded that PORT could improve local control but did not affect overall survival, possibly because of lack of effect on systemic disease. PORT is not recommended for patients with N0 or N1 disease, but may have some benefit in patients with N2 disease who are medically fit, and for patients with positive surgical margins.

Adjuvant chemotherapy was not standard of care until the last decade, since older adjuvant chemotherapy regimens studied did not show a survival benefit. From 1996 to 2005, a series of randomized studies of adjuvant chemotherapy in NSCLC were performed, using platinum doublets and triplets. An absolute 5-year survival benefit of 5.4% with adjuvant chemotherapy was found in a pooled analysis by the LACE collaborative group. This analysis included the five largest clinical trials that used adjuvant cisplatin-based chemotherapy after surgical resection [International Adjuvant Lung Cancer Trial (IALT), intergroup JBR.10 trial, Adjuvant Navelbine International Trialists Association (ANITA), European Big Lung trial, and the Adjuvant Lung Project Italy (ALPI)]. The survival benefit from adjuvant chemotherapy was greatest with the regimen of cisplatin and vinorelbine, with the most significant effect seen in patients with stage II and III NSCLC. Adjuvant chemotherapy should be considered for patients with stage II and III disease. The role of adjuvant chemotherapy in stage IB disease is controversial. American Society for Clinical Oncology (ASCO) and National Comprehensive Cancer Network (NCCN) recommended careful consideration for adjuvant chemotherapy in stage IB rather than routine use. So far, no prospective studies have demonstrated overall improvement in survival with molecularly targeted therapies in patients with completely resected NSCLC. The ongoing ALCHEMIST study, an NCI-sponsored study, will evaluate the benefit of adding molecularly targeted therapies in this setting in molecularly defined subgroups.

2. **Stage III.** Stage IIIA includes T3 Nl or N2 nodal disease. Patients with superior sulcus syndrome without mediastinal lymph gland involvement or disease involving the spine are candidates for surgery following induction chemoradiation.

Among patients with stage IIIA, surgery is the standard therapy for those with T3N1, followed by adjuvant chemotherapy, whereas the role of surgery is controversial for patients with stage IIIAN2, with no survival improvement from surgery after chemoradiotherapy in two large studies, the Intergroup 0139 and the European Organization for Research and Treatment of Cancer (EORTC) 08941. At present, definitive chemoradiation is considered standard of care for patients with T4, N2, or N3 involvement. When mediastinal involvement is detected only at the time of resection, surgery should be followed by adjuvant chemotherapy with or without sequential RT. Patients with superior sulcus syndrome without mediastinal lymph gland involvement or disease involving the spine are candidates for surgery following induction chemoradiation.

RT alone is not an optimal therapy in patients with unresectable stage III NSCLC and good PS, as the 5-year survival rates are only 5%.

It has been shown that the addition of chemotherapy to RT improves survival in patients with stage III NSCLC over RT alone. Chemotherapy administered concurrent with radiation is superior to induction chemotherapy followed by sequential thoracic radiation, due to improved survival, though at the cost of increased toxicity with increased incidence of acute esophagitis and pneumonitis. Common regimens in use include cisplatin and etoposide concurrent with radiation and carboplatin and paclitaxel concurrent with thoracic radiation. The role of consolidation chemotherapy with docetaxel was evaluated by the HOG-LUN 01-24 trial, where three cycles of docetaxel versus observation were given after concurrent chemoradiation using cisplatin and etoposide with thoracic radiation to 59.4 Gy (1.8 Gy/fraction). The updated results showed no significant difference in survival between the two groups, but more toxicities on the docetaxel arm (*Ann Oncol* 2012;23:1730–1738). Currently, concurrent chemoradiation with cisplatin-based doublet is recommended in patients with good PS and unresectable stage III disease. Although consolidation chemotherapy (chemotherapy after chemoradiotherapy) is commonly used, it has not been shown to improve outcomes in randomized clinical trials. For patients with poor PS, thoracic radiation alone or sequential chemotherapy followed by radiation are administered for symptom palliation and survival prolongation. Given the high incidence of eventual brain metastasis in patients with stage III disease, the role of prophylactic cranial irradiation (PCI) has been examined in this patient population. Although PCI resulted in decreased incidence of brain metastasis, there was no survival benefit from PCI in these patients. The RTOG 1306 study is examining the role of induction-targeted therapy followed by chemoradiotherapy in patients with locally advanced NSCLC.

3. **Stage IV**

   a. **Initial therapy.** Systemic chemotherapy improves survival in patients with previously untreated NSCLC over best supportive care (BSC). Some of the commonly used combination regimens in the treatment of NSCLC are listed in Appendix II. It is important that both the patient and the physician realize that the goal of systemic chemotherapy is not to cure the disease but rather to achieve palliation of symptoms and prolongation of survival without unacceptable toxicity. Patients with squamous NSCLC should be considered for platinum-based doublet therapy. The chemotherapy options include a platinum agent in combination with either a taxane (paclitaxel, docetaxel), vinorelbine, or gemcitabine and produce identical improvement in survival with slight differences in toxicity profile (*N Engl J Med* 2002;346:92). Carboplatin is commonly used in the United States in view of its favorable toxicity profile. A recent phase III trial showed higher response rates and less neurotoxicities with albumin-bound paclitaxel (nab-paclitaxel) plus carboplatin when compared with solvent-based paclitaxel (sb-paclitaxel) plus carboplatin (*J Clin Oncol* 2012;30:2055). The combination of pemetrexed and a platinum doublet (cisplatin or carboplatin) is reasonable choice for patients with metastatic nonsquamous NSCLC. The addition of bevacizumab to carboplatin–paclitaxel regimen was associated with improved overall survival in patients with advanced nonsquamous NSCLC and no brain metastases (*N Engl J Med* 2006;355:2542). The addition of cetuximab to platinum-doublet chemotherapy is associated with modest survival benefit, which may be related to the expression of epidermal growth factor receptor (EGFR; *Lancet Oncol* 2012;13:33). If tolerated, systemic chemotherapy should be given for four to six cycles in the absence of progressive disease. There is no evidence to indicate that prolonged courses of doublet chemotherapy result in improved survival. In elderly and patients with poor PS (PS2), single-agent chemotherapy (gemcitabine, vinorelbine, or a taxane) is appropriate.

   b. **Molecularly targeted therapy.** Patients with known driver mutation(s) should be treated with single-agent target therapy.

      i. **EGFR.** Initial studies with first generation reversible EGFR tyrosine kinase inhibitors (gefitinib and erlotinib) were conducted in molecularly unselected patients with previously treated NSCLC. The response rates for gefitinib were 11% and 18%, respectively, in the two Iressa Dose Evaluation in Advanced Lung Cancer (IDEAL) trials. However, gefitinib was not found to improve survival compared with placebo in the Iressa Survival Evaluation in Lung Cancer (ISEL) study. Erlotinib, another EGFR TKI, was found to improve both PFS and OS compared with placebo in the BR.21 study, and was approved by the U.S. Food and Drug Administration (FDA) in previously treated molecularly unselected patients, based on the results of this study. Clinical predictors for response to EGFR TKI include adenocarcinoma histology, female gender, East Asian ethnicity, and never smoker or previous light smoker status. Presence of activating EGFR tyrosine kinase mutations in the tumor, including deletion in exon 19 and L858R mutation involving exon 21 render the receptor constitutively active and predict for response to EGFR TKI therapy.

Gefitinib was the first EGFR TKI to be compared with chemotherapy in the frontline setting in light or never smokers in the Iressa Pan Asia Study (IPASS). Subset analysis confirmed improved response rates (71.2% vs. 47.3%) and significant progression-free survival advantage in patients with EGFR mutations (mainly exon 19 deletion or the exon 21 L858R mutation) who were treated with gefitinib compared with chemotherapy (*J Clin Oncol* 2011;29:2866). The OPTIMAL and EURTAC trials confirmed the progression-free survival and objective response rate advantages of erlotinib (EGFR TKI) in EGFR-mutant patients. Afatinib is a second-generation irreversible EGFR inhibitor that also targets HER2 and HER4 and was recently approved by the FDA for treatment of patients with activating EGFR tyrosine kinase mutations, based on the results of the phase III Lux-Lung 3 trial. In this study, afatinib was compared with cisplatin and pemetrexed in the frontline setting and was associated with significant improvement in PFS (11.1 vs. 6.9 months; HR 0.58, p=0.001) (*J Clin Oncol* 2013;31:3327). Most recently, it has been shown that this effect was specifically more pronounced in the subset of patients with exon 19 deletions.

However, despite the initial response, virtually all patients with EGFR-mutant NSCLC eventually develop disease progression on EGFR TKI therapy. Mechanisms of secondary resistance include EGFR T790M mutation (50% of patients), PIK3CA mutations, and gene amplifications of MET and HER2. Studies of third-generation EGFR TKIs (AZD 9291 and CO 1686) designed to target the T790M mutation have shown very promising results so far.

ii. **Anaplastic lymphoma kinase (ALK) gene rearrangements**. EML4-ALK is a novel fusion gene that is present in 3% of patients with advanced NSCLC. Additional partners of ALK fusion that have been described include TGF, KIF5B, and KLC1. ALK gene fusions are more commonly seen in younger patients with adenocarcinoma histology who report no history of tobacco smoking and have wild-type EGFR.

Crizotinib produces an impressive response rate of 57% in patients with ALK FISH–positive tumors. In a randomized second-line clinical trial comparing crizotinib with docetaxel or pemetrexed in ALK-positive patients, crizotinib was associated with a significant improvement in median PFS (7.7 vs. 3 months; HR 0.49, p < 0.001). Among the patients randomized to chemotherapy in this trial, pemetrexed was associated with improved PFS compared with docetaxel (4.2 vs. 2.6 months) (*N Engl J Med* 2013;368:2385). Crizotinib is currently being compared to chemotherapy with platinum plus pemetrexed in patients with ALK-positive tumors, in the frontline setting.

Resistance mechanisms to ALK inhibitors can be categorized as ALK-dominant, due to an ALK-resistant mutation or ALK copy number gain, or ALK-nondominant due to a second oncogene. Ceritinib is a selective oral tyrosine kinase inhibitor of ALK, which is 20 times as potent as crizotinib in inhibiting ALK. Ceritinib has activity both in patients who are ALK-inhibitor naïve (Overall Response Rate, ORR 70%) and in patients who have received prior ALK-inhibitor treatment (ORR 55%). Ceritinib crosses the blood–brain barrier and may be a good option for patients with brain metastasis, with ORR of 54% in target brain lesions. In view of the impressive ORR, ceritinib received accelerated approval by the FDA. Several novel ALK inhibitors are in development.

iii. **Other targetable molecular alterations in NSCLC.** ROS1 gene rearrangements are seen in 2% of patients with lung adenocarcinoma, and are also observed more commonly in never smokers. Crizotinib is an inhibitor of ROS1, in addition to MET and ALK. The response rate to crizotinib in patients whose tumors carry ROS1 gene fusions is 57%. KIF5B-RET gene fusion occurs in

1% of lung adenocarcinomas and represents novel targets in lung adenocarcinoma. Patients whose tumors carry RET gene fusions tend to be never smokers and younger, with small poorly differentiated primary tumors with N2 nodal involvement. A phase II study of cabozantinib, an inhibitor of RET tyrosine kinase activity, is ongoing. In the preliminary report of the first three patients enrolled, two patients had partial response (PR) and the third had stable disease.

BRAF mutations are also seen in 2% of lung adenocarcinomas, with half of them comprising of BRAF V600E mutations, while the remainder are characterized as non-V600E mutations. The response to BRAF inhibitor dabrafenib in patients with BRAF V600E mutations is 40% based on preliminary data from the BRF113928 study.

HER2 mutations involving exon 20 occur in 1% to 2% of patients with NSCLC. These mutations tend to occur in never smokers, and mostly in women. Afatinib, an inhibitor of HER1, HER2, and HER4 is associated with 100% disease control rate in a four-patient case series of HER2 mutation–positive lung adenocarcinoma, while trastuzumab-based therapies resulted in 96% disease control rate in 15 patients. The largest study of patients with HER2 mutation–positive patients with lung cancer is ongoing, in which patients are being treated with neratinib, an inhibitor of HER2, in combination with temsirolimus, an inhibitor of mTOR.

KRAS mutations are the most frequently observed somatic molecular alterations in lung adenocarcinoma (30%), occurring mostly in codons 12 and 13. KRAS mutations have proven difficult to target. The Biomarker-integrated Approaches of Targeted Therapy for Lung Cancer Elimination (BATTLE) trial included 14 patients with mutations in either BRAF or KRAS treated with sorafenib, with a disease control rate of 79%. A phase II study randomized patients with KRAS-mutant NSCLC to receive second-line docetaxel alone versus docetaxel in combination with selumetinib, an inhibitor of MEK. The selumetinib had an improved response rate (16%) compared with the docetaxel arm (0%), but the study failed to meet its primary end point of improvement in OS with addition of selumetinib to docetaxel.

c. **Maintenance therapy.** Frontline platinum-based doublet therapy is usually administered for four to six cycles, following which patients with significant side effects, fatigue, and decline in PS can be observed with serial imaging studies, with institution of second-line therapy at the time of disease progression. On the other hand, patients with good performance status with no disease progression following frontline platinum-doublet therapy who desire additional treatment can be considered for maintenance therapy. When the maintenance agent used is the same one used in conjunction with platinum in the frontline setting, it is called "continuation maintenance," whereas if the agent used for maintenance was not included in frontline therapy, it is termed maintenance therapy. Pemetrexed is a well-tolerated agent that has been studied as both switch maintenance following platinum-doublet therapy (*Lancet* 2009;374:1432) and continuation maintenance in the PARAMOUNT trial following four cycles of cisplatin and pemetrexed (*J Clin Oncol* 2013;23:2895), with improvement in both PFS and OS.

d. **Second-line therapy.** Prior treatment, presence of driver mutations, and the patient's overall health are important factors that impact the subsequent therapies for patients developing progressive disease after first-line chemotherapy. Docetaxel improves survival compared to BSC and chemotherapy with vinorelbine or ifosfamide, and pemetrexed has been found to be equivalent to docetaxel in the second-line setting (*J Clin Oncol* 2004;22:1589). Erlotinib improved survival compared with BSC in unselected previously treated patients (*N Engl J Med* 2005;353:123). However, single-agent chemotherapy is preferable to EGFR TKI in patients without EGFR mutation. The future for NSCLC therapy will depend on our better understanding of the tumor signaling pathways and inhibition of these pathways with novel agents or immunotherapy.

    e. Role of surgery or RT in stage IV NSCLC. An isolated metastatic lesion (e.g., brain) can be surgically resected before systemic therapy. Surgical intervention is also indicated in certain situations (e.g., metastatic lesion in weight-bearing bones, stabilization of spine). RT is indicated for palliation of the following:

        i. Atelectatic lobe, especially in COPD patients. Re-expansion is expected in 60% to 70% of patients if atelectasis has been present for less than 2 weeks.

        ii. Hemoptysis, intractable cough, and pain.

        iii. Metastatic disease. Bone: RT is used to alleviate pain and prevent impending fracture or compression syndrome. In case of pathologic fracture, RT is used in conjunction with orthopedic fixation to maintain function and activity. Brain: for solitary brain metastasis, better survival and function is seen when the lesion is resected before RT.

D. Follow-up. The recommendations with regard to surveillance imaging for patients who have been treated for NSCLC with no evidence of clinical or radiographical disease are somewhat arbitrary. NCCN guidelines recommend history, physical exam, and chest CT (with or without contrast) every 6 to 12 months for 2 years, then history, physical exam, and noncontrast CT chest annually. Routine PET CT or brain MRI is not recommended.

E. Background. Lung cancer is the second most common cancer and the leading cause of death due to malignancy in both men and women in the United States. An estimated 228,000 new cases will be diagnosed in 2013, with 160,000 deaths.

    1. Risk factors

        a. Tobacco use. Cigarette smoking is responsible for 90% of lung cancer cases, and 1 out of 10 individuals who smoke will develop lung cancer. The risk of developing lung cancer is directly related to the duration of smoking and persists for a long time, even after stopping smoking.

        b. RT. Patients treated with thoracic RT for breast cancer or lymphoma were shown to have a higher incidence of lung cancer.

        c. Coexisting lung diseases. These include COPD, chronic infections (e.g., tuberculosis), and others (e.g., alpha-1 antitrypsin deficiency, diffuse pulmonary fibrosis).

        d. Genetic factors. Lung cancer can be familial, and people with first-degree relatives diagnosed with lung cancer are at higher risk of developing it. However, the underlying gene abnormalities are ill-defined.

        e. Environmental exposure to asbestos, arsenic, chromium, hydrocarbons, radon, and uranium in mining workers and, less clearly, silicosis in smokers.

        f. Age. Incidence of lung cancer increases with age.

    2. Screening. The National Lung Cancer Screening Trial (NLST) demonstrated a 20% relative reduction in lung cancer specific mortality in high-risk population (old adult with 30 pack-year history of smoking) with the use of screening low-dose CT, compared with chest X-ray (*N Engl J Med* 2011;365:395). Currently, most of the medical societies recommend annual screening for lung cancer with low-dose CT scan in high-risk groups after an informed risk–benefit discussion.

F. Research initiatives. There is an ongoing effort to identify driver mutations in NSCLC and develop molecularly targeted therapies (see section on Molecularly Targeted Therapy). The Cancer Genome Atlas (TCGA) group has recently published results of comprehensive genomic analyses of squamous cell NSCLC and adenocarcinoma histology. In addition, there is great interest in applying immunotherapy in the treatment of lung cancer, including the use of the anti-CTLA4 drug ipilimumab, blockers of PD1 and PDL1, and lung cancer vaccines. Early results from studies involving PD-1 /PDL1- inhibitors show a response rate of 20% with relatively few toxicities. Some of the responses appear to be very durable.

II. SCLC

A. Presentation

    1. Subjective. Small cell lung cancer is primarily a disease of smokers, and is characterized by rapid doubling time, and early propensity to metastasize to lymph nodes and distant sites. Presenting symptoms often include shortness of breath, wheezing, cough, hemoptysis, chest pain, and postobstructive pneumonia. As the mediastinal lymph nodes are involved very commonly, patients can present with SVC syndrome (10% of patients at the time of diagnosis), hoarseness from recurrent laryngeal nerve compression or invasion, and dysphagia. Thirty percent of patients at some point in their disease course will have brain metastases; 90% of such patients will be symptomatic from brain metastases. Patients may present with bone pain due to painful bony metastasis.

2. **Objective.** The importance of a good physical examination in these patients cannot be emphasized enough because more than two-thirds of patients have obvious distant metastases, some of which can be recognized in the physical examination. This may include hepatomegaly, subcutaneous nodules, focal neurologic signs, palpable adenopathy, palpable subcutaneous or breast metastatic deposits, and bony tenderness. The most common sites of extrathoracic disease include bone (19% to 38% of all presenting patients), liver (17% to 34%), bone marrow (17% to 23%), and CNS (0% to 14%). Patients with liver metastasis may have abnormalities on hepatic function profile. Bone marrow involvement may be present, and when severe, can result in cytopenias. Paraneoplastic syndromes are also much more common in SCLC than NSCLC.

B. **Workup and staging**
   1. **Workup.** The physician should aim for a cost-effective workup that adequately stages the tumor for necessary therapeutic decisions. The key question is whether the patient has limited or extensive-stage disease, with the former being treated with thoracic radiation in addition to chemotherapy and the latter treated initially with chemotherapy alone. Therefore, once metastasis has been documented with extensive-stage disease, there is no need to document any other metastatic locations unless they are symptomatic, requiring palliative therapy.

   The typical radiographic appearance of SCLC is small primary tumors with large hilar and mediastinal lymph node involvement. Pleural effusions occur less frequently, though if present, upstage the patient to the "extensive stage" category.

   Staging for SCLC includes a CT scan of the chest and abdomen with contrast, to evaluate for primary tumor, nodal metastasis, and metastasis to liver and adrenal glands. Given the high propensity for brain metastasis in these patients, brain imaging (CT with contrast or brain MRI) should be performed for all patients at presentation. When distant metastasis is not apparent on these imaging studies, a PET scan should be performed. PET scans have been shown to upstage limited stage–SCLC to extensive stage–SCLC in up to 19% of patients (*Cancer Imaging* 2012;11:253).

   2. **Staging.** The Veterans Administration Lung Group staging system currently in use in North America categorizes patients into limited-stage and extensive-stage disease. Limited stage is defined as tumor confined to one hemithorax and regional lymph nodes and is often subjectively defined by what can fit into one RT portal. Extensive stage is defined as any disease outside limited stage. Generally, 30% to 40% of patients will have limited-stage, and 60% to 70%, extensive-stage disease. The same TNM staging system for NSCLC can be used in SCLC.

C. **Therapy and prognosis**
   1. **Limited stage**
      a. **Therapy.** The current standard of care is combined-modality therapy with chemotherapy and RT.
         i. **Chemotherapy.** Although patients with SCLC respond to chemotherapy initially, almost all will relapse and die from the disease. Combination chemotherapy results in higher response rates and longer survival than does single-agent chemotherapy. The overall response rate to treatment for limited-stage SCLC is estimated to be 80% to 90%. The combination of cisplatin and etoposide (PE) has been repeatedly demonstrated to yield similar or improved results as compared with any other studied combination, and is easily one of the most commonly used chemotherapeutic regimens for patients with SCLC. In addition, this combination is tolerated well when administered in conjunction with thoracic radiation. We typically administer PE for four to six cycles for those patients who have no evidence of progressive disease. A meta-analysis indicated that carboplatin can replace cisplatin without differences in outcome (*J Clin Oncol* 2012;30:1692).

    ii. RT. Administration of thoracic RT in conjunction with systemic chemotherapy has been shown to improve survival. A meta-analysis of 13 trials including 2,140 patients with limited disease demonstrated a higher survival rate for combined-modality approach with the combination of chemotherapy and thoracic RT as compared with combination chemotherapy alone, with the 3-year survival increasing from 8.9% to 14.3% (*N Engl J Med* 1992;327:1618). The intergroup 0096 study demonstrated improved survival with 1.5 Gy twice daily thoracic radiation to a dose of 45 Gy in 3 weeks, compared with 1.8 Gy once daily radiation to a total dose of 45Gy in 5 weeks (26% vs. 16%) (*N Engl J Med* 1999;340:265). The schedule of RT and temporal coordination with chemotherapy may be of some importance, with early RT associated with improved survival compared with treatment starting at the third or fourth cycles of chemotherapy (*J Clin Oncol* 2004;22:4785).

    iii. PCI. For those limited-stage patients who demonstrate a complete response to induction chemotherapy, PCI should be considered to reduce the incidence of brain metastasis and improve survival. A meta-analysis of 987 patients demonstrated a 16% decrease in mortality, 5.4% increase in 3-year survival, decreased incidence of brain metastasis, and prolonged disease-free survival in limited-stage patients who received PCI after complete response to induction chemotherapy (*N Engl J Med* 1999;341:476). The EORTC 08993 randomized 286 patients with any response to induction chemotherapy to PCI or observation. PCI was associated with improved 1-year overall survival from 13.3% to 27.1% (*N Engl J Med* 2007;357:664). Late neurocognitive dysfunction may develop, and careful consideration is imperative when treatment is offered to the elderly and patients with poor PS. Administering PCI after chemoradiation and in low doses per fractions could further reduce the risk of neurologic sequelae.

    iv. Surgery. Surgery followed by adjuvant chemotherapy is an option for patients with very limited disease, defined as T1-2N0M0.

2. Extensive stage

    a. Therapy. The current standard of care is platinum-based chemotherapy doublet, which has a 60% to 80% response rate. The combination PE is a commonly used regimen in patients with extensive-stage SCLC. The COCIS meta-analysis showed no significant differences in outcomes for patients treated with etoposide and either cisplatin or carboplatin (*J Clin Oncol* 2012;30:1692). Maintenance chemotherapy has not been shown to improve overall survival.

    Although the JCOG 9511 study showed improved survival from the combination of cisplatin and irinotecan compared with PE, confirmatory studies in the United States showed no difference in outcomes from the two regimens (*Cancer* 2010;116:5710).

    i. Relapsed SCLC. In spite of a high response rate, most patients with SCLC eventually have relapse of the disease and die of progressive disease. There are two categories of relapsed SCLC: sensitive relapse, that is, those who relapse 3 months after the completion of therapy, and resistant relapse, that is, those who have progressive disease during initial chemotherapy or those who have relapse within 3 months of completion of therapy. Although the response rates for the subgroup of patients with sensitive relapse is approximately 25%, fewer than 10% of patients with resistant relapse respond to salvage therapy. A number of single agents have been reported to be active in this setting including irinotecan (16% to 47%), paclitaxel (29%), docetaxel (25%), oral etoposide (23%), gemcitabine (6% to 16%), vinorelbine (15%), and temozolomide (16%). Topotecan is the only approved regimen for salvage chemotherapy in sensitive relapse patients. A phase III trial comparing topotecan with cyclophosphamide, adriamycin, and vincristine (CAV) reported similar survival and response rates, but lesser toxicity with topotecan

(*J Clin Oncol* 1999;17:658). A randomized study comparing oral and intravenous topotecan showed similar outcomes, with median overall survivals of 33 and 35 weeks, respectively (*J Clin Oncol* 2006;25:2086).

D. Prognosis. Unfavorable prognostic factors include extensive stage, poor PS, older age, hyponatremia, male gender, and elevated serum lactate dehydrogenase (LDH) and alkaline phosphatase. Of these, stage and PS are most powerfully associated with prognosis. The most important risk factor for treatment-related mortality, which can approach 5% in aggressive limited-stage therapy, is PS. Additionally, amplification of the *c-myc* oncogene is linked with shorter survival.

The natural history of the progression of this disease is that of rapid growth and early dissemination. The median survival of patients with limited-stage SCLC is 15 to 20 months. The reported 5-year survival varies from 10% to 13%. Median survival in extensive stage is 8 to 13 months, but only 2 to 4 months if untreated. From 50% to 80% of patients who survive longer than 2 years will have metastases to the brain.

E. Background

1. **Epidemiology.** The incidence of SCLC has been declining over the last few decades, accounting for only 13% of all newly diagnosed lung cancer cases (*J Clin Oncol* 2006;24:4539). It is a disease of the elderly, with age peaks at 70 to 74 years in men and 60 to 69 years in women. In addition, there has been a dramatic increase in the incidence among women, with a current incidence ratio of 1:1 between men and women.

2. **Risk factors.** Almost all patients with this cancer have a history of tobacco abuse: only 2% of 500 patients treated at the National Cancer Institute in one series denied ever smoking. Exposure to radioactive radon in mining also may be a risk factor.

F. Follow-up

1. **Secondary malignancies.** These patients are at high risk of developing other malignancies related to smoking. The cumulative risk of a second malignancy 15 years after diagnosis of SCLC is 70%. Overall, in 20% of long-term survivors in one large analysis, secondary malignancies developed. The risk of having a second primary lung cancer increases with time (14.4% after 10 years). If a new lung mass develops in a long-term survivor, the physician must obtain a biopsy to rule out a new primary malignancy that may not be SCLC. Additionally, these patients are at increased risk for other tobacco-related malignancies such as cancer of the upper aerodigestive tract (12.6% after 10 years).

2. **Smoking.** These patients should be strongly encouraged to stop smoking. Once a smoker quits, the risk of any type of lung cancer begins to decline, but it takes at least a decade for such patients to approach a risk equivalent to that of a nonsmoker.

SUGGESTED READINGS

Gerber D, Schiller J. Maintenance chemotherapy for advanced non-small-cell lung cancer: new life for an old idea. *J Clin Oncol* 2013;31:1009–1020.

Govindan R, Ding L, Griffith M, et al. Genomic landscape of non-small cell lung cancer in smokers and never-smokers. *Cell* 2012;150:1121–1134.

Kris MG, Johnson BE, Berry LD, et al. Using multiplexed assays of oncogenic drivers in lung cancer to select targeted drugs. *JAMA* 2014;311:1998–2006.

Mok TS, Wu L-Y, Thongprasert S, et al. Gefitinib or carboplatin-paclitaxel in pulmonary adenocarcinoma. *N Engl J Med* 2009;361:947–957.

National Lung Screening Trial Research T; Aberle DR, Adams AM, et al. Reduced lung-cancer mortality with low-dose computed tomographic screening. *N Engl J Med* 2011;365:395–409.

Sequist LV, Yang JC-H, Yamamoto N, et al. Phase III study of afatinib or cisplatin plus pemetrexed in patients with metastatic lung adenocarcinoma with *EGFR* mutations. *J Clin Oncol* 2013;3327–3334.

Shaw AT, Kim D-W, Nakagawa K, et al. Crizotinib versus chemotherapy in advanced *ALK*-positive lung cancer. *N Engl J Med* 2013;368:2385–2394.

Turrisi AT 3rd, Kim K, Blum R, et al. Twice-daily compared with once-daily thoracic radiotherapy in limited small-cell lung cancer treated concurrently with cisplatin and etoposide. *N Engl J Med* 1999;340:265–271.

13 Breast Cancer

Foluso Ademuyiwa • Rama Suresh
• Mathew J. Ellis • Cynthia X. Ma

I. BACKGROUND

A. Epidemiology. In developed countries, breast cancer is the most commonly diagnosed malignancy in women and is the second leading cause of cancer death. In 2013, the number of new breast cancers in the United States was estimated at 232,340 and the number of deaths at 39,620. Analysis of the Surveillance, Epidemiology, and End Results (SEER) data showed that breast cancer incidence rates were stable between 1973 and 1980. In the early 1980s, the incidence rates increased steeply because of increased detection by screening mammography. More recently, between 2006 and 2010, the total incidence of breast cancer declined by 2.3%. The overall mortality from breast cancer has been falling by an average of 1.9% each year over the last 10 years owing to better screening and adjuvant treatment.

B. Identifiable risk factors. Many women with breast cancer do not have any of the known risk factors, and the relative risks associated with each known factor are often quite modest. However, these factors have been formulated into several models to predict overall risk, of which the Gail model is the one most often used in the United States (http://www.cancer.gov/bcrisktool/).

1. Demographic factors. Women are 100 times more likely to have breast cancer as compared with men. SEER data analysis indicates that the incidence of breast cancer increases sharply between the ages 35 and 75, starts to plateau between 75 and 80, and then decreases. In the United States, breast cancer incidence is the highest in whites.

2. Hereditary factors. Only approximately 10% of patients with breast cancer have first-degree relatives with the disease. The risk of a true hereditary breast cancer syndrome, where the inheritance pattern suggests the presence of a dominant cancer gene, is determined by the number of first- or second-degree maternal or paternal relatives with breast or ovarian cancer and their age at diagnosis. When a genetic anomaly can be detected, it is usually in either the *BRCA1* or the *BRCA2* gene. Women with a loss-of-function mutation in a *BRCA1* and *BRCA2* allele have a 65% and 45% cumulative risk of developing breast cancer respectively (*Am J Hum Genet* 2003;72:1117). *BRCA1* and *BRCA2* mutations are more common in Ashkenazi Jews, where 2% of the population are carriers. Importantly, ovarian cancer has also been strongly linked to *BRCA1* mutations (44% by age 70) and to a lesser extent to *BRCA2* mutations (11% by age 70), and all patients with *BRCA1* or *BRCA2* mutations should consider a prophylactic bilateral oophorectomy after childbearing has been completed. Although an occasional case of primary peritoneal adenocarcinoma despite bilateral oophorectomy is described, the incidence is low, particularly if the surgeon was careful to remove all ovarian and fallopian tube tissue. A hysterectomy is not medically necessary since there is no increased risk of endometrial cancer. Both *BRCA1* and *BRCA2* are also general cancer predisposition genes with an increase in carriers of male breast, prostate, stomach, and pancreatic cancers. Other less common familial syndromes associated with inherited breast cancer risk include Li–Fraumeni and Li–Fraumeni-like syndrome (TP53 and CHK2), Cowden syndrome (PTEN), Peutz–Jaegers syndrome (LKB1), and homozygotes with ataxia telangiectasia (ATM).

3. History of breast cancer. Women with a previous invasive breast cancer are at risk of developing second breast cancer at an annual rate of 0.5% to 0.7%. Women with a history of ductal carcinoma in situ (DCIS) are at an increased risk of developing ipsilateral and contralateral breast cancers, with a cumulative incidence of 4.1% after 5 years.

4. **Benign breast disease.** Nonproliferative breast lesions such as cysts and ductal ectasia do not increase the risk for cancer. Proliferative breast lesions with atypia such as atypical ductal hyperplasia carry a 4- to 6-fold increase in the risk of developing cancer. Proliferative lesions without atypia such as fibroadenoma, intraductal papilloma, sclerosing adenosis, and radial scar carry a 1.5- to 2-fold risk of cancer. LCIS is associated with a 1% annual risk of developing cancer in either breast.

5. **Endocrine factors.** Higher endogenous estrogen levels are associated with an increased risk of breast cancer (Multiple Outcomes for Raloxifene Evaluation (MORE) trial and the Nurses Health Study). Early menarche, late menopause, nulliparity, and later age at first full-term pregnancy increase the risk of breast cancer presumably by elevating endogenous estrogen levels. Oral contraceptives (OCP) were initially thought to increase breast cancer risk slightly, but subsequent studies have not confirmed this association (*N Engl J Med* 2002;346:2025). Randomized studies of hormone replacement therapy (HRT) in postmenopausal women show that HRT increases incidence of breast cancer, particularly when a combined estrogen–progestin formulation is used. In the Women's Health Initiative trial, there was a 1.24-fold increased risk with combined estrogen and progesterone but no increased risk with estrogen-alone preparations (*JAMA* 2003;289:3243; *JAMA* 2006;295:1647). The Million Women Study, however, showed that both estrogen-alone and combined estrogen and progesterone preparations increase the risk. The risk is higher with an estrogen and progesterone combination (hazard ratio of 2) as compared with estrogen alone (hazard ratio of 1.3) (*Lancet* 2003;362:419).

6. **Dietary factors.** Postmenopausal obesity is associated with an increased incidence and mortality from breast cancer, perhaps through increased levels of circulating estrogen as a result of aromatization of adrenal androgens in adipose tissue. Alcohol consumption, as low as 3 drinks/week, has shown to increase the risk of breast cancer. There have been mixed results regarding associations with dietary fat intake, vitamins E, C, and A, selenium, alcohol, and caffeine.

7. **Environmental factors.** Women exposed to chest wall radiation, especially as children, adolescents, and young adults, have been shown to be at substantially increased risk for developing breast cancer throughout their lives. This a particularly severe problem in young women who received mantle radiation for Hodgkin's disease, where the lifetime risk for breast cancer is at least 19% by age 50 (average population risk at that age is approximately 4%), and one suspects that the lifetime incidence may be even higher.

8. **Protective factors.** Physical activity appears to reduce the risk of postmenopausal breast cancer. In addition, breastfeeding has shown to have a protective effect. The estimated risk reduction is 4.3% with every 12 months of breastfeeding.

C. **Histopathology of breast cancer.** The in situ carcinomas of the breast are classified as ductal (DCIS), lobular (LCIS), or Paget's disease of the nipple, which may have an associated component of DCIS or invasive carcinoma. Most invasive breast cancers are adenocarcinomas, with invasive ductal carcinoma being the commonest (80%) and invasive lobular carcinoma occurring approximately 10% of the time. Less common histopathologic types represent the remaining 10% and include the medullary, tubular, mucinous, papillary, squamous cell, adenoid cystic, metaplastic, secretory, cribriform, mixed, and undifferentiated types. Paget's disease of the nipple is a specialized form of ductal carcinoma that arises from the main excretory ducts in the breasts and extends to involve the skin of the nipple and areola. The pathologic hallmark is the presence of malignant intraepithelial adenocarcinoma cells (Paget's cells) occurring singly or in small groups within the epidermis of the nipple. It can just involve the nipple/areolar complex or be associated with either DCIS or invasive carcinoma. Inflammatory carcinomas infiltrate widely throughout the breast tissue and involve the lymphatic structures in the dermis, producing swelling, erythema, and tenderness in the involved breast. The diagnosis is clinical and requires redness or erythema to be present. Peau d'orange can be present without erythema and should not be considered inflammatory breast cancer (IBC). Traditionally, the prognosis for IBC has been considered to be poor. However, HER2 gene amplification is present in approximately 50% of cases, and with the use of a specific monoclonal antibody such as trastuzumab, the prognosis has improved.

   D. Screening. American Cancer Society has the following recommendations for breast cancer screening.

   1. Starting at age 40, yearly mammograms should be done and continued for as long as a woman is in good health.

   2. Clinical breast examination by a health professional approximately every 3 years for women in their 20s and 30s and annually for women aged 40 and above.

   3. Women should practice breast self-awareness and report any changes to their healthcare provider. Breast self-examination is an option for women in their 20s.

   4. Women at increased risk for breast cancer based on certain factors such as those with genetic mutation should get a mammogram and a magnetic resonance imaging (MRI) every year.

   Full-field digital mammography is a technique similar to film mammography, but the images are captured electronically and stored in a computer. Digital mammography is more expensive, but has the advantage of easy storage and ability to manipulate the image for clearer definition. Studies have shown that the diagnostic accuracy is superior to that with film mammography in women with dense breasts, women under the age of 50, and premenopausal and perimenopausal women (*N Engl J Med* 2005;353:1773). US of the breast may help in women with dense breasts as an adjunct to screening mammography (*Ann Oncol* 2004;15(Suppl 1):15). MRI of the breast as a screening technique is recommended only for women who are at an increased risk (more than 20% lifetime risk) of breast cancer with or without *BRCA1* or *BRCA2* mutation. In those patients, MRI is recommended in addition to yearly mammography. In other patients, MRI of the breast is not recommended for routine screening (*N Engl J Med* 2004;351:427; *J Clin Oncol* 2005;23:8469). Ductal lavage is considered investigational and has, to date, not proved to be useful for screening or diagnosis.

II. PRESENTATION

   A. History. The most common symptom is a painless breast mass. Some patients may have pain associated with the mass, unilateral nipple discharge, skin changes over the breast mass, and nipple retraction. Patients who have had the breast mass for a longer time may present with an ulcerating mass, and patients with inflammatory disease will complain of a "warm or hot" breast and have obvious erythema.

   B. Physical examination. A careful examination of the area should be performed after the patient has disrobed to the waist. Inspection of the area should include nipple and areolar complex for ulceration, thickening, and nonmilky nipple discharge; the breast for size, symmetry, and visible masses; the skin for color and thickening called the *peau d'orange* or *orange-peel skin* appearance; and the axilla and supraclavicular area for visible enlarged lymph nodes. The inspection should be done with the patient sitting in four views: with the arm against the side, the arm above the head, the arm on the hip position, and leaning forward. For palpation of the patient's breast, the patient should be supine with her arms raised above head. The entire breast, including the tail of the breast, should be palpated using the palmar aspect of the fingers in concentric circles. If a mass is felt then its size, shape, location, tenderness, consistency, and mobility should be noted. If nipple discharge is elicited by pressing the areolar area, the color, consistency, and quantity of any discharge should be recorded. The axilla, infraclavicular, and supraclavicular area should be palpated for lymph nodes in the sitting posture with the arm muscles relaxed.

III. WORKUP AND STAGING OF BREAST CANCER

   A. Evaluation of a breast mass. Although the physical characteristics on examination can make a physician suspect breast cancer, a biopsy provides definitive pathologic diagnosis. Mammogram helps evaluate the mass as well the rest of the ipsilateral breast and the contralateral breast. DCIS is usually an incidental finding on mammography as a cluster of microcalcifications. Suspicious lesions on mammogram should be biopsied by a core needle technique. Palpable masses may be biopsied by core needle, and although fine needle aspiration can also be used, core biopsies have the advantage of distinguishing between invasive disease, which require lymph node evaluation and DCIS, where nodal exploration can often be avoided. Incisional or excisional biopsy for diagnosis is rarely necessary and should be discouraged because once the diagnosis has been established by core biopsy, many patients can have their definitive breast surgery in a single procedure. If the mass is not palpable, biopsy can be conducted using the needle localization technique under mammographic guidance, US-guided core needle biopsy, or a stereotactic core biopsy using a special mammographic machine and table to localize the lesion. When the lesion is visible only by MRI, it may be used to guide the biopsy in some centers. If the biopsy result is benign and the lesion is considered to be of relatively low risk for cancer radiologically, then close follow-up (6 months) may be recommended. If the biopsy result is benign and the lesion is suggestive of cancer, this is considered nonconcordant, and a wire-localized surgical biopsy should be considered. If there are atypical epithelial changes in the biopsy, a surgical biopsy is often conducted because a more advanced lesion is ultimately present in a significant number of cases. Ultrasonography (US) can help differentiate solid from cystic lesions. A simple cyst should resolve with aspiration, and the aspirate should not be hemorrhagic. A cystic lesion should be biopsied if the aspirate produces hemorrhagic fluid, the lesion does not resolve, or recurs after aspiration. If there is a palpable mass, it needs to be core-biopsied to rule out malignancy, regardless of radiologic studies. MRI has 88% sensitivity, 67% specificity, and a 72% positive predictive value (superior to mammography) in breast cancer detection. It does not obviate the need for a subsequent biopsy of a mass as it is not specific enough to exclude a malignancy (*JAMA* 2004;292:2735). MRI is particularly useful in detecting the extent of tumors that are mammographically subtle or occult (e.g., lobular carcinomas). It is useful in the setting of adenocarcinoma of unknown primary site involving the axillary lymph node, where the detection of breast cancer by MRI can help direct further treatment. It is also useful to evaluate ipsilateral multifocal cancer in patients who are considering breast conservation therapy, and contralateral breast cancer when clinically suspected. MRI of the breast can also differentiate scar tissue from cancer, and can be used to detect local recurrence and residual cancer in patients with positive margin. MRI can also help assess response to neoadjuvant chemotherapy.

Pathologic evaluation should include standard tumor, node, metastasis (TNM) staging according to the latest American Joint Committee on Cancer (AJCC) criteria, estrogen receptor (ER), progesterone receptor (PgR), and HER2 measurements, tumor grade by Scarff-Bloom-Richardson (SBR) or Nottingham score, and the margin status. ER is expressed in approximately 75% of all breast cancers and is a predictor of responsiveness to endocrine therapies. About 20% to 25% of all breast cancers overexpress HER2 (a transmembrane tyrosine kinase receptor), a poor prognostic factor that is associated with high-grade disease, and a response to trastuzumab and other HER2-targeting agents. HER2 status can be measured by immunohistochemistry (IHC) or in situ hybridization (ISH). The most common form of ISH testing is using fluorescent in situ hybridization (FISH).

B. Staging of breast cancer. The AJCC staging system uses the TNM classification. The stage of the tumor has a strong influence on prognosis and treatment. The breast cancer staging may be summarized as follows: T1 (≤2 cm), T2 (>2 to 5 cm), T3 (>5 cm), T4 (direct extension to the chest wall, skin ulceration, or skin nodules), N1 microscopic (N1mic—>0.2 mm or more than 200 cells), N1 (1 to 3 axillary lymph nodes involved), N2 (4 to 9 axillary lymph nodes involved), N3 (10 or more axillary lymph nodes involved or infraclavicular lymph, or supraclavicular lymph node involvement), M1 (distant metastases). The staging groups include IA (T1N0M0), IB (TaN1micMO or T1N1micMO), IIA (T0-1N1M0 or T2N0M0), IIB (T2N1M0 or T3N0M0), IIIA (T0-3N2M0 or T3N1M0), IIIB (T4N0-2M0), IIIC (TanyN3M0), IV (M1). The 5-year overall survival rates for stages I, IIA, IIB, IIIA, IIIB, and IV are 95%, 85%, 70%, 52%, 48%, and 18% respectively (*Semin Radiat Oncol* 2009;19:195).

C. Staging workup of breast cancer

1. **Clinical examination.** A good clinical examination is required with careful inspection and palpation of the local lymph nodes, including supraclavicular and cervical nodes, skin, both breasts, abdomen, and spine.

2. **Laboratory tests.** Laboratory tests help physicians focus their workup for metastasis. An abnormal complete blood count (CBC) should prompt evaluation of the bone marrow for metastatic disease. Elevated levels of liver enzymes may suggest liver metastasis, and an elevated calcium/alkaline phosphatase level suggests bone metastasis. Levels of tumor markers CA 15-3, CA 27-29, and carcinoembryonic antigen (CEA) can be elevated in breast cancer. CA 15-3 and CA 27-29 have been evaluated for their ability to help in diagnosis, determine prognosis, predict recurrence of breast cancer after curative therapy, and monitor treatment response. The American Society of Clinical Oncology (ASCO) recommended in 2007 that there is not enough evidence to routinely use tumor markers to monitor for recurrence after primary breast cancer therapy. There is some evidence suggesting their use in the metastatic setting to monitor tumor response in select patients (*J Clin Oncol* 2001;19:1865).

3. **Radiologic tests.** Radiologic studies complete the clinical staging for breast cancer by detecting metastatic disease. A chest radiograph is fairly routine for almost all patients with invasive breast cancer, and a computed tomographic (CT) scan is recommended in patients who have stage III disease, localizing symptoms, or abnormal laboratory values suggesting liver disease. In stage II breast cancer, the use of CT is more controversial, but it is often ordered when the lymph nodes are positive. A bone scan should be obtained in patients with stage III disease, or localizing symptoms, or abnormal alkaline phosphatase. The role of fluorodeoxyglucose-positron emission tomography (FDG-PET) scan in staging breast cancer is evolving. It may be useful to detect occult systemic metastasis but care should be taken to never consider a patient to have advanced disease on the basis of PET alone without other corroboration, preferably by biopsy, because the false-positive rate associated with inflammatory conditions is high. Cardiac systolic function should be evaluated with multiple gated acquisition (MUGA) scan or echocardiogram before and during treatment with trastuzumab.

IV. THERAPY AND PROGNOSIS

A. **Ductal carcinoma in situ.** DCIS is a direct precursor of invasive breast cancer. The incidence of DCIS has increased with screening mammography where it is often diagnosed through the presence of a cluster of microcalcifications in more than 90% of the cases. Uncommonly, patients may have a mass, nodule, or other soft tissue changes. Although MRI may detect some foci that are not visible by mammography, it may also miss some mammographically visible foci. The pathologic subtypes of DCIS are the comedo, cribriform, micropapillary, papillary, and solid subtypes. Prognostically, they can be divided into comedo and noncomedo subtypes, the former being more often associated with subsequent recurrence. The modified Van Nuys prognostic index system (VNPI, Table 13-1), which takes into account several factors to predict the likelihood of recurrence after local excision, may be useful in clinical decision making.

1. **Local treatment**
   a. **Surgery.** Options include local excision and mastectomy. Although mastectomy yields a high cure rate at 98%, it may be considered unnecessarily aggressive

TABLE 13-1	Modified Van Nuys Prognostic Index		
Score	1	2	3
Size (mm)	≤15	16–40	>41
Margins (mm)	≥10	1–9	<1
Pathology	Non-high grade without necrosis	Non-high grade with necrosis	High grade with or without necrosis
Age (yr)	≤61	40–60	≤39

5-year disease-free survival for VNPI 4 to 6 = 100%, VNPI 7 to 9 = 100%, VNPI 10 to 12 = 97.6%.
10-year disease-free survival for VNPI 4 to 6 = 100%, VNPI 7 to 9 = 97.7%, VNPI 10 to 12 = 97.6%.
Adapted with permission from Silverstein MJ. Ductal carcinoma in situ: USC/Van Nuys prognostic index and the impact of margin status. *Breast* 2003;12:457–471.

surgery for a preinvasive condition when the amount of breast tissue involvement is low. As an alternative, patients may undergo breast-conserving therapy (BCT). Those who undergo BCT should consider adjuvant radiation therapy. Although a previous study suggested that a wide margin (>10 mm) is necessary to achieve the lowest chance of local recurrence (*J Clin Oncol* 2001;19:2263), this may be excessive, particularly since there is controversy regarding what constitutes a negative margin. Axillary lymph node involvement is rare (only 3.6%) and so is not routinely biopsied.

   b. Radiation therapy. The NSABP (National Surgical Adjuvant Breast Project) B17, EORTC (European Organisation for Research and Treatment of Cancer) 10853, and the UK/Australia/New Zealand (UK/A/NZ) trials showed that adjuvant radiation therapy after BCT for DCIS reduces the relative risk of local recurrence by 50% without improving overall survival (OS) and is usually recommended. In patients with a small, low VNPI DCIS, omitting adjuvant radiation therapy is controversial, but can be considered in motivated patients, particularly in the setting of older patients with small, low-grade ER+ lesions.

   c. Systemic therapy. In patients undergoing BCT and radiation therapy, the NSABP B24 study showed that tamoxifen reduces the relative risk of ipsilateral invasive breast cancer by 44% and noninvasive cancer by 18%, but the benefit was limited to ER+ DCIS. The risk of invasive ipsilateral recurrence at 15 years is 8.5% with tamoxifen compared with the 10% with placebo in addition to BCT and radiation, without a significant effect on OS. The NSABP B35 trial is looking at tamoxifen versus anastrozole in postmenopausal women with DCIS undergoing BCT and adjuvant radiation therapy. There is no role for chemotherapy in this disease.

B. Lobular carcinoma in situ. LCIS is a histologic biomarker that identifies women at increased risk for subsequent development of an invasive cancer in either breast (approximately 1% per year to a maximum risk of approximately 17.6% by year 25). It is usually not detected clinically and is an incidental finding in patients undergoing breast biopsy. Since the increased risk of breast cancer persists beyond 20 years, lifelong follow-up is suggested. Most of the subsequent cancers are infiltrating ductal (rather than lobular) carcinomas.

   1. Local treatment. LCIS can be managed by close follow-up with clinical breast examination every 6 to 12 months and annual mammogram. It is usually multicentric and bilateral, and there is no evidence that re-excision to obtain histologically negative surgical margins is beneficial. Bilateral prophylactic mastectomy can be considered in select patients who are unwilling to accept the risk of bilateral breast cancers, unable to follow up closely, or take prophylactic endocrine therapy. There is no role for radiation therapy.

   2. Systemic therapy. The NSABP tamoxifen prevention trial (NSABP P1) showed that the use of tamoxifen at 20 mg daily for 5 years is associated with a decrease in the risk of developing breast cancer by 56% in women with LCIS (*J Natl Cancer Inst* 1998;90:1371). The NSABP P2 trial showed equivalent benefit with raloxifene 60 mg daily for 5 years when compared with tamoxifen. There was decreased risk of thrombotic events and uterine cancer with raloxifene. There is no role for chemotherapy.

C. Treatment of early-stage invasive breast cancer (stages I to III). A multidisciplinary approach that includes surgery, radiation therapy, chemotherapy, hormone therapy, and anti-HER2 agents, such as trastuzumab and pertuzumab is used to treat these patients.

   1. Local treatment
   a. Surgery
      i. Primary tumor surgical approaches. Lumpectomy/BCT with adjuvant radiation therapy and modified radical mastectomy (with or without reconstructive surgery) shows similar survival and local control (*N Engl J Med* 1995;332:907). Radical mastectomy is no longer performed after the NSABP B04 trial showed that the procedure is not superior and has more morbidity than total mastectomy without muscle resection. The selection of a surgical approach depends on the size of the tumor in relation to the size of the breast, patient preference, and the presence or absence of contraindication to BCT.

The absolute contraindications are multicentric disease (two or more primary tumors in separate quadrants), extensive malignant-appearing microcalcifications, persistent positive margins despite repeat re-excision surgery after BCT, and previous breast or mantle irradiation. The relative contraindications include pregnancy, history of collagen vascular disease, and large pendulous breasts because of the risk of marked fibrosis and osteonecrosis after adjuvant radiation in these patients. Tumors more than 5 cm and focally positive margins are also relative contraindications to BCT, although for unifocal large T2 and T3 breast masses, neoadjuvant systemic therapy to improve the chance of breast-conserving surgery (BCS) can be considered. The age of the patient is not a criterion for selection of the type of local surgery. Family history of breast cancer is not a contraindication to BCT. In patients who are positive for *BRCA1* or *BRCA2* mutation, bilateral mastectomy is often recommended because of the very high risk for second breast cancer. If the patient still chooses to undergo BCT, very close follow-up with MRI and mammography is recommended.

ii. **Axillary lymph node surgical approaches.** Axillary lymph node status is one of the most important prognostic factors in breast cancer, and so axillary lymph node dissection (ALND) is important diagnostically and therapeutically. The sentinel lymph node (SLN) is the first lymph node that drains the tumor. In an effort to decrease the chances of arm lymphedema with ALND, SLN biopsy was evaluated in patients with a clinically negative axilla. ASCO has endorsed SLN biopsy as an alternative to full ALND in this setting (*J Clin Oncol* 2005;23:7703). SLN biopsy has been evaluated in women with T1 and T2 disease, without multifocal involvement and without clinically positive axillary lymph nodes (*N Engl J Med* 1998;337:941). Vital blue dye and/or technetium-labeled sulfur is injected in and around the tumor or biopsy site. The ipsilateral axilla is explored, and the first lymph node that has taken up the dye or radioactive material is excised and examined pathologically. The negative predictive value of this procedure in experienced hands is 93% to 97%. If the SLN is negative, further exploration of the axilla is not required. The management of a positive SLN biopsy is controversial. Based on Z0011 data, when less than three SLNs are positive in the setting of lumpectomy for T1 or T2 tumor without palpable lymph nodes before surgery and anticipated adjuvant radiation therapy, ALND may not be necessary. ALND remains a standard in most patients with clinically positive lymph nodes and in those with more advanced disease and those undergoing a mastectomy.

iii. **Breast-reconstruction techniques.** If a patient undergoes mastectomy, her options for breast reconstruction are a prosthetic device such as a saline or silicone implant under the pectoralis muscle and autogenous tissue reconstruction using myocutaneous flaps such as a transverse rectus abdominis myocutaneous (TRAM) flap or a latissimus dorsi flap. To improve cosmesis, the patient may elect to undergo another surgery to reconstruct the nipple/areolar complex. The only contraindication to reconstructive surgery is comorbid conditions that would make it difficult to do a longer surgery or reduce the vascular viability of a tissue flap (small vessel disease). Surgery to the contralateral breast may be needed to achieve a symmetrical appearance. Postmastectomy surveillance for reconstructed breasts has usually been performed by physical examination.

iv. **The role of neoadjuvant systemic therapy.** Neoadjuvant systemic therapy is considered in patients with locally advanced breast cancer. Tumor regression increases the opportunities for BCT. There is no difference in survival if the chemotherapy is given before or after the surgery. In addition, pathologic response to neoadjuvant therapy provides prognosis prediction. Patients with a pathologic complete response (pCR) experience excellent long-term outcome.

b. **Adjuvant radiation therapy.** Adjuvant radiation is indicated for women treated with BCT, but also in some patients after mastectomy if the tumor was T3 or T4, with positive margin, or with more than 3 positive lymph nodes or node-negative but triple negative pathology. Patients who had a mastectomy with T1-2 and 1-3 positive lymph nodes or T3N0 disease should be referred to radiation oncologists to discuss potential risks and benefits of radiation. Adjuvant radiation halves the rate of disease recurrence and reduces the breast cancer deaths by about a sixth (*Lancet* 2011;378:1707). The benefit is seen in both node-positive and node-negative patients. The conventional whole breast radiation delivers a dose of 4,500 to 5,000 cGy to the breast over 5 to 6 weeks. A radiation boost of 1,000 to 1,500 cGy to the tumor bed is often administered. For patients found to have negative axillary nodes by sentinel lymph node biopsy (SLNB) or ALND, regional nodal irradiation is not recommended. Patients with positive axillary nodes may benefit from regional nodal irradiation in addition to irradiation of the intact breast. In patients with four or more positive axillary nodes, the radiation field should include the supraclavicular nodes, and the upper internal mammary nodes should also be considered. In patients with 1 to 3 positive nodes, radiation to the supraclavicular area and internal mammary is optional, but is often performed because subset analyses of chest wall radiation studies have suggested there may be a survival benefit for nodal radiation in this subgroup. The internal mammary nodes must be irradiated if they are clinically or pathologically positive. Partial breast radiation with interstitial implants has been studied in early-stage breast cancer patients after BCT as an alternative to whole breast irradiation. Although the early results are promising, long-term results are still awaited.

The risk of local recurrence in postmastectomy patients is high when the tumor is more than 5 cm, there are positive margins, more than four positive nodes, lymphovascular invasion, and the patient is young, and premenopausal with ER− tumor. In these patients, chest wall, axillary, and supraclavicular radiation should be administered to reduce locoregional recurrence. In patients with fewer positive nodes, the axilla and supraclavicular area should be evaluated. The internal mammary nodes should be evaluated in all the patients receiving postmastectomy radiation therapy and should be treated if the nodes are clinically or pathologically positive. Adjuvant radiation therapy is given after completing all adjuvant chemotherapy as concurrent therapy increases the side effects of radiation therapy.

2. **Systemic therapy**

   a. **Adjuvant systemic therapy.** Adjuvant systemic therapy addresses the possibility of occult micrometastasis, which can, with time, grow into overt metastatic disease. Over the last three to four decades, stepwise improvements in adjuvant systemic therapy regimens have improved OS in early-stage breast cancer. The decision on the systemic therapy regimen is based on clinical (such as age, menopausal status, comorbidity) and pathologic parameters including tumor stage, grade, and ER and HER2 status. Adjuvantonline.com is a website that enables the treating oncologist to give an approximate average estimate of the benefit from adjuvant chemotherapy (of various types) and endocrine therapy. More recently, several multigene assays for prognosis assessment, including Oncotype DX (Genomic Health), Mammaprint (Agendia), and Prosigna (Nanostring), are available for clinical use. These tests offer the potential to avoid chemotherapy in the low-risk patient population.

      i. **Adjuvant endocrine therapy.** ER and PgR status of the tumor is routinely identified by immunohistochemical staining of breast cancer tissue. Estrogen binds to the receptor and stimulates cell proliferation, survival, and angiogenesis. The goal of adjuvant endocrine therapy is to suppress these tumor-promoting effects. ER and PgR are both prognostic factors as positivity indicates better prognosis. However, these biomarkers are much stronger predictive factors since the outcome of endocrine therapy is dependent on the level of ER expression. The value of PgR expression remains to be debated and does not provide useful clinical information independent of the ER status. ER–, PgR+ breast cancer should be treated as if it were ER+.

In premenopausal women, ovaries are the main source of estrogen production. Before the menopause, estrogen can be targeted either by tamoxifen, or by suppression of estrogen levels, or using both approaches in combination. Estrogen suppression can be achieved with luteinizing hormone-releasing hormone (LHRH) agonists (goserelin and leuprolide), or oophorectomy. In postmenopausal women, the predominant source of estrogen is peripheral conversion of adrenal androgens to estrogen by the enzyme aromatase. The action of estrogen can therefore be blocked by tamoxifen, or estrogen synthesis can be inhibited with a third-generation aromatase inhibitor (letrozole, anastrozole, and exemestane).

The Early Breast Cancer Trialists Collaborative Group (EBCTCG) meta-analysis of trials in women with early-stage breast cancer showed that after a median of 15 years of follow-up, tamoxifen reduced annual breast cancer mortality in women with ER+ breast cancer by 31%, and the annual breast cancer recurrence rate by 41%. This effect was irrespective of age, chemotherapy use, menopausal status, PgR status, involvement of axillary lymph nodes, tumor size, or other tumor characteristics (*Lancet* 2005;365:1687). It also showed that tamoxifen given for 5 years is better than tamoxifen given for 1 to 2 years. The benefits of tamoxifen persisted long after the course of therapy was finished. In fact, the rate of benefit at 15 years is the same as at 5 years. The Adjuvant Tamoxifen: Longer Against Shorter Trial (ATLAS) recently showed that continuing tamoxifen for 10 years rather than stopping after 5 years was associated with a further reduction in risk of mortality and recurrence (*Lancet* 2013;381:805).

The NSABP B-14 trial that evaluated only patients with node-negative, ER+ breast cancer in the 15-year follow-up report, showed that tamoxifen reduced breast cancer recurrence in the ipsilateral breast, contralateral breast, and distant sites by 42% and also reduced mortality by 20% (*Lancet* 2004;364:858).

In patients receiving adjuvant chemotherapy, the Intergroup trial 0100/SWOG-8814 showed that tamoxifen should be administered after the completion of chemotherapy (*Lancet* 2009;374:2055). The meta-analysis shows that chemotherapy and endocrine therapy are complementary adjuvant treatments in ER+ patients with independent and additive benefits but the question of which patients with ER+ disease require chemotherapy remains controversial, particularly in the setting of low-risk ER+ HER2– disease in older patients.

For ER+ premenopausal patients, the EBCTCG meta-analysis also showed that ovarian ablation/suppression reduced breast cancer mortality but appears to do so only in the absence of other systemic treatments (*Lancet* 2005;365:1687). Oophorectomy may be considered in women with hereditary breast cancer syndromes who are at an increased risk of development of ovarian malignancies and desire oophorectomy. The potential additive role of ovarian ablation to chemotherapy and/or endocrine therapy has been explored in the TEXT and SOFT trials and shows clinical benefit with the addition of ovarian suppression to endocrine therapy.

The use of aromatase inhibitors (AIs) as adjuvant hormonal therapy either instead of tamoxifen or in sequence with tamoxifen has been recommended in postmenopausal women on the basis of ATAC, MA17, IES, and BIG 1-98 trials. ASCO recommended in 2004 that an AI be considered as part of adjuvant hormone therapy for all postmenopausal women with ER+ breast cancer. The ATAC (5 years of anastrozole vs. 5 years of tamoxifen) and BIG 1-98 (5 years of letrozole vs. 5 years of tamoxifen) trials have shown that

AI improved disease-free survival (DFS) in comparison with tamoxifen. The MA17 trial (5 years of letrozole after 5 years of tamoxifen vs. 5 years of tamoxifen alone) showed improved DFS and improved OS in the node-positive subset with adding letrozole to 5 years of tamoxifen. The IES trial (2 to 3 years of exemestane following 2 to 3 years of tamoxifen for a total of 5 years of hormone therapy vs. 5 years of tamoxifen) has demonstrated improvement in both DFS and OS with exemestane. The optimal timing or duration of AI has yet to be established. In general, for all hormone receptor-positive post-menopausal women, 5 years of AI or sequential therapy of 2, 3, or 5 years of tamoxifen followed by 2, 3, or 5 years of AI, up to a total period of 10 years is recommended. In the BIG 1-98 trial, sequential therapy with 2 to 3 years of letrozole followed by tamoxifen to complete a total of 5 years of therapy was as effective as 5 years of letrozole or the sequential therapy of tamoxifen followed by letrozole, which were all superior to 5 years of tamoxifen. AIs as single agents are contraindicated in premenopausal women as inhibition of the aromatase enzyme can lead, by a feedback mechanism, to stimulation of the ovaries to produce more estrogen (*J Clin Oncol* 2005;23:619). These agents should only be combined with LHRH agonists in the adjuvant setting in clinical studies. The main side effects of AI include hot flashes, myalgias, arthralgias, and osteoporosis, whereas the main side effects of tamoxifen include thromboembolic events, uterine cancer, weight gain, hot flashes, and, rarely, visual changes.

ii. **Adjuvant chemotherapy.** The EBCTCG meta-analysis published the following conclusions on adjuvant chemotherapy (*Lancet* 2012;379:432). Adjuvant chemotherapy benefits early-stage breast cancer patients irrespective of age (up to at least 70s), nodal status, tumor diameter or differentiation (moderate or poor; few were well differentiated), estrogen receptor status, or tamoxifen use. In the meta-analysis comparing different adjuvant regimens, standard CMF (cyclophosphamide, methotrexate, fluorouracil) was equivalent to standard 4 cycles of AC (Adriamycin and cyclophosphamide) but inferior to anthracycline-based regimens with substantially higher cumulative doses than 4 AC (such as CAF or CEF for 6 cycles). The addition of 4 cycles of taxane to a fixed anthracycline-based regimen, extending treatment duration, reduced the breast cancer mortality. The breast cancer mortality was reduced by, on average, about one-third with taxane-plus-anthracycline-based or higher-cumulative-dosage anthracycline-based regimens (not requiring stem cells).

A key issue to understand is that although the reduction in annual odds of recurrence may be impressive, in low-risk groups the absolute benefit can be very small and not worth the cost of the intervention to the patient. For example, a patient with a 90% chance of being free of disease at 10 years without systemic treatment can expect only a very small absolute benefit, even from an agent that reduces the risk of recurrence by 50%.

Decision making for chemotherapy in patients with **ER+ HER2−** breast cancer is challenging as a subgroup of these patients may not benefit from chemotherapy. In general, chemotherapy is offered if node-positive or node-negative but with "high-risk features," for example, high-grade, size greater than 2 cm, or young age (which is a strong adverse risk factor for ER+ disease). Multigene assays could assist in the decision-making process. Oncotype DX test is a reverse transcriptase-polymerase chain reaction (RT-PCR) assay of 21 selected genes (16 "cancer" genes and 5 reference genes) using paraffin-embedded tumor tissue that gives rise to a recurrence score (RS) that separates tumors into low-, intermediate-, and high-risk categories in patients with node-negative and ER+ breast cancer. For patients whose tumors have a high recurrence risk score by Oncotype DX, chemotherapy should also be offered. Patients whose tumors have a low recurrence risk score can be potentially treated with adjuvant hormone therapy alone. In patients whose tumors are at intermediate risk, the treating medical oncologist should have a careful discussion of the benefit and risk of adjuvant chemotherapy with the patient (*N Engl J Med* 2004;351:2817). In the TAILORx trial, intermediate-risk patients are offered a treatment randomization to endocrine therapy versus endocrine therapy plus chemotherapy. For those with ER+ disease and 1 to 3 lymph nodes involved, the ongoing trial, RxPONDER, is evaluating the additional benefits of chemotherapy in those with a low- to intermediate Oncotype DX score. The Oncotype DX assay is not of value in patients with ER– disease as all tumors are typed to be high-risk (*N Engl J Med* 2006;355:560). Other available multigene assays include Mammaprint and Prosigna. Mammaprint is a 70-gene microarray assay that categorizes tumors into good and poor signature groups. The test is U.S. Food and Drug Administration (FDA)-approved and could be performed regardless of ER status for patients with early-stage breast cancer. Prosigna is also FDA-approved and provides a risk of recurrence score (ROR) based on PAM50 expression results using the nCounter System, and categorizes tumors into low-, intermediate-, and high-risk groups in patients with stage I to III breast cancer regardless of ER and HER2 status. PAM50 refers to the 50 genes and 5 control genes that predict the intrinsic molecular subtypes of breast cancer, including the luminal A, luminal B, HER2-enriched, and basal-like subtypes. These tests offer the potential to avoid chemotherapy in the low-risk patient population and are used by medical oncologists in clinical practice. The value of these tests in chemotherapy decision making are being validated in prospective clinical trials.

For **ER– HER2**– breast cancer, chemotherapy should be considered even when the tumor is more than 0.5 cm as these tumors tend to be aggressive and chemotherapy is the only available systemic therapy.

The common regimens used in high-risk node-negative breast cancer are shown in Table 13-2, with TC ×4 cycles being one of the most commonly used regimens because it was shown to be superior to AC ×4 cycles with no cardiac toxicity or leukemia toxicity associated with Adriamycin. For node-positive breast cancer, the recommendation is often a regimen that contains both an anthracycline and a taxane. However, the best regimen is unclear, but reasonable choices include dose-dense AC ×4 followed by paclitaxel ×4, dose-dense AC ×4 followed by weekly paclitaxel × 12 weeks, FEC ×3 followed by docetaxel 100 mg/m^2 ×3, or TAC ×6.

TABLE 13-2	Common Neo/Adjuvant Chemotherapy Regimens
Regimen	**Dosage**
CMF every 28 d ×6 cycles (Bonadonna regimen)	Cyclophosphamide 100 mg/m^2 PO days 1–14; methotrexate 40 mg/m^2 i.v. on days 1 and 8 5FU 600 mg/m^2 i.v. on days 1 and 8
CMF every 21 d ×6 cycles (i.v. regimen)	Cyclophosphamide 600 mg/m^2 i.v. on day 1 Methotrexate 40 mg/m^2 i.v. on day 1; 5FU 600 mg/m^2 i.v. on day 1
FAC every 28 d ×6 cycles	5FU 400 mg/m^2 i.v. on days 1 and 8 Doxorubicin 40 mg/m^2 i.v. on day 1 Cyclophosphamide 400 mg/m^2 i.v. on day 1
CAF every 21 d ×6 cycles	Cyclophosphamide 500 mg/m^2 i.v. on day 1 Doxorubicin 50 mg/m^2 i.v. on day 1 5FU 500 mg/m^2 i.v. on day 1

TABLE 13-2   Common Neo/Adjuvant Chemotherapy Regimens *(Continued)*

Regimen	Dosage
FEC 100 every 21 d ×6 cycles	5FU 500 mg/m^2 i.v. on day 1 Epirubicin 100 mg/m^2 on day 1 Cyclophosphamide 500 mg/m^2 on day 1
AC every 21 d ×4 cycles	Doxorubicin 60 mg/m^2 on day 1 Cyclophosphamide 600 mg/m^2 on day 1
TAC every 21 d ×6 cycles	Docetaxel 75 mg/m^2 i.v. on day 1 Doxorubicin 50 mg/m^2 i.v. on day 1 Cyclophosphamide 500 mg/m^2 i.v. on day 1
FEC 100 every 21 d ×3 cycles and then Docetaxel 100 every 21 d ×3 cycles	5FU 500 mg/m^2 i.v. on day 1 Epirubicin 100 mg/m^2 i.v. on day 1 Cyclophosphamide 500 mg/m^2 i.v. on day 1 Docetaxel 100 mg/m^2 i.v. on day 1
TC every 21 d ×4 cycles	Docetaxel 75 mg/m^2 i.v. on day 1 Cyclophosphamide 600 mg/m^2 i.v. on day 1
AC every 2 wk ×4 cycles followed by single-agent paclitaxel every 2 wk ×4 cycles (dose-dense AC + T)	Doxorubicin 60 mg/m^2 i.v. on day 1 Cyclophosphamide 600 mg/m^2 i.v. on day 1 Paclitaxel 175 mg/m^2 i.v. on day 1
AC every 3 wk ×4 cycles and then weekly Paclitaxel + trastuzumab ×12 cycles	Doxorubicin 60 mg/m^2 i.v. on day 1 Cyclophosphamide 600 mg/m^2 i.v. on day 1 Paclitaxel 80 mg/m^2 i.v. every week Trastuzumab 4 mg/kg i.v. loading dose and then 2 mg/kg i.v. weekly
AC every 3 wk ×4 cycles followed by docetaxel every 3 wk ×4 cycles with trastuzumab given for 1 year	Doxorubicin 60 mg/m^2 i.v. on day 1 Cyclophosphamide 600 mg/m^2 i.v. on day 1 Docetaxel 100 mg/m^2 i.v. on day 1 Trastuzumab 4 mg/kg i.v. loading dose and then 2 mg/kg i.v. weekly
TCH every 3 wk ×6 cycles, then trastuzumab given for 1 year	Docetaxel 75 mg/m^2 i.v. on day 1 Carboplatin AUC 6 i.v. on day 1 Trastuzumab 8 mg/kg i.v. loading dose and then 6 mg/kg i.v. on day 1 every 3 wk
TCHP (pertuzumab) every 3 wk ×6 cycles, surgery, then completion of trastuzumab for a total 1 year	Docetaxel 75 mg/m^2 i.v. on day 1 Carboplatin AUC 6 i.v. on day 1 Pertuzumab 840 mg i.v. loading dose and then 420 mg on day 1 every 3 wk Trastuzumab 8 mg/kg i.v. loading dose and then 6 mg/kg i.v. on day 1 every 3 wk
FEC every 3 wk ×3 cycles then docetaxel + trastuzumab and per-tuzumab every 3 wk for 3 cycles fol-lowed by surgery, then completion of trastuzumab for a total of 1 year	5FU 500 mg/m^2 i.v. on day 1 (cycles 1–3) Epirubicin 100 mg/m^2 i.v. on day 1 (cycles 1–3) Cyclophosphamide 600 mg/m^2 i.v. on day 1 (cycles 1–3) Docetaxel 75–100 mg/m^2 i.v. on day 1 (cycles 4–6) Pertuzumab 840 mg i.v. loading dose and then 420 mg on day 1 every 3 wk (cycles 4–6) Trastuzumab 8 mg/kg i.v. loading dose and then 6 mg/kg i.v. on day 1 every 3 wk (cycles 4–until end of 1 year)

i.v., intravenous; PO, orally.
This is a list of some of the common regimens used. There are other regimens reported that have not been included in this list.

iii. Adjuvant HER2 targeted therapy. In patients whose tumors overexpress HER2 as assessed by FISH or are designated 3+ by IHC, trastuzumab, a humanized monoclonal antibody to HER2, improves DFS by approximately 50%. This has been shown by the combined analysis of the North Central Cancer Treatment Group (NCCTG) N 9831 and NSABP B31 trials (AC ×4 cycles, weekly paclitaxel ×12 cycles, and trastuzumab for 1 year either concurrently with Taxol or sequentially after paclitaxel), HERA trial (chemotherapy of choice followed by trastuzumab for 1 or 2 years), and the BCIRG 006 trial (AC ×4 cycles followed by docetaxel ×4 cycles and trastuzumab for 1 year starting weekly during docetaxel and then every 3 weeks) as well as docetaxel, carboplatin, and trastuzumab [TCH] ×6 cycles followed by trastuzumab for 1 year. The NCCTG 9831/NSABP B31 trial also showed an improvement in OS by 33% (*N Engl J Med* 2005;353:1673).

In the NCCTG 9831/NSABP B31 study, concurrent paclitaxel plus trastuzumab treatment had a better DFS but a higher congestive heart failure incidence (4.1%) as compared with sequential therapy with Taxol followed by trastuzumab (1.2%). Close follow-up of the cardiac function (echocardiogram or MUGA scan) is recommended while the patient is receiving adjuvant trastuzumab. In the study, all patients with cardiac dysfunction recovered their cardiac function after discontinuing trastuzumab.

The results of the HERA trial show that 2 years of adjuvant trastuzumab is not superior to 1 year of treatment. Other trials also exploring shorter durations of adjuvant trastuzumab have shown that 1 year is the optimal duration.

iv. Sequence of adjuvant chemotherapy and radiation therapy. The administration of radiation therapy concurrently with chemotherapy increases the side effects of radiation therapy and is not recommended. In terms of optimal sequencing, a randomized clinical trial addressing this question showed that giving chemotherapy first followed by radiation therapy reduced recurrence rate for all sites from 38% to 31% and improved OS from 73% to 81%. There was a slight increase in local recurrence rate in the chemotherapy-first arm, but it was not statistically significant (*N Engl J Med* 1996;334:1356). Radiation therapy can be delayed up to 6 months postsurgery to allow completion of adjuvant chemotherapy. After completing chemotherapy, radiation therapy can be given concurrently with adjuvant trastuzumab with no increase in side effects including cardiac toxicity, although pneumonitis is a concern with patients receiving chest wall radiation.

b. Neoadjuvant systemic therapy. Neoadjuvant systemic therapy is routinely recommended in the treatment of locally advanced breast cancer and inflammatory breast cancer (a subset of stage II (T3N0), stage III A, stage III B, stage IIIC) to reduce tumor size and facilitate surgical excision. However, it is sometimes recommended for patients with earlier stage cancer to assess tumor responsiveness to systemic therapy and prognosis. In addition, neoadjuvant setting provides a unique opportunity for novel therapeutics development.

i. Neoadjuvant chemotherapy. Neoadjuvant chemotherapy will facilitate tumor regression to allow surgical resection with clear margins and is an in vivo test of the cancer cell sensitivity to the regimen used. Several studies have shown that patients with pathologic complete response (pCR) in the breast and axilla (more so axillary pCR) are associated with better DFS and OS in those with HER2+ and ER/PgR/HER2- (triple negative) breast cancer. Whether increasing the pCR rate will increase the DFS and OS rate is currently being investigated. In addition, residual cancer burden (RCB: 0, 1, 2, and 3) post neoadjuvant chemotherapy correlates with long-term outcome. Fewer than 5% of breast cancers progress while receiving neoadjuvant chemotherapy.

The same chemotherapy regimens used in neoadjuvant setting are recommended in the adjuvant setting. Trastuzumab-containing regimens are used in patients with HER2+ breast cancer. In addition, pertuzumab, a humanized monoclonal antibody that targets a different epitope of HER2 than trastuzumab to inhibit the formation of the HER2:HER3 dimerization, has received FDA approval to combine with trastuzumab-containing chemotherapy as neoadjuvant treatment for HER2+ breast cancer based on improved pCR rate observed in two neoadjuvant trials (*Lancet Oncol* 2012;13:25).

The pCR rate differs according to the subtypes of breast cancer. HER2+ breast cancer achieves over 50% pCR rate with trastuzumab-containing regimens. Triple negative breast cancer has a pCR rate of around 20% to 40% with an anthracycline- and taxane-containing regimen. ER+ HER2– breast cancer has the lowest pCR rate (less than 10%), especially for those with lower-grade and ER-rich tumors.

    ii. Neoadjuvant endocrine therapy. Neoadjuvant endocrine therapy with an aromatase inhibitor is an alternative for postmenopausal women with ER+ HER2– disease and offers similar benefits to chemotherapy with an improvement in breast conservation rates. The AI is generally offered for 4 to 6 months preoperatively. In carefully selected patients (ER-rich tumors), a 60% response rate and a 50% rate of conversion to breast conservation can be expected (*J Clin Oncol* 2001;19:3808). Studies are ongoing to assess whether pathologic tumor stage, and Ki67, a marker of proliferation, post neoadjuvant endocrine therapy could identify a subset of patients for whom chemotherapy is not necessary.

V. FOLLOW-UP. There are data to recommend monthly self-breast examination; annual mammography to the preserved and contralateral breast; and careful history and physical examination every 3 to 6 months for 3 years, then every 6 to 12 months for years 4 and 5, and then annually. Data are not sufficient to recommend routine bone scans, chest x-rays, blood counts, tumor markers, liver US, or CT scans. CT and bone scans should be done only for suggestive symptoms (*J Clin Oncol* 1999;17:1080).

In patients taking tamoxifen, yearly pelvic examination by a gynecologist is recommended. There is no evidence for endometrial cancer screening on a regular basis. In women with irregular or excessive bleeding or pelvic pain, a careful pelvic examination, US, and endometrial biopsy should be performed. While on tamoxifen, yearly ophthalmologic evaluation is recommended to identify corneal, macular, and retinal changes.

In patients taking AI, an initial bone density scan is recommended. Patients with normal bone mineral density (BMD) can be followed up clinically with only sparing use of repeat scans. Osteopenic patients should be offered calcium and vitamin D supplements and yearly BMD and lifestyle advice including exercise. Osteoporotic patients should be offered a bisphosphonate as well and followed up closely. Fasting lipid levels should also be followed up because AIs do not protect from heart disease, and in low-risk breast cancer patients, cardiovascular disease is the most common cause of death.

Physicians should also monitor their patients for long-term side effects from treatment, including sexual dysfunction, premature ovarian failure, infertility in younger patients, cognitive dysfunction, lymphedema, decreased arm mobility, postmastectomy pain syndrome, cardiac dysfunction, psychological stress, and second cancers (soft tissue sarcoma from RT, acute leukemia/myelodysplasia (MDS) from chemotherapy).

VI. LOCOREGIONAL RECURRENT BREAST CANCER. Locoregional recurrence can present as a breast lump or nipple discharge following BCT, chest wall rash, or nodules following mastectomy or enlargement of axillary, supraclavicular, or internal mammary lymph nodes.

Breast cancer can recur locally after BCT and mastectomy. In patients who undergo mastectomy, recurrence is usually within the first 3 years of surgery, but in patients who undergo BCT, tumor can recur even at 20 years postsurgery (*Cancer* 1989;63:1912). In patients who undergo BCT, the locoregional recurrence rate is higher in women who do not undergo adjuvant RT, and have positive margins, high-grade tumor, and lymphovascular invasion.

When a patient has cancer in the ipsilateral breast after BCT, it could either be a locally recurrent tumor or a second primary. Mastectomy is recommended for these patients. Radiation therapy is limited by earlier whole breast radiation therapy and other contraindications to RT. Systemic therapy is based on the size, nodal status, hormone receptor status, HER2/neu status and other tumor characteristics, and follows treatment principles similar to a first diagnosis of early-stage breast cancer. A small study (IBCSG 27-02, BIG 1-02, NSABP B-37) showed that chemotherapy improved clinical outcomes for patients with isolated local and regional recurrences.

When cancer recurs in the chest wall after mastectomy, 20% to 30% of patients have metastatic disease at the time. In patients with isolated chest wall recurrence, full-thickness chest wall resection can palliate symptoms, improve survival, and even result in cure (*Am Surg* 2005;71:711). Node-negative patients at the first presentation and those patients with a DFS of more than 24 months before chest wall recurrence had a better prognosis with outcomes improved by chest wall radiation therapy and systemic chemotherapy (*Ann Surg Oncol* 2003;10:628). Endocrine therapy or a change in endocrine therapy should also be considered for ER+ chest wall recurrences.

VII. METASTATIC BREAST CANCER. The most common sites for breast cancer to metastasize are the lung, liver, and bones. Metastatic breast cancer (MBC) is incurable except perhaps in a very small percentage of patients, who are chemotherapy naïve, receive multiagent chemotherapy, and may remain in durable remission for unexpectedly long periods of time, with the median OS for MBC being 2 to 3 years, although with the advent of newer therapies, the survival has been prolonged, particularly in ER+ breast cancer. Patients with bone or lymph node metastasis usually have longer survival than patients with visceral metastasis. Treatment aims to control the cancer, palliate symptoms, improve quality of life, and prolong survival. The choice of treatment in these patients is dependent on the hormone receptor status, HER2 status, site and extent of disease, prior therapy, as well as the patient's performance status and comorbidities.

A. Local treatment

1. Surgery. In patients with solitary/limited metastasis of the lung, liver, brain, and sternum, case reports and retrospective studies have suggested improved survival with surgical resection; however, these are uncontrolled patient series, and there are no definitive data. Patients should be chosen carefully on the basis of operative morbidity, disease-free interval since their primary tumor, the possibility of achieving negative margins, extent of metastasis, performance status, and comorbidities.

In patients who present with metastatic disease at the time of diagnosis, most oncologists do not routinely recommend primary breast tumor surgery. Surgery is done to palliate any symptoms related to the primary tumor. Retrospective studies have suggested improved survival with removal of the primary tumor in patients with metastatic disease, but this remains controversial. ECOG 2108 is an ongoing prospective trial evaluating the role of early local therapy for the intact tumor in patients with MBC.

Spinal cord compression from metastasis is a medical emergency and has improved outcomes with neurosurgical decompression of the spinal cord followed by radiation therapy as compared with radiation therapy and steroids alone (*Lancet* 2005;366:643).

Prophylactic pinning and rod placement of long bones with more than 50% destruction of the cortical bone is done to prevent fractures, which can lead to a poor quality of life and decrease in survival.

2. Radiation therapy. Radiation therapy is used to palliate symptoms and can help with pain in patients with bone metastasis and chest wall metastasis. Some patients can have significant mediastinal and hilar adenopathy or lung metastasis causing obstruction of the bronchus leading to collapse of a lung lobe or postobstructive pneumonia, and may benefit from palliative radiation therapy. In these cases, in patients with spinal cord compression, who are not candidates for neurosurgery, radiation therapy is used to relieve the cord compression.

In patients with unresectable brain metastasis, whole-brain radiation therapy (WBRT) is shown to help improve symptoms and improve median survival from 4 to 6 months. Stereotactic radiosurgery is used in patients with limited brain metastasis that is in an inaccessible place, as a boost to WBRT, and in patients with recurrences after WBRT. In patients with HER2+ brain metastasis, lapatinib, a HER2 kinase inhibitor, in combination with capecitabine has shown efficacy.

Radioactive isotopes such as ^{89}Sr and ^{153}Sm can be used to palliate bone pain from multifocal osteoblastic bone metastasis.

B. **Systemic therapy.** Endocrine therapy is recommended as first-line therapy in patients with hormone receptor–positive tumor, if they have bone, lymph node, soft tissue, or asymptomatic visceral metastasis. Chemotherapy is recommended in patients with hormone receptor–negative tumor or symptomatic visceral metastasis. Trastuzumab, pertuzumab, lapatinib, or TDM-1 are additional options if the tumor overexpresses HER2.

1. **Hormone therapy.** In premenopausal patients, options include tamoxifen (±LHRH agonists) and oophorectomy (±AIs). A nonsteroidal AI (anastrozole or letrozole) is often used as first-line hormonal therapy for postmenopausal patients. Subsequent options include steroidal AI (exemestane), tamoxifen, fulvestrant, and megestrol acetate. Exemestane in combination with everolimus (Afinitor), an inhibitor against mTOR, has shown to improve the PFS (10.6 months with combination therapy vs. 4.1 months with exemestane alone) in AI-resistant postmenopausal women with ER+ HER2–advanced breast cancer refractory to nonsteroidal AIs (*N Engl J Med* 2012;366:520), leading to FDA approval for its application in AI-resistant population. Estradiol 2 mg TID is an option in patients with acquired AI-resistant disease, although the mechanism of action of estrogen is not clear.

   When the tumor progresses through one endocrine agent, further endocrine therapy is recommended as long as the patient does not have symptomatic visceral disease or rapidly progressing disease. Second- and third-line endocrine therapy agents are chosen from a different drug class. With each subsequent endocrine therapy, the response rate and time to progression (TTP) decrease. Chemotherapy should be started when the disease eventually becomes resistant to hormone therapy, while considering the patient's performance status and comorbidities.

2. **Chemotherapy.** Although combination chemotherapy is associated with better response rate, better TTP, it has not shown to improve OS and is associated with more side effects compared with sequential single-agent therapy. Therefore, single-agent sequential therapy is often preferred except in the setting of rapidly progressive visceral metastasis.

   Anthracyclines (doxorubicin, liposomal doxorubicin, epirubicin, mitoxantrone) and taxanes (paclitaxel, docetaxel, nab-paclitaxel) are the two most active drug classes against breast cancer. Although these drugs are often used in the adjuvant setting, they may be reused at relapse, particularly if there has been an interval of more than a year since completion of the adjuvant therapy. When anthracyclines are used, liposomal doxorubicin is preferred as it has lower cardiac toxicity and has similar antitumor activity in the metastatic setting. Capecitabine, as an oral agent, is often used when the disease has recurred or progressed after anthracyclines and taxanes. The other active drugs include cytoxan, methotrexate, vinorelbine, eribulin, gemcitabine, and oral etoposide and platinum (carboplatin and cisplatin). The list of chemotherapeutic regimens is given in Table 13-3.

   Approximately 25% of MBC overexpress HER2. The combination of chemotherapy with trastuzumab was associated with higher response rates, longer TTP, and a statistically significant improvement in OS. Pertuzumab (Perjeta) in combination with trastuzumab and a taxane has shown to improve PFS (18.5 vs. 12.4 months) and OS than trastuzumab in combination with a taxane (*N Engl J Med* 2012;366:109), and therefore has been FDA-approved as first-line therapy for HER2+ MBC. Lapatinib (Tykerb) is a dual tyrosine kinase inhibitor that blocks both HER1 and HER2. It is FDA-approved in combination with capecitabine for the treatment of patients with metastatic HER2+ breast cancer with prior therapy including an anthracycline, a taxane, and trastuzumab. In patients with HER2+ brain metastasis, this combination has also shown efficacy. Data from EMILIA trial showed that T-DM1 (Kadcyla), trastuzumab linked to the cytotoxic agent mertansine (DM1), improved survival by 5.8 months with better tolerability compared with the combination of lapatinib and capecitabine (*N Engl J Med* 2012;367:1783), which led to the FDA approval of T-DM1 in patients with metastatic HER2+ breast cancer who had prior trastuzumab and a taxane. Subsequent therapies for HER2+ breast cancer include a switch to alternate chemotherapy, and trastuzumab should be continued upon tumor progression. The use of trastuzumab in combination with anthracyclines has been associated with

TABLE 13-3	Metastatic Breast Cancer Chemotherapy Regimens

Regimen	Dosage
Doxorubicin every 3 wk	40–75 mg/m² i.v. on day 1
Pegylated liposomal doxorubicin every 3–4 wk	45–60 mg/m² i.v. on day 1
Epirubicin every 3 wk	60–90 mg/m² i.v. on day 1
Paclitaxel every week	80–100 mg/m² i.v. on day 1
Docetaxel every 3 wk	80–100 mg/m² i.v. on day 1
Abraxane every 3 wk	260 mg/m² i.v. on day 1
Abraxane weekly on 3 wk off 1 wk q 28 d	125 mg/m² i.v. on days 1, 8, and 15 i.v.
Capecitabine on 2 wk off 1 wk every 3 wk	850–1,250 mg/m² PO b.i.d. on days 1–14
Gemcitabine weekly on 3 wk off 1 wk every 28 d	725 mg/m² i.v. on days 1, 8, and 15
Eribulin weekly on 2 wk off 1 wk every 3 wk	1.4 mg/m² i.v. days 1 and 8
Vinorelbine weekly	30 mg/m² i.v. on day 1
Ixabepilone and capecitabine every 3 wk	Ixabepilone 40 mg/m² i.v. on day 1
	Capecitabine 1,250 mg/m² PO b.i.d. on days 1–14
Etoposide on 2 wk off 1 wk every 3 wk	50 mg PO every day
Gemcitabine and paclitaxel every 21 d	Gemcitabine 1,250 mg/m² i.v. days 1 and 8
	Paclitaxel 175 m/m² i.v. day 1
Capecitabine and docetaxel every 21 d	Capecitabine 1,250 mg/m² PO b.i.d. on days 1–14
	Docetaxel 75 mg/m² i.v. on day 1
Capecitabine and paclitaxel every 21 d	Capecitabine 850 mg/m² PO b.i.d. on days 1–14
	Paclitaxel 175 mg/m² i.v. on day 1
Capecitabine and Navelbine every 21 d	Capecitabine 1,000 mg/m² PO b.i.d. on days 1–14
	Navelbine 25 mg/m² i.v. on days 1 and 8
CMF every 28 d (PO regimen)	Cyclophosphamide 100 mg/m² PO days 1–14
	Methotrexate 40 mg/m² i.v. on days 1 and 8
	5FU 600 mg/m² i.v. on days 1 and 8
CMF every 21 d (i.v. regimen)	Cyclophosphamide 600 mg/m² i.v. on day 1
	Methotrexate 40 mg/m² i.v. on day 1
	5FU 600 mg/m² i.v. on day 1
FAC every 28 d	5FU 400 mg/m² i.v. on days 1 and 8
	Doxorubicin 40 mg/m² i.v. on day 1
	Cyclophosphamide 400 mg/m² i.v. on day 1
CAF every 21 d	Cyclophosphamide 500 mg/m² i.v. on day 1
	Doxorubicin 50 mg/m² i.v. on day 1
	5FU 500 mg/m² i.v. on day 1
FEC 100 every 21 d	5FU 500 mg/m² i.v. on day 1
	Epirubicin 100 mg/m² on day 1
	Cyclophosphamide 500 mg/m² on day 1
AT every 21 d	Doxorubicin 60 mg/m² i.v. on day 1
	Paclitaxel 200 mg/m² i.v. on day 1
Docetaxel and doxorubicin every 21 d	Docetaxel 75 mg/m² i.v. on day 1
	Doxorubicin 50 mg/m² i.v. on day 1

i.v., intravenous; PO, orally; b.i.d., twice a day.
This is a list of some of the common regimens used. There are other regimens reported that have not been included in this list.

severe cardiac toxicity in up to 27% of patients, and therefore should not be combined with anthracyclines (*N Engl J Med* 2001;349:783). Other options include the combination of lapatinib and trastuzumab (*J Clinc Oncol* 2010;28:1124). The commonly used regimens for HER2+ MBC are listed in Table 13-4. In the subgroup of HER2+ breast cancer that is also ER+, with low volume disease, the combination of hormonal therapy with or without trastuzumab is also acceptable. The combination of letrozole and lapatinib (*Oncologist* 2010;15:122) has also been approved as first-line therapy for metastatic ER+ HER2+ breast cancer.

C. **Follow-up while on treatment.** Monitoring treatment can be done by physical examination if there is palpable adenopathy or chest wall or soft tissue nodules. Significant cancer-related symptoms such as pain can also be monitored. Monitoring of tumor markers is useful only if elevated (*J Clin Oncol* 1999;17:1080). Tumor marker levels may not correlate with tumor burden (by imaging). The tumor marker may be spuriously elevated due to cytolysis. The tumor marker level may be lower with clearly progressive disease

---

TABLE 13-4   **Metastatic Breast Cancer Overexpressing HER2**

Regimen	Dosage
Pertuzumab + trastuzumab + docetaxel (or paclitaxel) every 21 d	Pertuzumab 840 mg i.v. day 1 followed by 420 mg i.v.
	Trastuzumab 8 mg/kg i.v. day 1 followed by 6 mg/kg i.v.
	Docetaxel 75–100 mg/m^2 i.v. day 1 or
	Paclitaxel 80 mg/m^2 day 1 weekly
T-DM1 (Ado-trastuzumab emtansine) every 21 d	T-DM1 3.6 mg/kg i.v. day 1
Lapatinib + capecitabine every 21 d	Lapatinib 1,250 mg PO daily days 1–21
	Capecitabine 1,000 mg/m^2 PO twice daily days 1–14
Trastuzumab + lapatinib	Lapatinib 1,000 mg PO daily
	Trastuzumab
Other trastuzumab-containing regimens	
Paclitaxel + trastuzumab	
Docetaxel + trastuzumab	
Vinorelbine + trastuzumab	
Gemcitabine + trastuzumab	
Capecitabine + trastuzumab	
Liposomal doxorubicin + trastuzumab	
Cisplatin + trastuzumab	
Cisplatin + docetaxel + trastuzumab	
Carboplatin + docetaxel + trastuzumab	
Carboplatin + paclitaxel + trastuzumab	
Cisplatin + gemcitabine + trastuzumab	
Paclitaxel + gemcitabine + trastuzumab	
Epirubicin + cyclophosphamide + trastuzumab	

This is a list of some of the common regimens used. There are other regimens reported that have not been included in this list.

because the tumor has changed and is secreting lower levels of the marker. The physical examination and radiologic findings should then determine treatment decisions. Imaging (CT, MR, and bone scans) should be done periodically to assess response to treatment. Little data are available regarding the use of PET scans to monitor treatment. Recently, studies looking at circulating tumor cell (CTC) levels have been published. High levels of CTC before starting treatment have been associated with poorer DFS and OS (*N Engl J Med* 2004;351:781). When the CTC level has not declined after 3 to 6 weeks of starting a new regimen, those patients are unlikely to benefit from chemotherapy.

- **D. Duration of chemotherapy treatment.** Randomized studies have shown that OS is not significantly different whether chemotherapy is continued until disease progression or withheld after an optimum number of cycles (approximately 6 cycles). Patients who tolerate chemotherapy well may accept continued treatment, and randomized trials suggest that this may be the best option in terms of progression-free survival and quality of life (*N Engl J Med* 1987;317:1490). However, when toxicity is a problem, chemotherapy "holidays" may improve the quality of life, after which treatment can be resumed even if disease progression has not yet occurred.

- **E. Bone metastasis.** Pamidronate (90 mg, i.v. q 3 to 4 weeks), zoledronic acid (4 mg, i.v. q 3 to 4 weeks), and denosumab (120 mg, s.q. q 4 weeks) are FDA-approved drugs for use in patients with bone metastasis to palliate pain and prevent skeletal complications, although they have not shown an improvement in OS. While administering these drugs, the serum creatinine, electrolytes, calcium, and magnesium levels should be monitored. The drugs should be continued as long as the patient receives treatment for MBC. These drugs are being studied in clinical trials to see if they prevent bone metastasis.

VIII. FUTURE DIRECTIONS. Major advances have been made in the diagnosis and treatment of breast cancer, resulting in a decrease in mortality from breast cancer over the last four decades. However, a significant number of breast cancer patients experience disease relapse and death. More effective treatments are needed. Targeted therapies directed at cancer-specific alterations hold promise of personalized cancer treatment with better tolerability than that with chemotherapy. Every effort should be made to enroll patients in clinical trials.

Patients differ in their ability to tolerate treatment, and tumors differ in regard to how they proliferate, metastasize, and respond to treatment. New technologies such as gene expression profiling, genomic sequencing, genetic polymorphism studies, and proteomics are being used to help us understand these important differences at a molecular level.

While we are making an effort to better understand and treat breast cancer, efforts are also being made to improve the quality of life of patients undergoing treatment for breast cancer. Research is ongoing in the field of antiemetics, memory loss, fatigue, postmenopausal symptoms, and other symptoms related to the treatment of this disease.

SUGGESTED READINGS

Baselga J, Cortés J, Kim SB, et al. Pertuzumab plus trastuzumab plus docetaxel for metastatic breast cancer. *N Engl J Med* 2012;366:109–119.

Davies C, Pan H, Godwin J. Long-term effects of continuing adjuvant tamoxifen to 10 years versus stopping at 5 years after diagnosis of oestrogen receptor-positive breast cancer: ATLAS, a randomised trial. *Lancet* 2013;381:805–816.

Early Breast Cancer Trialists' Collaborative Group (EBCTCG). Comparisons between different polychemotherapy regimens for early breast cancer: meta-analyses of long-term outcome among 100,000 women in 123 randomised trials. *Lancet* 2012;379:432–444.

Early Breast Cancer Trialists' Collaborative Group (EBCTCG). Effects of chemotherapy and hormonal therapy for early breast cancer on recurrence and 15-year survival: an overview of the randomised trials. *Lancet* 2005;365:1687–1717.

Fan C, Oh DS, Wessels L, et al. Concordance among gene-expression-based predictors for breast cancer. *N Engl J Med* 2006;355:560–569.

Verma S, Miles D, Gianni L, et al. Trastuzumab emtansine for HER2-positive advanced breast cancer. *N Engl J Med* 2012;367:1783–1791.

14 Thymoma and Mesothelioma

Eric Knoche • Siddartha Devarakonda • Daniel Morgensztern

I. THYMOMA

A. Subjective complaints. The clinical presentation for patients with thymic neoplasms can range from an incidental radiographic finding to a symptom related to local extension or to a severe complication related to a variety of paraneoplastic syndromes. Up to 50% of patients present with an asymptomatic anterior mediastinal mass on the chest radiograph. The most common symptoms include cough, chest pain, and dyspnea. Other symptoms include hemoptysis, hoarseness, and dysphagia. Systemic complaints such as weight loss, fatigue, fever, and night sweats are less common and are more typical of lymphoma. The most common paraneoplastic syndrome is myasthenia gravis (MG), which occurs in approximately one-third of the patients. Among patients with MG, 10% to 15% are found to have thymoma during further investigation. Pure red cell aplasia (PRCA) occurs in approximately 5% to 10% of patients with thymoma, but half of the patients with PRCA have thymoma. This syndrome is suspected in patients with isolated anemia and low reticulocyte count. Hypogammaglobulinemia is present in up to 10% of the patients. The association of thymoma with combined B and T cell immunodeficiency is termed Good's syndrome. This condition is characterized by an increased susceptibility to infections by encapsulated bacteria and opportunistic infections (*J Clin Pathol* 2003;56:12). Several other paraneoplastic syndromes have been described in association with thymoma (Table 14-1).

B. Objective findings. At an early stage, patients often have a completely normal physical examination. The thoracic expansion of the tumor with invasion or compression of the superior vena cava may cause the characteristic findings of facial and upper extremity swelling, whereas invasion of the innominate vein will cause left arm edema. Phrenic nerve invasion is also possible and may result in decreased breath sounds on the affected side. Some patients develop ocular findings such as ptosis or diplopia.

II. WORKUP AND STAGING

A. Imaging studies. Most cases of thymoma are detected initially by standard chest radiographs. On the posteroanterior (PA) view, there is usually a round or oval lesion, with a smooth or lobulated border, near the junction of the heart and great vessels. Although the tumor may be primarily located in the midline, it also usually extends into one of the hemithoraces. The trachea is rarely displaced, and the presence of an elevated hemidiaphragm may suggest the invasion of a phrenic nerve. A small percentage of tumors have calcification in the periphery or within the tumor. On the lateral view, the mass causes opacification of the anterior cardiac window. Further evaluation is obtained with a computed tomography (CT) scan of the chest, which will best visualize and evaluate the extent of the mass. Although CT scan is unreliable for the detection of mediastinal invasion, highly

TABLE 14-1	Paraneoplastic Syndromes Associated with Thymoma
Endocrine	Addison's disease, Cushing's syndrome, panhypopituitarism, and thyroiditis
Cardiovascular	Myocarditis, pericarditis
Hematologic	Agranulocytosis, hypogammaglobulinemia, pernicious anemia, and red cell aplasia
Neuromuscular	Myasthenia gravis, limbic encephalopathy, polymyositis, and radiculopathy
Rheumatologic	Rheumatoid arthritis, scleroderma, Systemic lupus erythematosus, and Sjögren's syndrome
Miscellaneous	Alopecia areata, sarcoidosis, and ulcerative colitis

suggestive findings of invasion include complete obliteration of fat planes, encasement of mediastinal vessels, and pericardial or pleural thickening. The tendency to metastasize to the posterior basilar pleural space is unique of thymomas. Magnetic resonance imaging (MRI) is useful for the investigation of vascular invasion. Thymic tumors often express somatostatin receptors and may be detected by an indium-labeled octreotide scan.

B. **Biopsy.** The diagnosis of thymoma is usually made clinically, particularly in patients with paraneoplastic syndrome. When the tumor is small and confined to the thymus, surgical excision may facilitate diagnosis, treatment, and staging. Biopsy has an important role in patients with large and invasive tumors that may require a nonsurgical approach or neoadjuvant treatment, as well as in cases where lymphoma remains a strong possibility, because this malignancy is not primarily treated with surgery. The histopathologic diagnosis may be obtained through a fine needle aspiration (FNA) or surgical biopsy with success rates of approximately 60% and 90%, respectively. The sensitivity and specificity of FNA is limited due to the benign appearance of many thymomas when evaluated at a single cell level. There is limited data to support the concerns over seeding thymic tumors to the pleural space during the biopsy procedure. There are no reports of tumor seeding through the needle tract or biopsy site, and the pattern of spreading to the pleural space appears to be inherent of this malignancy, regardless of previous biopsy.

C. **Pathology.** The term thymoma should be restricted to neoplasms of thymic epithelial cells. Therefore, other tumors that may also involve the thymus such as seminomas and lymphomas should not be considered variants of thymoma. Most of the thymomas arise in the upper portion of the anterior mediastinum, corresponding to the location of the normal thymus gland. Rare locations include the posterior mediastinum, lower neck, perihilar tissues, lung parenchyma, and pleura (possibly arising from ectopic thymic tissue, which can be distributed throughout the mediastinum). Grossly, thymomas are largely or entirely solid, separated in lobules by connective tissue septa, and usually well-encapsulated. Microscopically, thymomas are composed of a mixture of neoplastic epithelial cells and a lymphocyte infiltrate. After many years of debate and several proposed schemes, the World Health Organization (WHO) developed a standard and unified classification for thymic epithelial neoplasms in 1999 (Table 14-2). In this report, two major types of thymoma were identified on the basis of the characteristics of the malignant epithelial cells, which could have a spindle or oval shape (resembling medullary cells) in type A or epithelioid appearance (resembling cortical cells) in type B. Tumors with both characteristics were designated as AB. Type B tumors were further subdivided into three groups, B1 to B3, depending on the progressive increase of the epithelial-to-lymphocyte ratio and the degree of atypia. An additional category, type C, was reserved for patients with thymic carcinoma, where there are overt characteristics of malignancy. There is a significant correlation between the WHO subtype and paraneoplastic syndromes, with MG occurring most commonly in subtype B and PRCA in subtype A.

D. **Staging.** The most commonly used staging system is the one proposed by Masaoka et al., in 1981 (Table 14-3). In this system, four clinical stages are created on the basis of the degree of invasion through the capsule and into the surrounding structures.

TABLE 14-2	WHO Classification of Thymomas
WHO scheme	**Other histologic classifications**
Type A	Medullary, spindle cell
Type AB	Mixed
Type B1	Lymphocyte-rich, predominantly cortical, organoid
Type B2	Cortical
Type B3	Epithelial, atypical, squamoid, well-differentiated thymic carcinoma
Type C	Thymic carcinoma

WHO, World Health Organization.

TABLE 14-3	Masaoka Staging System for Thymoma

Stage	Description
I	Completely encapsulated tumor
IIa	Microscopic transcapsular invasion
IIb	Macroscopic invasion into fatty tissue or grossly adherent to but not through the mediastinal pleura or pericardium
III	Macroscopic invasion into neighboring organs (pericardium, great vessels, lung)
IVa	Pleural or pericardial metastases
IVb	Lymphatic or hematogenous metastases

III. THERAPY AND PROGNOSIS
A. Resectable disease

1. **Surgery.** Surgery is a treatment of choice for thymoma and should be offered to all patients except those with clinically grossly unresectable disease or where it is spread beyond the thorax. As surgery may precipitate respiratory failure in a patient with MG, any patient with diagnosed or suspected thymoma should be tested for anti-acetylcholine receptor levels prior to surgery to rule out MG. If present, MG should be treated prior to the surgery. In patients with grossly encapsulated lesions, the procedure of choice is a complete excision with total thymectomy. Patients with gross fixation of the tumor to nonvital adjacent structures such as lung, pleura, or pericardium should undergo the resection of the adjacent involved tissues. The presence of intrapulmonary metastasis does not constitute a contraindication for the surgery if accomplished by lobectomy. The role for pneumonectomy in this setting is questionable. Patients with unilateral phrenic nerve involvement should undergo surgery with curative intent, provided that they can tolerate the loss of function in that hemidiaphragm, which can be particularly problematic in patients with MG. The operative mortality is approximately 2.5%, and overall survival for patients with resected thymoma is usually very good (Table 14-4). Patients with stage III or IV are considered unresectable when there is extensive involvement of the trachea, great arteries, or heart, extensive bilateral pleural metastases, or distant metastases. The role of debulking or subtotal resection in advanced stages remains controversial. Patients with relapsed disease following a complete resection should be considered for a second operation.

2. **Adjuvant therapy.** Adjuvant radiation therapy is not indicated for R0 resections in stage I disease, should be considered for R0 resections in stages II to IV, and is indicated in cases of R1 resection. In the case of R2 resections, patients should be considered for the addition of chemotherapy to the adjuvant radiotherapy.

B. Locally advanced disease

1. **Neoadjuvant therapy.** Although the use of preoperative single modality radiation therapy has not been associated with survival benefit, several studies suggest improvement in both resectability and survival with the use of multimodality treatment in patients with Masaoka stage III and IV patients. The National Comprehensive Cancer

TABLE 14-4	Overall Survival for Resected Thymomas	
Masaoka stage	5-year survival (%)	10-year survival (%)
I	92	88
II	82	70
III	68	57
IV	60	38

Network currently recommends chemotherapy as the initial treatment for patients with locally advanced thymomas followed by surgical evaluation. In the case of resectable disease, the treatment of choice is surgery followed by adjuvant radiation therapy. Unresectable tumors should be treated with chemoradiotherapy (*J Natl Compr Cancer Netw* 2013;11:562).

C. Advanced disease. Thymomas are sensitive to chemotherapy, and several chemotherapeutic drugs, either as a single drug or in combination regimens, have been shown to be active. The intergroup phase II trial evaluated the PAC regimen (cisplatin 50 mg/m^2, doxorubicin 50 mg/m^2, and cyclophosphamide 500 mg/m^2 every 3 weeks) in 30 patients with metastatic or recurrent thymoma and thymic carcinoma (*J Clin Oncol* 1994;12:1164). The overall response rate was 50% with median survival of 38 months and a 5-year estimated survival of 32%. PAC is currently the standard treatment for thymoma. The combination of cisplatin (60 mg/m^2 on day 1) and etoposide (120 mg/m^2 on days 1 to 3) resulted in a 56% response rate and median survival of 4.3 years (*J Clin Oncol* 1996;14:814). For patients with thymoma and positive indium-labeled octreotide scan, octreotide 0.5 mg subcutaneously three times daily for up to 1 year resulted in a 12.5% response rate. When combined with prednisone (0.6 mg/kg/day), octreotide showed a 31% response rate with median survival of 15 months (*Cancer* 2002;94:1414).

D. Prognosis. Prognosis is usually related to the stage at presentation, presence or absence of complete resection, and the histologic subtype. Most of the thymomas are slow-growing encapsulated tumors that can be cured by surgical resection. Staging, regardless of the system used, remains the single most important prognostic determinant, and the outcomes are significantly better in patients undergoing complete resection. There is a linear progression of malignancy among the WHO histologic subtypes, with A and AB thymomas behaving as benign tumors, B1 and B2 as low-grade tumors, and B3 as an aggressive tumor similar to thymic carcinoma. This correlation is reflected in both the likelihood of invasion and the overall survival.

IV. THYMIC CARCINOMA. Thymic carcinomas are rare tumors characterized by overt histologic and cytologic features of malignancy such as nuclear atypia, increased mitotic activity, and necrosis. Tumors are usually located in the anterosuperior mediastinum, and patients usually present with symptoms of local invasion such as dyspnea, cough, and chest pain. Most of the patients present with advanced disease with invasion of contiguous mediastinal structures and lymphadenopathy seen in approximately 80% and 40% of patients, respectively. Paraneoplastic syndromes are rarely seen. Owing to the paucity of cases, the optimal treatment remains undefined. Surgical resection is the mainstay of treatment, but complete resection is possible in only a few patients in view of the advanced stage. Adjuvant radiation therapy should be considered in patients with stage II to IV undergoing R0 resection. In the case of R1 or R2 resection, patients should receive adjuvant chemoradiotherapy. In patients with advanced disease, a small study including 23 patients with thymic carcinoma showed a 22% response rate, 5-month progression-free survival (PFS), and 20-month median survival with the combination of carboplatin and paclitaxel (AUC 6 and 225 mg/m^2 on day 1) (*J Clin Oncol* 2011;29:2060), which has become the regimen of choice for thymic carcinoma.

V. TARGETED THERAPY. The most frequent alterations in thymomas occur on the locus of the major histocompatibility complex (chromosome 6p). Abnormalities effecting *EGFR* gene amplification and overexpression, *HER2* overexpression, *c-KIT* overexpression, *BCL2* overexpression, *TP53* overexpression, and *PI16INK4A* loss of expression have been identified. Approximately 12% of patients with thymic carcinoma harbor c-KIT mutations, and several studies have shown response to tyrosine kinase inhibitors including imatinib, sorafenib, and sunitinib, occasionally lasting more than 12 months (*Ann Oncol* 2012;23:2409).

VI. BACKGROUND. Thymomas are the most common primary tumors of the anterior mediastinum in adults. Most of the patients are between the ages of 40 and 60 at the time of diagnosis, and there is no sex predilection. The overall incidence is 0.15 cases per 100,000 person-years.

VII. MESOTHELIOMA

A. Presentation

1. **Subjective.** The symptoms of mesothelioma are usually insidious and nonspecific. Therefore, a delay in diagnosis is typical. The median time between the onset of symptoms and the diagnosis is 2 to 3 months. The most common presenting complaints are dyspnea and nonpleuritic chest wall pain. Constitutional symptoms such as weight loss and fatigue are more frequent in the later stages of the disease but may occur in approximately one-third of the patients at presentation. Some patients may be asymptomatic, and their disease is first noticed incidentally on a routine chest radiograph.

2. **Objective.** Common findings on physical examination include signs of unilateral pleural effusion including dullness to percussion and decreased air entry in the involved lung base. Fixed hemothorax, characterized by the lack of expansion of the chest, is present in large tumors and usually represents a late finding. Occasionally, patients with advanced disease may have palpable supraclavicular lymph nodes or a palpable chest wall mass. Clubbing is rare. Some patients may have no physical signs owing to the presence of a localized pleural mass without effusion.

B. Workup and staging

1. **Imaging studies.** Radiographic evaluation begins with a PA and lateral chest radiograph, which usually demonstrates a unilateral pleural effusion and occasionally a pleural-based mass. Approximately 20% of the patients have radiologic evidence of asbestos exposure on chest radiograph such as pleural plaques. CT scan often shows an effusion with or without pleural mass and allows the evaluation of tumor extent. In some patients, mesothelioma produces a localized lobular thickening, whereas in others, it causes a rind of tumor encasing the lung. MRI may help to further define the local extension of pleural mesothelioma to the chest wall and diaphragm. Positron emission tomography (PET) scan can be used to differentiate between benign and malignant pleural masses. This functional imaging modality may also allow the detection of lymph node or extrathoracic involvement.

2. **Diagnosis.** Despite the presence of typical, clinical, or radiographic findings, the definitive diagnosis of mesothelioma should be made by pathologic evaluation. The initial diagnostic procedure is usually a thoracentesis. Cytology of the pleural fluid does not always provide a definitive diagnosis because the yield can be low. Furthermore, when abnormal cells are present, it is often difficult to differentiate mesothelioma cells from reactive mesothelial cells and other malignancies such as adenocarcinoma. The diagnostic value of cytology may improve with the use of immunohistochemical (IHC) stains. When the cytology is inconclusive, patients should undergo a pleural biopsy. Histology samples may be obtained either by a CT-guided biopsy or through direct thoracoscopy.

3. **Pathology.** Mesothelioma is classified into three histologic subtypes: epithelial, sarcomatoid, and mixed. The epithelial type is the most common, comprising 50% to 60% of all cases. The sarcomatoid type is present in approximately 15% of cases and is characterized by spindle cells that are similar to fibrosarcomas. The mixed or biphasic subtype contains features of both epithelioid and sarcomatoid elements. Because the diagnosis of mesothelioma may not be easily accomplished from the pathologic specimen, IHC studies are commonly used to differentiate between mesothelioma and metastatic or primary lung adenocarcinomas. Stains that are typically positive in mesothelioma include epithelial membrane antigen (EMA), Wilms' tumor antigen-1 (WT1), cytokeratin 5/6, calretinin, and mesothelin. Negative stains include carcinoembryonic antigen (CEA), thyroid transcription factor-1 (TTF-1), B72.3, CD15, MOC-31, Ber-P4, and Bg8. Electron microscopy should be reserved for difficult cases with equivocal IHC results. The epithelial form is composed of polygonal cells with long microvilli, prominent desmosomes, and abundant tonofilaments. The electron microscopy on the sarcomatoid variant reveals elongated nuclei and abundant rough endoplasmic reticulum.

4. **Serum markers.** Soluble mesothelin-related protein (SMRP) is a soluble form of mesothelin, which is elevated in most of the patients with mesothelioma. SMRP levels correlate with disease progression or response to therapy, and may be useful in in the early detection for patients at risk.

5. **Staging.** Although several staging systems have been proposed for mesothelioma, none achieved universal acceptance. The International Mesothelioma Interest Group (IMIG) proposed a new staging system for mesothelioma (Table 14-5). This tumor (T), lymph node (N), and metastases (M) staging system includes T descriptors that are much more detailed than in previous systems. In addition, the descriptors for nodal involvement are the same as those used in the staging of non–small cell lung cancer. This new system allowed a more accurate staging of mesothelioma patients according to prognosis. Median survival by stage was 35 months, 16 months, 11.5 months, and 5.9 months for stages I through IV, respectively.

C. **Treatment.** Mesothelioma is an essentially incurable disease, and the primary goal of therapy is to improve the quality of life and prolong survival. In most cases, the tumor spreads along the serosal surface and infiltrates the underlying vital thoracic organs, preventing a complete surgical resection. Furthermore, mesothelioma often arises from multiple sites in the parietal pleura. Patients are commonly elderly with significant co-morbidities, and the insidious symptoms frequently delay the diagnosis. The choice of treatment is determined by the stage of the disease and the patients' comorbidities.

1. **Surgery.** There are three main surgical procedures used in the management of patients with mesothelioma: pleurodesis, pleurectomy with decortication (PD), and extrapleural pneumonectomy (EPP). Pleurodesis is commonly used in the treatment of persistent dyspnea caused by large pleural effusions. This procedure is effective in preventing fluid accumulation and should be performed early during management. As the disease progresses, the tumor grows along the visceral pleura and encases the lung, preventing the re-expansion. The resultant trapped lung is usually refractory to pleurodesis. PD refers to the surgical removal of the visceral, parietal, and pericardial pleura from the lung, apex to diaphragm, without the removal of the lung. A complete resection is possible only in very early stages of the disease, and most of the patients develop a disease recurrence. EPP is the most aggressive procedure and involves the en bloc resection of the visceral and parietal pleura, lung, pericardium, and ipsilateral diaphragm. EPP achieves the greatest degree of cytoreduction and, because the lung has been removed, higher doses of adjuvant radiation to be delivered to the ipsilateral hemithorax. A retrospective study compared the two surgical modalities in 663 consecutive patients operated between 1990 and 2006. EPP was associated with increased operative mortality (7% vs. 4%) and decreased survival in a multivariate analysis adjusting for age, gender, histology, stage and addition of chemotherapy, and/or radiation therapy (HR 1.4; 95% confidence interval 1.18 to 1.69; p < 0.001) (*J Thorac Cardiovasc Surg* 2008;135:620). Although both PD and EPP are performed with curative intent, neither appears to provide a significant improvement in survival when used as a single modality therapy.

2. **Radiation therapy.** Mesothelioma cells are relatively sensitive to radiation therapy. However, owing to the diffuse nature of the cancer, the dose of radiation for mesothelioma is limited by the need to irradiate the entire hemithorax, which includes vital organs such as lung, heart, esophagus, and spinal cord. Radiation therapy has minimal effects on increasing survival. There are three main indications for the use of radiation therapy: palliation of pain, prophylaxis against needle tract metastases, and adjuvant therapy. Most of the patients treated with palliative radiation therapy achieve a short-lived pain control. Because mesothelioma is characterized by direct local invasion, it often invades tracts after local procedures. In these cases, radiation may be used as a prophylactic measure. Owing to the high rates of local relapse after surgery, radiation therapy has been used in the adjuvant setting in an attempt to eradicate residual tumor. Studies in patients undergoing EPP have shown decreased local relapse with disease palliation, but no definitive survival improvement.

TABLE 14-5	IMIG Staging for Mesothelioma

T: Tumor

T1	Tumor limited to the ipsilateral parietal pleura, including mediastinal and diaphragmatic pleura
	T1a—No involvement of the visceral pleura
	T1b—Tumor involving visceral pleura
T2	Tumor involving each of the ipsilateral pleural surfaces (parietal, mediastinal, diaphragmatic, and visceral pleura) with at least one of the following features:
	• Involvement of the diaphragmatic muscle
	• Extension of tumor from visceral pleura into the underlying pulmonary parenchyma
T3	Locally advanced but potentially resectable tumor
	Tumor involving all the ipsilateral pleural surfaces (parietal, mediastinal, diaphragmatic, and visceral pleura) with at least one of the following:
	• Involvement of the endothoracic fascia
	• Extension into the mediastinal fat
	• Solitary, completely resectable focus of tumor extending into the soft tissues of the chest wall
	• Nontransmural involvement of the pericardium
T4	Locally advanced technically unresectable tumor
	• Tumor involving all of the ipsilateral pleural surfaces (parietal, mediastinal, diaphragmatic, and visceral) with at least one of the following features:
	• Diffuse extension or multifocal masses of tumor in the chest wall, with or without associated rib destruction
	• Direct transdiaphragmatic extension of tumor to the peritoneum
	• Direct extension of tumor to the contralateral pleura
	• Direct extension of tumor to one or more mediastinal organs
	• Direct extension of tumor into the spine
	• Tumor extending through to the internal surface of the pericardium with or without a pericardial effusion, or tumor involving the myocardium

N: Lymph nodes

NX	Regional lymph nodes cannot be assessed
N0	No regional lymph node metastases
N1	Metastases in the ipsilateral bronchopulmonary or hilar lymph nodes
N2	Metastases in the subcarinal or the ipsilateral mediastinal lymph nodes, including the ipsilateral internal mammary nodes
N3	Metastases in the contralateral mediastinal, contralateral internal mammary, ipsilateral, or contralateral supraclavicular lymph nodes

M: Metastases

MX	Presence of distant metastases cannot be assessed
M0	No distant metastasis
M1	Distant metastases present

Stage groupings:

Stage	Ia	T1a	N0	M0
	Ib	T1b	N0	M0
Stage	II	T2	N0	M0
Stage	III	T3	N0–2	M0
		T1–2	N1–2	M0
Stage	IV	T4	Any N	M0
		Any T	N3	M0
		Any T	Any N	M1

3. **Chemotherapy.** Chemotherapy has been used in the neoadjuvant or adjuvant setting in patients treated with multimodality treatment or as single modality in advanced cases where the role of chemotherapy remains palliative, because even trimodality therapy does not appear to achieve cure or significantly prolong survival. Among several regimens, the combination of pemetrexed and cisplatin emerged as the standard of care after a phase III study showed improved survival compared with single agent cisplatin (*J Clin Oncol* 2003;21:2636). In this study, 456 patients were assigned to cisplatin alone (75 mg/m^2 day 1 every 3 weeks) or in combination with pemetrexed (500 mg/m^2 day 1 every 3 weeks). The combination arm resulted in significant benefit including improved response rate (41% vs. 16%, $p <0.0001$), median time to progression (5.7 months vs. 3.9 months, $p = 0.001$), and median survival (12.1 months vs. 9.3 months, $p = 0.02$). Carboplatin combined with pemetrexed is an acceptable alternative for patients who cannot tolerate cisplatin. This combination yielded median survival of 12.7 months in a first-line phase II study (*Clin Lung Cancer* 2010;11:30) and showed no response differences when compared with cisplatin with pemetrexed. Patients who cannot tolerate pemetrexed may be candidates for the combination of gemcitabine and cisplatin with comparable survival data (*Br J Cancer* 2002;86:342). Single-agent options include pemetrexed or vinorelbine in either first- or second-line settings.

4. **Targeted therapy.** Several novel approaches for the systemic treatment of mesothelioma have been recently investigated. A phase II trial of cisplatin, pemetrexed, and bevacizumab failed to reach a 33% improvement in PFS at 6 months compared with the historical control of 48%. (*Lung Cancer* 2012;77:567). The addition of bevacizumab to carboplatin and pemetrexed led to a median PFS of 6.9 months, which also failed to reach the primary end point of increase from the historical 6 months to a meaningful 9 months (*Br J Cancer* 2013;109:552). The Cancer and Leukemia Group B conducted a phase II study evaluating the role of gefitinib, an oral epidermal growth factor receptor (EGFR) tyrosine kinase in previously untreated patients with mesothelioma (*Clin Cancer Res* 2005;11:2300). Among the 43 enrolled patients, the response rate was 4% and median survival 6.8 months. EGFR expression was not correlated with response or survival. The tyrosine kinase inhibitor sunitinib targets the receptors of Vascular endothelial growth factor VEGF and Platelet-derived growth factor PDGF. A phase II study investigated sunitinib in patients progressive after systemic chemotherapy. Median time to progression was 3.7 months and median overall survival was 8.2 months (*J Thorac Oncol* 2012;9:1449). Other investigational therapeutic strategies include proteasome inhibitors, mTOR inhibitors, HDAC inhibitors, and immune modulators such as thalidomide (*J Natl Compr Cancer Netw* 2012;10:42).

D. **Prognosis.** The prognosis for patients with mesothelioma is poor, with median survival of approximately 12 months from diagnosis. Factors associated with poor prognosis include advanced stage, poor performance status, male sex, chest pain, weight loss, thrombocytosis, leukocytosis, anemia, older age, and sarcomatoid histology. Two prognostic systems have been developed on the basis of data collection from patients enrolled into large cooperative group trials. In the European Organization for Research and Treatment of Cancer (EORTC) study, the risk factors identified were Eastern Cooperative Oncology Group (ECOG) performance status 1 or 2, white blood cells more than 8,300/μL, hemoglobin decrease equal to or greater than 1 g/dL, probable or possible diagnosis, and sarcomatoid histology (*J Clin Oncol* 1998;16:145). Patients were subdivided into two prognostic groups: good prognosis with up to two risk factors and poor prognosis with three or more risk factors. Outcomes were significantly better for patients in the good prognosis category, with improved median survival (10.8 months vs. 5.5 months), 1-year overall survival (40% vs. 12%), and 2-year survival (14% vs. 0%). In the Cancer and Leukemia Group B (CALGB) study, the significant risk factors included poor performance status, chest pain, dyspnea, platelet count greater than 400,000/μL, weight loss, serum lactate dehydrogenase (LDH) greater than 500 IU/L, pleural involvement, anemia, leukocytosis, and age above 75 years (*Chest* 1998;113:723).

There were six identified prognostic subgroups with median survival times ranging from 1.4 to 13.9 months.

E. Background. Malignant mesothelioma is an aggressive tumor of the serosal surfaces. The incidence is increasing worldwide as a result of widespread exposure to asbestos. There are approximately 2,500 new cases per year in the United States. The main risk for the development of mesothelioma is exposure to asbestos. Although approximately 80% of patients with mesothelioma have a history of asbestos exposure, only approximately 10% of those exposed will develop mesothelioma.

SUGGESTED READINGS

Thymoma

Detterbeck FC, Parsons AM. Thymic tumors. *Ann Thorac Surg* 2004;77:1860–1869.

Duwe BV, Sterman DH, Musani AI. Tumors of the mediastinum. *Chest* 2005;128:2893–2909.

Ettinger D, Riely GJ, Akerley W, et al. Thymomas and thymic carcinomas. *J Natl Compr Cancer Netw* 2013;11:562–576.

Eng TY, Fuller CD, Jagirdar J, et al. Thymic carcinoma: state of the art and review. *Int J Radiat Oncol Biol Phys* 2004;59:654–664.

Giaccone G. Treatment of malignant thymoma. *Curr Opin Oncol* 2005;17:140–146.

Giaccone G, Wilmink H, Paul MA, et al. Systemic treatment of malignant thymoma: a decade of experience at a single institution. *Am J Clin Oncol* 2006;29:336–344.

Johnson SB, Eng TY, Giaccone G. Thymoma: update for the new millennium. *Oncologist* 2001;6:239–246.

Kelly RJ, Petrini I, Rajan A, et al. Thymic malignancies: from clinical management to targeted therapies. *J Clin Oncol* 2011;29:4820–4827.

Suster S, Moran CA. Thymoma classification: current status and future trends. *Am J Clin Pathol* 2006;125:542–554.

Thomas CR, Wright CD, Loehrer PJ. Thymoma: state of the art. *J Clin Oncol* 1999;17: 2280–2289.

Mesothelioma

Ceresoli GL, Zucali PA, Menconboni M, et al. Phase II study of pemetrexed and carboplatin plus bevacizumab as first line therapy in malignant pleural mesothelioma. *Br J Cancer* 2013;109:552–558.

Curran D, Sahmoud T, Therasse P, et al. Prognostic factors in patients with pleural mesothelioma: the European Organization for Research and Treatment of Cancer experience. *J Clin Oncol* 1998;16:145–152.

Dowell JE, Dunphy FR, Taub RN, et al. A multicenter phase II study of cisplatin, pemetrexed, and bevacizumab in patients with advanced malignant mesothelioma. *Lung Cancer* 2012;77:567–571.

Flores RM, Pass HI, Seshan VE, et al. Extrapleural pneumonectomy versus pleurectomy/decortication in the surgical management of malignant pleural mesothelioma: results in 663 patients. *J Thorac Cardiovasc Surg* 2008;135:620–626.

Herndon JE, Green MR, Chahinian AP, et al. Factors predictive of survival among 337 patients with mesothelioma treated between 1984 and 1994 by the cancer and leukemia group B. *Chest* 1998;113:723–731.

Krug LM. An overview of chemotherapy for mesothelioma. *Hematol Oncol Clin North Am* 2005;19:1117–1136.

Masaoka A, Monden Y, Nakahara K, et al. Follow-up study of thymomas with special reference to their clinical stages. *Cancer* 1981;48:2485–2492.

Pistolesi M, Rusthoven J. Malignant pleural mesothelioma: update, current management, and newer therapeutic strategies. *Chest* 2004;126:1318–1329.

Robinson BWS, Lake RA. Advances in malignant mesothelioma. *N Engl J Med* 2005;353:1591–1603.

Schirosi L, Nannini N, Nicoli D, et al. Activating c-KIT mutations in a subset of thymic carcinomas and response to different c-KIT inhibitors. *Ann Onc* 2012;23:2409–2414.

Volgelzang NJ, Rusthoven JJ, Symanowsky J, et al. Phase III study of pemetrexed in combination with cisplatin versus cisplatin alone in patients with malignant pleural mesothelioma. *J Clin Oncol* 2003;21:2636–2644.

Zauderer MG, Krug LM. Novel therapies in phase II and III trials for malignant pleural mesothelioma. *J Natl Compr Canc Netw* 2012;10:42–47.

15 Esophageal and Gastric Cancer

Maria Baggstrom • A. Craig Lockhart

I. ESOPHAGEAL CANCER

A. Subjective. Patients with esophageal cancer often do not have symptoms until the esophageal lumen is greatly narrowed. The most common symptom for patients with esophageal cancer is dysphagia. Ninety-five percent of symptomatic patients will report dysphagia. It typically begins with solid food only but often progresses to occurring with liquids as the esophageal lumen becomes blocked by the cancer. Other common symptoms include weight loss (50%), regurgitation (40%), pain on swallowing (20%), and cough (20%).

B. Objective. Physical examination findings are varied. It may be normal, show cachexia only, or there may be evidence of metastases such as supraclavicular lymphadenopathy, hoarseness from recurrent laryngeal nerve involvement, pleural effusion, hepatomegaly, or bony tenderness.

C. Workup. Symptoms or signs suggesting esophageal cancer should prompt further evaluation. The most important test is an esophagogastroduodenoscopy (EGD). This test allows visualization, localization, and biopsy of an esophageal lesion. If an esophageal cancer is found, a complete blood count (CBC), comprehensive metabolic panel (CMP), and a computed tomography (CT) of the chest and abdomen are indicated.

CT is an excellent initial staging tool, but depending on the CT results as well as the tumor location, further specialized testing may be necessary. If the patient does not have evidence of metastasis on CT, consultation with a thoracic surgeon and a radiation oncologist should follow.

In the absence of metastatic disease and if the patient is considered a candidate for curative surgery, an endoscopic ultrasound should be performed. This procedure, involving insertion of an ultrasound probe into the esophagus and stomach, allows the most precise assessment of depth of tumor involvement, length of esophagus affected, and magnitude of lymph node metastases, particularly paraesophageal and celiac nodes. A biopsy of suspicious lymph nodes can be done during the study.

Positron emission tomography (PET) scans are an important part of the staging evaluation of patients without clear evidence of metastasis on CT. FDG (2-fluoro-2-deoxy-D-glucose)-avid lymph nodes located in regions where therapy would be altered should be biopsied to confirm metastasis.

A primary tumor located above the carina increases the risk for tracheoesophageal fistula, indicating the need for bronchoscopy. Patients with tracheoesophageal fistulas often present with postprandial coughing and may sometimes have aspiration pneumonias.

D. Staging. Esophageal cancer staging depends on the tumor, node, metastases (TNM) system established by the American Joint Commission for Cancer (AJCC) and the International Union Against Cancer (UICC). The most recent edition of the AJCC for the staging of esophageal cancers includes tumors that include the gastroesophageal junction and tumors extending to the proximal 5 cm of the stomach.

E. Therapy

1. Therapy for localized esophageal cancer

a. General considerations. The treatment of esophageal cancer requires a multidisciplinary approach. It frequently involves a combination of surgery, radiation, chemotherapy, and supportive treatments. The functional status of the patient and location of the tumor play a key role in determining the management of the patient. Patient comorbidities may preclude the use of potentially curative therapies.

b. Surgery. Surgery is considered the standard therapy for stage I, II, and III esophageal cancers located outside the cervical esophagus. If an early-stage cancer is located in the cervical esophagus, however, the preferred treatment is a combination of chemotherapy and radiation.

The best chance for surgical cure involves removal of the entire tumor and draining lymph nodes with adequate proximal and distal margins. The three most frequently used approaches for resection are: (a) the Ivor Lewis approach, in which a laparotomy and right thoracotomy are performed for esophageal resection and gastric mobilization with an anastomosis in the upper thorax; (b) transhiatal esophagectomy, through a cervical and abdominal approach with cervical anastomosis; and (c) left thoracoabdominal approach, with an anastomosis below the aortic arch. After an esophagectomy, most patients are reconstructed with a primary esophagogastric anastomosis in the neck or chest.

Esophageal resection is a major surgery with a mortality rate of approximately 4% in experienced hands. Other complications of the surgery may include anastomotic leak, chylothorax, damage to the left recurrent laryngeal nerve, severe hemorrhage, and pulmonary embolus.

The cure rates from surgery are dependent on the stage of the cancer. Thirty percent to fifty percent of patients with stage I esophageal cancer will be cured by surgery alone. For patients with stage IIA and IIB disease, the 5-year survivals following surgery are 15% to 30% and 5% to 15%, respectively. Locoregional relapse after surgical resection ranges from 15% to 25%.

c. **Neoadjuvant and adjuvant therapy.** In patients with locally advanced cancers, neoadjuvant and adjuvant treatment with chemoradiotherapy have been shown to improve outcomes in randomized phase III trials.

The most prominent study evaluating neoadjuvant chemoradiotherapy is the CROSS trial (*N Engl J Med* 2012;366:2074). In the CROSS study, 368 patients with resectable esophageal cancers of both histologic subtypes (squamous and adenocarcinoma) were randomly assigned to immediate surgery or weekly administration of neoadjuvant carboplatin (doses titrated to an area under the curve of 2 mg/mL/min) and paclitaxel (50 mg/m^2) for 5 weeks and concurrent radiotherapy (41.4 Gy in 23 fractions, 5 days/ week), followed by surgery. Median overall survival was 49.4 months in the chemoradiotherapy–surgery group versus 24 months in the surgery group (hazard ratio [HR], 0.657; 95% confidence interval [CI], 0.495 to 0.871; P=0.003). For patients with locally advanced but surgically resectable esophageal cancers, neoadjuvant chemoradiotherapy is recommended by the National Comprehensive Cancer Network (NCCN).

Postoperative chemoradiotherapy has a role in the treatment of selected patients with esophageal cancer (*New Engl J Med* 2001;345:725). The SWOG 9008/INT 0116 randomized 556 patients with resected adenocarcinoma of the stomach or gastroesophageal junction, stage IB through IVM0, to surgery plus postoperative chemoradiotherapy or surgery alone. The adjuvant treatment consisted of 425 mg of fluorouracil/m^2/day, plus 20 mg of leucovorin/m^2/day, for 5 days, followed by 4,500 cGy of radiation at 180 cGy per day, given 5 days per week for 5 weeks, with modified doses of fluorouracil and leucovorin on the first 4 and the last 3 days of radiotherapy. The median overall survival in the surgery-only group was 27 months, compared with 36 months in the chemoradiotherapy group; the HR for death was 1.35 (95% confidence interval, 1.09 to 1.66; P=0.005). The HR for relapse was 1.52 (95% CI, 1.23 to 1.86; P<0.001). Since approximately 20% of the patients in this study had lesions at the gastroesophageal junction, this approach is commonly applied to patients with adenocarcinomas of the distal esophagus who have not received preoperative therapy. Patients with gross or microscopic residual disease following surgery are felt to benefit from combined modality chemoradiotherapy. Adjuvant chemoradiotherapy in patients with squamous cell cancers without residual disease after resection is less defined. In the current NCCN Guidelines, observation is recommended for those with squamous cell carcinoma.

d. **Therapy for unresectable locally advanced esophageal cancer.** The standard of care for unresectable locally advanced esophageal cancer is concurrent chemoradiotherapy.

Herscovic et al., randomized 120 patients to radiation alone (64 Gy) or cisplatin 75 mg/m^2 on day 1 and 5-FU 1,000 mg/m^2/day continuous intravenous infusion on days 1 to 4 to be repeated in weeks 1, 5, 8, and 11 along with 50 Gy of radiation over 5 weeks. The median survival for the chemoradiotherapy arm was 14.1 months versus 9.3 months in the radiation-alone arm. The 5-year survival for chemoradiotherapy was 27%, as compared with 0% in the radiation-alone group (*N Engl J Med* 1992;326:1593). Eighty-five percent of the patients had squamous cell esophageal cancers; therefore, there is more clinical data to apply this approach in patients with tumors that have squamous cell histology. However, this approach is also often used in patients with adenocarcinomas who are not candidates for curative surgery.

e. **Endoscopic treatment of superficial esophageal cancers.** Patients who undergo frequent endoscopic evaluations because of a history of Barrett's Esophagus, high-grade dysplasia, or long-standing acid reflux are sometimes found to have superficial esophageal cancers. Esophagectomy has been the standard treatment for these conditions with high cure rates but also significant impact on quality of life. More recently, endoscopic approaches (e.g., endoscopic mucosal resection [EMR], photodynamic therapy [PDT], and laser therapy) have increased in use for selected patients with encouraging results. These approaches should be considered only in patients who have a very low risk of lymph node metastases (T stage less than T1b) or are poor candidates for esophageal surgery.

2. **Therapy for metastatic esophageal cancer**
   a. **General considerations.** Metastatic esophageal cancer is incurable, and the toxicity of therapy must be weighed against its potential benefit. Palliative therapy for swallowing and nutritional support are especially important. There are a number of options for palliation of swallowing. These include esophageal dilatation, stent placement, brachytherapy, external beam radiation, and laser therapy. In regard to nutritional support, patients with metastatic esophageal cancer frequently require a gastrostomy tube.
   b. **Chemotherapy.** Several chemotherapeutic agents have activity in esophageal cancer. Unfortunately, no large phase III trials comparing chemotherapeutic regimens have been performed in recent years. The agents that have the most activity in esophageal cancer are cisplatin, carboplatin, 5-FU, paclitaxel, docetaxel, vinorelbine, oxaliplatin, and irinotecan. In general, platinum-based doublets have the highest response rate and are typically used as first-line therapy. It is a common practice, and listed in the NCCN, that patients with metastatic cancers of the esophagus, regardless of histology, can be treated similarly to patients with gastric adenocarcinomas. For patients with metastatic adenocarcinoma of the esophagus, it is recommended that the tumor be tested for HER2-neu status to determine whether trastuzumab should be added to chemotherapy (*Lancet* 2010;376:687). NCCN currently lists platinum-based and 5-FU–based chemotherapeutic regimens as category 1 recommendations (strongest recommendation). There are three category 1 regimens, epirubicin cisplatin, 5-FU (ECF), docetaxel, cisplatin, 5-FU (DCF), and fluorouracil with cisplatin. Three-drug regimens should be reserved for patients with excellent performance status, good organ function, and easy access to medical care.

F. **Course of the disease.** Metastatic esophageal cancer has a poor prognosis with a median survival of approximately 10 months despite systemic chemotherapy. Three fourths of the patients have mediastinal node involvement or distant spread at the time of diagnosis. Death often occurs from progression of their metastatic disease or aspiration pneumonia from local disease.

G. **Complications.** Complications of the esophageal cancer include hemorrhage, obstruction, tracheoesophageal fistula, and aspiration pneumonia.

H. **Epidemiology.** Esophageal cancer is a commonly found neoplasm and is the seventh most common cause of cancer death in the world. There is vast geographic variation in the incidence of this cancer. The incidence in the United States is about 5 per 100,000, although in African American men, it may be as high as 18 per 100,000, whereas China and Iran have an incidence of 20 per 100,000. In parts of Africa, Central America, and Western Asia, the incidence is only 1.5 per 100,000.

The two most common pathologic subtypes of esophageal cancer are squamous cell carcinoma and adenocarcinoma. Other histologic types such as sarcomas, small cell carcinomas, and lymphomas are extremely rare. Of the two most common histologies, squamous cell tumors make up 98% of malignancies in the upper and middle one-third of the esophagus, whereas adenocarcinoma is found predominantly in the lower third. Previously, squamous cell carcinoma was the most frequent subtype, but over the past 30 years, the incidence of adenocarcinoma has been increasing rapidly in the Western world. The reason for this shift is unknown. In non-Western countries, squamous cell cancers represent the majority of esophageal cancers, with adenocarcinomas remaining relatively unusual.

The incidence of esophageal cancer increases with age and is rarely found among patients younger than 40 years. Squamous cell carcinoma affects African American men six times more than it affects White men, whereas adenocarcinoma affects Whites four times as much. All subtypes of esophageal cancers affect men three times as often as they do women.

Several factors can increase the risk of developing esophageal cancer. The long-term use of tobacco and alcohol are predisposing factors for development of squamous cell carcinoma of the esophagus. Dietary factors such as inadequate vegetable and fruit intake may also increase the risk of the development of this cancer. Nitrosamines and their precursors (found in pickled vegetables, moldy or fermented foods, and smoked fish) are known to promote cancerous changes in the esophagus. Tylosis, a rare genetic syndrome, carries the highest risk of developing squamous cell carcinoma from chronic inflammation and stasis (1,000-fold risk). It is an autosomal dominant trait characterized by hyperkeratosis of the palms and soles that may produce defective vitamin A metabolism. Other conditions associated with esophageal cancer are head and neck malignancies, celiac disease, and gastroesophageal reflux disease.

Barrett's esophagus increases the risk of adenocarcinoma by 30 to 125 times that of the healthy patient population. In this disorder, the normal squamous epithelium of the esophagus is destroyed by chronic gastroesophageal reflux of acid, pepsin, and bile, and is ultimately replaced by a specialized intestinal columnar epithelium.

I. **Research initiatives.** The role of many targeted therapies is currently being studied. Optimizing neoadjuvant chemoradiation is also an important area of research.

II. GASTRIC CANCER

A. **Subjective.** Gastric cancer usually presents with nonspecific constitutional symptoms. The most common is weight loss that occurs in approximately 80% of patients. Other common symptoms include anorexia, early satiety, fatigue, vague stomach pain, dysphagia (from gastroesophageal [GE] junction tumors), GI bleeding, and vomiting (from gastric outlet obstruction).

B. **Objective.** The physical findings in gastric cancer are typically manifestations of metastatic disease. Several eponymic terms have been created to describe specific sites of metastatic gastric cancer. Virchow's node describes metastasis to the left supraclavicular node. Sister Mary Joseph's node is a periumbilical lymph node metastasis. A Krukenberg tumor is a gastric cancer metastatic to the ovaries. Blumer's shelf describes a "drop metastasis" into the perirectal pouch. Other common physical findings in patients with metastatic gastric cancer include cachexia, palpable abdominal masses, hepatomegaly from metastatic involvement and malignant ascites.

C. **Workup.** EGD is useful for the evaluation of suspected gastric cancer. This technique allows visualization of lesions and easy biopsy. EGD is used in the Japanese screening program for gastric cancer, which is credited with the increased proportion of early gastric cancers diagnosed in that country.

Once a diagnosis of gastric carcinoma is made, further staging is necessary. As in esophageal cancer, CT scans and PET/CT are used to evaluate for metastatic disease. In cases where surgical resection for cure is being considered, endoscopic ultrasound may be used to evaluate the tumor depth and involvement of local lymph nodes. Unfortunately, metastatic peritoneal deposits may not be seen on routine imaging, and a diagnostic laparotomy is necessary to rule this out before embarking on definitive therapy.

Gastric cancer is staged according to the AJCC TNM criteria.

D. Therapy

1. Localized gastric adenocarcinoma

a. Surgery. Surgery is the most effective curative therapy for gastric cancer. In the United States, patients with resected stage I cancer have a 5-year survival of 58% to 78%. For stage II, survival ranges from 20% to 34%, and for stage III from 8% to 20%.

Patients with cancers localized to the distal stomach may be cured with subtotal gastrectomy. Other sites are usually treated with total gastrectomy. With surgical resection, the standard of care surgery should include a D2 lymph node dissection that removes the perigastric nodes along the greater and lesser curvature (the N1 group of nodes) as well as the nodes along the left gastric artery, the common hepatic artery, the celiac artery, and the splenic artery (the N2 group of nodes). The tail of the pancreas and the spleen are sometimes removed additionally in a D2 dissection, although this procedure has been noted to increase morbidity and mortality (*Lancet Oncol* 2010;11:439).

The NCCN Guidelines recommend a D2 resection along with an examination of at least 15 lymph nodes. In Asian countries, D2 dissections are routinely completed. In the United States, D2 resections are less commonly achieved owing to concerns about greater morbidity. Patients should therefore be referred for surgery at centers with experience in these procedures.

b. Neoadjuvant and adjuvant therapy. Adjuvant therapies have been tried in an attempt to improve survival following resection. Adjuvant radiotherapy alone has not shown benefit. Adjuvant chemoradiotherapy, however, clearly has benefit for some patients. This is based on the Intergroup 116 (INT-116) study. In this study, 556 patients with at least stage IB gastric carcinoma, who had undergone definitive resection to negative margins, were randomized to observation or 5 months of therapy. The adjuvant therapy consisted of one cycle consisting of 5-FU (425 mg/m^2) plus leucovorin (20 mg/m^2) daily for 5 days. One month of rest followed this cycle of chemotherapy. Combination chemoradiotherapy was then started. Radiation dose of 4,500 cGy was given over 5 weeks with 5-FU (400 mg/m^2) and leucovorin (20 mg/m^2) on days 1 to 4 and for the last 3 days of radiation. A 1-month rest then followed. Then 5-FU (425 mg/m^2) plus leucovorin (20 mg/m^2) on days 1 to 5 was repeated monthly for two cycles. Adjuvant therapy increased overall survival from 27 months to 36 months (*p*<0.005) (*N Engl J Med* 2001;345:725). In the INT-116 study, a D2 resection was recommended for the study participants; however, only 10% of the patients received this type of surgery.

Adjuvant chemotherapy studies had not clearly shown a benefit until the recent CLASSIC study was reported (*Lancet* 2012;379:315). In this study, 1035 patients with stage II-IIIB gastric cancers who had undergone a D2 gastrectomy with curative intent were randomized to adjuvant chemotherapy of eight 3-week cycles of oral capecitabine (1,000 mg/m^2) twice daily (on days 1 to 14 of each cycle) plus intravenous oxaliplatin (130 mg/m^2) (on day 1 of each cycle) for 6 months versus surgery only. Three-year disease-free survival was 74% (95% CI 69 to 79) in the adjuvant group and 59% (53 to 64) in the surgery-only group (HR 0·56, 95% CI 0·44 to 0.72; *p*<0·0001). Therefore, adjuvant chemoradiotherapy is considered standard of care for patients who have had completely resected stage IB or more advanced gastric adenocarcinoma where adjuvant chemotherapy without radiation can be considered for patients who have had a D2 resection. For patients who had positive margins at resection, combination chemoradiation is also considered standard of care.

Neoadjuvant/perioperative chemotherapy has been tested to make unresectable cancers operable and to improve overall survival. The most prominent trial is the MAGIC trial, where 503 patients with at least stage II adenocarcinoma of the stomach, gastroesophageal junction, and distal esophagus were randomized to surgery alone or chemotherapy, in addition to surgery (*N Engl J Med* 2006;355:11). The chemotherapeutic regimen was ECF (epirubicin 50 mg/m^2 on day 1, cisplatin 60 mg/m^2 on day 1, and 5-FU 200 mg/m^2 by c.i.v.i. on days 1 to 21) every 3 weeks for three cycles before surgery and then three cycles after surgery.

The chemotherapy arm showed a statistically significant downsizing of the tumor as well as significant improvement in survival. The 5-year survival was 36% in the chemotherapy arm versus 23% in the surgery-only arm. Interestingly, only 42% of the patients randomized to chemotherapy were able to complete the three postoperative cycles. On the basis of the results of Intergroup 116, the CLASSIC and the MAGIC trials, it is clear that surgery alone is not sufficient therapy for gastric cancer. What remains unclear is the role for adjuvant or neoadjuvant versus perioperative therapy and the role of radiation therapy RT. Currently, NCCN recommends (with equal category 1 ratings) perioperative chemotherapy in patients who have not had surgery or adjuvant chemoradiotherapy in patients who have had surgery. Adjuvant chemotherapy as a single modality can be considered in patients who have undergone a D2 resection.

c. **Therapy for medically unresectable patients.** Combination chemoradiation is considered a standard of care for medically unresectable localized gastric adenocarcinoma. It typically combines 5-FU with 4,500 to 5,000 cGy of radiation, but a taxane-based regimen can also be considered. Combination chemotherapy as a single modality is also a consideration. Notably, only a very small percentage of patients can be cured with chemoradiotherapy alone.

2. **Metastatic gastric adenocarcinoma**

a. **Chemotherapy.** Chemotherapy has been shown to improve survival and quality of life in patients with metastatic gastric carcinoma. Several chemotherapeutic agents have activity in gastric cancer, including 5-FU, cisplatin, oxaliplatin, irinotecan, capecitabine, anthracyclines, and taxanes. In a recent Cochrane meta-analysis, combination chemotherapy appears to offer a small survival benefit over single-agent chemotherapy. Commonly used combination chemotherapeutic regimens include CF (cisplatin 100 mg/m^2 on day 1 every 4 weeks, and infusional 5-FU 1,000 mg/m^2/day on days 1 to 5 every 4 weeks), DCF (docetaxel 75 mg/m^2 on day 1 every 3 weeks, cisplatin 75 mg/m^2 on day 1 every 3 weeks, and infusional 5-FU 750 mg/m^2/day on days 1 to 5 every 3 weeks), ECF (epirubicin 50 mg/m^2 on day 1 every 3 weeks, cisplatin 60 mg/m^2 on day 1 every 3 weeks, and infusional 5-FU 200 mg/m^2/day continuously), EOF (epirubicin 50 mg/m^2 on day 1 every 3 weeks, oxaliplatin 130 mg/m^2 on day 1 every 3 weeks, and infusional 5-FU 200 mg/m^2/day continuously), EOX (epirubicin 50 mg/m^2 on day 1 every 3 weeks, oxaliplatin 130 mg/m^2 on day 1 every 3 weeks, and capecitabine 625 mg/m^2 p.o. b.i.d. continuously), FOLFOX (oxaliplatin 85 mg/m^2 on days 1 and 15 every 4 weeks, leucovorin 400 mg/m^2 on days 1 and 15 every 4 weeks, 5-FU bolus 400 mg/m^2 on days 1 and 15, 5-FU infusion 800 mg/m^2/day on days 1, 2, 15, and 16 every 4 weeks), and FOLFIRI (irinotecan 180 mg/m^2 on days 1 and 15 every 4 weeks, leucovorin 400 mg/m^2 on days 1 and 15 every 4 weeks, 5-FU 1,200 mg/m^2/day on days 1,2,15, and 16 every 4 weeks). Despite interesting phase III trials comparing combination chemotherapies such as the TAX 325, which showed an increased time to tumor progression for DCF compared with CF (*J Clin Oncol* 2007;25:3205) and the REAL-2 trial, with least equivalence of EOX, ECF, EOF, and ECX (*N Engl J Med* 2008;358:36), there is no clear standard of care first-line combination chemotherapy. Also, there is no clear standard of care for second-line chemotherapy regimens. Randomized trials have shown a survival benefit for second-line therapy in selected patients versus best supportive care. Common regimens in this setting include irinotecan or docetaxel.

b. **Targeted therapies.** HER2-neu, also known as ERBB2, a member of the ERBb family of receptors associated with tumor cell proliferation, apoptosis, adhesion, migration, and differentiation, is overexpressed in approximately 20% of gastric cancers and is a clinically validated cancer target. Trastuzumab, a monoclonal antibody against HER2, was investigated in combination with chemotherapy for first-line treatment of HER2-positive advanced gastric or gastroesophageal junction cancers in the ToGA study (*Lancet* 2010 28;376:687). Patients with HER2 overexpressing gastric or gastroesophageal junction cancers were randomly assigned to study treatment with capecitabine plus cisplatin or fluorouracil plus cisplatin given every 3 weeks for six cycles or chemotherapy in combination with intravenous trastuzumab. Median overall survival was 13.8 months (95% CI 12 to 16) in those assigned to trastuzumab plus chemotherapy compared with 11.1 months (10 to 13) in those assigned to chemotherapy alone (HR 0.74; 95% CI 0.60 to 0.91; p=0.0046). Therefore, HER2 testing is recommended for all patients with metastatic gastroesophageal cancers.

Antiangiogenic therapies have a proven role in a variety of malignancies and recent clinical trials in patients with gastric and gastroesophageal junction adenocarcinomas have validated the use of this treatment strategy in these cancers. Ramucirumab is a monoclonal antibody VEGFR-2 antagonist that is FDA approved for treatment of patients with gastric and gastroesophageal junction adenocarcinomas. The RAINBOW study (Lancet Oncology 2014 - 15(11):1224–35) was a randomized phase 3 trial comparing ramucirumab plus paclitaxel versus placebo plus paclitaxel in patients with previously treated advanced gastric or gastroesophageal junction adenocarcinomas. Patients receiving the combination regimen had improved overall survival (median 9.6 months versus 7.4 months; hazard ratio 0.807 [95% CI 0.678-0.962]; p=0.017). In the REGARD study (Lancet 2014 - 383(9911):31–9), patients with previously treated advanced gastric or gastroesophageal junction adenocarcinomas were randomized to receive ramucirumab monotherapy or placebo. The patients receiving ramucirumab had improved median overall survival (5.2 months versus 3.8 months; hazard ratio 0.776, [95% CI 0.603-0.998]; p=0.047). Therefore, ramucirumab in combination with paclitaxel or as monotherapy, is considered a standard second-line treatment option for patients with advanced gastric cancers.

   c. **Other palliative procedures.** Debulking/diverting surgery may improve quality of life in selected patients with discrete obstructing tumors. Radiotherapy may palliate bleeding or painful metastases. Other procedures are similar to those discussed earlier for esophageal cancer.
E. **Course of the disease.** The median survival of patients with metastatic gastric cancer is approximately 10 months. Common sites of metastasis include the liver, peritoneum, and lymph nodes.
F. **Complications.** Gastric cancer can lead to hemorrhage, gastric obstruction, and malignant ascites. Anastomotic leaks are the most common complication of gastrectomy. Development of B12 deficiency following gastric surgery is also a concern.
G. **Pathology.** Ninety percent of gastric carcinomas are adenocarcinomas. The rest are non-Hodgkin's lymphomas (NHLs) and leiomyosarcomas (gastrointestinal stromal tumors [GIST]).

   Two classification systems for gastric adenocarcinoma are used. The Lauren classification divides gastric adenocarcinomas into the intestinal and diffuse types. The intestinal type arises from a background of intestinal metaplasia and shows differentiation resembling that of a colonic adenocarcinoma. Intestinal type is predominant in endemic areas, affects older patients, and often metastasizes first to the liver. The diffuse type is poorly differentiated, affects younger patients, and has a tendency to metastasize to the peritoneum, resulting in implants and malignant ascites. Patients with the intestinal type appear to have better outcomes overall.

   The Borrmann classification divides adenocarcinomas by their growth pattern. Types I and II are polypoid and heaped-up ulcers, respectively, and are associated with the intestinal type. Type III is an ulcerated infiltrating tumor, and type IV, diffusely infiltrating. This last type is also referred to as *linitis plastica* or leather bottle stomach and is associated with the diffuse type of adenocarcinoma. GE-junction tumors are usually the diffuse type. The boundaries between these groupings are not sharp, and some tumors are not easily categorized.
H. **Epidemiology.** Gastric cancer was once the most common malignancy in the United States, but its incidence has decreased since the 1930s. Worldwide, gastric cancer is surpassed only by lung cancer in frequency. It is the most frequent visceral cancer in Japan, where the incidence reaches 93.3 per 100,000. The high incidence in Japan has resulted in the creation of an endoscopic screening program, which is credited with the high frequency of early-stage cancers (50%) in Japanese patients. In contrast, more than 80% of Western patients have advanced cancers at diagnosis.

The intestinal and diffuse types of gastric cancer differ in regard to epidemiology and risk factors. The intestinal type is associated with consumption of large amounts of salt and preserved foods, and possibly with *Helicobacter pylori* infection. These irritants lead to intestinal metaplasia of the stomach, which can then transform into frank malignancy. Other predisposing factors include achlorhydria associated with pernicious anemia and previous partial gastrectomy for peptic ulcer. It is thought that the lack of stomach acid in these conditions predisposes to intestinal metaplasia. Despite this, long-term use of H_2 blockers does not appear to be a risk factor.

The intestinal type of gastric cancer is more prevalent in Japan, where preserved and salty foods are widely consumed. The decrease in the incidence of gastric cancer in the United States may relate to the availability of refrigeration and a dietary shift toward fresh foods. Asian patients may have genetic predispositions increasing cancer risk as well, as the rate decreases in Japanese immigrants in the United States who adopt local diets, but remains elevated as compared with the U.S. populace as a whole. The diffuse type is more sporadic and is not associated with diet. It is the most common form found in the United States.

I. **Research areas.** The role of many targeted therapies is currently being studied. Using molecular genomics to improve the classification of the different tumors as well as to guide therapy is an active area of research.

SUGGESTED READINGS

Bang YJ, Van Cutsem E, Feyereislova A, et al. Trastuzumab in combination with chemotherapy versus chemotherapy alone for treatment of HER2-positive advanced gastric or gastro-oesophageal junction cancer (ToGA): a phase 3, open-label, randomised controlled trial. *Lancet* 2010;376(9742):687–697.

Bang YJ, Kim YW, Yang HK, et al. Adjuvant capecitabine and oxaliplatin for gastric cancer after D2 gastrectomy (CLASSIC): a phase 3 open-label, randomised controlled trial. *Lancet* 2012;379(9813):315–321.

Cunningham D, Allum WH, Stenning SP, et al. Perioperative chemotherapy versus surgery alone for gastric cancer. *N Engl J Med* 2006;355:11.

Herskovic A, Martz K, al-Sarraf M, et al. Combined chemotherapy and radiotherapy compared with radiotherapy alone in patients with cancer of the esophagus. *N Engl J Med* 1992;326:1593.

Macdonald J, Smalley SR, Benedetti J, et al. Chemoradiotherapy after surgery compared with surgery alone for adenocarcinoma of the stomach or gastroesophageal junction. *N Engl J Med* 2001;345:725.

Songun I, Putter H, Kranenbarg EM, et al. Surgical treatment of gastric cancer: 15-year follow-up results of the randomised nationwide Dutch D1D2 trial. *Lancet Oncol* 2010;11(5):439–449.

van Hagen P, Hulshof MC, van Lanschot JJ, et al. Preoperative chemoradiotherapy for esophageal or junctional cancer. *N Engl J Med* 2012;366(22):2074–2084.

16 Colorectal Cancer
Ashley Morton • Benjamin Tan

I. PRESENTATION

A. **Subjective.** Colorectal cancer (CRC) is diagnosed as a result of a positive screening test or workup of a symptomatic patient. Symptoms associated with CRC include rectal bleeding, abdominal pain, changes in bowel habits, weight loss, fatigue, anorexia, and abdominal distention. Patients could also present with bowel obstruction, perforation, peritonitis, or fever. A thorough family history and past medical/oncologic history should be done to exclude any familial colorectal cancer syndromes.

B. **Objective.** Physical examination should always include a thorough abdominal and rectal examination and may reveal abdominal tenderness, hepatomegaly, ascites, a palpable mass, palpable adenopathy, and gross blood or heme-positive rectal examination. Extracolonic manifestations in patients with hereditary colorectal cancer syndromes should also be noted.

II. WORKUP AND STAGING

A. **Initial evaluation.** Patients found to have a pedunculated or sessile polyp or mass in the colon or rectum require careful pathologic review of the excised specimen and precise marking of the polyp site. If invasive cancer is detected, additional workup should include a complete blood count, chemistry panel with liver function tests, carcinoembryonic antigen (CEA), and computed tomography (CT) of the chest, abdomen, and pelvis. Although routine positron emission tomography (PET) scan is not standard, it may be valuable in assessing the extent of metastatic disease in a patient considered for potentially curative resection. For rectal cancer, important clinical factors such as tumor distance from anal verge, presence of circumferential, obstructing, and tethered tumors should be recorded.

B. **Surgical principles.** Surgery remains the primary modality for cure in patients with colorectal cancer. Select patients with synchronous or metachronous solitary or limited hepatic and pulmonary metastatic disease should still be considered for potentially curative resection of both the primary and metastatic sites. The extent, type, and timing of resection are dependent on the location of the tumor and presence of bleeding, obstruction, or perforation and the presence of polyposis. The number of lymph nodes harvested and examined ($\geq$12 recommended) impacts staging accuracy and prognosis.

Laparoscopic colectomy has been associated with higher cancer-related survival, reduced relapse rates, decreased morbidity, blood loss, and hospital stays compared with open colectomy (*Lancet* 2002;359:2224).

C. **Pathology**

1. **Pathological review** of the surgical or biopsy specimen should include histologic type, tumor size and differentiation, depth of invasion, number and location of lymph nodes involved and examined, presence of extranodal deposits, nonregional lymph nodes and distant metastases, perineural and lymphovascular invasion, and margins (proximal, distal, and radial).

2. **Additional data.** DNA mismatch repair (MMR) proficiency or deficiency determination and the presence of any KRAS, NRAS, BRAF, and other somatic mutations would be necessary for treatment options.

D. **Staging.** Five-year survival rates for 109,953 colorectal cancer patients using the 7th edition of the New American Joint Committee on Cancer (AJCC) based on Surveillance, Epidemiology, and End Results (SEER) data from 1992 to 2004 (*J Clin Oncol* 2010;28:265) are shown in Table 16-1.

E. **Prognostic factors**

1. **Tumor grade.** Low-grade tumors are significantly associated with better survival in stages II, III, and IV, but not in stage I, colon cancer.

2. **Histologic subtype.** Adenocarcinoma comprises >85% of CRC, while mucinous and signet ring types occur in 12% and 1%, respectively. Patients with signet ring cell carcinomas had the worse prognosis compared with adenocarcinomas and mucinous types (5-year overall survival (OS) 36%, 66%, and 62%, respectively).

3. **Tumor location.** Sigmoid colon cancers confer the best 5-year survivals (70%) compared with tumors in the right colon (64%), transverse colon (65%), and the left colon (65%).

4. **Number of positive lymph nodes.** Worse survival rates are seen in patients with more lymph nodes involved with cancer. Further subcategorizing lymph node involvement to N2 (4-5 LN+), N3 (6-8 LN+), and N4 ($\geq$9 LN+) could provide a more accurate prognosis among stage III CRC patients with 5-year OS of 52%, 43%, and 27%, respectively.

5. **Lymphovascular involvement** is associated with worse prognosis.

6. **Molecular markers** including microsatellite instability, KRAS, NRAS, BRAF, and PIK3CA also carry predictive and prognostic information. The majority of KRAS mutations occur on codons 12 and 13 of exon 2, and are present in approximately 40% of colorectal cancers. KRAS is the best predictor for resistance for EGFR targeting agents. An additional 15% to 18% of CRC will harbor other KRAS and

TABLE 16-1	Five-Year Survival Rates for Colorectal Cancer

TN	M	AJCC 7th	5-yr OS colon (%)	5-yr OS rectal (%)
T1-2 N0	M0	I	76.3	77.6%
T3 N0	M0	IIA	66.7	64
T4a N0	M0	IIB	60.6	55.7
T4b N0	M0	IIC	45.7	44.7
T1-2 N1	M0	IIIA	71.1	72.1
T1-2 N2	M0	IIIA/IIIB	61.5	56.1
T3 N1	M0	IIIB	54.9	52.4
T3 N2a	M0	IIIB	42.8	42.5
T3 N2b	M0	IIIC	30.4	32
T4a N1	M0	IIIB	47	48.2
T4b N1	M0	IIIC	27.9	24.3
T4a N2	M0	IIIC	26.6	34.3
T4b N2	M0	IIIC	15.8	15.6
Any T	Any N	IV	8	

T1, tumor invades submucosa; T2, tumor invades muscularis propria; T3, tumor invades through the muscularis propria into the subserosa or into nonperitonealized pericolic tissues; T4a, tumor perforates visceral peritoneum; T4b, tumors invading adjacent organs; N0, no regional lymph node (LN) metastasis; N1, 1–3 + LN; N2a, 4–6 + LN; N2b, ≥7+ LN; M0, no distant metastasis; M1, distant metastasis.

NRAS mutations (most NRAS mutations occur on codon 61 of exon 2), 5% to 8% of CRC will harbor BRAF V600E mutations, and 9% to 15% of CRC will have a PIK3CA mutation (68.5% located on exon 9 and 20.4% on exon 20) (*PLoS One* 2013;8:e81628; *Lancet Oncol* 2010;11:753). KRAS and BRAF are mutually exclusive and should be tested independently. KRAS mutations are strongly associated with PIK3CA mutations. Adjuvant aspirin therapy may improve overall survival in PIK3CA-mutated tumors (*New Engl J Med* 2012;367:1596). NRAS and PIK3CA mutations may inhibit response to anti-EGFR therapy, despite KRAS wild-type status. BRAF-mutated tumors are associated with poorer prognosis.

III. TREATMENT BY STAGE

A. **Stage I colon cancer (T1–T2, N0 M0).** Since surgical resection confers a high cure rate for patients with stage I cancer, no adjuvant therapy is recommended.

B. **Stage II colon cancer (T3–T4, N0 M0).** Although the American Society of Clinical Oncology does not recommend the routine use of adjuvant therapy for stage II CRC patients, "high-risk" patients including those with inadequately sampled nodes, T4 lesions, perforation, obstruction, or poorly differentiated histology should be considered for chemotherapy (*J Clin Oncol* 2004;22:3408).

   1. The **IMPACT B2 Study** reported a 2% to 3% absolute difference in 5-year disease-free survival (DFS) (76% vs. 73%) and OS (82% vs. 80%) in patients treated with adjuvant 5-fluorouracil (5-FU)-leucovorin chemotherapy versus observation (*J Clin Oncol* 1999;17:1356).

   2. The **QUASAR study** showed a significant improvement in recurrence rates (22.2% vs. 26.2%) and 5-year survival (80.3 vs. 77.4%, HR 0.83) with 5-FU versus observation.

   3. A systematic review of published literature included 37 randomized studies, and 11 meta-analyses with 20,317 patients demonstrated a 5% to 10% absolute improvement in DFS associated with adjuvant therapy, although this did not achieve statistical significance (*Cancer Prev Control* 1997;1:379).

   4. With more aggressive oxaliplatin-based adjuvant chemotherapy, patients with stage II colon cancer treated on the **MOSAIC study** had an absolute 4-year DFS benefit of 3.8% (85.1% vs. 81.3%) compared with those treated with 5-FU/leucovorin alone (*N Engl J Med* 2004;350:2343). In high-risk stage II patients, the benefit is higher at 5.4%. However, no overall survival advantage was observed with the addition of oxaliplatin.

5. Defective MMR is predictive of lack of efficacy of 5-FU adjuvant therapy in colon cancer (*J Clin Oncol* 2010;28:3219). A 12-gene recurrence score may predict recurrence risk in stage II colon cancer and potential benefit from oxaliplatin-based adjuvant therapy (*J Clin Oncol* 2013;31:4512). A careful assessment of risk of recurrence based on tumor and patient characteristics, and a thorough discussion with the patient regarding the absolute and relative benefits and toxicities are necessary during consideration of adjuvant therapy in patients with stage II CRC.

C. **Stage III colon cancer (any T, N1–N2, M0).** Adjuvant oxaliplatin-based chemotherapy is standard for patients with stage III CRC.

1. Stage III CRC patients treated with FOLFOX4 on the **MOSAIC** study had an 8.7% absolute benefit in 3-year DFS (77.9% vs. 72.8%) and 4-year DFS (69.7% vs. 61%) compared with 5-FU/leucovorin. For patients with N2 disease, the absolute benefit is 12%.

2. The **NSABP C-07** confirmed the efficacy of oxaliplatin, with bolus 5-FU showing a significant improvement in 3-year DFS (76.5% vs. 71.5%) compared with bolus 5-FU/LV.

3. **Capecitabine plus oxaliplatin** is also another recommended option for adjuvant treatment. A large multicenter, randomized trial compared XELOX versus 5-FU/LV. The 3-year DFS rate was 70.9% with XELOX and 66.5% with 5-FU/LV; 5-year OS for XELOX and 5-FU/LF were 77.6% and 74.2%, respectively (*J Clin Oncol* 2011;29:146).

4. **Elderly age** should also be considered when choosing adjuvant treatment. In the **NSABP-07 trial**, patients <70 years old had improved OS with FLOX compared to FU/LV (HR 0.80), with 5-year OS 81.8% for FLOX and 78.8% with FU/LV. In patients >70 years old, OS did not vary significantly by treatment type, but nominal OS at 5 years was 4.7% worse with FLOX (71.6%) versus FULV (76.3%). Additionally, toxicity and dose intensity varied by age. Furthermore, **MOSAIC** included patients younger than 75 years of age.

5. For patients unsuitable for oxaliplatin-based therapy, capecitabine or 5-FU with leucovorin are alternative therapies. In the **X-ACT** study, adjuvant capecitabine resulted in a trend toward improved 3-year DFS (64.2% vs. 60.6%) and OS (77.6% vs. 81.3%) compared with Mayo Clinic schedule of 5-FU/LV (*N Engl J Med* 2005;353:2696).

6. Irinotecan-based therapies cannot be considered for the adjuvant treatment of stage III CRC based on three large randomized trials (ACCORD, PETACC-3, and CALGB 89803) showing no benefit over 5-FU alone.

7. **Targeted agents in the adjuvant setting.** Adjuvant bevacizumab or cetuximab were shown to be of no benefit in stage III colorectal cancer. **NSABP-08** is a phase III trial that showed no benefit with the addition of bevacizumab to FOLFOX in the adjuvant setting (*J Clin Oncol* 2010;29:11), whereas N0147 demonstrated no benefit with the addition of cetuximab to adjuvant chemotherapy (*JAMA* 2012;307:1383).

D. **Metastatic colorectal cancer—first-line therapy.** The goal of therapy, whether potentially curative versus palliative, may help determine the choice of regimen used for initial therapy for patients with metastatic CRC. More aggressive regimens associated with the best response rates (RR) may be favored for patients with limited metastatic sites potentially amenable to resection or patients with rapidly growing symptomatic visceral metastases, whereas the toxicity profiles of equally effective regimens may determine the choice of palliative therapy for patients with widely metastatic CRC. KRAS and BRAF status will also be important in selecting appropriate therapy.

1. **Chemotherapy backbone**

a. Oxaliplatin-based (FOLFOX) or irinotecan-based 5-FU regimens (FOLFIRI) are appropriate first-line treatments for metastatic CRC. The **N9741 study** demonstrated the superiority of FOLFOX over irinotecan with bolus 5-FU (IFL) in terms of RR (45% vs. 31%) and OS (19.5 months vs. 14.8 months) (*J Clin Oncol* 2004;22:23). Two studies have shown equal efficacy between FOLFOX and FOLFIRI regimens (*J Clin Oncol* 2004;22:229; *J Clin Oncol* 2005;22:4866). Capecitabine combination therapies have also been studied in the CAIRO2 and TREE-2 studies.

b. In a phase III trial, triplet therapy of FOLFOXIRI showed improved RR (60% vs. 34%), median PFS (9.8 months vs. 6.9 months; HR 0.63), and median OS (22.6 months vs. 16.7 months) compared with FOLFIRI in unresectable metastatic colorectal patients (*J Clin Oncol* 2007;25:1670).

    c. Single-agent capecitabine or 5-FU may be appropriate initial therapy for those with significant comorbidities precluding more aggressive treatment.

  2. **Chemotherapy with targeted agents**

    a. **Bevacizumab** is the first antiangiogenic drug approved for cancer treatment. When added to chemotherapy, this anti-vascular endothelial growth factor (anti-VEGF) antibody significantly improved outcomes. Hurwitz demonstrated a 4.7-month survival advantage with bevacizumab + IFL compared with IFL alone (20.3 months vs. 15.6 months). Furthermore, RR (45% vs. 35%) and duration of response (10.4 months vs. 7.1 months) are superior in the bevacizumab arm. Moreover, when bevacizumab is combined with 5-FU/LV alone, median survival of 18.3 months was achieved with RR of 40% (*J Clin Oncol* 2005;23:3502). Bevacizumab with FOLFOX or FOLFIRI also resulted in high RR and relatively long survivals (TREE-2 and BICC-C trials).

    b. Comparison between XELOX and FOLFOX with bevacizumab versus placebo was evaluated in a phase III trial. Median PFS improved to 9.4 months with bevacizumab versus 8 months in placebo group (HR 0.83 to 0.72), and median OS 21.3 months versus 19.9 months (*J Clin Oncol* 2008;26:2013).

    c. In KRAS wild-type tumors, **cetuximab and panitumumab**, anti-epidermal growth factor receptors, have also been combined with oxaliplatin and irinotecan-based chemotherapy in the first-line CRC setting.

    d. **CRYSTAL** compared **FOLFIRI + cetuximab** versus FOLFIRI alone. In an all-randomized patient population, RR improved to 46.9% from 38.7%; median PFS 8.9 months versus 8.1 months; and median OS 19.6 months versus 18.5 months. Upon further review, a post hoc analysis for KRAS wild-type subpopulation was noted to have improved OS to 23.5 months versus 19.5 months with RR 57% versus 39% (*J Clin Oncol* 2011;29:2011). **OPUS** assessed overall RR with FOLFOX4 + Cetuximab versus FOLFOX4 alone, and noted improvement (46% vs. 36%). In KRAS wild-type tumors, clinical significance was noted with the addition of cetuximab to 61% versus 37% (*J Clin Oncol* 2009;27:663).

    e. **PRIME** evaluated **panitumumab** with FOLFOX4 and noted improved PFS when compared with FOLFOX4 alone (10.1 months vs. 7.9 months). OS was 26 months with panitumumab arm and 20.2 months with FOLFOX alone. But mutated KRAS tumors had a significant reduction of PFS with the combination therapy. Interestingly, 17% of the patients in this trial had KRAS wild type (WT) tumors on exon 2, but were noted to have other RAS mutations and were associated with inferior PFS and OS with the panitumumab + FOLFOX (*N Engl J Med* 2013;369:1023).

E. **Maintenance therapy**

  1. Once maximal response to 1st line therapy has been achieved, maintenance therapy should be considered. Optimox1 and Optimox2 evaluated a "stop-and-go" approach to chemotherapy administration. Duration of disease control, resulted in Opitmox2, was longer within the maintenance arm of 5FU/LV at 13.1 months, while the chemotherapy-free interval arm was 9.2 months. OS improved by 4.3 months with maintenance 5FU (JCO December 1, 2009 vol. 27 no. 34 5727-5733).

  2. CAIRO3 supports maintenance therapy with cabecitabine + bevacizumab after XELOX versus observation with PFS 7.4 months versus 4.1 (Koopman, M. JCO 31, 2013 (suppl; abstr 3502).

F. **Metastatic colorectal cancer— second-line and subsequent therapy**

  1. For patients who received oxaliplatin-based therapy, irinotecan-based therapy can be considered after progression, and vice versa, with a median OS of 21 months (*J Clin Oncol* 2004;22:229). Bevacizumab is approved for second-line therapy when combined with FOLFOX. This regimen improved OS (12.5 months vs. 10.7 months) compared with FOLFOX alone in patients who progressed after first-line therapy with irinotecan (*J Clin Oncol* 2007;25:1539).

  2. **Bevacizumab beyond first progression (ML18147)** is associated with significantly prolonged PFS and OS (5.9 months and 11.9 months), when compared with patients who had chemotherapy alone (4.3 months and 10.6 months) (*Ann Oncol* 2013;24:2342).

3. **Ziv-Aflibercept,** a VEGF Trap, prevents activation of VEGF receptors, therefore inhibiting angiogenesis. VELOUR tested second-line aflibercept with FOLFIRI in patients who failed oxaliplatin-based regimens (irinotecan-naive patients). FOLFIRI + ziv-aflibercept had OS of 13.5 months versus 12.1 months in FOLFIRI + placebo; RR 19.8% and 11.1% (*Eur J Cancer* 2014;50:320).

4. **Single-agent cetuximab or panitumumab** have been compared with best supportive care and are appropriate third or later line therapies for those with KRAS wild-type tumors. Regorafenib, an oral multiple kinase inhibitor, can be considered if all other standard therapies fail. In refractory colon cancer, the phase III CORRECT trial compared regorafenib versus placebo and found that the OS was slightly improved by 1.4 months (6.4 months vs. 5.0 months). PFS was also modest at 1.9 months versus 1.7 months (*Lancet* 2013;381:303).

G. **Liver dominant or liver-only metastatic disease may be amenable to regional therapies**

1. **Principles.** Liver metastases can be found in approximately 80% of CRC patients; about 25% to 50% are encountered at initial presentation. Alternative treatment regimens should be considered to prolong survival rates.

   a. Isolated liver lesions may be amenable to surgical resection (usually up to five, in one lobe of the liver) and is the standard curative treatment.

   b. Systemic chemotherapy and/or transarterial administration of chemotherapy (with either vascular occlusive agents or hepatic chemoperfusion) may produce further tumor response and improved survival.

H. **Rectal cancer.** A multimodality approach, including colorectal surgery, radiation oncology, and medical oncology, is necessary for the optimal treatment of patients with rectal cancer. Initial workup should include a transrectal ultrasound to assess depth of invasion and lymph node involvement, CT or MRI to assess distant metastases, and biopsy to rule out other rectal tumors such as squamous cell carcinoma, melanoma, sarcoma, or lymphoma). Low anterior resection (LAR) is suitable for tumors located in the middle and upper third of the rectum, whereas an abdominoperineal resection (APR) may be necessary for low-lying rectal cancer. T stage and grade, lymphovascular involvement, lymph node metastases, and achievement of a negative radial margin are important prognosticators and predictive of local and distant recurrences. Total mesorectal excision (TME) in conjunction with LAR or APR has been advocated as the optimal surgical procedure for rectal cancer. A sharp (rather than blunt or avulsive) dissection is performed to remove the entire rectum. This technique has been shown to achieve a higher negative radial margin rate than blunt dissection (93% vs. 80%). Laparoscopic procedures are safe in the hands of experienced surgeons.

1. **T1–T2 N0 rectal cancer.** Transrectal ultrasound staged rectal lesions confined to the submucosa may be treated with full thickness local resection. Regional lymph node involvement occurs in 10% to 15% of these patients. T1 tumors invading the deepest part of the submucosa (SM3) carry a significantly higher risk of lymph node involvement than more superficial lesions (SM1 or SM2). Lesions invading the muscularis propria (T2) have a higher incidence of lymph node involvement (12% to 22%). If pathologically confirmed, patients require additional chemoradiotherapy. Preoperative radiation may be indicated for low-lying rectal lesions in an attempt to convert an APR to a potential sphincter-preserving LAR.

2. **Locally advanced T3–T4 or N1 rectal cancer.** Neoadjuvant chemoradiation is a standard treatment for locally advanced rectal cancer. 5-FU–based infusional chemoradiation is associated with lower local recurrence rate (6% vs. 13%), reduced acute and long-term toxicities, improved compliance, and promotes higher sphincter preservation, but achieved similar 5-year OS compared with postoperative therapy (*N Engl J Med* 2004;351:1731). The degree of downstaging achieved with neoadjuvant therapy also provides prognostic information. Resection is generally done 6 to 10 weeks after chemoradiation, and the decision to administer adjuvant chemotherapy is based on the initial clinical staging.

IV. COMPLICATIONS

  A. Cancer-related. Bowel obstruction, hemorrhage, abdominal pain, perforation, fistula formation, peritonitis, anemia, and malnutrition. Extensive liver metastases hepatomegaly, liver failure, or jaundice.

  B. Treatment-related

    1. Surgical and radiation complications. Common bowel dysfunction after surgery includes stool frequency, episodic frequency, pressure sensation, urgency, nocturnal movements, and soilage. Anastomotic stricture, leak, ulceration, bleeding obstruction, infection, bladder, and sexual dysfunction may occur.

    2. Chemotherapy and targeted therapy

      a. Fluoropyrimidines -5-FU or capecitabine may cause myelosuppression, mucositis, diarrhea, excessive lacrimation, skin discoloration, dehydration, palmar–plantar erythrodysesthesia (PPE), and rare cardiotoxicity. Patients with dihydropyrimidine dehydrogenase (DPD) deficiency may have severe myelosuppression, ataxia, and diarrhea.

      b. Oxaliplatin may cause cold-induced peripheral neuropathy, laryngodysesthesias, myelosuppression, nausea, and fatigue.

      c. Irinotecan causes acute and delayed diarrhea, nausea, vomiting, myelosuppression, and alopecia. Patients with the UGT1A1 7/7 polymorphism may require irinotecan dose reductions owing to increased risk for grade 4 to 5 neutropenia.

      d. Bevacizumab can cause common side effects such as epistaxis, hypertension, and proteinuria. Rarer side effects include arterial thrombotic events (ATEs) such as myocardial infarction or stroke, perforation, wound dehiscence, and reversible leukoencephalopathy, among others.

        i. Should any of these issues occur while on bevacizumab therapy, dose holding or discontinuation may be warranted. Brain metastasis must be treated prior to considering bevacizumab. Grade 3 venous thromboembolic events may be resumed WITH CAUTION (after a 2-week holding period) after therapeutic dose anticoagulation therapy is provided and the patient has no hemorrhagic complications. In patients with arterial thrombus (TIA, MI, CVA), bevacizumab should not be administered for at least 6 months and should then be reevaluated. Reasons for permanent discontinuation include: Gastrointestinal perforation, surgery (at least 28 days prior to and after elective surgery) and wound-healing complications, hemorrhage, hypertensive crisis, nephrotic syndrome, non-GI fistula formation, reversible posterior leukoencephalopathy syndrome (RPLS), severe/life-threatening thrombosis. Hold when 24-hour urine protein ≥2 grams.

      e. Cetuximab/Panitumumab can cause acneform rash/folliculitis, trichomegaly, paronychial inflammation, xerosis, diarrhea, fatigue, hypomagnesemia, and rare pulmonary toxicities.

        i. Management of rash will vary for each patient. Moisturizers and sunscreen may reduce severity. Folliculitis usually occurs within 1 to 3 weeks. If it is restricted to facial area only or there is mild-to-severe reaction, topical antibiotics, such as clindamycin 2%, may be used. Topical steroids such as hydrocortisone 1% may also improve symptoms. Oral therapy with minocycline may be added to the topical regimen. Referral to a dermatologist may be necessary if symptoms worsen or are severe at baseline.

V. FOLLOW-UP.
After curative resection and completion of therapy, a history, physical examination, and CEA determination is recommended every 3 months for the first 2 years, then every 4 to 6 months until the 5th year. Colonoscopy is recommended 1 year after diagnosis or 1 year from surgical resection, and repeated in 1 year if abnormal; otherwise, repeated in 2 to 3 years. For patients without prior full colonoscopy (i.e., due to obstructing lesion or emergent surgery), colonoscopy in 6 months is recommended.

VI. EPIDEMIOLOGY AND SCREENING

  A. CRC ranks fourth in frequency among men and women, with approximately 140,000 new cases per year. It is the second leading cause of cancer deaths in the United States.

In regard to mortality rates, it ranks second in men and women. Median age of diagnosis is 69, and the median age at death is 74. Patients with average risk (age ≥50, no prior history or adenoma, no Inflammatory bowel disease (IBD)) should have a colonoscopy done at age 50 (90% of cases occur after age 50). If no polyps are seen, colonoscopy should be repeated in 10 years. If polyps are seen, polypectomy should be done. Alternatively, fecal occult blood tests (FOBT) annually with flexible sigmoidoscopy every 5 years or double-contrast barium enema every 5 years could be performed.

B. If there is a family history of colon cancer in a first-degree relative (parent, sibling, child), risk increases about twofold. If an adenoma is diagnosed under age 60, screening should begin at age 40, or 10 years earlier than the youngest cancer in the family. According to the American Cancer Society and the American College of Gastroenterology, screening for African Americans should begin at age 45.

VII. RISK FACTORS. The lifetime risks for developing CRC are as follows:

A. General population 5%.

B. Personal history 15% to 20%.

C. Inflammatory bowel disease 15% to 40%.

D. Hereditary nonpolyposis colorectal cancer (HNPCC) 70% to 80%—or Lynch syndrome. HNPCC is characterized by early onset of colon cancer and adenomas but not polyposis. HNPCC is autosomal dominant with 80% penetrance and is due to a mutation in MMR genes MLH1, MSH2, MSH6, PMS1, PMS2, and MSH3. Extracolonic manifestations include endometrial, ovarian, gastric, urogenital, bile duct, and sebaceous gland (Muir–Torre) cancer.

E. Familial adenomatous polyposis (FAP) >95%. FAP is characterized by the presence of thousands of polyps with an autosomal dominant inheritance with high penetrance and a prevalence of 1 in 8,000. The APC suppressor gene is located on chromosome 5q21, which is important in cell adhesion, signal transduction, and transcriptional activation in its interaction with beta catenin and the Wnt pathway. Cyclin D1 and c-myc are downstream targets. Cancer occurs at a median age of 39, and >90% will develop adenomas by age 30. Extracolonic manifestations include cholangiocarcinoma, duodenal carcinoma, gastric cancer, desmoid tumors, osteomas, thyroid cancer, and brain tumors.

F. Other risk factors include age >50, high red meat intake and low fiber diets, Peutz–Jeghers syndrome, juvenile polyposis, immunosuppression, smoking, alcohol, and others.

VIII. PATHOGENESIS. There are three major pathways to CRC: Chromosomal instability (CIN) pathway, mutator-phenotype/DNA MMR pathway, and hypermethylation phenotype hyperplastic/serrated polyp pathway (CIMP+).

A. Chromosomal instability or suppressor pathway accounts for 85% of sporadic CRC, with an adenoma as the precursor lesion. FAP coli is the prototype for this model characterized by the loss of APC gene. A potential subtype of this model is characterized by the silencing of methylation of the DNA repair enzyme methylguanine DNA methyltransferase with serrated polyps as precursor lesions.

B. Microsatellite instability or mutator pathway accounts for 15% of sporadic CRC. HNPCC is the prototype for this model characterized by a loss of MMR genes (MLH1, MSH2, MSH6, etc).

C. Hypermethylation phenotype (CIMP+). Hyper- or hypomethylation can silence the expression of certain genes including MMR enzymes. A defect in the CpG islands causes particularly high-frequency methylation, therefore promoting silencing of enzymes such as MLH1.

IX. ANAL CANCER

A. Presentation. Bleeding, pain, constipation, tenesmus, diarrhea, discharge, and pruritus. Often, the symptoms are ascribed to other benign conditions such as hemorrhoids, fistula-in-ano, fissure, or anal condylomata. A careful history on risk factors also needs to be obtained.

Physical examination findings include a firm, indurated, or exophytic anal mass or inguinal lymphadenopathy. A careful digital examination and anoscope is necessary to evaluate the extent of the tumor. Women with anal cancer should also have a thorough gynecological examination. Diagnosis is made with incisional biopsy of the mass and any inguinal lymphadenopathy.

Pathology usually reveals squamous cell carcinoma or cloacogenic carcinoma. Adenocarcinomas involving the anus should be treated similar to rectal cancer. Rare cases of melanomas or neuroendocrine cancers may occur. Workup should include chest radiograph and CT or MRI of the abdomen and pelvis. HIV testing should be considered in high-risk individuals in addition to baseline laboratory tests.

B. Staging. Staging is based on the TNM system.

T_{is}, carcinoma in situ

T1, tumor is 2 cm or smaller

T2, tumor is between 2 cm and 5 cm

T3, tumor larger than 5 cm

T4, tumor of any size that invades adjacent organs such as the vagina, urethra, or bladder

N0, no regional lymph nodes involved

N1, metastases in unilateral internal iliac or inguinal lymph node

N3, metastases in perirectal and one inguinal lymph node and/or bilateral internal iliac or inguinal lymph nodes

M0/1, no or (+) distant metastases present

Stage I, T1, N0, M0

Stage II, T2, 3, N0, M0

Stage IIIA, T1–T3, N1, M0 or T4, N0, M0

Stage IIIB, T4, N1, M0 or any T, N2–N3, M0

Stage IV, any T, any N, M1

C. Prognosis. Prognosis is based on staging. T1 and T2 tumors have a 5-year survival of more than 80%, whereas T3 and T4 tumors have 5-year survivals of less than 50%. Inguinal lymphadenopathy and male sex also are related to a poorer prognosis. Tumors in the anal margin have a more favorable prognosis than do those in the canal.

D. Treatment. Standard therapy includes the Nigro protocol chemoradiation with mitomycin C and 5-FU. Higher DFS (73% vs. 51%) and lower colostomy rates (9% vs. 22%) are associated with chemoradiation compared with radiation alone. Five-year survival varied between 64% and 83% with combined-modality therapy. Patients with HIV/AIDS and anal cancer may be treated with the same Nigro protocol, but caution should be applied as they may not tolerate full doses of chemotherapy. Patients with T1 lesions may be considered for local excision alone or with chemoradiation.

E. Epidemiology and risk factors

1. **Epidemiology.** Anal cancer accounts for about 1.6% of all digestive system cancers in the United States. It is more common in men than in women. Its incidence generally increases with age, with peak incidence in the sixth and seventh decades of life. The incidence is increasing in men younger than 40 years.

2. **Risk factors.** Human papillomavirus (HPV) infection- HPV 16 and 18, women with HPV-related cervical cancer, smoking, HIV infection, and anal receptive sex.

SUGGESTED READINGS

Andre T, Boni C, Mounedji-Boudiaf L, et al.; Multicenter International Study of Oxaliplatin/5-Fluorouracil/Leucovorin in the Adjuvant Treatment of Colon Cancer (MOSAIC) Investigators. Oxaliplatin, fluorouracil, and leucovorin as adjuvant therapy for colon cancer. *N Engl J Med* 2004;350:2343–2351.

Benson AB, Schrag D, Somerfield MR, et al. American Society of Clinical Oncology recommendations on adjuvant chemothaerapy for Stage II colon cancer. *J Clin Oncol* 2004;22:3408–3419.

Nishihara R. Long-term colorectal cancer incidence and mortality after lower endoscopy. *N Engl J Medicine* 2013;369:1095–1105.

Ryan DP, Compton CC, Mayer RJ. Medical progress: carcinoma of the anal canal. *N Engl J Med* 2000;342:792–800.

Sauer R, Becker H, Hohenberger W, et al.; German Rectal Cancer Study Group. Preoperative versus postoperative chemoradiation for rectal cancer. *N Engl J Med* 2004;351:1731–1740.

HEPATOCELLULAR CARCINOMA

I. PRESENTATION

A. Subjective. Common symptoms of hepatocellular carcinoma (HCC) include anorexia, weight loss, increasing abdominal girth, and jaundice. Up to 25% of patients may be asymptomatic at presentation. Patients may present with paraneoplastic syndromes, including hypoglycemia, erythrocytosis, hypercalcemia, and dysfibrinogenemia or progressive signs of liver failure.

B. Objective. Hepatomegaly, ascites, fever, bleeding, and splenomegaly can be seen.

II. WORKUP AND STAGING.
High-risk patients (including those with cirrhosis—such as viral- or nonviral-induced—and hepatitis B carriers without cirrhosis) should have periodic screening with ultrasonography (USN) of the liver, alpha-fetoprotein (AFP), and albumin and alkaline phosphatase levels (*Cancer* 1996;78:977). There is some evidence from a study of screening in Chinese patients with hepatitis B infection or a history of chronic hepatitis that screening results in fewer patients dying from HCC (*J Cancer Res Clin Oncol* 2004;130:417). A rising AFP with negative liver imaging should result in more frequent radiographic follow-up.

Tissue diagnosis can be obtained by fine needle aspiration (FNA), core biopsy, or laparoscopic biopsy. The potential for tumor "spillage" appears to be very small. Although occasionally patients may be treated for HCC based on the clinical, radiologic, and biochemical features, generally an attempt should be made to obtain a tissue diagnosis. For example, while a serum AFP >400 ng/mL is sometimes considered diagnostic of HCC, such high values are seen only in a small number of patients with HCC. The American Association for the Study of Liver Diseases (AASLD) no longer includes AFP tests as part of the diagnostic evaluation. Magnetic resonance imaging (MRI) or four-phase computed tomography (CT) should be used to better define tumor extent. MRI with arterial phase enhancement may also be used for the evaluation of tumor extension (*Surg Oncol Clin N Am* 2007;16:343). Staging should also include chest imaging and complete blood count CBC and liver function tests.

The fibrolamellar histology is noteworthy for its higher likelihood of resectability and the lack of association with cirrhosis. The current American Joint Committee on Cancer/Union Internationale Contre Cancer (AICC/UICC) staging includes the presence or absence of cirrhosis/fibrosis, which are histologic features that predict prognosis after surgery.

III. MANAGEMENT.
Surgical resection represents the only known curative therapy. Child–Pugh classification and other scoring systems, which help predict liver function and reserves with surgery, have been used to identify patients eligible for resection (*J Hepatolbiliary Pancreat Surg* 2002;9:469).

A. According to the United Network for Organ Sharing (UNOS), transplant should be considered in those not eligible for resection and who fulfill all of the three Milan criteria: (1) Single tumor ≤5 cm or up to three tumors <3 cm; (2) Absence of macrovascular invasion; (3) No extrahepatic spread. The model for end-stage liver disease (MELD) may be useful for assessing placement on the liver transplant wait list. Four-year relapse-free survival up to 80% has been observed with carefully selected patients. After transplant, the survival may be as high as 92% in selected patients meeting the Milan criteria, with vascular invasion predicting lower survival (*Ann Surg Oncol* 2008;15:1001). Patients with unresectable but small tumors may be considered for tumor ablation followed by liver transplantation.

Other "local" therapies such as radiofrequency ablation (RFA), alcohol injection, cryotherapy, and chemoembolization may improve symptoms and control local disease in selected patients. RFA appears to be superior to percutaneous alcohol injection (PEI)

(*Hepatology* 2009;49:453; *Am J Gastroenterol* 2009;104:514; *J Hepatol* 2010;52:380), with 5-year survival rates of 70% in selected patients. The likelihood of success with these approaches may involve the expertise of the clinician, the number, size, and location of the tumors, as well as whether there is vascular involvement by the tumors. Several arterial-directed therapies are now widely available. All arterial-directed therapies are considered relatively contraindicated in patients who have bilirubin levels greater than 3 mg/dL, unless segmental therapy is used.

Stereotactic beam radiation therapy (SBRT) resulted in 2-year progression-free survival (PFS) of 33% in selected patients (*Cancer* 2012;118:5424). SBRT has also been used as bridging therapy for those with HCC and cirrhosis awaiting transplant (*J Surg Oncol* 2012;105:692; *Int J Radiat Oncol Biol Phys* 2012;83:895; *Liver Transpl* 2012;18:949).

B. Cytotoxic chemotherapy has traditionally been associated with low response rates and questionable disease control. An international Phase III placebo-controlled trial in which 602 patients with hepatocellular carcinoma were randomly assigned to receive sorafenib 400 mg twice daily or placebo demonstrated an overall survival (OS) benefit for those receiving sorafenib (10.7 vs. 7.9 months) (*N Engl J Med* 2008;359:378). Roughly 97% of patients in this study had Child–Pugh A liver function. Therefore, sorafenib should be used cautiously with Child–Pugh B liver function. Enrollment in clinical trials utilizing novel agents and approaches should be considered.

IV. EPIDEMIOLOGY. HCC is among the most frequent causes of cancer death worldwide, more commonly affecting men than women. In the United States, HCC is relatively less common, but is increasing in frequency, in part due to hepatitis C infection (*Am Intern Med* 2003;139:817). Among patients with hepatitis C–induced cirrhosis, 1% to 2% per year develop HCC. Although HCC in patients with hepatitis C occurs almost exclusively in patients with advanced fibrosis or cirrhosis, hepatitis B–induced HCC may occur without cirrhosis in a minority of patients. Other risk factors for HCC include cirrhosis due to other causes (alcohol, aflatoxin B), primary biliary cirrhosis, hereditary hemochromatosis, and non-alcoholic steatohepatitis (NASH) in patients with diabetes (*Hepatology* 2003;37:917).

CANCER OF THE GALLBLADDER

I. PRESENTATION

A. Subjective. Patients typically present with symptoms referable to the biliary tract, and often cholecystitis or biliary colic is suspected. Suspicion of malignancy should particularly be raised in older patients with weight loss and more continuous pain. In a retrospective study of 6,135 patients at a single institution and treated with curative resection, 47% of the gallbladder carcinomas were diagnosed incidentally during laparoscopic cholecystectomy (*J Surg Oncol* 2008;98:485).

B. Objective. Physical examination may reveal icterus, scratch marks from pruritis, and hepatomegaly.

II. WORKUP AND STAGING. A carbohydrate antigen 19-9 (CA19-9) greater than 20 μ/mL has a reported 79% sensitivity and 79% specificity. Approximately 93% of patients with gallbladder cancer where surgery is planned for benign disease will have carcinoembryonic antigen (CEA) greater than 4 ng/mL (*Int J Cancer* 1990;45:821).

An abnormality on USN may imply the need for CT, MRI, or magnetic resonance cholangiopancreatography (MRCP) for a better characterization of the extent of the disease. PET scanning may help identify regional lymph nodes and distant metastases (*J Am Coll Surg* 2008;206:57; *J Gastroenterol* 2010;45:560). Endoscopic retrograde cholangiopancreaticography (ERCP) with endoscopic USN may identify patients with unresectable disease, or allow for a tissue diagnosis. There is no clear risk of dissemination in obtaining cytology using ERCP and endoscopic USN.

Diagnosis is often made at the time of surgery, and definitive resection rather than cholecystectomy should be planned in suspicious, yet resectable cases. In addition to cytology specimens obtained with ERCP, percutaneous needle biopsy and core biopsy are used, although core biopsy, in particular, may carry significant "tracking" risk and should be reserved for unresectable cases (*Acta Cytol* 1995;39:494). Gallbladder cancer is typically adenocarcinoma, although other histologic subtypes occur infrequently. Higher grade tumors are associated with a worse prognosis, whereas the rare papillary tumors are associated with a better prognosis (*Cancer* 1992;70:1493). If no distant metastases are identified radiographically, laparoscopy should be considered to complete preoperative staging.

III. **MANAGEMENT.** Patients with incidentally found gallbladder tumors who are identified as having resectable disease should be considered for cholecystectomy, en bloc hepatic resection, lymphadenectomy, and possible bile duct resection. A similar approach is warranted for patients with preoperative radiographic staging, which reveals the possibility of resection of all radiographically evident tumors. If jaundice is present, the evaluation may include ERCP/percutaneous transhepatic cholangiography/MR cholangiography. If, at cholecystectomy, the gallbladder is removed intact, and a T1a tumor with negative margins is identified, no additional surgery is recommended. Lymph node involvement is very rare for T1. For T1b or greater disease, more extensive surgery has been recommended, although the evidence supporting radical resection for T1b tumors is not definitive (*Arch Surg* 2011;146:734; *World J Gastroenterol* 2012;18:4736).

In combining retrospective reviews, 5-year survival for patients with T1 tumors generally approaches 100%; whereas for T2, 70% to 90% survival may be expected (*Ann Surg* 1992;215:326; *Eur J Surg* 1997;163:419; *Surgery* 1994;115:751). Surgery remains the only curative therapy with 5-year survivals of 45% to 63% for patients with N1 disease.

In a small trial, adjuvant 5-fluorouracil (FU) and radiation demonstrated an improved 5-year survival compared with surgery alone (64% vs. 33%) (*Int J radiat Oncol Biol Phys* 2002;52:167) and, as a result, has been recommended for those with greater than T1 disease. However, studies of adjuvant therapy for biliary cancer often involved both bile duct and gallbladder cancers. In a meta-analysis of 6,712 patients, there was a trend toward OS improvement with adjuvant therapy that was greater for those with gallbladder compared with other biliary cancers (*J Clin Oncol* 2012;30:1934).

Patients with unresectable but not metastatic disease may benefit from combined chemotherapy and radiation therapy (RT), although this approach has not been extensively studied. Gemcitabine or capecitabine alone or in combination have been used in patients with metastatic disease. The overall prognosis from metastatic gallbladder cancer remains poor, with average survival of approximately 6 months for untreated patients and only approximately 5% of patients surviving 5 years. Biliary decompression may be necessary before initiation of chemotherapy and may also relieve obstructive symptoms. ABC-02 was a Phase III-controlled trial in which 410 patients with locally advanced or metastatic cholangiocarcinoma, gallbladder, or ampullary cancer received gemcitabine alone or in combination with cisplatin. OS was 11.7 months for the combination versus 8 months for gemcitabine alone (*N Engl J Med* 2010;362:1273).

IV. **EPIDEMIOLOGY.** Marked regional and ethnic differences are seen in the incidence of gallbladder cancer. For example, gallbladder cancer has been reported as the leading cause of cancer death in Chilean women. High rates are seen in other South American countries as well as in Central Europe, Israel, and in Native Americans, Japanese men, and others. In the United States, gallbladder cancer is the most common biliary tract cancer, and is more common in women than in men. There are approximately 2,800 deaths per year from gallbladder cancer.

Chronic inflammation, often due to gallstones, is associated with gallbladder cancer. In fact, 75% to 98% of gallbladder cancer patients will have had gallstones (*Cancer Treat Res* 1994;69:97). The so-called "porcelain gallbladder" will be associated with cancer in up to 25% of patients. Gallbladder polyps, particularly those greater than 1 cm and those in older patients, warrant special attention (*Br J Surg* 1992;79:227). There are associations between gallbladder cancers and anomalous biliary ductal malformations as well as with typhoid.

CHOLANGIOCARCINOMA

I. PRESENTATION

A. **Subjective.** Patients typically present with weight loss or symptoms related to biliary obstruction such as jaundice, pruritis, or fever from infection.

B. **Objective.** Physical examination may reveal icterus, a palpable gallbladder (Courvoisier's sign), and an enlarged liver.

II. **WORKUP AND STAGING.** Cholangiocarcinomas arise in the biliary tree and are classified as intrahepatic or extrahepatic tumors. Extrahepatic cholangiocarcinomas account for 90% of all cholangiocarcinomas and include hilar cholangiocarcinomas, which are commonly called Klatskin's tumors (*Ann Surg* 1996;224:463). Laboratory findings often reveal elevated liver function tests, CEA, and CA19-9. A variety of radiographic studies, such as USN and delayed contrast CT or MRI scanning, are used to define disease extent as well as chest imaging. Retrograde cholangiopancreatography with ERCP is used for stent placement and to obtain cytology for diagnosis. Cytology sampling has demonstrated 62% sensitivity. For hilar tumors, percutaneous transhepatic cholangiography may be used to define proximal bile duct involvement. MRI cholangiography, angiography, and endoscopic USN (which also define a mass for biopsy) have potential roles in defining disease extent and vascular involvement. Molecular testing has been shown to increase the sensitivity for diagnosis (*Gastroenterology* 2006;131(4):1064).

Adenocarcinoma is the most common histology. Subtypes include sclerosing, nodular, and papillary variants. Revised staging systems for intra- and extrahepatic cholangiocarcinomas incorporate features predictive of prognosis.

III. **MANAGEMENT.** Surgery offers the best chances of cure for those with disease confined to a localized portion of the liver. Involvement of both hepatic lobes indicates generally unresectable disease. Nodal involvement or more distant metastases are usually considered contraindications to curative surgery. In summarizing multiple series, the median and 5-year survival rates after surgery have ranged from 15 to 29 months and 13% to 42%, respectively. Either stents or surgery can be used to improve biliary drainage and reduce symptoms and potentially delay hepatic function deterioration. Silastic stents are changed regularly as metal stents do not require changing, but cannot be removed once obstructed.

For intrahepatic potentially resectable cholangiocarcinoma, a laparoscopy appears to improve detection of liver and peritoneal metastasis, and should be considered before resection. For intrahepatic cholangiocarcinomas, negative margin resection has been associated with an improved 5-year survival (39.8% vs. 4.7% for those with a positive margin) and lower recurrence rates (53.9% vs. 73.6%) (*Arch Surg* 2012;147:1107).

Optimal adjuvant postoperative therapy has not been determined, but for intrahepatic cholangiocarcinoma (particularly with positive tumor margins [R1] or residual local disease [R2] after resection), reasonable options include fluoropyrimidine-based chemoradiation or chemotherapy alone with fluoropyrimidine or gemcitabine-based combinations.

Local regional therapies for intrahepatic cholangiocarcinomas include RFA, transhepatic chemoembolization (TACE), drug-eluting spheres with TACE (DEB-TACE), and transarterial radioactive embolization with yttrium microspheres (TACE). Each of these approaches has been shown to be potentially effective in small series. For example, in a small series of patients with unresectable intrahepatic cholangiocarcinomas, OS was 38.5 months with RFA (*AJR Am J Roentgeno* 2011;196:W205).

For extrahepatic cholangiocarcinomas, radical surgery appears to result in 5-year survival rates of 20% to 42% for resected hilar tumors and 16% to 52% for resected distal cholangiocarcinoma (*World J Clin Oncol* 2011;2:94).

Retrospective series together do appear to support adjuvant chemotherapy or chemoradiation therapy, particularly for higher risk biliary cancers after resection.

Liver transplantation is a consideration for cholangiocarcinomas without distant spread. Five-year OS rates range from 25% to 42%. Neoadjuvant chemoradiation or adjuvant chemoradiation appear to be associated with an improved relapse-free survival compared with curative resection in select patients (*Ann Surg* 2005;242:451; *Arch Surg* 2011;146:683).

IV. **EPIDEMIOLOGY.** Cholangiocarcinomas are associated with conditions causing chronic inflammation such as primary sclerosing cholangitis, chronic bile duct calculi, choledochal cysts, and liver flukes. Viral hepatitis also appears to be a risk factor for intrahepatic cholangiocarcinomas.

Cholangiocarcinomas are more common in Southeast Asia and China, and the incidence and mortality from cholangiocarcinomas is rising (*J Gastroenterol Hepatol* 2002;17:1049).

SUGGESTED READINGS

Hepatocellular Carcinoma

Goudolesi GE, Roayaie S, Munoz L, et al. Adult living donor transplantation for patients with hepatocellular carcinoma: extending UNOS priority criteria. *Ann Surg* 2004;239:142–149.

Greten TF, Papendorf F, Bleck JS, et al. Survival rate in patients with hepatocellular carcinoma: a retrospective analysis of 389 patients. *Br J Cancer* 2005;92:1862–1868.

Groupe d'Etude et de Traitement du Carcinome Hepatocellulaire. A comparison of lipidol chemoembolization and conservative treatment for unresectable hepatocellular carcinoma. *N Engl J Med* 1995;332:1256–1261.

Llovet JM, Real MI, Montana X, et al. Arterial embolization or chemoembolization versus symptomatic treatment in patients with unresectable hepatocellular carcinoma: a randomized controlled trial. *Lancet* 2002;359:1734–1939.

Llovet JM, Ricci S, Mazzaferro V, et al. Sorafenib in advanced hepatocellular carcinoma. *N Engl J Med* 2008;359:378–390.

Mazzaferro V, Ragalia E, Doci R, et al. Liver transplantation for the treatment of small hepatocellular carcinoma in patients with cirrhosis. *N Eng J Med* 1996;334:693–699.

Cancer of the Gallbladder

de Aretexaba XA, Roa IS, Burgos LA, et al. Curative resection in potentially resectable tumors of the gallbladder. *Eur J Surg* 1997;163:419.

Daines WP, Rajagopalan V, Groosbard ML, et al. Gallbladder and biliary tract carcinoma: a comprehensive update, part 2. *Oncology (Huntington)* 2004;18:1049.

Lazcano-Ponce EC, Miquel JF, Munoz N, et al. Epidemiology and molecular pathology of gallbladder cancer. *CA Cancer J Clin* 2001;51:349.

Matsumoto Y, Fugii H, Aoyama H, et al. Surgical treatment of primary carcinoma of the gallbladder based on histologic analysis of 48 surgical specimens. *Am J Surg* 1992;162:239.

Shirai Y, Yoshida K, Tsukaka K, et al. Inapparent carcinoma of the gallbladder: an appraisal of a radical second operation after simple cholecystectomy. *Ann Surg* 1992;215:326.

Tsukaka K, Kurosaki I, Uchida K, et al. Lymph node spread from carcinoma of the gallbladder. *Cancer* 1997:80:661.

Valle J, Wasan H, Palmer DH, et al. Cisplatin plus gemcitabine versus gemcitabine for biliary tract cancer. *N Engl J Med* 2010;362:1273–1281.

Cholangiocarcinoma

Heimbach JK, Haddock MG, Alberts SR, et al. Transplantation for hilar cholangiocarcinoma: 5-year follow-up of a prospective phase II study. *Gastrointest Endosc* 2004;60:68–75.

Jarnagin WR, Fong Y, DeMatteo RP, et al. Staging resectability and outcome in 255 patients with hilar cholangiocarcinoma. *Ann Surg* 2001;234:507–517; discussion 517–519.

Klatskin G, Adenocarcinoma of the hepatic duct at its bifurcation within the porta hepatic: an unusual tumor with distinctive clinical and pathologic features. *Am J Med* 1965;38:241.

Lee CC, Wy CY, Chen JT, et al. Comparing combined hepatocellular-cholangiocarcinoma and cholangiocarcinoma: a clinicopatholigic study. *Hepatogastroenterology* 2002;49:1487.

Rajagopalan V, Daines WP, Grossbard ML, et al. Gallbladder and biliary tract carcinoma: a comprehensive update, part 1. *Oncology* 2004;18:889–896.

Sudan D, DeRoober A, Chinnakotla S, et al. Radiochemotherapy and transplantation allow long-term survival for nonresectable hilar cholangiocarcinoma. *Am J Transplant* 2002;2:774–779.

18 Pancreatic Cancer

Andrea Wang-Gillam

CANCER OF THE PANCREAS

I. PRESENTATION

  A. Subjective. Typical presenting symptoms include painless jaundice, weight loss, abdominal pain, back pain, nausea, vomiting, and pruritus. Infrequently, new-onset diabetes develops prior to the diagnosis of pancreatic cancer.

  B. Objective. Physical examination findings may include sclerotic icterus, jaundice, ascites, left supraclavicular adenopathy (Virchow's node), periumbilical adenopathy (Sister Mary Joseph's node), or perirectal drop metastases (Blumer's shelf).

II. WORKUP AND STAGING.
Pancreatic ductal adenocarcinoma is the most common histology of pancreatic cancer. Neuroendocrine tumors in the pancreas are uncommon (less than 5%) and carry a much better prognosis than ductal adenocarcinoma. The treatment for pancreatic neuroendocrine tumors is completely different from that for adenocarcinoma, so it is crucial to distinguish between the two histologies at the time of diagnosis. Metastatic disease to the pancreas is rare.

The golden standard diagnostic procedure for pancreatic cancer is to perform an upper endoscopic ultrasound-guided fine needle aspiration (EUS-FNA) of the primary pancreatic cancer, especially in patients without frank metastasis. Although the brushing is commonly collected in patients undergoing endoscopic retrograde cholangiopancreatography for obstructive jaundice, the sample yield for a positive cytology varies. In patients with metastatic disease, it is reasonable to obtain a biopsy from the easily accessible metastatic sites. Tumor marker CA 19-9 is not used for diagnosis because it can be positively elevated in patients with benign conditions such as biliary obstruction. Additionally, about 10% of patients with pancreatic cancer have normal CA 19-9 because of being Lewis-negative phenotypes.

Given the vague symptoms and lack of an effective screening method, only 10% to 20% of patients with pancreatic cancer have resectable disease at the time of diagnosis; therefore, the classic pathological staging of tumor, node, metastasis (TNM) system is not practical for the majority of pancreatic cancer patients. Clinical staging based on the radiographic findings is the preferred staging method, and it classifies patients into four categories: resectable, borderline resectable, locally advanced, and metastatic disease. To optimally delineate the vasculature involvement of the tumor, which is the main determinate for surgical resection in localized cancer, the preferred imaging tool is a computed tomography (CT) scan (a triple-phase, high-speed helical scanning) with contrast enhancement, which is commonly referred to as "pancreatic protocol" CT. Staging with laparoscopy may be needed to evaluate peritoneal metastasis. In fact, up to 37% of cases with apparent locally advanced disease have peritoneal metastases seen upon laparoscopy (*Gastrointest Surg* 2004;8:1068).

III. MANAGEMENT

  A. Resectable disease. Surgery remains the only modality clearly established to cure pancreatic cancer. Unfortunately, only 10% to 20% of patients present with apparently resectable disease. The Whipple procedure is indicated for tumors in the head of pancreas, while distal pancreatectomy is reserved for tumors in the body and tail of the pancreas. The clinical outcome is superior if surgery is performed in a high-volume surgery center. Among all pathological features of the resected tumor, the positive malignant lymph node appears to be the strongest predictor for outcome.

  In light of a distal recurrence rate of 70%, adjuvant therapy is recommended to patients with adequate recovery from curative resection. Adjuvant therapies have evolved over the years; however, a controversy remains regarding radiation therapy (RT), and RT

TABLE 18-1	Key Adjuvant Trials in Pancreatic Cancer							
	CONKO-001		RTOG-9704 Head of pancreas		ESPAC-3		JSPAC-01	
	Surgery	Gem	5FU	Gem	5FU	Gem	S1	Gem
Median OS (m)	20.2	22.8	17.1	20.5	23.0	23.6	NR	25.9
2-year survival (%)	42	47.5	N/A	N/A	48.1	49.1	70	53
5-year survival (%)	10.4	20.7	18	22	N/A	N/A	N/A	N/A
10-year survival (%)	7.7	12.2	N/A	N/A	N/A	N/A	N/A	N/A

OS, overall survival; m, months; Gem, gemcitabine; 5FU, 5-fluorouracil; NR, not reached; N/A, not available.

is not part of adjuvant care for these patients in Europe. At present, four large randomized phase III adjuvant trials in pancreatic cancer have demonstrated the benefit of adjuvant therapy (see Table 18-1). The CONKO-001 study was the first randomized phase III trial to demonstrate the survival benefit from a course of 6 months of gemcitabine as adjuvant therapy (*JAMA* 2013;310:1473). The 5-year and 10-year overall survival rates were superior in the gemcitabine arm compared with surgery alone (20.7% vs. 10.4% and 12.2% vs. 7.7%, respectively). The disease-free survival was also favorable in the gemcitabine arm (13.4 months vs. 6.7 months; hazard ratio, 0.55; P<0.001). The ESPAC-3 trial was initially designed to randomly assign pancreatic cancer patients post surgical resection to receive 5-FU plus folinic acid or gemcitabine or surgery alone. The surgery arm was discontinued because of the benefit of adjuvant gemcitabine therapy reported in the CONKO-001 study. In the ESPAC-3 study, the median survival was 23 months for patients receiving the 5-FU plus folinic acid compared with 23.6 months for those receiving gemcitabine (*JAMA* 2010;304:1073). Both the CONKO-001 and the ESPAC-3 studies were conducted in Europe where RT was not part of adjuvant regimen.

In North America, the Radiation Therapy Oncology Group (RTOG) conducted a study (RTOG-9704) of pancreatic cancer patients postresection who were randomly assigned to receive either gemcitabine followed by 5-FU and radiation followed by gemcitabine or 5-FU followed by 5-FU and radiation followed by 5-FU. The two treatment arms differed on the systemic therapy components. The study reported superior survival in patients with pancreatic head tumors treated with the gemcitabine-based regimen (20.5 months vs. 16.9 months, hazard ratio, 0.82; P=0.09) (*JAMA* 2008;299:1019). More recently, Japanese researchers reported the preliminary results of their trial using S1 or gemcitabine as adjuvant therapy in the pancreatic cancer at the 2013 American Society of Clinical Oncology (ASCO) meeting, and so far, the survival benefit in this trial has surpassed all previous adjuvant studies with a 2-year survival rate of 70% in the S1 arm and 53% in the gemcitabine arm. Currently, S1 is available only in Asia.

B. **Borderline resectable and locally advanced pancreatic cancer.** Borderline resectable disease is an emerging entity. It is distinguished from locally advanced disease by having less involvement of the tumor vasculature. For example, if the tumor abuts the superior mesentery artery (SMA), it is considered borderline resectable because there is still a chance for resection, despite the fact that the risk for a positive margin is high. If the tumor encases the SMA, then it is considered locally advanced because the chance of resection with a clean margin is zero; so by definition, patients with locally advanced disease are not candidates for curative resection. The detailed radiographic differences of vascular involvement between borderline resectable and locally advanced pancreatic cancer can be found on the National Comprehensive Cancer Network (www.nccn.org).

Because of the 70% distant recurrent rate in patients who undergo curative resection, it is logical to consider systemic therapy prior to surgery. The rationales for exploring this approach include identifying patients with rapidly progressive disease so that they may avoid an unnecessary operation, eliminating micrometastases, improving the effectiveness of RT (because surgery may interfere with the effectiveness of postoperative RT as a result of vascular damage from surgery), and downstaging tumors to decrease the risk of positive surgical margins. This upfront systemic therapy approach to managing borderline resectable pancreatic cancer is gaining acceptance in the oncology community. Although the optimal upfront therapy remains undefined, aggressive chemotherapy regimens with proven survival benefits in the metastatic setting, such as 5FU, oxaliplatin, irinotecan (FOLFIRINOX), or gemcitabine and nab-paclitaxel, have been extrapolated to this setting. Concurrent chemotherapy and RT has also been used in this setting.

The standard treatment for patients with locally advanced pancreatic cancer is systemic chemotherapy. The benefit of concurrent chemotherapy and RT in this setting was initially reported in the Groupe Cooperateur Multidisciplinaire en Oncologie (GERCOR) study (*J Clin Oncol* 2007;25:326). The study reviewed the outcome of patients with locally advanced pancreatic cancer who were enrolled in phase II or III GERCOR studies and had achieved stable disease after 2 to 3 months of systemic therapy. It compared the survival of those who received chemotherapy with that of those who received chemotherapy and RT after being treated with systemic therapy for a period of 3 months. The addition of RT to the chemotherapy regimen increased survival by more than 3 months (15.0 months vs. 11.7 months; P=0.0009); however, this study was criticized because of its retrospective nature. More recently, a large randomized prospective phase III study for patients with locally advanced pancreatic cancer disease was completed. The study has a 2 × 2 factorial design for which patients were first randomized to receive gemcitabine or gemcitabine plus erlotinib for 4 months; then they were randomized again to continue on chemotherapy alone or receive chemotherapy and RT. The preliminary results of this study were presented at the 2013 ASCO Annual Meeting, and no survival difference between the chemotherapy alone and chemotherapy and RT arms was observed. Additionally, patients who received gemcitabine plus erlotinib did not have any additional survival benefit but experienced slightly more toxicity. This large prospective study provides level I evidence that concurrent chemotherapy and RT does not provide any additional benefit in locally advanced disease.

C. **Metastatic pancreatic cancer.** Patients with metastatic pancreatic cancer have a poor prognosis, with survival of less than 1 year. Gemcitabine has been the cornerstone of frontline therapy for the past decade. It was compared with 5-FU in patients with advanced pancreatic cancer, and the median survival favored gemcitabine (5.65 months vs. 4.41 months, P=0.0022). Clinical benefit was defined as improvement for ≥4 weeks in pain, analgesic use, weight loss, or performance status without worsening of another one of these symptoms. The likelihood of clinical benefit favored gemcitabine (24% vs. 5%). As a consequence of this study, gemcitabine was soon established as standard therapy (*J Clin Oncol* 1997;21:3402).

While targeted agents have flourished in multiple cancer types, the success of this approach in pancreatic cancer has been more elusive. Erlotinib (an epidermal growth factor receptor inhibitor) combined with gemcitabine was tested in patients with advanced pancreatic cancer. A small but statistically significant survival benefit was observed in patients receiving gemcitabine plus erlotinib compared with those receiving gemcitabine alone (6.24 months vs. 5.91 months, hazard ratio, 0.82; P=0.038). Interestingly, the development of a rash appeared to be a positive prognostic factor for patients receiving erlotinib; patients who developed grade 0, 1, and 2+ rash had median survivals of 5.3, 5.8, and 10.5 months, respectively (*J Clin Oncol* 2007;25:1960).

More recently, two regimens have become standard of care in the frontline setting for metastatic pancreatic cancer (Table 18-2). A phase III study of FOLFIRNIOX or gemcitabine in patients with metastatic pancreatic cancer with good performance status demonstrated the survival benefit of FOLFIRINOX (11.1 months vs. 6.8 months; P<0.001). Median progression-free survival was also favorable in patients who received FOLFIRINOX (6.4 months vs. 3.3 months; P<0.001). The response rate was also significantly

Table 18-2	Two Key FrontLine Trials in Advanced Pancreatic Cancer			
	ACCORD		**MPACT**	
Objective response	FOLFIRINOX (n=171)	Gem (n=171)	Nab-paclitaxel/ gem (n=431)	Gem (n=430)
Complete response	0.6%	0%	<1%	0%
Partial response	31% (25–39)	9.4% (6–15)	23%	7%
Stable disease	38.6%	41.5%	27%	28%
Disease control	70.2%	50.9%	48%	33%
Progression-free survival (m)	6.4	3.3	5.5	3.7
Overall survival (m)	11.1	6.8	8.5	6.7

higher in the FOLFIRINOX arm (31.6% vs. 9.4%; P<0.001); however, the aggressive FOLFIRINOX regimen results in moderate toxicities including neutropenia, fatigue, and diarrhea (*N Engl J Med* 2011;364:1817).

The combination of nab-paclitaxel plus gemcitabine as the frontline therapy has gained popularity after nab-paclitaxel was approved in pancreatic cancer by the Food and Drug Administration. A randomized phase III study (MPAC) of nab-paclitaxel plus gemcitabine versus gemcitabine as the frontline therapy in patients with metastatic pancreatic cancer yielded a median overall survival of 8.5 months in the combination arm compared with 6.7 months in the gemcitabine alone arm. The 1-year survival rate was higher in those who received the combination therapy compared with those who received gemcitabine alone (35% vs. 22%; P<0.001). The severe side effects of the combination regimen include neutropenia and neuropathy (*N Engl J Med* 2013;369:1691). At present, multiple novel agents are being combined with nab-paclitaxel plus gemcitabine in clinical trials.

Despite the poor prognosis associated with pancreatic cancer, about 40% of patients who progress on frontline therapy are able to receive second-line therapy. So far, in patients progressed on gemcitabine-based therapy, 5-FU and oxaliplatin (OFF regimen) have shown to provide a survival benefit compared with those who received best supportive care (4.82 months vs. 2.30 months; P=0.008) (*Eur J Cancer* 2011;47:1678). The OFF regimen was further tested against FF (5FU-folinic acid) in a randomized phase III trial in patients with metastatic disease, and the survival was superior in patients who received OFF (5.89 months vs. 3.09 months; P=0.01). The study was reported in the abstract form. For patients who progressed on frontline FOLFIRINOX or a FOLFIRINOX-like regimen, a gemcitabine-based regimen has been the natural choice for second-line therapy, but there are no studies yet to support this approach given the fairly recent adoption of FOLFIRINOX. Beyond two lines of therapy, there is no standard of care available. These patients, in general, should be referred for clinical studies.

IV. **EPIDEMIOLOGY.** Pancreatic cancer is the fourth most common cause of cancer death in the United States. It is projected to be the second most common cancer-related death by 2030. Approximately 46,000 patients were diagnosed with pancreatic cancer in 2013, and about 40,000 died the same year, underscoring the extremely poor prognosis associated with this disease. While the majority of pancreatic cancers are sporadic, 10% of cases are hereditary. An increased risk for pancreatic cancer is seen in populations that have hereditary pancreatitis, hereditary breast cancer (BRCA and PALB2 mutations), Peutz–Jeghers syndrome, familial atypical multiple mole melanoma (FAMMM) syndrome, and Lynch syndrome.

V. **FUTURE DIRECTIONS.** New strategic approaches in targeting pancreatic cancer are under investigation. Strategies that disrupt dense stroma are a current center of focus. Additionally, clinical trials that use immunotherapy have gained recent momentum. Because more than 90%

of pancreatic tumors harbor a KRAS mutation and direct targeting of KRAS has not been successful, targeted agents that inhibit KRAS downstream mediators are currently being evaluated in clinical studies.

SUGGESTED READINGS

Callery MP, Chang KJ, Fishman EK, et al. Pretreatment assessment of resectable and borderline resectable pancreatic cancer: expert consensus statement. *Ann Surg Oncol* 2009;250(1):96–102.

Lim KH, Chung E, Khan A, et al. Neoadjuvant therapy of pancreatic cancer: the emerging paradigm? *Oncologist* 2012;17(2):192–200.

Oettle H, Neuhaus P, Hochhaus A, et al. Adjuvant chemotherapy with gemcitabine and long-term outcomes among patients with resected pancreatic cancer: the CONKO-001 randomized trial. *JAMA* 2013;310(14):1473–1481.

Neoptolemos JP, Stocken DD, Bassi C, et al; European Study Group for Pancreatic Cancer. Adjuvant chemotherapy with fluorouracil plus folinic acid vs gemcitabine following pancreatic cancer resection: a randomized controlled trial. *JAMA* 2010;304(10):1073–1081.

Regine WF, Winter KA, Abrams RA, et al. Fluorouracil vs gemcitabine chemotherapy before and after fluorouracil-based chemoradiation following resection of pancreatic adenocarcinoma: a randomized trial. *JAMA* 2008;299(9):1019–1026.

Conroy T, Desseigne F, Ychou M, et al; Groupe Tumeurs Digestives of Unicancer; PRODIGE Intergroup. FOLFIRINOX versus gemcitabine for metastatic pancreatic cancer. *N Engl J Med* 2011;364(19):1817–1825.

Von Hoff DD, Ervin T, Arena FP, et al. Increased survival in pancreatic cancer with nab-paclitaxel plus gemcitabine. *N Engl J Med* 2013;369(18):1691–1703.

Kidney Cancer
Daniel Morgensztern • Bruce Roth

I. PRESENTATION

A. Subjective. Symptoms from renal cell carcinoma (RCC) can be caused by local tumor growth, paraneoplastic syndromes, or distant metastases. The classic triad of flank pain, gross hematuria, and palpable abdominal mass is present in less than 10% of patients and indicates locally advanced disease. Paraneoplastic syndromes occur in approximately 20% of patients at presentation and up to 40% during the course of their disease. Hypercalcemia, the most common paraneoplastic manifestation of RCC, occurs in approximately 15% of patients and may be due to bone metastases or production of parathyroid hormone-related protein (PTHrP). Nonmetastatic hepatic dysfunction, also known as Stauffer's syndrome, is characterized by elevated alkaline phosphatase, elevated prothrombin time, and hypoalbuminemia, with some patients also having elevated bilirubin and liver transaminases. Most patients have associated fever, weight loss, neutropenia, and thrombocytopenia. Symptoms improve or resolve in the majority of patients undergoing nephrectomy. Although erythrocytosis occurs in up to 5% of patients owing to increased production of erythropoietin, anemia is a far more common manifestation, usually with parameters of anemia of chronic disease. Hypertension may occur in up to 40% of patients with RCC and is usually caused by either renin secretion by the tumor or secondary to compression of the renal artery and parenchyma. Constitutional symptoms including fever, weight loss, and fatigue occur in approximately one-third of the patients at presentation. The most common sites of metastases are the lungs, bone, and liver. More recent patient series have shown an increased percentage of asymptomatic patients with incidental diagnosis during radiological investigation of unrelated problems.

B. Objective. Hematuria and flank mass are the most common objective findings in RCC. Scrotal varicoceles are usually left-sided or bilateral owing to higher pressure in the left renal vein, and decompress in the supine position. The presence of unilateral right-sided varicoceles or the lack of reduction in the supine position is suspicious for inferior vena cava (IVC) thrombus, which may be caused by RCC.

II. EVALUATION OF A RENAL MASS. Patients with unexplained hematuria, flank pain, or mass suggesting RCC should be evaluated with a radiographic study, preferably computed tomography (CT) scan. Magnetic resonance imaging (MRI) or magnetic resonance angiography (MRA) may be used for further evaluation of the collecting system or IVC involvement. Because of the increased background activity of healthy renal tissue and fluorodeoxyglucose (FDG) excretion in the urine, positron emission tomography (PET) scan has limited value in the RCC diagnosis. With the presumptive diagnosis of RCC by the characteristic radiographic appearance, most patients without metastases undergo resection, which provides both diagnosis and treatment. In patients that are unfit for surgery, renal biopsy of small masses may be performed with minimal risk of tumor spreading, and such patients may be offered cryoablation.

III. PATHOLOGY. RCC is not a single disease but rather a heterogeneous group of cancers originating in the renal tubular epithelium, with distinct morphology, biology, and response to therapy. Clear cell is the most common subtype, representing approximately 75% of the cases. These tumors arise in the proximal tubule and frequently have loss of 3p25, which is the locus of the von Hippel–Lindau (VHL) gene. These tumors have a vascular stroma with frequent development of hemorrhagic areas. Papillary carcinomas represent approximately 15% of RCCs, also arise in the proximal tubule, are more commonly bilateral and multifocal compared with other subtypes, and may be subdivided into type 1 and type 2, which may be associated with mutations in c-met or fumarate hydratase, respectively. Chromophobe tumors represent approximately 5% of the RCC cases, arise in the distal nephron, may be associated with a higher incidence of liver metastases compared with other histologies, and have an overall better prognosis compared with clear cell carcinomas. Collecting duct carcinomas account for approximately 1% of the cases and usually behave aggressively, with metastases at presentation. Renal medullary carcinomas are aggressive tumors associated almost exclusively with sickle cell trait. Renal oncocytomas are benign tumors (*Semin Cancer Biol* 2013;23:3).

IV. WORKUP AND STAGING. The initial workup for patients with a suspicious renal mass incudes history and physical examination, complete blood count, metabolic panel, urinalysis, and chest imaging. MRI of the abdomen may be performed to rule out IVC involvement. If a central mass is present suggesting urothelial carcinoma, patients should have urine cytology performed. Since most metastases to the bones or brain are symptomatic at presentation, bone scan and brain MRI are performed only when clinically indicated.

The current staging for RCC divides the T stage into T1 (tumor ≤7 cm limited to the kidney; T1a ≤4 cm, T1b >4 to 7 cm), T2 (tumor >7 cm limited to the kidney), T3 (tumor extending into major veins or perinephric tissues), and T4 (tumor invades beyond the Gerota's fascia including the ipsilateral adrenal gland). N stage is divided into N0 (no regional lymph node metastases) and N1 (metastasis in regional lymph nodes), whereas M stage is divided into M0 or M1 on the basis of the absence or presence of distant metastases. Stages I and II are defined by the presence of T1 and T2, respectively, without lymph node or distant metastases. The presence of T3 or N1 defines stage III, whereas stage IV is defined by T4 or M1.

V. TREATMENT

A. Localized disease (stage I). The standard therapy for localized disease is surgical resection, with either a radical nephrectomy or nephron-sparing surgery. Radical nephrectomy involves the complete removal of the Gerota's fascia and its contents including the kidney perirenal fat, regional lymph nodes, and ipsilateral adrenal gland. More recently, adrenalectomy has been indicated predominantly for patients with large upper pole lesions or abnormal gland by CT imaging, in an attempt to avoid the complications from adrenal insufficiency (*J Urol*

2009;181:2009). Regional lymphadenectomy provides prognostic information but does not have an established therapeutic role. The main complication from radical nephrectomy is the development of chronic kidney disease, which increases the risk of cardiovascular events and overall mortality. With the use of modern imaging techniques, there has been a stage migration, with most patients being currently diagnosed with stage T1a. Nephron-sparing surgery, or partial nephrectomy, is indicated for patients with T1a disease and selected cases of T1b. This approach, however, is not indicated for patients with stage II or III disease. Both radical and nephron-sparing nephrectomies can be performed through a laparoscopic approach, depending on the size of the primary tumor. Patients with stage T1a disease that are not candidates for even nephron-sparing surgery may be treated with ablative therapy, including either cryoablation or radio frequency ablation (RFA), which should be preceded by a biopsy to establish the histological diagnosis for future therapies, if needed. Patients with T1a disease and decreased life expectancy or high surgical risk may be offered surveillance based on the fact that for such small tumors, the probability of benign tumor is 20%, only 20% to 30% of the tumors within this size range are potentially aggressive variants, and the risk of development of metastasis is overall low (*J Urol* 2009;182:1271).

B. **Locally advanced disease (stages II, III, and T4).** Patients with stage II and III RCC should be treated with radical nephrectomy. Following complete surgical resection, for patients with locally advanced RCC, the estimated risk for relapse at 5 years ranges from 11% in T2N0 to 66% in T4N1. Randomized clinical trials comparing immunotherapy, using either interferon alpha (IFN-α) or interleukin-2 (IL-2), failed to improve the disease-free survival (DFS) or overall survival (OS) compared with observation. A new generation of adjuvant trials using vascular endothelial growth factor (VEGF) or mammalian target of rapamycin (mTOR) inhibitors is currently accruing patients, with DFS as the primary end point (*Oncologist* 2014;19:1). At this time, however, there is no established role for adjuvant therapy in patients with resected RCC. Surveillance in these patients should include history, physical examination, metabolic panel, and imaging every 6 months for the first 2 years, and annually starting in the third year.

C. **Metastatic disease.** The standard approach for patients with metastatic disease is systemic therapy, although surgery may have a role in selected cases.

1. **Resection of solitary metastases.** Patients with oligometastatic disease may still be cured with surgery, particularly those with single site and metachronous presentation. In a retrospective series of 278 patients with recurrent RCC between 1980 and 1993, the 5-year OS for the 141 patients undergoing curative resection for their first metastasis was 44%. Furthermore, resections of subsequent second and third metastases after the initial curative intent resection had an OS of 45%, which was similar to those undergoing the initial resection (*J Clin Oncol* 1998;16:2261).

2. **Cytoreductive nephrectomy.** The removal of the primary cancer followed by INF-α has been associated with a significant improvement in the median OS compared with INF-α alone in two identical large randomized trials including a total of 331 patients (13.6 vs. 7.8 months, p = 0.002) (*J Urol* 2004;171:1071). Patients considered for cytoreductive nephrectomy should have resectable primary tumor, good performance status, and adequate organ function. Although the role for cytoreductive nephrectomy is established for patients treated with subsequent immunotherapy, its use in patients treated with VEGF-targeted therapy has not been prospective established. Optimal candidates for this approach would include patients with small volume metastatic disease, an easily resectable primary tumor, no significant comorbidities that would place them at an increased risk of surgery/general anesthesia, or whose dominant symptoms are from the primary lesion, either bleeding or pain.

3. **Systemic therapy.** The main options for systemic therapy in patients with metastatic RCC are immunotherapy and targeted therapy with VEGF and mTOR inhibitors.

   Immunotherapy with cytokines has been used for several years with IL-2 and IFN-α as the main drugs. High-dose IL-2 is usually administered as 600,000 to 720,000 IU/kg intravenously over 15 minutes every 8 hours for up to 14 doses over 5 days as tolerated, with a second cycle starting after 5 to 9 days of rest, with responding patients restarting the therapy in 6 to 12 weeks. In a retrospective evaluation of 255 patients treated in seven phase II trials, the overall response rate (RR) was 14%, with 12 (5%) patients achieving complete response (CR). Toxicities were mostly related to capillary leak syndrome, including hypotension in 96% of patients and arrhythmias (*J Clin Oncol* l995;13:688). In an updated analysis of 259 patients treated with high-dose IL-2 at the National Cancer Institute between 1986 and 2006, 23 patients (9%) achieved CR and 30 patients (12%) achieved partial response (PR). Although all patients with PR eventually developed disease recurrence with a median of 15 months, only 4 of the 23 CR patients developed recurrence by the time of the last follow-up, with the median OS not reached (*Cancer* 2008;113:293). Administration of high-dose IL-2 should be restricted to a small subset of metastatic patients, including those with nonvisceral metastatic disease, good performance status, optimal end-organ function, and those with dominant clear cell histology. It should be administered by oncologists and staff with extensive experience in the management of side effects of this therapy in high-volume centers. Treatment with IFN-α is associated with fewer response rates and rare durable benefit. Therefore, IFN-α is not currently indicated as single-agent therapy for patients with metastatic RCC. In a retrospective evaluation of 463 patients from six clinical trials treated with first-line IFN-α, five factors were used to create a risk model, known as the Memorial Sloan Kettering Cancer Center (MSKCC) model: Karnofsky performance status (KPS) <80%, Lactate dehydrogenase (LDH)>1.5 times the upper limit of normal (ULN), serum hemoglobin lower than the lower limit of normal (LLN), serum calcium >10 mg/dl, and time from initial diagnosis to treatment of less than 1 year. The median and 3-year OS for patients with good risk (0 factors), intermediate risk (1–2 factors), and high risk (3–5 factors) were 30 months and 45%, 14 months and 17%, and 5 months and 2%, respectively. The median PFS for low-, intermediate-, and high-risk groups was 8.3, 5.1, and 2.5 months, respectively (*J Clin Oncol* 2001;20:289).

More recent studies have shown promising activity from targeting the programmed death 1 (PD1) and its ligand (PDL1) in patients with RCC. In a phase I study, 9 out of 33 patients (27%) responded to treatment with the anti-PD1 monoclonal antibody nivolumab (BMS936558). Among the 8 responding patients with at least 1 year of follow-up, 5 had continued response lasting more than 1 year. Furthermore, 9 patients (27%) had stable disease (SD) lasting 24 weeks or more (*N Engl J Med* 2012;366:2443).

4. **Targeted therapy.** Several drugs have been approved for the treatment of metastatic RCC including the VEGF monoclonal antibody bevacizumab, multitarget tyrosine kinase inhibitors, and mTOR inhibitors.

Bevacizumab is a monoclonal antibody that binds circulating VEGF, preventing its interaction with the VEGF receptor. Two large randomized clinical trials initially showed a significant benefit from the combination of bevacizumab and IFN-α compared with IFN-α alone. Nevertheless, the updated results from the CALGB 90206 trial showed no significant benefit from the combination arm (18.3 months vs. 17.4 months) (*J Clin Oncol* 2010;28:2137). The approved VEGF tyrosine kinase inhibitors include sunitinib, sorafenib, pazopanib, and axitinib. The two mTOR inhibitors approved for the treatment of metastatic RCC are the intravenous temsirolimus and the oral everolimus.

In a retrospective analysis of 645 patients with metastatic RCC treated with sunitinib, sorafenib, or the combination of bevacizumab plus IFN-α between 2004 and 2008, six prognostic factors were used to group patients into three risk categories. The prognostic factors were hemoglobin less than LLN, serum-corrected calcium higher than ULN, KPS <80%, time from diagnosis to initiation of therapy less than 1 year, absolute neutrophil count higher than ULN, and platelets higher than ULN. The median and 2-year OS for patients within the favorable (0 factors), intermediate (1–2 factors), or poor (3–6 factors) categories were not reached and were 75%, 27 months and 53%, and 8.8 months and 7%, respectively (*J Clin Oncol* 2009;27:5794). Another prognostic score was used in an ARCC trial, which randomized patients to temsirolimus, IFN-α or both. The inclusion criteria specified that patients were previously untreated and had three or more unfavorable risk factors (KPS 60–70, hemoglobin <LLN, corrected calcium >10 mg/dl, LDD >1.5 times ULN, less than 1 year from diagnosis, and metastases to more than one organ site). The study showed improved median OS for temsirolimus alone compared with IFN-α and increased toxicity without survival benefit from the combination (*N Engl J Med* 2007;356:2271).

5. **Treatment of nonclear RCC.** Both immunotherapy and VEGF-targeted therapies may be less effective in patients with non-clear cell RCC and those with any histology associated with sarcomatoid variant, with the latter being an aggressive form with poor prognosis. There is far less data on the use of these agents with nonclear cell histology, since such patients were generally excluded from the randomized trials cited above that resulted in the approval of these agents. Although chemotherapy has a limited role in patients with metastatic RCC, gemcitabine, doxorubicin, and capecitabine may have a limited role in those with sarcomatoid variant. A meta-analysis of 7,771 patients with RCC enrolled into 49 studies included 1,244 patients (16%) with non-clear histology, having a significantly lower RR, median PFS, and OS compared with the clear cell histology (*Eur Urol* 2014; in press).

The initial therapy for patients with metastatic RCC depends on the histology and risk category. Temsirolimus is indicated mainly for poor-prognosis patients according to the ARCC trial, and high-dose IL-2 may be used in selected patients. Subsequent therapy after first-line therapy includes everolimus and axitinib. Following cytokine therapy, the main options for clear cell RCC include sunitinib, sorafenib, axitinib, and pazopanib. For patients with nonclear RCC, there are no clear recommendations, with essentially all approved drugs being acceptable.

VI. BACKGROUND

A. **Epidemiology.** Approximately 65,000 cases of RCC occur in the United States each year, resulting in 14,000 deaths (*Ca Cancer J Clin* 2014;64:9). The median age at diagnosis is 64 years, and the male-to-female ratio is approximately 1.5 to 1. The incidence of RCC is higher in Europe and North America compared with Asia and South America.

B. **Risk factors.** There are several established and suspected risk factors for the development of RCC (*Hematol Oncol Clin North Am* 2011;25:651). Cigarette smoking is an established risk factor for the development of RCC, with a strong dose dependence and decreased risk after smoking cessation. Obesity increases the risk for RCC in both men and women, with the increase in obesity rates providing a possible explanation for the steady increase in the incidence of RCC. Hypertension is another established risk factor for RCC, independent from obesity. There are several familial syndromes associated with increased risk for developing RCC, including VHL (associated with clear cell carcinoma), hereditary papillary cell carcinoma (associated with papillary type I RCC), hereditary leiomyomatosis RCC (caused by abnormalities in the fumarate hydratase and associated with papillary type II RCC, cutaneous and uterine leiomyomas), Birt–Hoggs–Dubé syndrome (associated most commonly with chromophobe tumors or oncocytomas, fibrofolliculomas, and pulmonary cysts), and tuberous sclerosis complex (associated with bilateral renal angiomyolipomas and less frequently clear cell carcinomas).

SUGGESTED READINGS

Cho E, Adami H-O, Lindblad P. Epidemiology of renal cell carcinoma. *Hematol Oncol Clin North Am* 2011;25:651–665.

Flanigan RC, Mickisch G, Sylvester R, et al. Cytoreductive nephrectomy in patients with metastatic renal cancer: a combined analysis. *J Urol* 2004;171:1071–1076.

Heng DY, Xie W, Regan NM, et al. Prognostic factors for overall survival in patients with metastatic renal cell carcinoma treated with vascular endothelial growth factor targeted agents: results from a large multicenter study. *J Clin Oncol* 2009;27:5794–5799.

Moch H. An overview of renal cell cancer: pathology and genetics. *Semin Cancer Biol* 2013;23:3–9.

Topalian SL, Hodi FS, Brahmer JR. Safety, activity and immune correlates of anti-PD-1 antibody in cancer. *N Engl J Med* 2012;366:2443–2454.

Vera-Badillo FE, Templeton AJ, Duran I, et al. Systemic therapy for non-clear cell carcinomas: a systematic review and meta-analysis. *Eur Urol* 2014 (in press).

20 Bladder Cancer
Daniel Morgensztern • Bruce Roth

I. PRESENTATION

A. **Subjective.** The most common presenting symptom of bladder cancer is hematuria, which is usually gross, intermittent, and total (present during the entire urine stream). Virtually all patients with bladder cancer have at least microscopic hematuria. Since the hematuria is usually intermittent, further evaluation after the first episode should be pursued even if the repeated subsequent urinalyses are negative. In a prospective study evaluating 1,930 patients with either microscopic or gross hematuria, 230 patients (11.9%) had bladder cancer, including 47 (4.8%) with microscopic and 183 (19.3%) with gross hematuria (*J Urol* 2000;163:524). Irritative lower urinary tract symptoms including frequency, urgency, and dysuria may indicate the presence of microscopic hematuria, and should prompt additional workup. Obstructive lower urinary tract symptoms such as incomplete emptying and decreased force of the urinary stream may occur in patients with tumor located at the bladder neck or prostatic urethra. Symptoms related to distant metastases are uncommon at presentation.

B. **Objective.** Most patients have no disease-specific findings in the physical examination. With more advanced disease, a pelvic mass may become palpable.

II. WORKUP AND STAGING

A. **Workup.** Evaluation of patients with hematuria includes urinalysis, cystoscopy, and imaging of the upper urinary tracts. Hematuria is considered to be clinically significant when there are more than three red blood cells (RBCs) per high power field (HPF). The gold standard for the diagnosis of bladder cancer is cystoscopy with transurethral resection of the bladder tumor (TURBT). Urine cytology, which has a low sensitivity but a very high specificity, should also be performed to increase the detection of upper urinary malignancies. Imaging studies help define the extent of the tumor and the presence of additional synchronous lesions. The most commonly used imaging test is CT urography, although intravenous pyelogram (IVP) may also be used in selected cases.

B. **Pathology and staging**

1. **Pathology.** Urothelial or transitional cell carcinomas are the most common histologic subtypes of bladder cancer, representing more than 90% of cases in the Western countries. The most common non-urothelial malignancies are squamous cell carcinomas, adenocarcinoma, and small cell carcinomas. Pathologic features such as identification of the "nested" variant of urothelial carcinoma, as well as the presence of sarcomatoid or plasmacytoid elements predicts for a more aggressive clinical course.

2. **Staging.** Bladder cancer may be broadly subdivided into three categories including non-muscle–invasive, muscle-invasive, and metastatic tumors. Noninvasive tumors belong to stages 0 to I and are divided into Ta (noninvasive papillary carcinoma), T1 (invasion of the subepithelial connective tissue), and Tis (carcinoma in situ). Stage II is defined as invasion of the muscularis propria, and stage III indicates the invasion of perivesical tissue, either microscopically or macroscopically as a vesical mass or invasion of adjacent organs. Invasion of the pelvic or abdominal wall indicates T4b, which is classified as stage IV. Involvement of regional or iliac lymph nodes and the presence of distant metastases also indicate stage IV. The prognosis and goals of therapy are distinct for each category, ranging from prevention of relapse in non-muscle–invasive tumors to palliation in those with metastatic disease.

III. NON-MUSCLE–INVASIVE BLADDER CANCER.
Approximately 75% of the bladder tumors are non-muscle–invasive. The treatment of choice for these tumors is TURBT with bimanual examination under anesthesia. The resection should sample the muscle to evaluate for invasion.

Without additional therapy after a complete TURBT, more than half of the patients will have recurrence, with 10% of recurrences progressing to muscle-invasive disease. The most important factor for progression to muscle invasion is the tumor grade. Other risk factors for recurrence and progression include tumors larger than 3 cm, multifocal tumors, stage T1, and sessile lesions. Most patients with metastases have concurrent or prior diagnosis of muscle-invasive tumor, with the development of metastasis in patients without history of previous muscle invasion being rare. The use of immediate intravesical chemotherapy using mitomycin, thiotepa, or epirubicin decreases the risk of recurrence (*J Urol* 2004;171:2186). The International Bladder Cancer Group recommends immediate intravesical chemotherapy for patients with low risk disease (solitary and primary tumor, low grade Ta). The most commonly used drug in this setting is mitomycin. Patients with intermediate (multiple or recurrent low grade tumors) or high risk (T1, Tis, or grade 3) should be treated with Bacillus Calmette–Guerin (BCG) with six weekly instillations starting after bladder healing from surgery (*J Urol* 2011;186:2158). Maintenance BCG is usually offered to patients after the 6-week induction. BCG has been associated with decreased risk for both recurrence and progression. A large randomized trial conducted by the European Organization for Research and Treatment of Cancer (EORTC) showed that there was no benefit from maintenance BCG for 3 years compared to 1 year in patients with intermediate risk. For patients with high risk, 3 years of BCG decreased the risk of recurrence but not progressions or deaths (*Eur Urol* 2013;63:462). BCG is contraindicated in patients with bleeding, urethral stricture, active tuberculosis, urinary tract infection, immunosuppression, and within 14 days from TURBT (*Semin Oncol* 2012;39:559). Patients that are at high risk for progression, including those with multiple recurrences and high-grade T1, should be considered for immediate cystectomy.

IV. **MUSCLE-INVASIVE DISEASE.** The standard therapy for patients with muscle-invasive bladder cancer is radical cystectomy with removal of the bladder, adjacent organs, and pelvic lymph node dissection followed by urinary diversion through an ileal conduit or an internal urinary reservoir. The survival after radical cystectomy depends on the tumor extension and lymph node status. For patients who refuse cystectomy or who have comorbidities that prohibit a major surgical intervention, "bladder-sparing" approaches utilizing a combination of radiotherapy and chemotherapy have been studied and found to be effective (*J Clin Oncol* 1998:16;3576).

   A. **Neoadjuvant chemotherapy** theoretically provides benefit via the treatment of occult metastatic disease and has been tested in multiple trials. The Southwest Oncology Group (SWOG) 8710 randomized 317 patients to muscle-invasive bladder cancer stages T2–T4a to radical cystectomy alone or preceded by three cycles of methotrexate 30 mg/m^2 on days 1, 15, and 22, vinblastine 3 mg/m^2 on days 2, 15, and 22, and doxorubicin 30 mg/m^2 plus cisplatin 70 mg/m^2 on day 2 (M-VAC) (*N Engl J Med* 2003;349:859). The median overall survival by intention-to-treat analysis was increased in the neoadjuvant M-VAC arm (77 vs. 46 months, $p = 0.06$). The BA06 30894 trial randomized 900 patients with muscle-invasive bladder cancer staged T2–T4a to three cycles of neoadjuvant cisplatin 100 mg/m^2 on day 2 and methotrexate 30 mg/m^2 plus vinblastine 3 mg/m^2 on days 1 and 8 (CMV) followed by definitive standard management according to enrolling site (radical cystectomy or radiation therapy) or local therapy alone (*Lancet* 1999;354:533). The 10-year overall survival increased from 30% in the control group to 36% in the neoadjuvant CMV (hazard ratio [HR] 0.84, $p = 0.037$). In a meta-analysis including 3,005 patients enrolled into 11 randomized trials comparing neoadjuvant chemotherapy to local therapy alone, the former was associated with an increase in the 5-year overall survival from 45% to 50% (HR 0.86, $p = 0.02$) (*Lancet* 2003;361:1927). Since the combination of cisplatin and gemcitabine (GC) has been associated with similar outcomes compared to M-VAC in patients with advanced disease, it is also commonly used in the neoadjuvant setting despite the lack of prospective data, particularly since retrospective analyses have shown similar rates of pathologic complete response and survival between the two regimens (*Cancer* 2008;113:2471; *Urology* 2012;79:384).

   B. **Adjuvant chemotherapy.** Due to the lack of completed randomized studies with adequate sample sizes, there is no level I evidence of benefit with this approach, with conflicting results from the reported studies (*Eur Urol* 2012;62:523). The ABC meta-analysis evaluated data from 491 patients in six trials, showing a 25% reduction in the risk of death with adjuvant chemotherapy, with most of the benefit observed in patients with pathological T3–T4 disease or lymph node involvement (*Eur Urol* 2005;48:189). More recently, updated data from an EORTC intergroup randomized phase III trial demonstrated that immediate postoperative chemotherapy in high risk individuals resulted in a 22% reduction in the risk of death, although this was non-statistically significant given the size of the trial (660 patients). Therefore, patients who did not undergo neoadjuvant chemotherapy should at least have a discussion regarding the use of adjuvant chemotherapy, particularly in patients with high risk features such as extravesical involvement or positive lymph nodes.

C. **Radiation therapy.** In many countries, external-beam radiation is considered standard therapy for muscle-invasive bladder cancer. In the BA06 30894 trial, the local therapy consisted of radiation, surgery, or both at the discretion of the treating physicians. Radiation was used in 50% of the patients, including 42% as the only modality for local therapy. Although the local therapies were not compared, there was no evidence for a preferential benefit from neoadjuvant chemotherapy in either group. Due to the high risk for local relapse in patients with pathological T3 or T4 disease, these patients may be considered for adjuvant radiotherapy. Since neoadjuvant radiation therapy does not improve survival compared to surgery alone, it is not indicated in this setting.

D. **Bladder preservation** options are alternatives to radical cystectomy in selected patients with stage T2 or T3a who are not fit for surgery or who are not interested in such an aggressive approach, which is associated with a significant morbidity. These patients may be treated with transurethral resection (TUR) alone, TUR followed by adjuvant chemotherapy, radiotherapy, or chemoradiotherapy. Another option is partial cystectomy, which allows the complete resection of the bladder tumor with wide surgical margins. In medically operable patients, trimodality therapy with maximal TUR followed by chemoradiotherapy appears to be associated with the best outcomes. The presence of persistent or recurrent muscle-invasive bladder cancer after any form of bladder preservation represents a formal indication for radical cystectomy (*BJU Int* 2013;112:13).

V. **METASTATIC DISEASE.** A number of single agents have been found to produce a significant number of partial remissions. Unfortunately, these remissions tend to be brief, in the range of a few months. These findings led investigators to pursue combinations of active single agents, and these efforts have led to a number of active combinations in the treatment of bladder cancer. The most active classes of drugs for bladder cancer are cisplatin, taxanes, and gemcitabine, which form the backbone for most of the chemotherapy regimens.

The currently recommended regimens for patients with advanced bladder cancer and eligible for cisplatin therapy include GC and dose-dense M-VAC (DD-MVAC). A large clinical trial randomized 405 patients to GC (gemcitabine 1,000 mg/m^2 on days 1, 8, and 15 plus cisplatin 70 mg/m^2 on day 2) to standard dose M-VAC for a maximum of six cycles (*J Clin Oncol* 2000;18:3068). The study showed no significant differences in response rate (55% in both arms), time to progression (7.4 months in both arms), and median overall survival (13.8 months with GC and 14.8 months in MVAC). Since GC was associated with lower rate of toxicities, it became a more commonly used regimen than M-VAC. The EORTC 30924 randomized 263 patients with untreated unresectable or metastatic bladder cancer to standard M-VAC or DD-MVAC (methotrexate 30 mg/m^2 on day 1, vinblastine 3 mg/m^2 on day 2, doxorubicin 30 mg/m^2 on day 2, and cisplatin 70 mg/m^2 on day 2, with granulocyte colony stimulating factor on days 3 to 7, repeating every 15 days) (*Eur J cancer* 2006;42:50). DD-MVAC was associated with increased response rates (64% vs. 50%, $p = 0.009$), median progression-free survival (9.5 vs. 8.1 months, HR 0.73, $p = 0.017$), and 5-year overall survival (21.8% vs. 13.5%, $p = 0.042$). Several drugs have activity in patients with bladder cancer and may be used in the second-line setting, including taxanes, ifosfamide, pemetrexed, and gemcitabine, if not previously used.

Patients that are not candidates for cisplatin may be treated with gemcitabine combinations, most commonly with either carboplatin or taxanes (*Int J Urol* 2014;21:630).

Biological agents targeting epidermal growth factor receptor (EGFR), HER-2, and angiogenesis, either alone or in combination with chemotherapy have shown promising preliminary results but until data from randomized clinical trials become available to demonstrate their benefit, the standard of care for bladder cancer remains chemotherapy alone. Recent data has also suggested significant activity of agents that inhibit the programmed cell death (PD-1) pathway (*J Clin Oncol* 2014;32:325s) and a large number of clinical trials confirming preliminary results are currently underway.

VI. FOLLOW-UP. Specific follow-up recommendations depend on the clinical presentation of disease. Patients with noninvasive bladder cancer should have a repeated cystoscopy and urine cytology at 3 months for the first year of follow-up. After that, those with low grade cTa may have increasing intervals between the cystoscopies, whereas patients with T1, Tis, or high grade tumors should have cystoscopy and urine cytology every 3 to 6 months for the first 2 years. Patients with high grade tumors should be considered for imaging of the upper urinary tract with IVP, CT urography, or MRI urogram every 1 to 2 years. Patients with muscle-invasive bladder cancer treated with either radical cystectomy or bladder preservation should have urine cytology, chemistry, and imaging of the chest, abdomen, and pelvis every 3 to 6 months for 2 years, with further evaluations as indicated. Patients with associated Tis in the bladder or prostatic urethra should have urethral wash cytology every 6 to 12 months (*J Natl Compr Cancer Netw* 2013;11:446).

VII. BACKGROUND

   A. Epidemiology. Bladder cancer is relatively common, with approximately 75,000 cases diagnosed in the United States in 2014. The median age at diagnosis is 65 years, and this disease is uncommon in patients younger than 40. It is more common in men than in women (3:1) and in Caucasians. Superficial tumors account for 75% of disease at diagnosis, whereas muscle-invasive disease accounts for 20% to 25%.

   B. Risk factors. The most well-defined risk factor for bladder cancer in the United States is cigarette smoking, responsible for about 50% of cases. Other risk factors include exposure to occupational carcinogens such as polycyclic aromatic hydrocarbons (PAHs) and benzene, and occupational exposure accounts for another 25% of cases in the United States. Chronic cystitis from prolonged indwelling catheters or in spinal cord patients is associated with an increased risk for bladder cancer, with a higher percentage of squamous histology. Infection with *Schistosoma haematobium*, a parasite found mostly in Africa, Middle East, and India, increases the risk of bladder cancer, primarily associated with squamous histology. Iatrogenic bladder cancer may occur due to pelvic radiation therapy or prolonged exposure to cyclophosphamide.

SUGGESTED READINGS

Brausi M, Witjes JA, Lamm D, et al. A review of current guidelines and best practice recommendations for the management of nonmuscle invasive bladder cancer by the International Bladder Cancer Group. *J Urol* 2011;86:2158–2167.

Clark PE, Agarwal N, Biagioli MC, et al. Bladder cancer. *J Natl Compr Canc Netw* 2013;11:446–475.

Smith ZL, Christodouleas JP, Keefe SM, et al. Bladder preservation in the treatment of muscle-invasive bladder cancer (MIBC): a review of the literature and practical approach to therapy. *BJU Int* 2013;112:13–25.

Khadra MH, Pickard RS, Charlton M, et al. A prospective analysis of 1,930 patients with hematuria to evaluate current diagnostic practice. *J Urol* 2000;163:524–527.

Grossman H, Natale R, Tangen C, et al. Neoadjuvant chemotherapy plus cystectomy compared with cystectomy alone for locally advanced bladder cancer. *N Engl J Med* 2003;349:859–866.

Meeks JJ, Bellmunt J, Bochner BJH, et al. A systematic review of neoadjuvant and adjuvant chemotherapy for muscle-invasive bladder cancer. *Eur Urol* 2012;62:523–533.

Powles T. Inhibition of PD-L1 by MPDL3280A and clinical activity with metastatic urothelial bladder cancer. *J Clin Oncol* 2014;32:325s.

Shipley WU, Winter KA, Kaufman DS, et al. Phase III trial of neoadjuvant chemotherapy in patients with invasive bladder cancer treated with selective bladder preservation by combined radiation therapy and chemotherapy: initial results of Radiation Therapy Oncology Group 98-03. *J Clin Oncol* 1998;16:3576–3583.

Sio TT, Ko J, Gudena VK, et al. Chemotherapeutic and targeted biological agents for metastatic bladder cancer: a comprehensive review. *Int J Urol* 2014;21:630–637.

Von der Maase H, Hansen SW, Roberts JT, et al. Gemcitabine and cisplatin versus methotrexate, vinblastine, doxorubicin, and cisplatin in advanced or metastatic bladder cancer: results of a large, randomized, multinational, multicenter, phase III study. *J Clin Oncol* 2000;17:3068–3077.

21 Prostate Cancer
Ramakrishna Venkatesh • Seth Strope • Bruce Roth

I. PRESENTATION

A. Subjective. Prostate cancer rarely causes symptoms early in the course of the disease as most of the adenocarcinomas arise in the periphery of the gland away from the urethra.

In the prostate-specific antigen (PSA) era, the most common finding is the **absence** of symptoms. The presence of symptoms due to prostate cancer often suggests locally advanced or metastatic disease. Growth of prostate cancer around or into the urethra, or involvement of bladder neck can result in decreased urinary force of stream, frequency, urgency, nocturia, or hematuria. However, many of these symptoms are not specific and may occur with benign prostatic hyperplasia and aging. Involvement of ejaculatory ducts can cause hemospermia, and extraprostatic disease involving the branches of pelvic plexus can cause erectile dysfunction (ED).

Metastatic disease can cause a wide variety of symptoms related to the sites of metastases. Bone is the favored site of metastasis, with pain being a common, and at times, debilitating symptom. Men with spinal metastases may live for years; therefore, careful and thoughtful serial histories and examinations are mandatory. The most devastating consequences of bone involvement are pain, fractures, and spinal cord or nerve root compression. Spinal cord compression is usually accompanied by back pain that is often made worse by coughing, sneezing, or straining (and other activities that increase intradural pressure). Unlike nonmalignant causes of back pain, the back pain of metastatic prostate cancer is usually worse at night. If a peripheral nerve is pinched by tumor, the back pain may radiate around to the front of the patient in the thorax or abdomen or down the legs. Patients with early spinal cord compression will have weakness, with progression to paralysis occurring, on the one hand, over a period of weeks to even months. On the other hand, late spinal cord compromise leads to loss of sensation distal to the level of metastasis, urinary retention, and incontinence in a matter of minutes to hours. The classic symptoms of cauda equina syndrome are low back pain, bilateral sciatica, sensory and motor deficits, including sacral and perianal anesthesia, and loss of sphincter control of bladder and anus. Delays in management result in permanent loss of sensation, motor function, and continence.

Fatigue is a prominent complaint of patients, but it may occur for very different reasons depending on the state of the tumor and the patient. If due to advanced or metastatic disease, it may be an indicator of bone marrow infiltration by tumor with associated anemia. Liver involvement occurs in only 15%, usually at the end of life. Hepatic metastases are usually due to poorly differentiated adenocarcinomas or to tumors with small cell (neuroendocrine) differentiation.

Androgen deprivation therapy (ADT) and/or chemotherapy can cause anemia, but the former is usually mild, whereas the latter may be moderate or severe. Lower limb edema can result from pelvic lymph node involvement, compression of iliac veins, and/or deep vein thrombosis (DVT).

Shortness of breath may be due to chemotherapy treatment, anemia, pulmonary embolism, and/or lung metastases, but the latter occurs late in only 15% of patients. Later in the course of the disease, older men complain of fatigue and gradually fail to thrive at home, with debilitating bone pain, weakened legs, decreased activity, poor appetite, weight loss, and other symptoms of advanced metastatic disease.

B. Objective. With the widespread use of PSA screening and early detection programs, the most common finding on examination of the prostate is the **absence** of findings. Despite the lead time bias that PSA screening introduces, physicians must be able to perform an excellent digital rectal examination (DRE) to diagnose and clinically stage localized prostate cancer. Attention should be directed to defining the presence or absence of a nodule and its location with respect to the right or left lobe and median raphe. Clearly, the absence of a nodule does not preclude the diagnosis of prostate cancer, and simply hardness of the prostate may indicate the presence of tumor. As patients become more obese, the DRE becomes more difficult to perform, but one should try to define extracapsular extension and/or involvement of the seminal vesicles. The sensitivity and specificity of the DRE is modest to poor, depending on the examiner, which can lead to both over- and underdiagnosis.

As with all cancer patients, the oncologist must do a careful, comprehensive physical examination, with special attention to signs of anemia, lymphadenopathy, bone tenderness, neuropathy, and lower extremity edema. For men treated with ADT, the testicular examination ought to show atrophy, whereas its absence should alert the physician that the patient does not have castrate levels of testosterone. Because of the potential for extended periods of good quality of life (QOL) and survival, even with metastatic disease, prostate cancer remains one of several neoplasms that physicians must rule out in the evaluation of carcinoma of unknown primary tumor.

II. **WORKUP AND STAGING.** Autopsy studies have shown localized prostate cancer in approximately 30% of men older than 50 years and 70% of men older than 80 years. However, with the availability of serum PSA and transrectal ultrasonogram-guided needle biopsy of the prostate, clinically organ-confined prostate cancer is increasingly diagnosed, with continuing uncertainty regarding the clinical significance of some tumors. Defining the grade of the tumor and anatomic stage are critical in understanding the prognosis and formulation of a treatment plan. Various predictive models (e.g., Partin table, Kattan nomograms) have been developed and are available for use in clinical practice for counseling patients and for planning a rational management plan. Most of these validated models include prognostic variables such as PSA, Gleason score, and clinical stage of the cancer.

A. **Laboratory testing**

1. **PSA.** PSA is a serum marker that is central to the diagnosis and management of prostate cancer. The use of PSA testing has helped to identify cases of prostate cancer that are or will become clinically significant, rather than simply identifying cases of cancer that are unlikely to be detected until autopsy. PSA is directly associated with tumor volume and clinical stage. Normal PSA ranges depend on factors such as age and race, and PSA level is affected by prostatic biopsy but not significantly by DREs.

Absolute PSA levels and the rate of change of those levels with respect to time can predict the likelihood of organ-confined disease and influence opinions on the likelihood of a cure. PSA levels greater than 10 μg/L are associated with increased risk for extracapsular extension. The positive predictive value for a PSA between 4 and 10 ng/mL in patients with normal DRE is only 30% approximately. To improve the performance of the PSA test, modifications, such as PSA velocity, PSA density, and free-to-total PSA ratio have been used. Some physicians advocate the use of free PSA versus bound PSA to quantify further the risk of cancer and need for biopsy; higher percentage free PSA levels are associated with more favorable histopathologic features in prostate tumors. A cutoff of 25% free PSA detects 95% of cancer while avoiding 20% of unnecessary biopsies.

PSA kinetics has been explored to improve PSA testing. A study showed men whose PSA level increased by more than 2.0 ng/mL during the year before diagnosis of prostate cancer were at high risk for cancer-specific death even if they had "favorable" clinical parameters (such as a PSA level <10 ng/mL and Gleason score <6 at diagnosis) and that they should undergo radical prostatectomy (RP). For these men, active surveillance may not be an appropriate option. Their increased risk also makes them candidates for enrollment in clinical trials examining various combination treatment strategies. Physicians must use caution when using such measures because men with tumors with Gleason scores of 8, 9, and 10 may be so poorly differentiated that they do not synthesize and secrete large amounts of PSA.

2. **Complete blood count and chemistries.** The laboratory workup should include a complete blood count and comprehensive metabolic panel. Widely metastatic disease may cause anemia or thrombocytopenia because of marrow infiltration, but most patients will have normal peripheral counts and normal chemistries at the time of diagnosis. Abnormal tests should prompt investigation, especially in patients thought to have only localized disease. For example, an elevated alkaline phosphatase may be due to bone metastases and, therefore, a bone scan should be done to rule out this possibility.

B. **Imaging.** Computed tomography (CT), magnetic resonance imaging (MRI), and bone scans are important in the assessment of advanced disease, but they are not indicated in the standard workup of low risk prostate cancer because of their low sensitivity and high cost. Physicians should adopt a symptom-directed approach to the use of imaging of low risk disease. Patients with high risk disease are more likely to have benefit from routine imaging, and many physicians use CT of the abdomen and bone scan as adjuncts to clinical staging in this group. Imaging in these patients may help to identify those with lymph node involvement, but sensitivity is poor even in this risk group. It has been suggested that MRI of the prostate can be used to categorize risk further in intermediate risk tumors by identifying seminal vesicle involvement and extraprostatic extension before surgery. Additionally, MRI is a possible adjunct for patients considering active surveillance to help rule out larger tumors that may have been missed in the initial prostate biopsy. Current imaging studies (CT, MRI, or positron emission tomography [PET] scan) cannot accurately show metastatic disease in most patients with newly diagnosed prostate cancer.

C. **Pelvic lymphadenectomy.** Pelvic lymphadenopathy is rarely performed in isolation in current practice. It can be safely omitted at the time of surgical therapy in patients with low risk of lymph node spread (PSA <10, Gleason 6, and T1c cancer). In an occasional patient with high risk disease, laparoscopic pelvic lymphadenectomy should be considered to rule out metastatic disease before definitive therapy. However, most of these high risk patients will receive either surgical resection or multimodality therapy with radiation and androgen deprivation.

D. **Staging.** The first purpose of a staging system is to provide a well-accepted classification where health care workers from around the world may interpret the extent of disease of the patient. However, in addition, the clinical and/or pathologic stage of the prostate cancer patient may guide discussions about the optimal modality for treatment. The clinical or pathologic stage of the patient is the stage that is defined at the time of initial diagnosis.

To answer queries from patients about prognosis and treatment options, one must weigh the clinical and/or pathologic tumor, node, metastasis (TNM) staging, Gleason grade, and serum PSA level in the context of the general health of the patient. The oncologist should give estimates of both prostate cancer–specific survival and overall survival. The median age at diagnosis for U.S. men is declining, but is still approximately 68 years, and the average man lives to 75 years at this time. In the future, men will get diagnosed earlier and will live longer, leading to more treatment, more "cures," more PSA relapses, and longer times with side effects from therapies for recurrent disease.

1. Prostate cancer is staged according to the AJCC Cancer Staging Manual 7th edition. T stage is divided into T1 (clinically undetectable tumor by palpation or imaging), T2 (tumor confined to the prostate; T2a—one-half or less of a lobe, T2b—more than one-half of one lobe, T2c—bilateral lobe involvement), T3 (Extension through the prostate capsule; T3a—extracapsular extension; T3b—seminal vesicle invasion), and T4 (invasion of adjacent structures such as rectum, levator muscles, and pelvic wall). N1 is defined as the involvement of regional lymph nodes and M1 as metastases to non-regional lymph nodes, bones, or other sites. In addition to the TNM status, both PSA (<10, ≥10 to <20, ≥20) and Gleason score (G1 ≤6, G2 7, G3 >7) are used in the final staging. Stage I is defined by the presence of T1–T2a plus G1. Stage IIA is defined by T1–T2b plus PSA <20 and Gleason ≤7, and stage IIB is defined as T2c or T1–T2 with PSA >20 or Gleason score >7. Stage III is defined by the presence of T3 and stage IV by the presence of T3 and T4, N1 or M1.

2. **Histologic grade** is best determined with the Gleason scoring system. The Gleason grade is a classification of gland formation from a relatively low power view. It is not a histologic classification in the basic sense, such as a comment on nucleoli, nuclear-to-cytoplasmic ratio, and so on. The tumor pattern is graded from 1 for well-differentiated to grade 5 for poorly differentiated pattern. Gleason score is the sum of the scores for the primary and secondary Gleason patterns seen on the biopsy or prostatectomy specimen. If there is a tertiary pattern 5 on a biopsy, that score is reported as the secondary pattern to better describe the disease risk. Because the prognosis varies according to the primary and secondary Gleason grades, each should be assessed along with the sum score. Most men have intermediate-range Gleason scores (Gleason 6 or 7), and it is important to recognize that Gleason scores from transrectal ultrasonogram-guided biopsies may underscore a tumor. Pathologic review from subsequent prostatectomy may increase Gleason scores; for example, a "Gleason 3 + 3 = 6" may be upgraded to a "Gleason 3 + 4 = 7."

3. **The combination of clinical stage, Gleason score, and PSA level** allows physicians to prognosticate most accurately. Patients may be classified as low risk (PSA ≤10, Gleason score <7 and stage up to T2a), intermediate risk (PSA 10–20, Gleason score 7, stage T2b) or high -risk (PSA >20, Gleason score >7, stage T2c). Histologic grade is a good predictor of the outcome, but is not as good as the Gleason sum score. Patients with well-differentiated, moderately differentiated, and poorly differentiated tumors had 15-year death rates for untreated disease of 9%, 28%, and 51%, respectively.

III. TREATMENT

A. **Localized disease (T1 to T2 N0 M0).** The discussion of treatment options for localized disease should include risks and benefits of surgery, radiation (either external beam or brachytherapy), or active surveillance. The 5-year disease-free survival for both RP and radiation therapy (XRT) is approximately 60% to 70%. Recently, the PIVOT study showed no benefit for surgical intervention compared to observation for low risk disease. These results contrast to the SPOG-4 trial where a survival benefit was seen for prostatectomy versus observation.

1. **RP.** The optimal post-RP outcome for the patient is to be cancer-free (with undetectable serum PSA) and to recover preoperative urinary and erectile function. Anatomic RP, also known as **radical retropubic prostatectomy**, is the most common technique for resection currently and allows for the possibility of nerve-sparing techniques that increase the likelihood of preserving potency as well as total continence. The procedure is performed through a midline lower abdominal incision and may involve pelvic (hypogastric and obturator) lymph node dissection. External iliac nodes are not generally removed to reduce the risk of future lower extremity edema. Nerve-sparing techniques allow preservation of neurovascular bundles if uninvolved by tumor. RP is likely curative for organ-confined prostate cancer and rarely curative in lymph node–positive/metastatic disease.

   a. **Laparoscopic radical prostatectomy (LRP) with or without robotic assistance.** Surgeons have demonstrated that LRP with or without robotic assistance can be performed with excellent results. LRP is technically demanding, requiring a significant learning curve. The average intraoperative blood loss is less with robotic or laparoscopic approach. The perceived advantages that laparoscopic or robotic prostatectomy with a magnified surgical image would markedly improve patient outcomes has not been realized. However, the short-term outcomes of robotic RP are no worse than open prostatectomy. Robotic prostatectomy is more expensive than RP. To date, no prospective randomized trials have compared the two approaches. As with open surgical procedures, laparoscopic outcomes, including surgical margin status, continence, and potency, reflect technique more than approach.

2. **Pelvic lymphadenectomy** does not provide additional curative benefit, but may provide prognostic information. However, more recently, some authors have recommended extended pelvic lymph node dissection for high risk disease patients to adequately

stage the disease with potential therapeutic benefit. Pelvic lymphadenectomy can be especially useful in patients with high risk or locally advanced disease in which future hormonal therapy will be an important consideration.

3. **Radiation therapy.** Radiation therapy for the prostate is a continually evolving field as new and better technologies make it possible to deliver higher doses of targeted local radiation, sparing normal tissues, with less local toxicity.

   a. **External-beam radiation.** At least two prospective studies have shown that a dose of 78 to 79 Gy is better than 70 Gy. Advanced computer modeling has led to the development of intensely modulated radiation therapy (IMRT). This technique uses complicated tools that precisely control both the dose of radiation and the tissue targeted. Outcomes for T1/T2 disease are similar to those seen with surgery, with 87% of patients free of local recurrence at 10 years.

   b. **Brachytherapy.** An alternative to external-beam therapy is interstitial XRT with seed implants (brachytherapy). High-dose-rate (HDR) brachytherapy has been reported to be associated with lesser incidence of dysuria, frequency, and rectal pain compared to the low-dose-rate brachytherapy.

4. **Active surveillance (AS).** Active surveillance may be a safe alternative to immediate treatment in compliant men with a low risk of cancer progression. The goal of AS is to avoid overtreatment for most patients while administering curative therapy to those in need of more aggressive treatment. Additional baseline reevaluation, including imaging study of the prostate (MRI with spectroscopy) and ultrasonogram-guided systematic needle biopsy can be considered prior to starting AS. If these studies confirm a low risk cancer, and the patient chooses AS, checkups with DRE and PSA every 3 to 6 months indefinitely are recommended, with repeat imaging and biopsy 12 to 18 months after the baseline evaluation and then every 2 to 3 years.

5. **Cryotherapy.** With better ultrasonographic imaging along with real-time monitoring of freezing and improvements in the cryotherapy technology with smaller cryoprobes, interest in cryotherapy has been rekindled. With the "third generation" cryotherapy technology, the reported morbidity is significantly less compared to the older generation cryotechnology. Cryotherapy is currently limited to patients who are poor candidates for RP or XRT and who have poor sexual function. It can also be used as salvage therapy for locally recurrent prostate cancer following RP or failed brachytherapy or external-beam XRT. However, currently the role of cryotherapy as a primary treatment of prostate cancer continues to be controversial.

B. **Locally advanced disease (T3 N0).** For high risk patients with locally advanced disease, both surgery and radiation therapy may be used as standard therapy.

1. **Surgery.** Radical prostatectomy can be successfully employed in patients with clinical stage T3 disease. Patients should be counseled on the possibility of adverse findings at final pathology including positive margins, extracapsular disease, and seminal vesical invasion. Should these pathologic findings exist, patients are candidates for adjuvant XRT. Current ASTRO/AUA guidelines recommend providing adjuvant XRT to these patients based on improved biochemical recurrence free survival in three randomized clinical trials. The role of adjuvant versus salvage XRT is not known. However, the efficacy of salvage radiation therapy is greatest when XRT is given at a PSA level less than 0.5.

2. **Radiation.** The combination of hormone therapy with radiation alone in locally advanced disease (intermediate and high risk disease) has also been evaluated. The combination of XRT and hormonal therapy in high risk disease has been shown to result in superior survival when compared with XRT alone, and there appears to be a benefit for ADT in intermediate risk disease as well. The duration of ADT (4 months vs. 36 months) and the role of ADT with higher doses of XRT (greater than 72 Gy) remain to be determined. An additional unanswered question is the role of whole pelvic versus prostate-only XRT. The combination of hormonal therapy with brachytherapy in locally advanced disease has not yet shown convincing evidence of survival benefit.

3. **Increasing PSA after prostatectomy or radiation.** Asymptomatic progressive increase in PSA is a common problem in patients with prostate cancer after XRT or surgery. Prognostic factors to consider in this setting are doubling time of PSA, time from definitive therapy to increase in PSA, age of the patient, and comorbidities. Many methods have been used to predict failure, and most physicians consider higher risk patients to be those with seminal vesicle involvement, aggressive histology (Gleason greater than 6), and PSA greater than 10. D'Amico et al. reported that PSA doubling time of less than 6 months is highly predictive of disease progression compared to doubling time of more than 10 months.

Local control after initial failure can be attempted. XRT may provide additional local control after RP, but it has not shown survival benefit and may be associated with higher rates of radiation-related complications. Salvage prostatectomy after XRT is an option, but is associated with higher surgical complication rates. Other surgical options in this setting include cryotherapy and brachytherapy, but no conclusive clinical trials supporting use of these modalities are available.

Most men who have increasing PSA levels after initial management are given medical therapy (see Section III.C). Ongoing trials will attempt to determine whether combined hormonal and XRT is beneficial in patients with increasing PSA after definitive surgery.

C. **Metastatic disease (N+ or M+)**
1. **Initial therapy (hormone-sensitive disease).** Medical or surgical castration remains the first-line therapy for metastatic disease, as it is associated with a response rate greater than 80% and can often reduce PSA levels to undetectable levels. In the recent past, metastatic prostate cancers have remained sensitive to the effects of hormonal blockade for an average of 12 to 18 months. Currently, with lead time bias of diagnosis, more widespread use of PSA as a serum marker, improved imaging, and early hormonal intervention, men can respond to androgen deprivation for 2 or more years, with some living up to a decade.

Given the psychological impact of surgical castration, most men in the United States prefer medical androgen blockade to bilateral orchiectomy. However, surgery is certainly the most cost-effective treatment. Gonadotropin-releasing hormone (GnRH) agonists are the most commonly employed first-line agents. Because these agents are agonists, they will initially increase serum testosterone levels and could result in progression of pain, disease, and even spinal cord compression. Therefore, before GnRH injection, treatment with an androgen receptor antagonist (bicalutamide 50 mg daily; nilutamide 150 mg daily, or flutamide 250 mg three times a day) is warranted. Routinely, these drugs are started 2 weeks before injections and are prescribed for 1 month. Then, leuprolide acetate (Lupron) may be given as 4-month (30 mg), 3-month (22.5 mg) or 1-month (7.5 mg) intramuscular injections. Another GnRH agonist, goserelin (Zoladex), is introduced as a depot injection into the anterior abdominal wall, subcutaneously, every 3 months (10.6 mg) or every month (3.6 mg). The most common side effects are hot flashes and ED. However, over the first year of ADT, many men will become anemic and fatigued, lose muscle mass and gain fat tissue, and lose bone density. Combined androgen blockade (CAB), with both a GnRH agonist and an androgen-receptor blockade (ARB), is not substantially better than GnRH agonist alone.

Failure of first-line ADT is often marked by an asymptomatic rise in PSA, although symptoms of urinary track outlet obstruction, bone pain, and so on may be observed as well. This transition may be referred to as **castrate-independent** disease, but the androgen receptor is still present and can still respond to androgens. Therefore, it is important to maintain patients on ADT with GnRH agonists. If the patient was treated with a GnRH agonist alone, then one may add an ARB. If the patient was managed with CAB, then it is wise to stop treatment with the ARB, to rule out "antiandrogen withdrawal syndrome." Only approximately 10% of these patients will respond, but sometimes it may take 6 weeks to observe a decrease in PSA levels. Some data suggest that in tumors of a subset of patients, mutations of the androgen receptor result in flutamide acting as an agonist, instead of an antagonist of the androgen receptor.

Eventually, second-line hormonal therapy will no longer work and this stage may be treated with inhibitors of adrenal androgen synthesis (ketoconazole, hydrocortisone, or the combination), estrogens, and progestins. Although randomized trials have not shown a clear benefit to the use of third-line hormonal therapy, there is clearly a subset of patients that respond.

2. **Hormone refractory disease.** Once the tumor has progressed through ADT plus antiandrogen therapy, it is considered to be castration-recurrent prostate cancer. Nevertheless, the tumor can still respond to androgens, so it is important to maintain castrate levels of testosterone.

   Abiraterone (1,000 mg daily) combined with prednisone (5 mg b.i.d) showed improved outcomes compared to prednisone alone. There was a trend toward improved survival in the phase III randomized study in the pre-docetaxel setting (*N Engl J Med* 2013;378:138). The agent was approved by the FDA for use in this setting. Side effects of abiraterone include hypertension, hypokalemia, peripheral edema, atrial fibrillation, congestive heart failure, liver injury, and fatigue.

   The second agent being tested in this setting is enzalutamide. A randomized study for FDA approval has been completed in the setting prior to docetaxel chemotherapy, and preliminary results were reported at the Genitourinary Cancer Symposium in February of 2014. Approval for the agent is pending the final review of the full trial.

   Importantly, both enzalutamide and abiraterone were tested in men who were asymptomatic or mildly symptomatic. This study population is different from that of the docetaxel trials where men were symptomatic from their metastatic disease. Also, both studies enrolled men with metastatic disease. PSA progression alone was not an indication for starting either medication.

   Sipuleucel-T is an alternative for men with asymptomatic or minimally symptomatic metastatic castration refractory prostate cancer. It was FDA-approved in this setting from a phase III trial showing an extension in survival to 25.8 months in the treatment arm compared to 21.7 months in the control arm. Side effects included chills, pyrexia, and headache (*N Engl J Med* 2010;363:411).

   Chemotherapy was tried in metastatic prostate cancer for four decades and was considered a failure. However, the improvement with antiemetics, supportive care, pain control, and hematopoietic growth factors finally allowed for adequate trials in this elderly group of men. In a randomized trial, the anthracycline, mitoxantrone, plus prednisone proved to be superior to prednisone alone in terms of QOL, but not in survival. Nevertheless, this regimen became the control group for future chemotherapy trials. Finally, the taxanes and other microtubule inhibitors showed activity in prostate cancer in the late 1990s. Then, two randomized, controlled, prospective, multicenter studies were performed testing docetaxel-based chemotherapy versus mitoxantrone plus prednisone in castrate-independent, metastatic prostate cancer. For the first time, docetaxel-based therapy resulted in superior median and overall survival rates. Docetaxel plus prednisone was approved by the U.S. Food and Drug Administration (FDA) and is considered the standard of care in the United States. Current studies are designed to ask whether the addition of antiangiogenesis agents will improve outcome. The prominent side effects of docetaxel include fatigue, aches and pain in muscles and joints, nail changes, diarrhea, and sequelae of bone marrow suppression. Due to the possible side effects, docetaxel should be used in patients who have symptomatic castration-resistant prostate cancer.

   ^{223}Ra is an alternative therapy for men with hormone-recurrent prostate cancer who are not candidates for chemotherapy. ^{223}Ra admits alpha particles and is absorbed by bone. In a phase III study of men with symptomatic bone metastases, the median overall survival was 14 months for men treated with ^{223}Ra and 11.2 months for the placebo arm. Some men in the trial had received prior docetaxel therapy.

The medication is not for use in men with visceral metastases. Side effects included nausea, diarrhea, vomiting, and swelling of the lower extremities.

3. **Approved agents after chemotherapy.** Multiple agents are approved for use in patients who have disease recurrence or progression after docetaxel-based chemotherapy. Cabazitaxel with prednisone was FDA-approved based on a phase III randomized study showing prolonged overall and progression-free survival. (*Lancet* 2010;376:1147). This agent has a high risk of neutropenia, and also patients with severe neuropathy are not candidates for this therapy.

Additionally, enzalutamide and abiraterone are approved for use in the post-docetaxel setting for men with symptomatic castration-resistant metastatic prostate cancer. Both agents showed prolongation in survival in randomized phase III trials.

4. **Preservation of bone health.** Both zoledronic acid and denosumab are effective agents for preservation of bone health in men with metastatic castration-recurrent prostate cancer. Zoledronic acid is a bisphosphonate and is administered intravenously. In a randomized study, men with asymptomatic or mildly symptomatic bone metastases had a significant reduction in skeletal-related events (33% zoledronic acid, 44% placebo). Denosumab is a RANK ligand inhibitor that was compared to zoledronic acid in a double-blind placebo-controlled study. The incidence of skeletal related events was similar for the two agents, but time to first event was delayed by 3.6 months in the denosumab arm. Denosumab is administered subcutaneously.

IV. COMPLICATIONS

A. Complications of therapy

1. **Complications of surgery.** The complications of RP are predominantly urinary incontinence and impotence, but the nerve-sparing and retropubic approach has decreased complication rates. In the best series, an estimated 8% of men will have stress incontinence after surgery, with only 1% to 2% requiring more than one pad daily. Larger, population-based studies, unfortunately, have shown higher complication rates. Patients are less likely to complain about urinary incontinence to their surgeons, and in some reports, 11% of men after prostatectomy were using two or more pads per day.

Impotence is still a major problem, and the rate of total impotence increases with advanced disease, advanced age, and poor surgical technique. An estimated 20% to 80% of men who are fully potent before surgery will retain potency after the procedure, but the erections may not be of the same quality. In men younger than 50 years, some degree of potency is preserved in an estimated 91%, even if one neurovascular bundle is excised. However, in men older than 70 years, potency rates decrease to approximately 25% with excision of the neurovascular bundles. It is important to make men aware of available therapies designed to restore potency, both pharmacologic and nonpharmacologic. Sensation to the penis is preserved after RP (through the pudendal nerve), although the autonomic innervation of the corporal bodies are damaged. Medications such as sildenafil, vardanafil, and tadalafil may help men regain erectile function and improved sexual activity and QOL.

The reported blood transfusion rate for robotic or laparoscopic prostatectomy is 1% to 2% compared to 5% to 10% for open RP. Other rare complications include DVT (1% to 3%) and rectal injury (less than 1%). The risk of postoperative mortality after RP is relatively low (less than 0.5%) for otherwise healthy older men up to age 79. In one large study, 61,039 patients with prostate cancer had undergone RP as the principal procedure at 1,552 U.S. hospitals. The post-RP mortality rate was 0.11% (66 deaths). Procedure-specific volumes predominantly affected the odds of in-hospital mortality from RP.

2. **Complications of XRT.** Toxicities of XRT most commonly involve the rectum and the bladder. An estimated 60% of patients will have moderate rectal symptoms including pain, tenesmus, or diarrhea. Others will have symptoms of cystitis, hematuria, impotence, incontinence, or difficulty with urination around the period of XRT. Most of these symptoms resolve on completion of the therapy. Less than 1% of conventional

XRT patients require hospitalization for local toxicities including rectal pain, rectal/urinary bleeding, or other urinary complaints.

3. **Complications of hormone deprivation therapy and antiandrogens.** Men who are contemplating treatment with ADT should be made aware of the potential side effects of therapy. Decreased total and free serum testosterone levels lead to hypogonadism, impotence, and decreased libido. In addition, over the first year or so, the patient will notice decreased muscle mass and increased adipose tissue, especially centripetally. A decrease in bone mineral density may lead to osteoporosis. An increase in estrogen to testosterone ratio may result in hot flashes, sweats, and gynecomastia. Endocrine changes may result in an increase in components of the metabolic syndrome, such as hyperglycemia, hyperinsulinemia and insulin resistance, dyslipidemia (hypertriglyceridemia and low high density lipoprotein [HDL] cholesterol levels). These metabolic changes may lead to an increased risk of cardiovascular disease. As we detect more men with prostate cancer at younger ages and these men live longer, the metabolic consequences of ADT will work against the very benefits of treatment.

4. **Complications of chemotherapy.** Docetaxel has a complicated structure that is poorly soluble in water. Therefore, it is formulated in polysorbate-60, and the side effects of treatment may be due to both the chemotherapy agent and its solvent. Allergic reactions such as shortness of breath, facial flushing, fever, chest pain, dizziness, lightheadedness, or skin rash may occur, but are rare with premedication with dexamethasone. Musculoskeletal and bone and joint symptoms of pain and stiffness are among the most common reported by patients.

5. **Complications of bisphosphonate and RANK ligand inhibitor therapy.** Hypocalcemia, arthralgias, and osteonecrosis of the jaw may occur with these therapies. Preexisting dental problems significantly increase the risk of osteonecrosis of the jaw.

V. BACKGROUND. Prostate cancer is the most common malignancy and the second most common cause of cancer-related death in men in the United States. The lifetime risk of a prostate cancer diagnosis is approximately 16%, but the lifetime risk of prostate cancer death is only 3.4%. With the unproven, yet widespread use of PSA screening, the clinical presentation of prostate cancer has changed from advanced to localized disease in more than 80% at the time of diagnosis. The current challenge of research is to use this lead time bias to our advantage to achieve better overall survival and QOL with new treatments. However, the price of early detection and screening is "overdiagnosis," which results in diagnosis, treatment, side effects, and anxiety in tens of thousands of men who would not have manifested symptoms of prostate cancer within their lifetime.

With improved understanding of the molecular aberrations and their influence on clinical outcomes, it is likely that we will individualize therapy for this common malignancy.

SUGGESTED READINGS

Albertsen PC, Fryback DG, Storer BE, et al. Long-term survival among men with conservatively treated localized prostate cancer. *JAMA* 1995;274:626–631.

Andriole GL, Crawford ED, Grubb RL 3rd, et al. Prostate cancer screening in the randomized prostate, lung, colorectal, and ovarian cancer screening trial: mortality results after 13 years of follow-up. *J Natl Cancer Inst* 2012;104(2):125–132.

Bianco FJ Jr, Scardino PT, Eastham JA. Radical prostatectomy: long-term cancer control and recovery of sexual and urinary function ("trifecta"). *Urology* 2005;66(Suppl 5):83–94.

Bolla M, Gonzalez D, Warde P, et al. Improved survival in patients with locally advanced prostate cancer treated with radiotherapy and goserelin. *N Engl J Med* 1997;337:295–300.

Catalona WJ, Carvalhal GF, Mager DE, et al. Potency, continence and complication rates in 1,870 consecutive radical retropubic prostatectomies. *J Urol* 1999;162:433–438.

Catalona WJ, Partin AW, Slawin KM, et al. Percentage of free PSA in black versus white men for detection and staging of prostate cancer: a prospective multicenter clinical trial. *Urology* 2000;55:372–376.

D'Amico AV, Huy-Chen M, Renshaw AA, et al. Identifying men diagnosed with clinically localized prostate cancer who are at high risk for death from prostate cancer. *J Urol* 2006;176:S11–S15.

D'Amico AV, Moul JW, Carroll PR, et al. Surrogate end point for prostate cancer-specific mortality after radical prostatectomy or radiation therapy. *J Natl Cancer Inst* 2003;95:1376–1383.

de Bono JS, Oudard S, Ozguroglu M, et al. Prednisone plus cabazitaxel or mitoxantrone for metastatic castration-resistant prostate cancer progressing after docetaxel treatment: a randomised open-label trial. *Lancet* 2010;376:1147–1154.

Kantoff PW, Higano CS, Shore ND, et al. Sipuleucel-T immunotherapy for castration-resistant prostate cancer. *N Engl J Med* 2010;363:411–422.

Messing EM, Manola J, Sarosdy M, et al. Immediate hormonal therapy compared with observation after radical prostatectomy and pelvic lymphadenectomy in men with node-positive prostate cancer. *N Engl J Med* 1999;341:1781–1788.

Pagliarulo V, Bracarda S, Eisenberger MA, et al. Contemporary role of androgen deprivation therapy for prostate cancer. *Eur Urol* 2012;61(1):11–25.

Pilepich MV, Caplan R, Byhardt RW, et al. Phase III trial of androgen suppression using goserelin in unfavorable-prognosis carcinoma of the prostate treated with definitive radiotherapy: report of radiation therapy oncology group protocol 85-31. *J Clin Oncol* 1997;15:1013–1021.

Ryan CJ, Smith MR, deBono JS, et al. Abiraterone in metastatic prostate cancer without previous chemotherapy. *Engl J Med* 2013;368:138–148.

Schroder FH, Hugosson J, Roobol MJ, et al. Screening and prostate-cancer mortality in a randomized European study. *N Engl J Med* 2009; 360(13):1320–1328.

Valicenti RK, Thompson I, Albersen P, et al. Adjuvant and salvage radiation therapy after prostatectomy: American Society for Radiation Oncology/American Urological Association Guidelines. *Int J Radiat Oncol Biol Phys* 2013;86(5):822–828.

Wilt TJ, Brawer MK, Jones KM, et al. Radical prostatectomy versus observation for localized prostate cancer. *N Engl J Med* 2012;367(3):203–213.

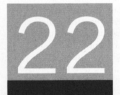

22 Testicular Cancer and Germ Cell Tumors

Daniel Morgensztern • Bruce Roth

I. PRESENTATION

A. Subjective. Patients with testicular cancer most commonly present with a painless solid testicular mass. Less frequently, the testicular mass may become painful as the result of bleeding or infarction in the tumor. Symptoms from metastatic disease may be present in up to 25% of patients, including lower back pain from bulky retroperitoneal disease, bone pain, and pulmonary symptoms such as cough, dyspnea, and chest pain.

B. Objective. A thorough physical examination is essential in patients with suspected testicular cancer. This examination should include evaluation of the external genitalia and scrotum, palpation of each testis by bimanual technique, examination of lymph nodes, with particular attention to the supraclavicular areas, and breast examination for evidence of gynecomastia. If the examination reveals a suggestive scrotal mass, the next step in the workup is ultrasonography. A hypoechoic mass within the testicular parenchyma should be considered a neoplasm until proven otherwise.

II. WORKUP AND STAGING

A. Practical approach to a new testicular mass. The differential diagnosis for patients presenting with a testicular mass includes malignancy, hydrocele, varicocele, testicular torsion, and epididymitis. For suspicious testicular masses, further evaluation includes chest x-ray and serum concentrations of α-fetoprotein (AFP), beta-human chorionic gonadotropin (β-hCG), and lactate dehydrogenase (LDH). These tumor markers are useful for diagnosis, prognosis, and assessment of treatment outcome. Referral to urology for suspected testicular malignancy is indicated for radical inguinal orchiectomy, which should be performed before any further therapy in patients with high clinical suspicion for germ cell tumor (GCT). Both testicular biopsy and trans-scrotal surgical approach are contraindicated due to concerns of tumor seeding. If testicular GCT is confirmed pathologically, patients should have computed tomography (CT) of the chest, abdomen, and pelvis. Additional imaging such as bone scan may be obtained in individuals with pure seminoma histologically or the presence of an elevated serum alkaline phosphatase. CNS imaging with either CT or MRI is indicated in those with CNS symptoms, or those with pure choriocarcinoma histologically, large volume pulmonary metastases, or a baseline hCG of >100,000. Sperm banking should be considered before any therapeutic intervention that may compromise fertility, including surgery, radiation therapy, and chemotherapy. At least 70% of GCT patients are oligospermic prior to any intervention.

B. Pathologic classification of testicular tumors

1. **GCT.** Approximately (95%) of primary testicular tumors originate from germ cells. GCTs carry an excellent prognosis with more than 90% of patients cured, including 50% to 90% of those with advanced disease. GCTs are classified for clinical purposes into two major groups: seminomas or nonseminomas. Nonseminomas include embryonal carcinoma, teratoma, choriocarcinoma, and yolk sac tumor, and frequently contain more than one cell type. Approximately 50% of GCTs are of pure seminoma histology, 35% are nonseminomas, and 15% have features of both. Patients with mixed histology or elevated AFP should be treated as nonseminomas. Pathology reports should also include the presence or absence of vascular/lymphatic invasion (VI) of the primary tumor, which carries prognostic significance in early stage tumors.

   a. **Testicular intratubular germ cell neoplasia carcinoma (TIGCN).** TICGN, also known as testicular intraepithelial neoplasm (TIN) or carcinoma in situ (CIS) is a premalignant germ cell lesion with a 70% probability of progression to GTC within 7 years. It is often found in a normal-appearing testis biopsied for indications such as infertility evaluation, undescended testis, extragonadal germ cell tumors (EGGCTs), or when a contralateral testis contains a malignant GCT.

   b. **Seminomas.** Pure seminoma is the most common testicular tumor, representing approximately 50% of GCTs. They generally have a more favorable prognosis, being more likely confined to the testicle at presentation, and having a higher response rate to both first-line and salvage chemotherapy regimens than nonseminomas. Only tumors with pure seminoma histology, and without elevated AFP, are considered seminoma for management purposes. Syncytiotrophoblasts capable of producing hCG are present in roughly 20% of these tumors. Seminoma typically presents in patients approximately 10 years older than their nonseminoma counterparts.

   c. **Nonseminomas.** These are present in approximately 35% of all testicular tumors, and an additional 15% of GCTs with mixed histology are classified as nonseminoma. The peak age of incidence in is the 15- to 35-year range, where it represents the most common male malignancy. Nonseminomas often consist of mixed histology in any combination, and may also include histologic features of seminoma.

      i. **Yolk sac tumor.** Pure yolk sac tumors (formerly referred to as endodermal sinus tumors) are uncommon, and frequently associated with significantly elevated levels of AFP, and a tendency to develop hepatic metastases.

      ii. **Choriocarcinoma.** Pure choriocarcinoma may present with very elevated levels of hCG, frequently in the hundreds of thousands. These tumors, while rare, may have significant metastatic burden, possibly even with an occult primary lesion, and have a propensity to develop CNS metastases, where the lesions are at an increased risk of associated bleeding.

      iii. **Embryonal carcinoma.** There is no definitive tumor marker pattern seen in pure embryonal carcinoma, as these tumors may be associated with elevated levels of either hCG, AFP, or both.

iv. **Teratomas.** These tumors have elements from one or more germ layers in various stages of maturation. Histologically, teratomas are divided into three subgroups: mature teratoma, immature teratoma, and teratoma with malignant transformation (TMT). Both immature and mature teratomas may contain primitive or mature elements of ectodermal, endodermal, or mesodermal origin, but clinically there are no significant differences between them. However, the presence of teratoma with malignant transformation (which contains malignant degeneration along somatic lines) has negative prognostic significance.

v. **Other testicular tumors.** Approximately 5% of testicular tumors are not of germ cell origin. Sex cord stroma tumors account for approximately 5% of all testicular tumors and include interstitial tumors (Leydig cell tumors and Sertoli cell tumors), granulosa cell tumors, and sarcomas. Embryonal rhabdomyosarcomas of the paratesticular tissues, mesothelioma of the tunica vaginalis, and adenocarcinoma of the rete testis are extremely rare. Non-GCT testicular malignancies in men older than 50 years are most commonly lymphomas.

vi. **Occult testicular tumor presenting as carcinoma of unknown primary.** Metastatic disease alone may be the initial presentation in 5% to 10% of testicular GCTs. The testis may have a small asymptomatic tumor, CIS, scar, or residual testicular tumor detected only on ultrasonograph. Given the favorable prognosis of testicular cancer, serum tumor markers for GCTs should be part of the diagnostic workup in patients presenting with carcinoma of unknown primary, particularly in cases with midline distribution including retroperitoneal and mediastinal lymphadenopathy.

C. **Serum tumor markers.** Serum tumor markers are frequently elevated in GCTs. The three tumor markers that have been established in testicular GCTs are AFP, hCG, and LDH. Any elevation of AFP implies the presence of nonseminomatous elements, even if the pathology of the testicle is read as pure seminoma. Serum tumor markers are useful in patients with suspicious testicular lesions, providing both diagnostic and prognostic information. Patients with nonseminoma histology should have serum tumor markers, before retroperitoneal lymph node dissection (RPLND) in stages I and II, immediately before chemotherapy for stages II and III, before each chemotherapy cycle, at the end of treatment, and during surveillance.

1. **hCG** is produced by syncytiotrophoblasts. Levels less than 200 may be seen in patients with pure seminoma, but higher levels generally indicate the presence of nonseminomatous elements. Extremely high levels (perhaps in the hundreds of thousands to 1 million or greater) suggest choriocarcinoma. The half-life of hCG is 1 to 3 days. Because of the potential cross-reactivity of diagnostic tests for luteinizing hormone (LH) and hCG, a hypogonadal state (occasionally seen in patients post-orchiectomy and/or post-chemotherapy), elevated levels of LH may produce a "false-positive" hCG, although generally not in excess of a level of 20. Levels greater than this, particularly if they continue to rise, are indicative of recurrent testicular cancer.

2. **AFP** is produced exclusively in nonseminoma. It is elevated in approximately 50% of nonseminomas. The half-life of AFP is 5 to 7 days. AFP may also be elevated in hepatocellular disease of any etiology.

3. **LDH** is a relatively nonspecific tumor marker, but may be particularly helpful in the follow-up of patients with no elevations of hCG or AFP, such as in pure seminoma on marker-negative nonseminoma. Several large multivariate analyses have found it to be an independent prognostic variable.

D. **Staging.** In addition to traditional TNM (Tumor, Node, Metastasis) classification that assesses the primary tumor, lymph node involvement, and metastatic disease, the American Joint Committee on Cancer (AJCC) guidelines include measurement of serum tumor markers (S) in testicular GCT staging. Stage I is defined as disease limited to the testis; stage II, disease limited to retroperitoneal lymph nodes, and stage III is characterized

TABLE 22-1	International Germ Cell Cancer Collaborative Group Risk Classification	
Risk status	**Nonseminoma**	**Seminoma**
Good risk	Testicular or retroperitoneal primary No non-pulmonary visceral metastases S0 or S1	Any primary site No non-pulmonary visceral metastases Any S
Intermediate risk	Testicular or retroperitoneal primary No non-pulmonary visceral metastases S2	Any primary site Non-pulmonary visceral metastases Any S
Poor risk	Mediastinal tumor Non-pulmonary visceral metastases S3	None[a]

AFP, α-fetoprotein; hCG, human chorionic gonadotropin; LDH, lactate dehydrogenase.
[a]No patients with seminomas are considered to have poor risk.

by involvement of non-regional lymph nodes or distant metastases. T stage may be further subdivided into T1 (invasion of the tunica albuginea and no vascular or lymphatic invasion), T2 (vascular or lymphatic invasion, or involvement of the tunica vaginalis), T3 (invasion of the spermatic cord), or T4 (invasion of the scrotum). N stage may be subdivided into N0 (no regional lymph node metastases), N1 (metastasis to one or more lymph node measuring 2 cm or less), N2 (metastases to one or more lymph nodes measuring more than 2 cm and less than 5 cm), or N3 (lymph node measuring more than 5 cm). M stage can be further subdivided into M0 (no distant metastases), M1a (non-regional lymph nodes or pulmonary metastases), and M1b (distant metastases other than non-regional lymph nodes or pulmonary). The serum tumor marker (S) stage is divided into S0 (normal tumor markers), S1 (hCG <5,000 mIu/ml, AFP <1,000 ng/ml, and LDH <1.5 times the upper limit of normal [ULN]), S2 (hCG 5,000 to 50,000, AFP 1,000 to 10,000, or LDH 1.5 to 10 times ULN), and S3 (hCT >50,000, AFP >10,000, or LDH >10 times ULN). Stage IA is defined by T1N0M0, whereas IB is defined as T2–4N0M0. Stages IIA, IIB, and IIC are defined by the presence of N1, N2, or N3, respectively, without distant metastases. Stage III is defined by the presence of M1 or lymph node positive plus S2 or S3.

All patients with advanced disease requiring chemotherapy as initial treatment should be risk-stratified using the International Germ Cell Cancer Consensus Group (IGCCCG) classification system (Table 22-1). Patients with seminoma or nonseminoma are stratified into risk prognostic groups based on the primary site of tumor, presence of non-pulmonary metastatic disease, and serum tumor markers. Risk status is used to predict prognosis and to determine the appropriate first-line chemotherapy. Cure rates for patients with good risk, intermediate risk, and poor risk are 90%, 75%, and 45%, respectively.

E. **Fertility issues and sperm banking.** Infertility is associated both with disease and treatment. Approximately 70% of newly diagnosed patients are oligospermic at presentation prior to any therapy, and certainly treatments such as combination chemotherapy and abdominal/pelvic radiotherapy can compromise sperm counts to an even greater degree. Any patient considering active therapy of either of these two modalities should be counseled regarding sperm cryopreservation, as sterility following therapy may be permanent. It should also be recommended that patients use an approved form of contraception during chemotherapy and for a full year following its completion.

III. THERAPY

A. **Testicular seminoma**
1. **Stage I seminoma.** Despite normal CT scans, there is a 15% risk of occult metastatic disease in locoregional lymph nodes with subsequent disease progression if no adjuvant

treatment is given after orchiectomy in stage I seminoma. However, the cure rate in clinical stage I seminoma patients is greater than 99% regardless of management strategy, and adjuvant radiation, adjuvant chemotherapy, or surveillance with subsequent salvage therapy in the event of relapse representing acceptable standard management options. The main risk factors for relapse in stage I seminoma are tumor size >4 cm and invasion of rete testis (*J Clin Oncol* 2002;20:4448), as well as the presence of lymphovascular invasion.

  a. **Radiation therapy.** Adjuvant radiation therapy with 20 Gy, in 10 fractions of 2 Gy each to the infradiaphragmatic area with or without radiation to the ipsilateral inguinal lymph nodes, is associated with a relapse rate of 3% to 4%. Radiation toxicity includes dose-related gastrointestinal toxicity, impaired fertility, and possibly late malignancies. The few patients who relapse almost always have recurrent disease outside the radiation field, typically within 18 months of diagnosis of the primary tumor, and may still be salvaged with chemotherapy. Contraindications to adjuvant radiation include pelvic or horseshoe kidney, inflammatory bowel disease, or previous radiation, due to risk for excessive toxicity.

  b. **Surveillance.** Since 85% of patients are already cured with an orchiectomy alone, by definition, all of these patients will be overtreated with any additional therapy. The curability of advanced disease makes surveillance the most appropriate treatment option in these patients (*J Clin Oncol* 2013;31:3490). In a retrospective study including 1,344 patients with stage I seminoma undergoing surveillance after orchiectomy, there were 173 (13%) relapses at a median time of 14 months, with 92% occurring in the first 3 years. After a median follow-up of 52 months, there were no disease-related deaths, with 99% of patients alive without disease, 1 patient dying from treatment-related complications, and 16 (1%) from unrelated causes (*J Clin Oncol* 2014, in press). Pooled data from several large observational experiences has shown 5-year disease-specific survival of 99.7%.

  c. **Adjuvant carboplatin chemotherapy.** A third alternative is adjuvant chemotherapy with one cycle of carboplatin at area under the curve (AUC) of 7. The MRC TE 19/EORTC 30982 randomized 1,447 patients with resected stage I seminoma to adjuvant radiation therapy with 20 or 30 Gy or one cycle of single-agent carboplatin AUC7. The mature data from the trial showed a relapse-free rate at 5 years of 94.7% and 96% for the carboplatin and radiotherapy arms, respectively (*J Clin Oncol* 2011;29:957). This intervention, however, will unnecessarily expose 85% of patients not requiring any additional therapy to toxicity.

2. **Stage II seminoma.** One approach to the treatment of Stage IIA or IIB seminoma following orchiectomy is radiation therapy. The usual course of therapy includes the para-aortic lymph nodes and iliac chain nodes on the same side as the primary tumor (so-called inverted hockey stick field). This results in a relapse-free survival rate of 95% for stage IIA and 89% for stage IIB at 6 years. While some investigators have argued to eliminate the pelvic potion of the field (para-aortic strip only), this approach clearly results in a higher risk of recurrent disease in the pelvis.

   The other, more commonly utilized approach in the modern era is the use of combination chemotherapy with either three cycles of cisplatin plus etoposide and bleomycin (BEP), or four cycles of etoposide and cisplatin (EP) alone. See Table 22-2 for the common chemotherapy regimens.

3. **Stage IIC and III seminoma.** Patients with advanced seminoma require chemotherapy according to the risk stratification based on the IGCCCG classification. Patients with good risks may be treated with four cycles of EP or three cycles of bleomycin plus etoposide and cisplatin (BEP). Approximately 90% of patients have good risk and 10% intermediate risk, with 5-year overall survivals of 86% and 72%, respectively.

4. **Management of residual mass.** Following chemotherapy for seminoma, reassessment of serum tumor markers and CT scan of the chest, abdomen, and pelvis is recommended. The larger the volume of disease initially, the higher the likelihood that a residual mass will be present at the end of chemotherapy. In the vast majority

TABLE 22-2	Combination Chemotherapy Regimens Commonly Used in Testicular Germ Cell Cancer

BEP

Bleomycin, 30 units i.v. on days 1, 8, and 15 or on days 2, 9, and 16

Etoposide (VP-16), 100 mtg/m^2 i.v. days 1–5

Cisplatin, 20 mg/m^2 i.v. from days 1–5

EP

Etoposide (VP-16), 100 mg/m^2 on days 1–5

Cisplatin, 20 mg/m^2 i.v. on days 1–5

VeIP

Vinblastine 0.11 mg/kg i.v. on days 1–2

Ifosfamide 1,200 mg/m^2 i.v. on days 1–5

Cisplatin 20 mg/m^2 i.v. on days 1–5

Mesna 400 mg/m^2 i.v. daily every 8 h on days 1–5

VIP

Etoposide 75 mg/m^2 on days 1–5

Ifosfamide 1,200 mg/m^2 on days 1–5

Cisplatin 20 mg/m^2 on days 1–5

Mesna 400 mg/m^2 i.v. daily every 8 h on days 1–5

TIP

Paclitaxel, 250 mg/m^2 i.v. on day 1

Ifosfamide, 1,500 mg/m^2 i.v. daily on days 2–5

Mesna, 500 mg/m^2 i.v. before, and then 4 and 8 h after each dose of ifosfamide

Cisplatin, 25 mg/m^2 i.v. daily on days 2–5

All regimens are given on 21-day cycles

of cases, post-chemotherapy resection of residual masses should not be undertaken. These masses almost always are comprised of just necrosis/fibrosis, and these patients following either radiation or chemotherapy have dense desmoplastic reactions, vastly increasing the risk of perioperative complications, including vascular or renal injury. Patient who have normal tumor serum markers and either complete response or residual tumors measuring ≤3 cm do not need additional therapy. Patient with residual tumors larger than 3 cm should have a positron emission tomography (PET) scan at approximately 6 weeks after completion of chemotherapy to evaluate for the presence of residual tumor. In case of negative PET scan, no further therapy is required and the patients should undergo surveillance. However, since a positive PET scan usually indicates the presence of residual active disease, patients may require biopsy or resection. If resection is not possible or the serum tumor markers are elevated, the most appropriate treatment is with second-line chemotherapy.

B. **Testicular nonseminoma**

1. **Stage I.** For patients with disease confined to the testicle and whose serum tumor markers (if elevated pre-orchiectomy) normalize, 70% of these individuals are already cured of their disease with the orchiectomy and will never relapse. Therefore, any additional therapy (surgery, chemotherapy) will unnecessarily cause toxicity in these individuals. Additionally, in the 30% destined to relapse after orchiectomy, their close follow-up should have assured a relatively small tumor burden at relapse, which is associated with a >95% cure rate with subsequent chemotherapy. For that reason, active surveillance represents the best option for these patients. In a recent multicenter study evaluating 1,139 patients with nonseminoma undergoing surveillance after orchiectomy, there were 221 (19%) relapses, including 81 out of 183 (44%) patients

with LVI, 132 out of 934 (14%) without LVI, and 8 out of 21 (38%) with unknown LVI status. The median time to relapse and percentage of relapses within 3 years were 4 months and 98% for patients with LVI and 8 months and 93% for those without LVI. The overall 5-year disease-specific survival was 99.7% (*J Clin Oncol* 2014, in press). With the patterns of relapse, the authors suggested that the surveillance include physical examination and tumor markers every 2 months on the first year, every 3 months on the second year, and every 6 months from the third to fifth year. Chest radiograph and CT scan of the abdomen was recommended at 4, 8, 12, 18, and 24 months after orchiectomy, with consideration for repeating CT scan at 36 and 60 months.

Traditionally these patients were treated surgically with a full, bilateral retroperitoneal lymph node dissection, developed at a time when systemic curative chemotherapy had not been yet developed. Despite modifications to this approach over the past several decades (modified template dissections, nerve-sparing approaches, etc.), this procedure is being offered much less frequently. As a result, with the exception of high volume testicular cancer centers, fewer urologists are being trained in this technique and its utilization will continue to fade in the clinical stage I patient.

2. **Stage II.** Patients with stage IIA and negative serum tumor markers should be treated with NS-RPLND, whereas four cycles of EP or three cycles of BEP remains an alternative option. For patients with stage IIB and negative serum tumor markers, the primary option is chemotherapy with four cycles of EP or three cycles of BEP. In case of complete response or residual tumor less than 1 cm after chemotherapy, there is no need for additional therapy. However, tumors measuring 1 cm or more after chemotherapy should be treated with NS-RPLND. Patient with persistently elevated serum tumor markers should be treated with chemotherapy.

3. **Stages IIC and III.** Patients with advanced nonseminoma, similar to those with seminoma, should be classified according to the IGCCCG criteria as having either good, intermediate, or poor-prognosis disease.

   a. **Good-risk patients.** This category includes 56% of patients and is associated with a 5-year overall survival of 92%. The recommended treatment is four cycles of EP or three cycles of BEP, which have been shown to have similar efficacy. The substitution of carboplatin for cisplatin in either EP or BEP has been associated with inferior outcomes.

   b. **Intermediate- and poor-risk patients.** Intermediate- and poor-risk nonseminomas are present in 28% and 16% of patients, respectively, with 5-year overall survivals of 80% in the intermediate-risk group and 48% in the poor-risk group. Patients should be treated with four cycles of BEP chemotherapy. Clinical trials, if available, should be considered for poor-risk patients. If brain metastases are present, cranial irradiation should be offered prior to chemotherapy.

4. **Management of post-chemotherapy masses.** Patients with advanced nonseminoma treated with chemotherapy should have a repeated CT scan between 4 and 8 weeks following completion of chemotherapy. In the setting of normalized tumor markers, maximum shrinkage of disease in response to chemotherapy may not occur for up to a year following completion of chemotherapy, and no decision regarding subsequent resection of residual disease should be made until maximum shrinkage has occurred. At that time, if <90% volumetric reduction (compared to pre-therapy scans) has occurred, consideration should be given to resection of residual radiographic disease, because of the possible presence of teratoma. Teratoma is unresponsive to chemotherapy, does not secrete tumor markers, and is only surgically curable. There is no diagnostic study (including PET scan) that can differentiate between teratoma and scar tissue. At the time of resection, if only necrosis/fibrosis or teratoma are found, no other therapy is required. If viable germ cell tumor is resected, additional chemotherapy (generally two additional cycles of EP) is warranted.

C. **Management of recurrent disease after initial therapy.** Patients with early stage disease who develop recurrent disease or those with advanced stage who have relapse following first-line chemotherapy can still be cured with additional chemotherapy, with the

TABLE 22-3	Prognostic Model for Salvage Therapy

Factors	Points
Primary site	
Gonadal	0
Retroperitoneal	1
Mediastinal	3
Response to first-line therapy	
CR or PR with negative serum markers	0
PR with positive serum markers or SD	1
PD	2
Progression-free interval after first-line therapy	
>3 months	0
≤3 months	1
Serum hCG	
≤1,000	0
>1,000	1
Serum AFP	
Normal	0
≤1,000	1
>1,000	2
Liver, bone, or brain metastases	
No	0
Yes	1
Histology	
Pure seminoma	−1
Non-seminoma or mixed tumors	0

AFP, α-fetoprotein; hCG, human chorionic gonadotropin; CR, complete response; PD, progressive disease; PR, partial response; SD, stable disease. Final score and 2-year progression-free survival.
Very low (score = −1): 75.1%; low (0): 51%; intermediate (1): 40.1%; High (2): 25.9%; very high (3): 5.6%.

survival depending on several factors including primary site of disease, response to first-line therapy, progression-free survival, tumor markers, and presence of liver, bone, or brain metastases. The standard salvage chemotherapy regimens include vinblastine plus ifosfamide and cisplatin (VeIP) and paclitaxel plus ifosfamide and cisplatin (TIP). High-dose chemotherapy, usually with carboplatin plus etoposide, followed by auto-SCT is another option for patients with relapsed or recurrent GCTs. The large multicenter phase 3 IT-94 trial randomized 280 patients to chemotherapy alone of followed by auto-SCT and showed no significant differences in survival (*Ann Oncol* 2005;16:1152). In a retrospective analysis of 1,984 patients with GTC progressing after first-line chemotherapy, 604 patients (38%) achieved a 2-year progression-free survival using either conventional chemotherapy or high-dose salvage regimens followed by autologous stem cell transplant (auto-SCT). The 2-year progression-free survival ranged from 75% in patients with very low risk to 5.6% in those with high risk (Table 22-3) (*J Clin Oncol* 2010;28:4906). In a subset analysis of the study according to salvage treatment, the 2-year progression-free survival was significantly higher for the auto-SCT compared to standard chemotherapy for all patients (49.6 vs. 27.8%, p <0.001) and for each prognostic risk category. The 5-year overall survival also favored the auto-SCT group (53.2 vs. 40.8%, p <0.001), although it did not reach statistical significance for patients with low risk (*J Clin Oncol* 2011;29:2178).

Late relapses are defined as recurrences occurring 2 years or longer after the initial successful chemotherapy. These relapses occur in approximately 3% of patients, are more common in nonseminomas, and are typically associated with less responsiveness to chemotherapy and worse outcomes. Surgery is recommended for all lesions if technically feasible, with chemotherapy alone or followed by auto-SCT used in unresectable disease (*Hematol Oncol Clin North Am* 2011;25:615).

IV. BACKGROUND AND EPIDEMIOLOGY. While testicular GCTs account for only 2% of all cancers overall, they are the most common solid tumors in men between the ages of 15 and 34 years. The incidence worldwide has more than doubled in the last 40 years. The incidence of testicular GCTs is lower in African American and Asian populations than in Caucasians. A recent study has reported an increasing frequency of the disease in Hispanic adolescents and young adults in the United States for unclear reasons. Incidence rates climb rapidly and peak in young adults, followed by a decline and leveling off in the elderly. The median age at diagnosis of seminoma is approximately 10 years older than that of nonseminoma.

Several factors have been associated with the development of testicular cancer, including prior testicular cancer, family history, cryptorchidism, and Klinefelter's syndrome. Approximately one-third of testicular cancers developing in patients with a history of cryptorchidism 1 arise in the normally descended testicle. Additionally, first-degree relatives of testicular cancer patients have a higher incidence of nonmalignant urogenital abnormalities, such as hypospadias. These data suggest that what is inherited is a urogenital field defect, one outcome of which may be the malignant degeneration of germinal epithelium. The lifetime risk of a patient with testicular cancer developing a contralateral primary tumor is approximately 1.5%.

V. EGGCT. An extragonadal germ cell tumor can arise from residual germinal epithelium left behind during gonadal migration during embryogenesis, and can arise in the pineal gland, the mediastinum, or the retroperitoneum without evidence of a testicular primary lesion. These lesions characteristically develop in the midline. Primary mediastinal and primary retroperitoneal nonseminomas are associated with an inferior prognosis compared to testicular primaries.

SUGGESTED READINGS

Einhorn LH, Williams SD, Loeher PJ, et al. Evaluation of optimal duration of chemotherapy in favorable-prognosis disseminated germ cell tumors: a Southwestern Cancer Study Group protocol. *J Clin Oncol* 1989;7:387–391.

Gilligan TD, Seidenfeld J, Basch EM, et al. American Society of Clinical Oncology Clinical Practice Guideline on uses of serum tumor markers in adult males with germ cell tumors. *J Clin Oncol* 2010;28:3388—3404.

International Germ Cell Cancer Collaborative Group (IGCCCG). International germ cell consensus classification: prognostic factor-based staging system for metastatic germ cell cancers. *J Clin Oncol* 1997;15:594–603.

Kollmannsberger C, Tandstad T, Bedard PL. Patterns of relapse in patients with clinical stage I testicular cancer managed with active surveillance. *J Clin Oncol* 2014;e-pub ahead of print 8/18/2014.

Motzer RJ, Agarwal N, Beard C, et al. Testicular cancer. *J Natl Compr Canc Netw* 2009;7:672—693.

Nichols CR, Roth B, Albers P, et al. Active surveillance is the preferred approach to clinical stage I testicular cancer. *J Clin Oncol* 2013;31:3490—3493.

Oldenburg J, Fossa SD, Nuver J, et al. Testicular seminoma and non-seminoma: ESMO clinical practice guidelines for diagnosis, treatment and follow-up. *Ann Oncol* 2013;24(Suppl 6):125—132.

23 Ovarian Cancer

Sara S. Lange • Matthew A. Powell

I. EPITHELIAL OVARIAN CANCER

A. **Epidemiology and etiology.** Approximately 21,980 new cases of ovarian cancer are diagnosed each year in the United States and 14,270 deaths were estimated to occur in 2014, as a result of this disease. Ovarian cancer remains the fifth most common cause of cancer death in women and the leading cause of death from gynecologic cancer. It has been estimated that 1 woman in 70 in the United States will develop ovarian cancer in her lifetime and 1 in 100 will die from this disease. Most of the (85% to 90%) malignant ovarian tumors are epithelial in origin. The median age at diagnosis is 63 years and incidence is higher in women of white race. Risk factors include a strong family history, nulliparity, early menarche, late menopause, increasing age, white race, and residence in North America and Europe. Oral contraception usage and pregnancy are associated with a decreased risk, suggesting that continuous ovulation may lead to malignant changes. The etiology of malignant changes of the ovarian epithelium, which is contiguous with the peritoneal mesothelium, is unknown and likely a combination of genetic, environmental, and endocrine effects.

B. **Genetics/familial syndromes.** Familial ovarian cancer may be related to a breast–ovarian cancer syndrome caused by an inherited mutation in one of two genes, *BRCA1* and *BRCA2* on chromosome 17 and 13, respectively. Certain ethnic groups such as Ashkenazi Jewish women have an increased risk of a mutation in one of these two genes. Women with a *BRCA1* mutation are reported to have a 16% to 44% lifetime risk of ovarian cancer, whereas those with *BRCA2* mutations have a lower risk at 10%. Women with ovarian cancer due to these mutations tend to have a more indolent course than those with sporadic disease. Site-specific familial ovarian cancer and Lynch syndrome II in which multiple individuals within a family develop tumors in the colon, endometrium, and ovary are other types of familial ovarian cancers. Inheritance in familial ovarian cancer is in an autosomal dominant manner with multiple members in successive generations affected. There is sufficient evidence for prophylactic oophorectomy in women with a known mutation in *BRCA1* or *BRCA2* after completion of childbearing or 35 years of age so as to prevent the development of both ovarian and breast cancers. All patients with epithelial ovarian, tubal, and peritoneal cancer should be offered genetic counseling.

C. **Clinical presentation.** Women present with vague, nonspecific symptoms of abdominal bloating, distension, dyspepsia, early satiety, anorexia, weight loss, or constipation. Women are often treated for gastrointestinal problems such as gastritis, irritable bowel syndrome, and gall bladder disease. Physical examination findings may include ascites, pleural effusion, or an abdominal mass. Most patients with early-stage disease are asymptomatic and given the vague nature of the symptoms, approximately 80% present with advanced stage (metastatic) disease. The National Cancer Institute (NCI) does support annual screening through both CA-125 measurements and transvaginal ultrasonography for women at high genetic risk based on family history; however, in the general population no data exists that screening is effective in improving length and quality of life in women with ovarian cancer. Several biomarkers with potential application to ovarian cancer screening are under development but have not yet been validated or evaluated regarding their efficacy for early detection and mortality reduction.

Women found to have a mass or ascites on examination or by radiographic or ultrasonographic imaging should be evaluated to assess the possible risk of abnormality representing a malignancy. Appearance and size on ultrasonography or computed tomography (CT) scan combined with patient age and family history are factors that help determine the need for surgical evaluation. A complex mass with both solid and cystic components with septations and internal echoes is suggestive of cancer. Benign-appearing and indeterminate lesions can be followed for a brief period to evaluate for progression of disease. Serum CA-125 cancer antigen can occasionally be of aid in postmenopausal patients. CA-125 is elevated in more than 80% of patients with ovarian cancer but this test is neither sufficiently sensitive nor specific enough to be diagnostic as this may be elevated in a number of other benign and malignant conditions. CA-125 is most useful in following response to postoperative chemotherapy and detecting disease recurrence. No definitive tests are currently available and definitive diagnosis is often only possible with surgical evaluation.

D. **Surgical treatment.** Surgery is typically performed for histologic diagnosis, staging, and tumor cytoreduction. Exceptions to an immediate surgical approach are patients who are poor surgical candidates secondary to other comorbid diseases or performance status. In these patients, a confirmatory biopsy or cytology is obtained to establish a diagnosis followed by chemotherapeutic treatment. Preoperatively, patients should undergo all age-appropriate cancer screening (Pap smear, mammogram, and colorectal cancer screening) as well as additional tests depending on the clinical scenario (barium enema, colonoscopy, and/or cystoscopy). Laboratory assessment should include complete blood count, type and screen, electrolytes, renal and hepatic panel, electrocardiogram, and chest radiograph. Additional studies depend on the patient's medical condition(s). Given the likelihood of large and small bowel involvement requiring resection, a thorough bowel preparation is recommended. Staging of ovarian cancer is surgical and proper staging procedures should typically consist of the following: (a) midline abdominal incision; (b) evacuation of ascites or peritoneal washings for cytologic analysis; (c) resection of the primary ovarian tumor, total abdominal hysterectomy, and bilateral salpingo-oophorectomy; (d) biopsies of omentum or omentectomy; (e) biopsies of the pelvic and abdominal peritoneum, including pericolic gutters; and (f) retroperitoneal nodal sampling (pelvic and para-aortic), if indicated by lack of abdominal disease greater than 2 cm or if grossly involved with tumor. The surgical staging system established by the International Federation of Gynecology and Obstetrics is depicted in Table 23-1 and was recently updated as of January 2014 to improve utility and reproducibility across all ovarian tumor types (*Int J Gynaecol Obstet* 2014;124:1). Tumor debulking is a critical component of initial surgical management as women with residual disease of less than 1 cm have survival rates higher than those with residual disease.

Five-year survival in patients with early-stage disease (stage I or II) is often as high as 80% to 95%; however, patients with advanced disease (stage III or IV) have much lower survival rates of 30% to 40%.

TABLE 23-1	Updated FIGO Ovarian Cancer Staging
Stage	**Definition**
IA	Tumor limited to one ovary with intact capsule and no tumor on surface
IB	Tumor involves both ovaries
IC	Surgical spill (IC1), capsule rupture or tumor on ovarian surface (IC2), malignant cells on the ascites or peritoneal washings (IC3)
IIA	Extension or implant on uterus and/or fallopian tubes
IIB	Extension to other pelvic intraperitoneal tissues
IIIA1	Positive retroperitoneal lymph nodes (IIIA1(i) ≤10 mm, IIIA1(ii) >10 mm)
IIIA2	Microscopic extrapelvic peritoneal involvement
IIIB	Macroscopic extrapelvic peritoneal metastases ≤2cm
IIIC	Macroscopic extrapelvic peritoneal metastases >2cm
IVA	Pleural effusion with positive cytology
IVB	Metastases to liver, spleen or extra-abdominal organs including lymph nodes

E. Postoperative treatment

1. **Epithelial tumors of low malignant potential (LMP).** Also called borderline tumors, this subgroup represents approximately 10% to 15% of all epithelial ovarian tumors. The tumors are usually stage I (80%) and are characterized pathologically by epithelial cell stratification, increased mitoses, nuclear abnormalities, and atypical cells without stromal invasion. Surgical staging is usually recommended, but given that these tumors tend to occur in younger patients, conservation of fertility is often possible. Treatment is simple surgical resection. Chemotherapy does not appear to have a role in treating most of these tumors. However, LMP tumors are on rare occasions found to have invasive implants (metastases) in which case the patient should be treated similar to frankly invasive disease with adjuvant chemotherapy. By convention, however, the tumor is still considered LMP as the diagnosis is based on the primary tumor only. Recurrent disease is usually treated with repeat surgical debulking. The prognosis for patients without invasive implants is excellent with very few patients dying of disease, with the average time to recurrence being 10 years. Patients are often followed with serum CA-125 determinations every 3 to 12 months, but it is unclear if this provides any survival benefit. Additionally, patients have been known to recur with invasive disease.

2. **Early-stage disease.** Patients with stage IA or IB with grade 1 or 2 disease are considered low risk, with excellent survival chances (90% to 95%). Treatment with full surgical staging followed by close follow-up is typically all the treatment that is required. For those patients who wish to preserve fertility, a unilateral salpingo-oophorectomy with adequate staging may be considered in some patients with stage IA grade 1 disease. Patients with stage IC disease, stage I grade 3 disease, stage I grade 2, or stage II disease are considered at high risk for recurrence and are treated with platinum-based adjuvant chemotherapy to reduce the risk of relapse. With chemotherapy, disease-free survival is approximately 80%.

The number of chemotherapeutic cycles for treatment of early-stage disease is debatable and in 2006, the Gynecology Oncology Group GOG 157 showed that, compared to three cycles, six cycles of carboplatin and paclitaxel do not significantly alter the recurrence rate in high risk, early-stage ovarian cancer but are associated with more toxicity. However, some question the statistical power of this study as there was a strong trend toward decreased recurrence in stage I disease with six cycles ($p = 0.073$). Given these findings, in 2010, an exploratory analysis of the patients included in GOG 157 was undertaken to determine if there were subsets of patients with high risk early-stage ovarian cancers that may benefit from more cycles of chemotherapy (*Gynecol Oncol* 2010;116:301). The authors found that compared to three cycles, six cycles of adjuvant chemotherapy may decrease the recurrence of women with serous histologies, with a statistically significant difference at 2-year recurrence-free survivals (93% for 6 cycles vs. 80.8% for 3 cycles, p = 0.007). Unfortunately, this benefit did not extend to overall survival (OS). Additionally, the utility of subset analyses in shaping clinical treatments is debated, and a prospective randomized clinical trial would be necessary to confirm these findings.

F. Advanced disease. Most ovarian cancer patients present with advanced stage disease (stage III and IV). Maximal efforts for surgical cytoreduction of the tumor before chemotherapy should be made as studies have consistently demonstrated improved survival in those patients with an "optimal" cytoreduction. Optimal cytoreduction has been defined a variety of ways in the literature; currently, the GOG defines optimal cytoreduction as no residual tumor nodules with a diameter greater than or equal to 1 cm, but many are now using an international standard of no gross residual to be considered "optimal". Optimally cytoreduced patients (<2 cm) have a median progression-free survival (PFS) and OS of 22 months and 50 months, respectively (GOG 158), versus suboptimally cytoreduced patients with an 18-month PFS and 38-month OS (GOG 111). A study assessing survival rates at specific residual disease diameters to determine the optimal goal of primary cytoreduction found that patients with no gross disease or less than 1 mm had significantly longer overall median survival compared with patients with macroscopic residual disease greater than 1 mm (*Gynecol Oncol* 2006; 103:559). Patients with advanced stage disease will require postoperative adjuvant chemotherapy to treat residual disease. Taxane and platinum-based chemotherapy is the current standard of postoperative care and has been shown to extend PFS as well as OS. This current standard of care is based on clinical trials demonstrating similar efficacy of carboplatin/paclitaxel to cisplatin/paclitaxel with less chemotherapy-related toxicity and a shorter administration time. The regimen consists of intravenous administration of paclitaxel (175 mg/m^2) given over 3 hours and carboplatin dosed with an area under the curve (AUC) of 5 to 7.5, utilizing the Jeliffe formula to estimate creatinine clearance and the Calvert formula to determine AUC. This regimen is given every 3 weeks for a total of six cycles. Response rates (complete response [CR] + partial response [PR]) are approximately 80% with this combination, and more than 50% of patients will have a complete clinical response. Although most patients tolerate platinum- and taxane-based chemotherapy relatively well, some develop severe peripheral neuropathy and the use of docetaxel has been shown to result in less neuropathy with similar efficacy (*J Natl Cancer Inst* 2004;96:1682).

Recent clinical trials have investigated the success of maintenance chemotherapy in improving both PFS and OS. A Cochrane review from 2013 looked at eight trials including 1,644 women total, and determined that there was no significant difference in 3-, 5-, and 10-year PFS and OS between women who received maintenance chemotherapy and those that did not. The trials included regimens with platinum agents, doxorubicin, and paclitaxel. However, two well-designed phase III clinical trials (ICON7 and GOG218) investigated the use of bevacizumab, a VEGF monoclonal antibody, alongside standard chemotherapy in women with newly diagnosed advanced ovarian, primary peritoneal, and fallopian tube cancer. GOG 218 included a maintenance bevacizumab arm as well, and a significant improvement in PFS of 3.8 months was noted in the maintenance bevacizumab arm when compared to both the standard paclitaxel and carboplatin and the paclitaxel, carboplatin, and bevacizumab arm (*N Engl J Med 2011*;365:2473). ICON7 compared two arms, a standard carboplatin and paclitaxel arm with 6 cycles of therapy and the experimental carboplatin, paclitaxel, and bevacizumab arm, which included 5 to 6 cycles plus up to an additional 12 cycles of maintenance therapy (*N Engl J Med* 2011;365:2484). Bevacizumab did improve PFS; however, final analysis of OS revealed no clinically important improvement in the randomized population, with a 4.8-month improvement in mean survival time in a subgroup of women at high risk of progression. However, the use of bevacizumab did expand the number of toxic effects in both studies, including hypertension and bowel perforation. Currently, the NCCN considers the administration of chemotherapy plus bevacizumab in the first-line setting a reasonable option, but does not routinely recommend the drug at this time given the clear lack of OS benefit.

In 2013, the Japanese Gynecologic Oncology Group (JGOG) published its results of a prospective randomized clinical trial (JGOG 3016) comparing standard treatment with carboplatin and paclitaxel every 3 weeks to the experimental arm of carboplatin every 3 weeks concurrently with weekly paclitaxel. In both arms, the regimen was repeated every 3 weeks for up to nine cycles. The dose-dense therapy arm resulted in a significant improvement in PFS (28 months vs. 17.5 months) and OS (100.6 months vs. 62 months), with women who had >1cm of residual disease following surgical treatment showing the greatest benefit in PFS (17.6 months vs. 12 months) and OS (51 months vs. 33 months). However, this benefit did not extend to patients with mucinous or clear cell histologies. Also, there was a higher rate of treatment discontinuation and delay secondary to toxicity in the dose-dense arm. It should be noted that better survival outcomes with standard chemotherapy have been noted in other trials, as well as a potential difference in outcomes based on race, with Asian patients appearing to fare better in this trial than in other trials with a predominately Caucasian enrollment (*Lancet Oncol* 2013;14:1020).

Intravenous chemotherapy has been the standard treatment in the past; however, intraperitoneal chemotherapy (IP) has also been investigated over the last several decades. Three recent large prospective trials have shown survival improvements for those patients treated with IP (*N Engl J Med* 2006;354:34; *N Engl J Med* 1996;335:1950; *J Clin Oncol* 2001;19:1001). More recently, GOG 172 reported a PFS of 23.8 months for combination IP and intravenous chemotherapy versus 18.3 months for intravenous (IV) alone (*N Engl J Med* 2006;354:34). Similarly, OS was longer with the combined IP/IV therapy (65.6 months vs. 49.7 months). Patients who receive IP therapy do experience greater toxicity and even report worse quality of life in some studies; therefore, many oncologists are still slow to use this method of treatment. A small study recently published investigated the use of IP chemotherapy in the community-based practice setting. They identified 288 women with FIGO stage 2 or greater ovarian cancer diagnosed between 2003 and 2008 at three integrated delivery systems in the United States. They noted that 12.5% (n=36) of women received IP chemotherapy between 2003 and 2008, with a height of use at 26.9% of patients in 2006. These results demonstrate that the use of IP chemotherapy for newly diagnosed advanced ovarian cancer patients in the community setting was uncommon (*Front Oncol* 2014;4:43).

Second-look laparotomies are not recommended unless the patient is enrolled in a protocol as these studies have shown no impact on survival. Less commonly, radiation of the abdomen and pelvis is employed as treatment for advanced stage and/or recurrent disease. Following adjuvant chemotherapy, patients are monitored with physical examination, CA-125 measurements, and imaging studies (CT, magnetic resonance imaging [MRI], and positron emission tomography [PET]) as clinically indicated for recurrent disease.

G. Recurrent disease. Despite standard treatment with cytoreductive surgery and chemotherapy, up to 75% of patients experience recurrence and will eventually succumb to disease. Median survival following relapse from initial therapy is approximately 2 years. Patients found to progress with upfront therapy or with a recurrence should be offered additional treatments that will hopefully allow for control of their disease and maintain the best quality of life possible. One must realize that very few of these patients are ultimately cured of their disease, and enrollment in clinical trials at this point is strongly encouraged. The usual first sign of recurrence is a rising CA-125, which is usually followed by evidence of recurrence on examination or by a CT scan of the abdomen and pelvis. It is not clear if early retreatment (before the onset of symptoms or radiographic evidence of disease) of a patient with an elevating CA-125 has any effect on disease control or OS.

Treatment of recurrent or persistent disease is based on the timing and location of the recurrence. "Platinum-sensitive" patients are defined as experiencing a recurrence more than 6 months from the time of their initial CR. These patients can be successfully retreated with platinum-based regimens with reasonable responses (20% to 40%). ICON IV showed that in patients with platinum-sensitive disease, combination chemotherapy (platinum plus paclitaxel) led to higher CRs or PRs (66% vs. 54%) as well as PFS (13 months vs. 10 months) compared to platinum therapy alone for recurrent disease. Patients with a treatment-free interval of greater than 12 months received the greatest benefit from retreatment with combination platinum, paclitaxel therapy.

Patients having a recurrence before 6 months ("platinum-resistant") can be treated with a variety of agents. Many authorities recommend that single-agent therapy be used in this setting to minimize toxicity and to more easily identify non-responding agents. Given that there is no ideal second-line salvage agent(s), patients should be encouraged to participate in available study protocols. Second-line agents have an approximate response rate of 15% to 40%, depending on agent and amount of previous chemotherapeutic treatments. Treatment is usually continued until the CA-125 normalizes, toxicity precludes further therapy, or disease progression. Patients with progressive disease are then offered a different regimen usually with a differing side effect profile to minimize toxicity.

Generally speaking, because recurrent disease is typically not curable, symptom palliation and prevention of complications such as bowel obstruction remain the goals of management. Radiation and/or surgical resection have been used to successfully treat localized disease. Indications for repeat surgery (secondary debulking) are highly controversial and decisions must be individualized. In general, if the progression-free interval is greater than 1 year and the mass appears isolated, or if it is symptomatic (obstruction of bowel or kidney), surgical resection can result in prolonged survival.

Complications of therapy are primarily related to continued growth of the tumor (bowel obstruction) and toxicities of the chemotherapy. Bowel obstructions should initially be managed conservatively with intravenous fluids and gastric decompression. Studies such as abdominal plain films, small bowel follow-through, contrast enemas, and abdominal/pelvic CT may be necessary to further evaluate cause of obstruction. Persistent obstructions can be managed with chronic decompression (G-tube) or surgical exploration in cases where the imaging studies suggest a limited focus of obstruction. Toxicities of chemotherapy are related to the specific agents and are covered elsewhere in this text.

H. Future directions. A great deal of attention has been focused on identification of the genetic factors involved with ovarian cancer tumorigenesis with identification of potentially useful biomarkers. Inhibition of epidermal growth factor receptor (EGFR) and vascular epithelial growth factor (VEGF) has been studied both alone and in combination with chemotherapy. Treatment with VEGF inhibitors such as bevacizumab needs to be optimized in terms of length of maintenance treatment and identification of additional active drugs. Poly (ADP-ribose) polymerase (PARP) inhibitors, namely olaparib, have shown promise in phase I trials and randomized trials comparing the drug to liposomal doxorubicin. PARP inhibitors are thought to cause significant tumor lethality secondary to the cell's inability to repair spontaneous DNA damage without the PARP repair pathway. Identification of more specific tumor markers could potentially be used to identify disease at earlier, more treatable stages. Microarray gene expression profiles hold promise as prognostic tools for identification of gene targets and may shed light on mechanisms of drug resistance. Current clinical studies are examining new chemotherapeutic agents and novel combinations of known agents in efforts to improve survival of this devastating disease.

II. FALLOPIAN TUBE CARCINOMA. Fallopian tube carcinoma is a rare gynecologic malignancy that behaves biologically like serous epithelial ovarian carcinoma. Fallopian tube carcinoma is staged and treated in a manner similar to ovarian carcinoma. The classic presentation is intermittent, profuse, watery vaginal discharge (hydrops tubae profluens). The diagnosis is seldom made preoperatively but has been detected by Pap smear. Prognosis is related to stage of disease with long-term survival of approximately 50% for stages I and II. As with ovarian carcinoma, long-term survival is rare with advanced disease.

III. GERM CELL OVARIAN CANCERS. These cancers typically occur in young women, are highly curable, and account for approximately 3% of ovarian cancers. The majority present as early-stage lesions confined to one ovary except for dysgerminomas, which are bilateral in 15% of cases. Dysgerminoma, endodermal sinus tumor (yolk sac tumor), embryonal carcinoma, choriocarcinoma, immature (embryonal) teratoma, and malignant mixed germ cell tumors are the cell types seen. Fertility-sparing surgery is nearly always possible. Surgical cytoreduction appears to be important and is likely associated with increased survival. Most of these tumors will have a tumor marker available to follow (human chorionic gonadotropin [HCG], α-fetoprotein [AFP], lactate dehydrogenase [LDH], CA-125, or neuron-specific enolase [NSE]). Following surgery, most tumors are treated with chemotherapy except some well-staged IA/IB cancers. The BEP regimen is the most commonly used and consists of a 5-day regimen, although a 3-day regimen has also been studied (cisplatin 20 mg/m^2 IV days 1 to 5, bleomycin 30 units IV weekly, etoposide 100 mg/m^2 IV days 1 to 5—cycle repeated every 3 weeks). Some support observation only for localized, completely resected malignant germ cell tumors based on French survival data and pediatric oncology group trials.

IV. STROMAL TUMORS OF THE OVARY. Stromal tumors are classified by the World Health Organization (WHO) into five main classes: (a) granulosa-stromal cell tumors (adult and juvenile granulosa cell tumor and tumors in the thecoma/fibroma group); (b) Sertoli-stromal cell tumors (Sertoli, Leydig, or Sertoli–Leydig cell tumor); (c) gynandroblastoma; (d) sex cord tumor with annular tubules; and (e) unclassified. These tumors are rare and are usually of early stage and low grade, which make them readily curable with simple surgical resection. Primary metastatic or recurrent disease is usually treated with surgical cytoreduction followed by combination chemotherapy. The BEP regimen is most often used; however, recent data from Brown et al. suggest that taxanes demonstrate activity against ovarian stromal tumors and have less toxicity than BEP regimens.

SUGGESTED READINGS

Armstrong DK, Bundy B, Wenzel L, et al. Intraperitoneal cisplatin and paclitaxel in ovarian cancer. *N Engl J Med* 2006;354(1):34–43.

Bowles EJ, Wernli KJ, Gray HJ, et al. Diffusion of intraperitoneal chemotherapy in women with advanced ovarian cancer in community settings 2003-2008: The effect of the NCI clinical recommendation. *Front Oncol* 2014;34:43.

Burger RA, Brady MF, Bookman MA, et al. Incorporation of bevacizumab in the primary treatment of ovarian cancer. *N Engl J Med* 2011;365:2473–2483.

Chan JK, Tian C, Fleming GF, et al. The potential benefit of 6 vs. 3 cycles of chemotherapy in subsets of women with early-stage high-risk epithelial ovarian cancer: an exploratory analysis of a Gynecologic Oncology Group study. *Gynecol Oncol* 2010;116:301–306.

Katsumata N, Yasuda M, Isonishi S, et al. Long-term results of dose-dense paclitaxel and carboplatin versus conventional paclitaxel and carboplatin for treatment of advanced epithelial ovarian, fallopian tube, or primary peritoneal cancer (JGOG 3016): a randomised, controlled, open-label trial. *Lancet Oncol* 2013;14:1020–1026.

Kauff ND, Satagopan JM, Robson ME, et al. Risk reducing salpingoophorectomy in women with a *BRCA*1 or *BRCA*2 mutation. *N Engl J Med* 2002;346(21):1609–1615.

Ozols RF, Bundy BN, Greer BE, et al. Phase III trial of carboplatin and paclitaxel compared with cisplatin and paclitaxel in patients with optimally resected stage III ovarian cancer. *J Clin Oncol* 2003;21:3194–3200.

Ozols RF. Challenges for chemotherapy in ovarian cancer. *Ann Oncol* 2006;17(5):v181–v187.

Perren TJ, Swart AM, Pfisterer J, et al. A phase 3 trial of bevacizumab in ovarian cancer. *N Engl J Med* 2011;365:2484–2496.

Prat J. Staging classification for cancer of the ovary, fallopian tube and peritoneum. *Int J Gynaecol Obstet* 2014;124:1–5.

Rubin SC, Benjamin I, Behbakht K, et al. Clinical and pathological features of ovarian cancer in women with germ-line mutations of *BRCA*1. *N Engl J Med* 1996;335:1413–1416.

Young RC. Early-stage ovarian cancer: to treat or not to treat. *J Natl Cancer Inst* 2003;95:94–95.

24 Uterine, Cervical, Vulvar, and Vaginal Cancers

Lindsay M. Kuroki • Pratibha S. Binder • David G. Mutch

I. UTERINE NEOPLASIA

A. Premalignant disease of the endometrium

1. **Background.** Endometrial hyperplasia is a spectrum of proliferative disorders primarily of the endometrial glands, and to a lesser extent, the stroma. In the normal menstrual cycle, estrogen stimulation leads to growth and proliferation of the endometrium, whereas progesterone leads to predecidual changes and inhibition of endometrial proliferation. In the absence of progesterone, unopposed estrogen can lead to a spectrum of endometrial abnormalities varying from simple endometrial hyperplasia to endometrial malignancies. This often results from chronic anovulation (polycystic ovarian syndrome and perimenopause), obesity (high peripheral estrogen production), estrogen-producing ovarian neoplasms (granulosa cell tumor), exogenous estrogen administration (hormone replacement therapy), and the use of selective estrogen receptor modulators (SERMs) like tamoxifen that has estrogen-like properties on the endometrium.

2. **Presentation.** The majority of patients with endometrial hyperplasia remain asymptomatic and therefore these precursor lesions can go unrecognized for years. Some patients are diagnosed due to symptoms of abnormal or postmenopausal bleeding. Other patients may be diagnosed due to incidental abnormal findings on an ultrasound ordered for other reasons or abnormal endometrial cells noted on Papanicolaou (Pap) test. Normal menstrual cycles occur every 28 days (range 21 to 35 days) with a normal duration of 2 to 7 days and an average blood loss of less than 80 mL. Bleeding outside of these ranges or any postmenopausal bleeding should be evaluated. Any age group can be affected, but one should be especially concerned with abnormal bleeding in patients aged 35 years and older. Obesity, a history of anovulatory cycles, use of tamoxifen, and use of exogenous estrogens without concurrent progestational agents are known risk factors.

3. **Workup and staging.** Typically, the diagnosis can be made with an office endometrial (pipelle) biopsy. If this is nondiagnostic or technically not feasible, a dilation and curettage (D&C), with or without hysteroscopy can be performed to obtain more tissue for accurate histologic diagnosis. The International Society of Gynecological Pathologists classifies endometrial hyperplasia into four distinct categories based on a 1994 classification system looking at architectural structure and cytologic features: simple and complex hyperplasia, both with and without atypia.

4. **Therapy and prognosis**

   a. **Simple or complex hyperplasia without atypia.** Treatment is usually conservative and depends on the fertility desires of the patient. The risk of developing malignancy over a 13- to 15-year untreated period is 1% for simple and 3% for complex hyperplasia (Table 24-1).

      i. **Patients desiring pregnancy.** Treatment consists of inducing withdrawal bleed followed by ovulation induction with clomiphene citrate. Withdrawal bleed can be achieved with medroxyprogesterone acetate (Provera), 10 mg PO per day for 5 to 10 days (after a negative pregnancy test) followed by ovulation induction with clomiphene citrate, 50 mg PO on day 5 of bleeding to continue for a total of 5 days. If patient does not menstruate within a month, this cycle of treatment can be repeated with higher doses of clomiphene citrate after pregnancy test is negative.

      ii. **Patients not considering pregnancy.** Management usually consists of oral, intramuscular, or intrauterine progestins followed by repeat biopsy after 3 to 6 months. Accepted regimens include medroxyprogesterone 10 mg PO for 7 to 13 days/month, depot medroxyprogesterone 150 mg IM every month, oral contraceptive pills, and levonorgestrel intrauterine device (IUD). Regression of hyperplasia occurs in up to 92% of patients treated with levonorgestrel IUD.

TABLE 24-1	Comparison of Follow-up of Patients with Simple and Complex Hyperplasia and Simple and Complex Atypical Hyperplasia (170 Patients)			
Histology	**No. of patients**	**Regressed no. (%)**	**Persisted no. (%)**	**Progressed to carcinoma no. (%)**
Simple hyperplasia	93	74 (80%)	18 (19%)	1 (1%)
Complex hyperplasia	29	23 (80%)	5 (17%)	1 (3%)
Simple atypical hyperplasia	13	9 (69%)	3 (23%)	1 (8%)
Complex atypical hyperplasia	35	20 (57%)	5 (14%)	10 (29%)

Kurman RJ, Kaminski PF, Norris HJ. The behavior of endometrial hyperplasia: a long-term study of "untreated" hyperplasia in 170 patients. *Cancer* 1985;56:403–412.

b. **Simple or complex hyperplasia with atypia.** Twenty-three percent of untreated atypical hyperplasia progress to endometrial cancer (8% for simple atypical and 29% for complex atypical hyperplasia) over 11 years. More importantly, there is a 13% to 43% rate of concurrent endometrial cancer with atypical hyperplasia. In a Gynecologic Oncology Group (GOG 167) prospective cohort study of women with atypical endometrial hyperplasia, the rate of concurrent endometrial cancer was 43% for analyzed specimens, with 31% of these demonstrating myometrial invasion, and 11% invading the outer 50% of the myometrium (*Cancer* 2006;106:812). Due to these findings, patients with atypical hyperplasia should undergo D&C with or without hysteroscopy to rule out the presence of invasive cancer in the unsampled endometrium.

  i. **Patients desiring pregnancy.** Progestational agents including megestrol acetate 80 to 160 mg/day and levonorgestrel IUD have been used for treatment. The goal of therapy is complete regression of disease and reversion to normal endometrium followed by ovulation induction or assisted reproductive techniques for pregnancy. Repeat sampling with biopsy or D&C is recommended after 3 months of therapy.

  ii. **Patients not considering pregnancy. Medical treatment:** Regression is up to 90% with progestational agents including oral medroxyprogesterone (40 mg PO per day) and megestrol acetate (160 to 320 mg PO per day in divided doses) as well as levonorgestrel IUD (*Obstetric Gynecol* 2012;120:1160). Repeat biopsy or D&C to check for persistence or progression is recommended every 3 to 6 months till regression. **Surgical treatment:** Extrafascial hysterectomy with gross inspection and frozen section of the endometrium for evidence of endometrial cancer.

5. **Complications** are rare and minor, usually related to surgical complications of D&C including risk of anesthesia, infection, hemorrhage, and uterine perforation. An underlying concern is inappropriate surgical management due to misdiagnosed cancer.

6. **Follow-up.** Medically managed patients should be resampled at regular intervals (3 to 12 months) until regression of endometrial pathology. Those with normal histology can then either be taken off therapy or be cycled with progestational agents and should undergo periodic endometrial sampling. Follow-up interval for patients after hysterectomy is not well-established, but annual examinations should be adequate.

7. **Current focus.** The current focus is on determining molecular markers that predict progression to endometrial cancer and important prognostic factors in fertility-sparing medical management.

B. **Endometrial cancer**

1. **Background.** Endometrial cancer is the most common gynecologic malignancy in the United States with a rising incidence over the last 5 years. There were approximately 49,560 new cases and 8,190 deaths due to endometrial cancer in 2013 (*CA Cancer J Clin* 2013;63:11). Five-year survival for localized disease is 96%, whereas relative survival for all stages is approximately 82%. There are two morphologically and molecularly distinct histologic subtypes: type I and type II. Risk factors for type I endometrial cancer include unopposed exogenous estrogenic stimulation (estrogens or tamoxifen), chronic anovulation, obesity, diabetes mellitus, nulliparity, and late age of menopause (older than 52 years). Type II histology tends to be more sporadic and is not associated with clinical and physical factors mentioned above.

2. **Presentation.** More than 90% of patients are first seen with abnormal uterine bleeding. Patients with any postmenopausal bleeding or discharge deserve evaluation. Patients with abnormal pre- or perimenopausal bleeding, especially those with history of anovulatory cycles, older than 35 years, or morbidly obese warrant evaluation as well. Pap tests with atypical glandular cells of undetermined significance (AGUS) in patients of any age should be evaluated with a colposcopy, endocervical curettage, and endometrial biopsy. Pap test with endometrial cells on a postmenopausal patient should also be evaluated.

| TABLE 24-2 | FIGO Surgical Staging and Grade of Endometrial Cancer, 2009 |

Stage	Description
IA	Tumor limited to uterus, no or less than half myometrial invasion
IB	Tumor limited to uterus, equal to or more than half myometrial invasion
II	Cervical stromal invasion
IIIA	Uterine serosal and/or adnexal involvement
IIIB	Vaginal metastasis and/or parametrial involvement
IIIC1	Positive pelvic lymph nodes
IIIC2	Positive para-aortic lymph nodes (with or without pelvic nodes)
IVA	Bladder and/or bowel/rectal mucosal invasion
IVB	Distant metastases including intra-abdominal and/or inguinal lymph nodes

Grade	Description
1	Less than 5% of tumor is solid sheets of undifferentiated neoplastic cells
2	6%–50% of tumor is solid sheets of undifferentiated neoplastic cells
3	>50% of tumor is solid sheets of undifferentiated neoplastic cells

Cytology is mentioned separately and does not change stage.
FIGO, International Federation of Gynecology and Obstetrics.

3. **Workup and staging.** An office endometrial biopsy (pipelle) is an extremely sensitive method of obtaining a tissue diagnosis. A meta-analysis of 39 studies involving 7,914 women demonstrated a detection rate for endometrial cancer of 91% and 99.6% in pre- and postmenopausal women, respectively (*Cancer* 2000;89:1765). Patients with a nondiagnostic office biopsy, persistent bleeding abnormality despite a normal office biopsy, or those unable to undergo an office biopsy should undergo a fractional D&C, with or without hysteroscopy. All patients should be screened for other malignancies as appropriate for age and family history (Pap test, ultrasound, mammogram, and colorectal cancer screening). Cystoscopy, proctoscopy, and radiologic imaging may be necessary, as clinically indicated, if advanced stage is suspected. Surgical staging of endometrial carcinoma was adopted by the International Federation of Gynecologists and Obstetricians (FIGO) in 1988 and then revised in 2009 (Table 24-2). All patients who are medically able should first undergo surgical exploration with appropriate staging. Extrafascial hysterectomy with bilateral salpingo-oophorectomy, collection of peritoneal cytology, pelvic and para-aortic lymph node dissection, and biopsy of any suspicious areas are necessary for staging, except in small well-differentiated tumors without myometrial invasion. Omentectomy or omental biopsy is also indicated for high grade tumors and type II histology.

4. **Therapy and prognosis.** The first step of treatment is hysterectomy and surgical staging (abdominal, laparoscopic, or robotic). Total laparoscopic staging is being performed with increasing frequency for suspected early-stage endometrial cancer, and lymph node count and survival appear similar when compared to laparotomy. Hysterectomy removes primary tumor and intraoperative findings like size of tumor, myometrial invasion, and grade can help estimate risk or lymph node involvement and need for adjuvant therapy. Removal of adnexa is important due to the risk of metastasis to the ovary, synchronous ovarian cancers, and risk of future recurrence or primary cancer in the ovary. Lymphadenectomy is somewhat more controversial. Lymph node status is prognostically important and is essential in the decision of postoperative adjuvant therapy. But since there are rare but substantial risks and complications associated with the procedure, the benefit of lymphadenectomy is controversial in patients with low risk of positive nodes, high risk of morbid complication, and in patients that

TABLE 24-3 Treatment of Endometrial Cancer

Condition	Possible adjuvant therapies to consider
Stage IA or IB and grade 1 or 2	No further therapy or vaginal brachytherapy
Stage I and II with HIR	Vaginal brachytherapy vs. pelvic RT
	Vaginal brachytherapy with chemotherapy (currently under investigation, GOG 249)
Stage IIIA (serosal and/or adnexal involvement)	Systemic chemotherapy vs. Pelvic RT and VB or combination
Stage IIIB (vaginal involvement)	Systemic chemotherapy vs. Pelvic RT and VB or combination
Stage IIIC (microscopic nodal involvement)	Systemic chemotherapy vs. Pelvic RT with extended-field radiation to para-aortic region (if indicated) and systemic chemotherapy
Stage IIIC (macroscopic nodal), stage IV, and recurrent disease (extrapelvic)	Palliative RT vs. systemic chemotherapy vs. hormonal therapy vs. targeted therapies or combinations
Recurrent disease (pelvic)	Radiotherapy in the patient without earlier RT vs. possible surgical resection (exenteration) vs. chemotherapy or combinations
High intermediate risk	*Risk factors:*
Any age with three risk factors	**1.** *Moderately to poorly differentiated tumor*
Age >50 with two risk factors	**2.** *Lymph vascular space invasion*
Age >70 with one risk factor	**3.** *Outer ⅓ myometrial invasion*

RT, radiation therapy; VB, vaginal cuff brachytherapy; HIR, high–intermediate risk.

will receive adjuvant therapy due to other findings. Historically, radiation therapy (RT) had been the preferred choice of adjuvant therapy for patients with high risk of recurrence. However, the role of chemotherapy in all stages of endometrial cancer is evolving. While low risk stage I disease can be treated with surgery alone, adjuvant treatment for other stages is variable and includes vaginal brachytherapy (VB), external beam pelvic radiation therapy (EBRT), and chemotherapy (Table 24-3).

a. **Early stage.** Results from GOG 33 and GOG 99 helped define a high intermediate risk (HIR) category for patients with Stage I or II disease with a higher risk of recurrence (*Gynecol Oncol* 2004;92:744). GOG 99 and PORTEC-1 showed that EBRT compared to no adjuvant treatment decreased local recurrence in patients with HIR stage I or II disease, but survival benefit was not significant. PORTEC-2 compared EBRT to VB and showed both were comparable in local recurrence rate. Therefore, adjuvant radiation treatment is recommended based on HIR criteria and patient desires of further treatment to decrease risk of recurrence or treatment when recurrence occurs. The pooled data from two randomized controlled trials showed a significant decrease in progression-free survival (PFS), cancer-specific survival (CSS), and overall survival (OS) for HIR stage I and II patients treated with combination chemotherapy and pelvic RT compared to pelvic RT alone. Currently there are two randomized trials comparing concurrent chemoradiation followed by adjuvant chemotherapy (PORTEC-3) or VB followed by chemotherapy (GOG 249) to pelvic RT alone in the treatment of HIR early-stage endometrial cancer.

b. **Advanced stage.** Cytotoxic chemotherapy for advanced stage endometrial cancer includes the following agents (response rate): cisplatin (20% to 35%), carboplatin (30%), doxorubicin (Adriamycin; 20% to 35%), epirubicin (25%) and paclitaxel. The combination of doxorubicin (60 mg/m^2) plus cisplatin (50 mg/m^2) every 3 weeks showed an improved response rate of 42%, progression-free interval of 6 months, and median OS of 9 months in a randomized trial by the GOG (*J Clin Oncol* 2004;22:3902). Combination of doxorubicin (60 mg/m^2 × 7 cycles) and cisplatin (50 mg/m^2 × 8 cycles) (AC) was superior to whole abdominal radiation (WAI, 30 Gy in 20 fractions with a 15-Gy boost) in a phase III trial of 202 randomized patients with stage III/IV endometrial cancer optimally debulked to ≤2 cm of residual disease with PFS of 50% versus 38% and OS 55% versus 42%, respectively (*J Clin Oncol* 2006;24:36). In 2004, a GOG trial demonstrated improved survival in patients with advanced or recurrent endometrial cancer treated with TAP (paclitaxel, doxorubicin, cisplatin) as compared to cisplatin and doxorubicin alone, although with increased toxicity (*J Clin Oncol* 2004;22:2159). A phase III trial comparing TAP and PT (carboplatin/paclitaxel) is currently underway and preliminary results show that PT is non-inferior to TAP and has a more favorable toxicity profile. In GOG 184, patients with stage III/IV endometrial cancer were treated with pelvic RT followed by AC versus TAP. There was no patient outcome benefit by adding paclitaxel but the study showed that combination radiation and chemotherapy was a feasible treatment option with acceptable toxicity.

Treatment with chemotherapy, RT, and/or hormone therapy is acceptable in patients where surgical staging and debulking is not a medically feasible option. Hormone therapy is also often used for patients with advanced/recurrent disease who test positive for estrogen and progesterone receptors. Response rate with either medroxyprogesterone acetate, 200 mg daily, or megestrol acetate, 160 mg daily, is approximately 20%.

5. **Complications.** Complications of staging surgery include pain, hemorrhage, infection, and damage to surrounding structure including bowel, bladder, and blood vessels. Lymphocysts and lymphedema of the lower extremities are rare complications of lymphadenectomy. Immediate toxicities from chemotherapy include hematologic, GI, and infectious complications. Immediate and late effects of radiation are usually related to bowel and bladder dysfunction. Concurrent treatment with chemotherapy and radiation therapy is currently under investigation, and the toxicities of combination treatment remain a major concern.

6. **Follow-up.** Typically patients are evaluated with physical examination, Pap test, and pelvic examination every 3 months for the first year, every 3 to 4 months for the second year, every 6 months for third to fifth year, and then at 6 to 12 month intervals thereafter.

7. **Current focus.** Current efforts are directed toward elucidating molecular markers that are prognostic and important in understanding endometrial cancer tumorigenesis New advances focused on the etiologic heterogeneity and defects in molecular pathways has lead to better histologic classification and the identification of potential therapies targeting defects in these pathways. Therapies targeting aberrations P13K/AKT/mTOR pathways, tyrosine kinase pathways, and angiogenesis are being studied in preclinical and phase II trials. While single-agent treatment with these drugs have not shown promising results, combination treatment with currently used chemotherapy regimens are being evaluated. Improved prognosis in endometrial cancer patients being treated with metformin has been observed in retrospective studies. Research to identify the pathways associating metformin use with improved endometrial cancer prognosis is underway.

C. **Sarcomas**

1. **Background.** These are uncommon tumors arising from the mesenchymal components of the uterus and comprise of 3% to 8% of uterine tumors. The GOG has broadly classified them based on histology: (1) Non-epithelial neoplasms including endometrial stromal sarcoma (ESS), leiomyosarcoma (LMS), and smooth muscle tumor of uncertain malignant potential (STUMP) and (2) Mixed epithelial–nonepithelial tumors including adenosarcoma and carcinosarcoma. Homologous types contain sarcomatous components that are unique to uterine tissue, whereas heterologous types produce stromal components that are not native to the uterus.

TABLE 24-4	FIGO Surgical Staging of Uterine Sarcomas, 2009

Stage	Description
LMS	
IA	Tumor limited to the uterus, <5cm
.IB	Tumor limited to the uterus, >5cm
IIA	Adnexal involvement
IIB	Tumor extends to extra-uterine pelvic tissue
IIIA	Tumor invades abdominal tissue, one site
IIIB	Tumor invades abdominal tissue, > one site
IIIC	Metastasis to pelvic and/or para-aortic lymph nodes
IVA	Tumor invades bladder and/or bowel mucosa
IVB	Distant metastases
Endometrial stromal sarcoma/adenosarcoma	
IA	Tumor limited to endometrium/endocervix, no myometrial invasion
IB	Less than or equal to half myometrial invasion
IC	More than half myometrial invasion
IIA	Adnexal involvement
IIB	Tumor extends to extra-uterine pelvic tissue
IIIA	Tumor invades abdominal tissue, one site
IIIB	Tumor invades abdominal tissue, > one site
IIIC	Metastasis to pelvic and/or para-aortic lymph nodes
IVA	Tumor invades bladder and/or bowel mucosa
IVB	Distant metastases

FIGO, International Federation of Gynecology and Obstetrics.

2. **Presentation** varies depending on type of tumor. Carcinosarcomas usually present with postmenopausal bleeding, while ESS and LMS can present as abnormal bleeding, rapidly enlarging pelvic pain or pelvic pressure and pain. Uterine sarcomas are often incidental diagnoses on hysterectomy specimens, and reoperation for complete surgical staging is usually not recommended.

3. **Workup and staging.** Workup is similar to endometrial cancer and involves endometrial biopsy or core biopsy of any masses protruding through the cervix. Pelvic imaging can be performed to delineate the size and origin of protruding masses. Staging for LMS and ESS is summarized in Table 24-4, As more is discovered about the biology and activity of these rare cancers, uterine carcinosarcomas may be considered more closely related to poorly differentiated endometrial carcinomas, and therefore they are staged using the 2009 FIGO staging for endometrial cancer (Table 24-2). Patients should be treated primarily with surgical exploration with appropriate staging, as primary radiotherapy and chemotherapy have very disappointing results.

4. **Therapy and prognosis.** Although each histologic subtype of sarcoma behaves differently, in general, survival is poor, with more than half the number of patients dying of their disease. For stage I and II disease, adjuvant RT often improves local recurrences but has little impact on long-term survival. Cytotoxic chemotherapy may have a role in the adjuvant setting. Hormonal therapy with high dose progestin therapy (megestrol acetate, 240 to 360 mg p.o. daily) has shown activity against endometrial stromal sarcomas, especially those that are low grade. Advanced stage (III/IV) and recurrent disease have been treated with radiotherapy with minimal success. Chemotherapy is most often used in this setting since phase II trials have shown tolerable toxicities and improved response compared to historical data. Single agent doxorubicin (60 mg/m^2

IV q3 weeks) or ifosfamide (1.2 to 1.5 g/m^2 IV q.d. × 4 to 5 days) have shown activity against LMS with approximate response rates of 25% and 20%, respectively. Combination gemcitabine (900 mg/m^2 IV on day 1 and 8, q3 weeks) and docetaxel (75 mg/m^2 IV q3 weeks) showed favorable response rates for completely resected stage I–IV disease as well as advanced and recurrent disease (*Gynecol Oncol* 2009;112:563). For carcinosarcomas, ifosfamide plus MESNA, with or without cisplatin, showed response rates of 30% to 50% in patients with advanced, persistent, or recurrent disease (*Gynecol Oncol* 2000;79:147). The combination therapy produced higher response rates but greater toxicity and no survival advantage over single-agent ifosfamide (GOG117). This combination chemotherapy regimen had similar patient outcomes as WAI for stage I–IV disease in a phase III GOG trial (GOG 150). Survival in advanced disease patients was improved by the addition of paclitaxel (135 mg/m^2 IV q3 weeks up to 8 cycles to ifosfamide). A phase II trial also showed acceptable response rates with paclitaxel and carboplatin in the treatment of carcinosarcoma patients with advanced disease (*J Clin Oncol* 2010;28:2727). Surgical resection of recurrent sarcoma and chemotherapy has shown to be beneficial in other soft tissue sarcomas, and may provide a survival advantage in uterine sarcomas as well.

- **5. Current focus.** Recent chemotherapy trials for advanced or recurrent LMS have included doxorubicin, 40 mg/m^2, mitomycin, 8 mg/m^2, and cisplatin, 60 mg/m^2 q3 weeks; liposomal doxorubicin (Doxil), 50 mg/m^2 IV q4 weeks; and paclitaxel, 175 mg/m^2 i.v. over a 3-hour period q3 weeks. Further studies are underway to establish the use of paclitaxel and carboplatin in the treatment of advanced carcinosarcoma. Determining risk factors, prognostic factors, and the tumorigenesis for uterine sarcomas is also a focus for current research.

D. Gestational trophoblastic disease (GTD)

1. **Background.** Abnormal growth of the human trophoblast is called **GTD**. GTD encompasses a spectrum of abnormalities of trophoblastic tissue including classic (complete) hydatidiform moles, partial hydatidiform moles, invasive hydatidiform moles, choriocarcinoma, and placental site trophoblastic tumors. The most common abnormality, the hydatidiform mole, has two pathologic varieties—complete and partial mole. Complete moles are the most common subtype of GTD and typically occur as a result of dispermy, with both chromosomes paternal in origin resulting from fertilization of an empty ovum (46,XX). Partial moles are the result of fertilization of a normal egg by two sperms (69,XXY), resulting in an abnormal pregnancy with fetal parts usually identifiable. The reported incidence of mole varies widely throughout the world, with 1:1,500 pregnancies affected in the United States. Invasive mole is a pathologic diagnosis of a benign tumor that invades the uterine myometrium or on occasion metastasizes. The incidence is estimated at 1:15,000 pregnancies. Choriocarcinoma is a malignant tumor that has a propensity for early metastasis and an aggressive course, arising in 1:40,000 pregnancies. Fifty percent of choriocarcinomas develop after a molar gestation, 25% after a term pregnancy, and 25% after an abortion or an ectopic pregnancy. Placental-site trophoblastic tumor is the rarest variant, arising from the intermediate trophoblast, and is relatively chemotherapy resistant. The tumors often secrete human placental lactogen (HPL), which can be used as a tumor marker. GTD is more common in extremes of reproductive age (teenagers and women, aged 40 to 50 years).

2. **Presentation.** Most cases of malignant/persistent GTD are seen after a hydatidiform mole. Hydatidiform moles usually present with vaginal bleeding and a positive pregnancy test. Nearly all hydatidiform moles are now diagnosed by ultrasound examination, demonstrating the "snowstorm" appearance of the vesicle-filled intrauterine cavity. Occasionally, patients will have symptoms of preeclampsia, hyperthyroidism, and/or severe hyperemesis. Physical examination demonstrates uterine size larger than estimated gestational dates, bilateral ovarian enlargement (due to thecal lutein cysts), and usually an absence of fetal heart sounds or fetal parts. GTD can also occur after a normal pregnancy, abortion (spontaneous or induced), or ectopic pregnancy, and

the diagnosis is often easily missed in these patients. Presentation is the same in these patients, although the delay in diagnosis may lead to widely metastatic disease.

3. **Workup and staging.** After diagnosis of a molar pregnancy (usually by ultrasound), the patient should undergo chest radiograph (CXR; if positive, a metastatic workup should follow; see later), blood type and cross-matching, and serum quantitative b-human chorionic gonadotropin (HCG) evaluation. Mainstay of treatment is an ultrasound-guided suction D&C followed by sharp curettage. Intravenous oxytocin, 20 to 40 units/L or other uterotonic agents should be used shortly after the beginning of the procedure and continued for several hours to avoid excessive bleeding. Patients with Rh-negative blood should receive Rh immune globulin (RhoGAM), as indicated to prevent isoimmunization in future pregnancies. Patients are followed up after surgery with quantitative pregnancy tests (b-HCG) weekly until normal and then monthly for 1 year. Eighty percent of moles will resolve with D&C alone. **Persistent gestational trophoblastic neoplasia (GTN)** is diagnosed with any of the following conditions (note that histologic verification is not required): (a) after evacuation of a hydatidiform mole, the HCG level does not decrease appropriately (plateau or two consecutive weeks with an increasing titer), (b) metastatic disease is discovered, or (c) pathologic diagnosis of choriocarcinoma or placental-site trophoblastic tumor. Once the diagnosis of persistent GTN is made, a further metastatic workup should include a complete history and physical examination and computed tomography (CT) of the chest, abdomen, pelvis, and possibly head, if indicated. A pelvic ultrasound should also be performed to rule out an early pregnancy in patients with inadequate contraception. Complete blood count (CBC) and metabolic panel (hepatic and renal) are also indicated. An anatomic staging system (FIGO, 1992) does exist but is seldom clinically used. Prognosis and subsequent therapy are usually based on the World Health Organization (WHO) scoring system or the National Institutes of Health (NIH) system used by most U.S. trophoblastic disease centers (Table 24-5).

4. **Therapy and prognosis.** Therapy is directed by the NIH class or the WHO score. Prognosis is generally excellent, and the key is to limit toxicity of the therapy as much as possible. Therapy should be started immediately, as delays can be devastating. The primary therapy of malignant GTD is chemotherapy. Surgery is used to decrease the amount of chemotherapy required for remission or to remove resistant foci of disease. Treatment of nonmetastatic GTN includes hysterectomy for those no longer

---

TABLE 24-5	Prognostic Classification of Gestational Trophoblastic Neoplasia

I. Nonmetastatic disease
II. Metastatic disease
    A. Low risk/good prognosis GTN
        1. Short duration since last pregnancy event (<4 mo)
        2. Low pretreatment HCG (<40,000 mIU/mL serum)
        3. No brain or liver metastasis
        4. No prior chemotherapy
        5. Pregnancy event is not a term delivery
    B. High risk/poor prognosis GTN
        1. Long duration since last pregnancy event (>4 mo)
        2. High pretreatment HCG (>40,000 mIU/mL serum)
        3. Brain or liver metastasis
        4. Prior chemotherapy failure
        5. Antecedent term pregnancy

NIH, National Institutes of Health; HCG, human chorionic gonadotropin.

TABLE 24-6	Chemotherapeutic Regimens for Persistent GTN

Nonmetastatic and low risk metastatic GTN

Methotrexate, 30–50 mg/m^2 IM q wk (preferred method)

Methotrexate, 0.4 mg/kg IV/IM qd × 5 days, repeat every 2 weeks

Methotrexate, 1–1.5 mg/kg IM days (1, 3, 5, 7) + folinic acid, 0.1–0.15 mg/kg IM days (2, 4, 6, 8), repeat every 15–18 days

Actinomycin D, 10–13 μg/kg IV/day × 5 days, repeat every 14 days

Actinomycin D, 1.25 mg/m^2 IV q14 days (superior to weekly methotrexate in GOG 174)

Etoposide, 200 mg/m^2/day PO × 5 days q14 days

High risk metastatic GTN: EMA-CO regimen

EMA-CO regimen

Day 1, etoposide, 100 mg/m^2 IV (over 30 min); actinomycin D, 0.35 mg IV push; methotrexate 100 mg/m^2 IV push, then 200 mg/m^2 IV infusion over 12 h

Day 2, etoposide, 100 mg/m^2 IV over 30 min; actinomycin D, 0.35-mg IV push; folinic acid, 15 mg PO, IM or IV q12 h × 4 doses

Day 8, vincristine, 1 mg/m^2 IV plus cyclophosphamide, 600 mg/m^2 IV

Repeat entire cycle every 2 weeks. Patients with CNS metastasis should also receive radiation therapy and intrathecal methotrexate (12.5 mg on day 8) (*Gynecol Oncol* 1989;31:439).

Triple Agent (MAC) regimen

Day 1–5, methotrexate, 15 mg IM; actinomycin D 0.5 mg IV; cyclophosphamide 3 mg/kg IV

Repeat cycle every 15 days.

CNS, central nervous system.

desiring fertility and for all with placental site trophoblastic tumors. Chemotherapy is recommended for all patients, even if hysterectomy is performed, and is usually given as a single agent. Table 24-6 summarizes the chemotherapeutic regimens used to treat GTN. **Low risk metastatic GTN** is treated primarily with single-agent chemotherapy; both methotrexate and actinomycin D should be used individually before resorting to multi-agent chemotherapy. Single-agent actinomycin D IV q 14 days was found to have superior complete response rates than methotrexate IM weekly (GOG 174); however, all patients were eventually cured after switching to alternative single-agent or multi-agent regimens (*J Clin Oncol* 2011;29(7):825) **High risk metastatic disease** is treated with multi-agent chemotherapy with the addition of radiation if a brain metastasis is present and surgery to remove resistant foci in the uterus or chest, as needed. All patients receiving chemotherapy should be evaluated with appropriate laboratory studies (CBC, hepatic, and/or renal panel) for the specific regimens plus a serum β-HCG every cycle. Treatment should continue until three consecutive normal HCG levels are obtained. At least two courses should be given after the first normal HCG.

5. **Complications.** Complications are related mainly to the specific chemotherapeutic regimen used. Single-agent therapy is normally well-tolerated with minimal side effects. Any suspicious metastatic sites should not be biopsied due to risk of hemorrhage.

6. **Follow-up.** Patients should be monitored with serum HCG monthly for 1 year. Contraception is needed for a minimum of 6 months, but 12 months is preferred. If pregnancy should develop, an early ultrasound should be performed to document an intrauterine pregnancy.

7. **Current focus.** Chemotherapy for low-risk GTN is currently being studied by the GOG 275 in a randomized manner with multiday methotrexate regimen versus pulsed dactinomycin (1.25 mg/m^2 IV push q14 days). The predictive value of modeled HCG residual production is also being validated in patients treated in GOG 174.

II. UTERINE CERVIX NEOPLASIA

A. Preinvasive lesions of the cervix

1. **Background.** More than 2.5 million women in the United States have Pap test abnormalities with more than 200,000 new cases of dysplasia diagnosed annually. Human Papilloma Virus (HPV) has been detected in more than 90% of preinvasive and invasive carcinomas, and there is strong evidence that HPV is the etiologic factor in the vast majority of dysplasias and cervical cancers. HPV subtypes 16, 18, 45, and 56 are considered high risk (HR HPV); 31, 33, 35, 51, 52, and 58 are of intermediate risk; and 6, 11, 42, 43, and 44 are of low risk for progression to cancer. Other risk factors for the development of cervical dysplasia include smoking, multiple sexual partners, low socioeconomic status, young age at coitarche, presence of HR HPV, or immunodeficiency.

2. **Presentation.** Preinvasive lesions of the cervix are often asymptomatic, but can reliably be detected with cytology or biopsy. Median age is approximately 28 years and risk factors are often present.

3. **Screening.** The goal of screening programs is to identify women with preinvasive disease and manage them appropriately so as to decrease the incidence and mortality rate from cervical cancer. It is estimated that approximately 4 million women per year will have an abnormal Pap result in the United States. Communities that implement cervical cancer screening programs reduce deaths from cervix cancer by approximately 90%, making it one of the most successful cancer screening programs. Unfortunately, most women in whom cervical cancer develops have not been adequately screened. The American Cancer Society and the American College of Obstetrics and Gynecology recommend that annual cervical cytology screening (Pap test) and pelvic examination be initiated at age 21 regardless of onset of sexual activity. Exceptions to this are women with a history of **cervical intraepithelial neoplasia** (CIN) 2 or greater, diethylstilbestrol (DES) exposure, or who are immunocompromised. In 2012, the American Society for Colposcopy and Cervical Pathology (ASCCP) together with its partner organizations revised the consensus guidelines to reflect improved understanding of: (1) the natural history of HPV infection and cervical cancer precursors; and (2) future pregnancy implications of treatment for CIN among younger women. On the basis of these new guidelines, women aged 21 to 29 years should undergo Pap screening every 3 years. Because of the high prevalence of HPV in this age group, HPV testing should not be used for either co-testing or as a stand-alone test due to potential harm (e.g., psychosocial impact, discomfort from additional diagnostic/therapeutic procedures, and even longer term increased risk of pregnancy complications due to excision procedures). The preferred recommendation for women aged 30 to 64 years is cytology with HPV co-testing every 5 years. Alternatively, cytology alone every 3 years is acceptable.

4. **Terminology.** In 1988, the Bethesda system for the reporting of cervicovaginal cytologic results was developed in an effort to simplify and bring uniformity to the reporting of cytology results. This was revised in 1991 and 2001 for clearer terminology and larger application. Specimens are now specifically described in regard to specimen adequacy ("satisfactory" or "unsatisfactory"), presence of the transformation zone ("present" or "absent"), and evaluation of epithelial cell histology ("negative for intraepithelial lesion or malignancy" or abnormal) (Table 24-7). More recently in 2012, the Lower Anogenital Squamous Terminology (LAST) project incorporated changes in their classification terminology to reflect HPV-associated squamous lesions of the anogenital tract. Specifically, CIN2 is stratified based on p16 immunostaining—specimens that are p16-negative are referred to as **low grade squamous intraepithelial lesions (LSILs)** and those that are p16-positive are considered **high grade squamous intraepithelial lesions (HSILs)**.

5. **Workup. Colposcopy** is performed in specific circumstances for further evaluation of an abnormal Pap result. It is performed with a colposcope that allows magnification of the cervix, which is treated with a 4% acetic acid solution. Colposcopic characteristics of dysplasia include acetowhite changes, punctuations, and abnormal vascularity

TABLE 24-7	Bethesda System of Categorizing Epithelial Cell Abnormalities, 2001

Squamous cell

Atypical squamous cells (ASC)
  Of undetermined significance (ASCUS)
  Cannot exclude high grade squamous intraepithelial lesions (ASC-H)

Low grade squamous intraepithelial lesions (LGSIL)
  Encompassing moderate and severe dysplasia, carcinoma in situ, CIN 2, and CIN 3
  Squamous cell carcinoma

High grade squamous intraepithelial lesions (HGSIL)
  Encompassing moderate and severe dysplasia, carcinoma in situ, CIN 2, and CIN 3
  Squamous cell carcinoma

Glandular cell
  Atypical glandular cells (AGS)
    (Specify endocervical, endometrial, or not otherwise specified)
  Endocervical adenocarcinoma in situ (AIS)
  Adenocarcinoma

CIN, cervical intraepithelial neoplasia.

(mosaicism). Biopsies are performed of abnormal areas, and a histologic diagnosis is made (normal, inflammation, or CIN 1, 2, or 3). Endocervical curettage (ECC) is part of most routine colposcopic examinations, especially those with high grade cytologic abnormalities or if no ectocervical abnormalities are appreciated on colposcopy. The following is a highly simplified approach to managing the abnormal Pap test based on ASCCP guidelines and will not apply to all situations. For **atypical squamous cells of undetermined significance (ASCUS)**, HR HPV DNA testing is at least 80% effective in detecting **CIN 2 or 3 and therefore HPV testing** is commonly performed. Patients aged 25 and older with ASCUS who are HR HPV–positive should undergo colposcopy, whereas ASCUS HR HPV-negative patients may undergo screening again in 1 year. If the result is ASCUS or worse, colposcopy is recommended; if the result is negative, cytology testing at 3-year intervals is recommended. **Atypical squamous cells that cannot exclude HSIL (ASC-H)** represent approximately 15% of ASCUS Pap results with a much higher predictive value for detecting CIN 2 to 3. These patients as well as those with LGSIL and HGSIL cytology results need colposcopic examination. However, HR HPV testing is not indicated for ASC-H, LGSIL, and HGSIL cytology since the test is almost always positive and management decisions are not affected (i.e., colposcopy is needed for these groups regardless of HPV results). "Screen and treat" protocols are often implemented if there is a concern for noncompliance with follow-up and is acceptable for women with HSIL cytology. For women with all subcategories of AGC and AIS except atypical endometrial cells, colposcopy with ECC is recommended regardless of HPV result. Endometrial sampling should be performed in conjunction with colposcopy and ECC in women 35 years of age and older because they may be at risk for endometrial hyperplasia/carcinoma. Women with AGC not otherwise specified in whom CIN2+ is not identified, co-testing at 12 and 24 months is recommended. For women with AGC "favor neoplasia" or endocervical AIS cytology, if invasive disease is not identified during colposcopic workup, an excisional procedure is recommended. In addition to these diagnoses, a diagnostic cervical conization may also be necessary in the following situations: (1) inadequate colposcopy, (2) ECC results are positive for CIN3, (3) there is a high grade lesion on

Pap test not accounted for by colposcopy, or (4) a biopsy suggesting microinvasion. Cervical conizations are also sometimes therapeutic procedures depending on the extent of dysplasia or histologic abnormality.

6. **Therapy and prognosis.** Treatment of CIN is dependent on biopsy results. However, choice of therapy should take into consideration the patient's age, desire for subsequent fertility, and physician experience. No therapy is 100% effective and the risk and benefits should be thoroughly discussed. For CIN 1 preceded by ASCUS or LGSIL cytology, HPV 16/18 and persistent HPV can safely be monitored with co-testing at 12 months. If both the HPV test and cytology are negative, then age-appropriate retesting 3 years later is recommended. After two consecutive negative Pap tests, routine screening guidelines may be resumed. More than 60% of these abnormalities will spontaneously resolve. Repeated colposcopy should be performed if high grade lesions ($\geq$ ASC or HPV-positive) are present on Pap test. CIN2 remains the consensus threshold for treatment in the United States except in special circumstances (i.e., young women aged 21 to 24 with a histologic diagnosis of CIN2,3 not otherwise specified, and pregnant women, etc.). Treatment options (and their respective failure rates) for CIN include: electrocautery (2.7%), cryosurgery (8.7%), laser (5.6%), cold coagulation (6.8%), loop electrosurgical excisional procedure (LEEP) (4.3%), "cold" knife conization (CKC) (4%), and hysterectomy. LEEPs have gained widespread acceptance and use due to the fact that they are well-tolerated outpatient procedures that have diagnostic and therapeutic effects. For CIN2 lesions, it appears that 40% to 58% will regress if left untreated, while 22% progress to CIN3, and 5% progress to invasive cancer. The estimated spontaneous regression rate for CIN3 is 32% to 47%, with up to 40% progressing to invasive cancer if untreated. Management of AIS, however, remains controversial as many assumptions used to justify conservative management for CIN2 and 3 do not apply. For example, determination of depth of invasion is more obscure due to the extension of AIS into the endocervical canal. Furthermore, AIS can be multifocal and discontinuous. Therefore, negative margins on a specimen do not provide assurance of complete resection. Therefore, total hysterectomy remains the treatment of choice in women who have completed childbearing. Alternatively, women who desire fertility should be counseled that observation is an option, although it carries a less than 10% risk of persistent AIS. Should a patient forego conservative management, if the margins of the specimen are positive or ECC at time of excision contains CIN or AIS, re-excision is preferred.

7. **Complications.** Complications following an excisional procedure occur in about 1% to 2% of patients. Acute complications include bleeding, infection of the cervix or uterus, anesthesia risk, and injury to surrounding organs such as vaginal sidewall, bladder, and bowel. However, given that the majority of patients are of childbearing age, the more concerning issues to patients are long-term complications related to the integrity of the cervix and its impact on future pregnancy outcomes. Cervical stenosis after a LEEP has been reported between 4.3% and 7.7%. Not only does this impair complete examination of the transformation zone of the cervix, but it also occludes access to the uterine cavity leading to a hematometra or pyometra. In pregnancy, cervical scarring/stenosis may also inhibit the cervix from dilating normally during labor. Other obstetric complications following a LEEP, although controversial, include: increased risk for spontaneous abortion especially in women with a shorter time interval from LEEP to pregnancy, second trimester pregnancy loss, preterm premature rupture of membranes, and preterm delivery.

8. **Follow-up.** In general, women undergoing observation for CIN1-2 should have Pap tests every 6 months with repeat colposcopy for ASC or worse until 24 months, and then return to routine screening. Unfortunately, many women do not follow up promptly after abnormal cervical cytology. In a retrospective study of over 8,571 women with abnormal cervical cytology, 18.5% were lost to follow-up including 8% of those with HSIL. Follow-up rates were higher for those patients with higher degree of cytologic abnormality (OR 1.29, 95% CI 1.17 to 1.42), older patients (OR 1.03,

95% CI 1.02 to 1.030), and those receiving index Pap test at a larger health care facility (OR 1.13, 95% CI 1.01 to 1.27). For women with CIN1, if disease persists for 2 years, either continued follow-up or treatment is acceptable. For women treated for CIN2-3, co-testing at 12 months and 24 months is recommended. If both co-tests are negative, then retesting in 3 years is recommended, but if any test is abnormal then colposcopy with ECC is recommended. If CIN2 or 3 is identified at the margin of an excisional procedure or in an ECC sample obtained immediately after the procedure, follow-up with cytology and ECC is preferred 4 to 6 months after treatment. Alternatively, repeating the excisional procedure is also acceptable.

9. **Current focus.** New advances in HPV molecular testing are being developed and integrated into diagnostic and preventative strategies. Two HPV vaccines have been approved in the United States for administration to women aged 9 to 26 years. In June 2006, the U.S. Food and Drug Administration (FDA) approved Gardasil (Merck) as a quadrivalent prophylactic vaccine targeted against HPV subtypes 16/18 (responsible for 70% of cervical cancers worldwide) and 6/11 (responsible for 90% of genital warts). This recombinant vaccine is a mixture of virus-like particles derived from the L1 capsid proteins of the HPV types it is targeted against. It is administered IM in three doses at 0, 2, and 6 months. In 2007, a bivalent prophylactic vaccine, Cervarix also became available in the United States. Since their respective debuts, several randomized controlled trials (RCTs) have established their safety profiles and reported efficacy rates that nearly reach 100% against target HPV types when administered prior to HPV exposure. The Future II Study Group performed a combined analysis of four RCTs to assess the effect of prophylactic HPV vaccination on CIN2/3 and AIS (*Lancet* 2007;369:1861). In an intention-to-treat analysis, they noted an 18% reduction (95% CI 7 to 29) in the overall rate of CIN2/3 or AIS due to any HPV type compared to placebo. The Costa Rica Vaccine Trial was a community-based double-blind randomized controlled phase 3 trial of 7,466 women aged 18 to 25 years, who were randomized to receive either a bivalent HPV vaccine or hepatitis A vaccination (*J Infect Dis* 2013;208:385). CIN2+ cases were not significantly different between study groups, and similarly, the proportion of LEEPs done in all HPV-vaccinated women was 5% versus 5.7% in the placebo group with a relative reduction rate of 11.3% (p=0.24, 95% CI: −8.91, 27.8). However, in a subgroup analysis assessing patients who had no evidence of prior HPV exposure, the vaccinated group had a 45.6% rate reduction in LEEPs compared to the controls (p=0.08, 95% CI: −9.34, 73.90).

B. **Cervical cancer: Invasive disease**

1. **Background.** Cervix cancer is the third most common gynecologic malignancy in the United States, with approximately 15,000 new cases and 5,000 deaths per year. Worldwide, it is the second leading cause of death from cancer among women with approximately 200,000 deaths annually. Areas of the world that have implemented screening and treatment programs for preinvasive cervical lesions have decreased the mortality by approximately 90%. HPV infection has been well-established as the underlying etiology for the development of cancer with 70% of cases attributed to HPV genotypes 16 and 18.

2. **Presentation.** The majority of patients with cervical cancer present between ages 45 and 55 years with abnormal vaginal bleeding or discharge, which is often serosanguinous and foul smelling. Late symptoms or indicators of more advanced disease include flank or leg pain, dysuria, hematuria, rectal bleeding, obstipation, and lower extremity edema. Invasive cancer detected by Pap test is much less common. Visually, cervical cancer lesions are exophytic (most common), endophytic, or ulcerative. They are usually very vascular and bleed easily. Biopsies should be performed on all lesions with pathologic confirmation of disease before initiation of therapy.

3. **Workup and staging.** Women with biopsies suggesting microinvasive cervical cancer without a gross lesion on the cervix should undergo a large cone biopsy to fully evaluate depth of invasion. FIGO staging of cervical cancer is clinical and is determined mainly by physical examination, CXR, intravenous pyelography (IVP), cystoscopy,

TABLE 24-8	FIGO Staging of Cervix Cancer

Stage	Description
0	Carcinoma in situ, intraepithelial carcinoma
I	The carcinoma is confined to the cervix .
IA	Microscopic disease. All visible lesions are stage IB.
IA1	Invasion of stroma ≤3 mm in depth, and ≤7 mm width
IA2	Invasion of stroma >3 mm and ≤5 mm in depth, and ≤7 mm width
IB	Visible lesion confined to the cervix
IB1	Visible lesion(s) ≤4 cm
IB2	Visible lesion(s) >4 cm
II	The carcinoma extends beyond the cervix, but does not extend to the distal 1/3 vagina or pelvic sidewall
IIA	Upper 2/3 of vagina, but no obvious parametrial involvement
IIA1	Clinically visible lesion ≤4 cm
IIA2	Clinically visible lesion >4 cm
IIB	Obvious parametrial involvement, but not extending to the sidewall
III	The carcinoma involves the lower 1/3 of the vagina or extension to the pelvic sidewall. All cases of hydronephrosis or nonfunctioning kidney are included, unless they are known to be due to other causes
IIIA	Involvement of the lower 1/3 vagina, but not out to the pelvic sidewall
IIIB	Extension to the pelvic wall and/or hydronephrosis or nonfunctional kidney
IV	The carcinoma has extended beyond the true pelvis
IVA	Involvement of the mucosa of the bladder or rectum
IVB	Distant metastases

FIGO, International Federation of Gynecology and Obstetrics.

proctosigmoidoscopy, and results of cone biopsy (if necessary). CT, magnetic resonance imaging (MRI), lymphangiography, and positron emission tomography (PET) scans are used to guide treatment, but should not be used to change the stage. Table 24-8 summarizes FIGO staging of cervix cancer.

4. **Therapy and prognosis.** In general, all cancers of the cervix can be treated with RT. Specifics of therapy as well as the surgical alternative are as follows: **Stage IA1** may be treated with extrafascial hysterectomy or cervical CKC alone in a patient who strongly desires to preserve her fertility. If lymphovascular space invasion (LVSI) is present then modified radical or radical hysterectomy with lymphadenectomy (LND) or pelvic RT and implants is indicated. The risk of lymph node metastasis is very rare (0.2%) and prognosis is excellent with very few deaths due to disease. Patients with **stage IA2, IB1, and IIA** can be treated with either radical hysterectomy/trachelectomy with pelvic lymphadenectomy or RT; both have similar efficacies. Although controversial, lesions larger than 4 cm (stage 1B2) should be managed with primary radiotherapy except when on a study protocol or if a contraindication to RT exists (e.g., adnexal mass, inflammatory bowel disease, or earlier RT). Surgically managed patients with positive margins, positive lymph nodes, or other high risk factors should be offered adjuvant chemoradiation. Radiosensitivity can be enhanced by cisplatin through the formation of DNA-platinum adducts. Other high risk factors include LVSI plus one of the following: (1) deep one-third penetration of tumor; (2) middle-third penetration and clinical tumor larger than 2 cm; (3) superficial penetration and larger than 5 cm tumor; or (4) tumor larger than 4 cm and middle or deep one-third invasion in the absence of LVSI. **Stage IB2, IIB–IVA** lesions are treated primarily with RT usually

with whole pelvis radiation (5,040 cGy) given as 180- to 200-cGy daily fractions with one to three brachytherapy applications. Patients should be given weekly cisplatin chemotherapy (40 mg/m^2 IV) as a radiation-sensitizing agent. A CBC with differential, basic metabolic panel (electrolytes and renal panel), and magnesium levels are usually obtained weekly prior to administration of chemotherapy. **Stage IVB** is usually treated with palliative doses of radiation to minimize symptoms of pain or vaginal bleeding. Chemotherapy in this setting does not have a significant impact on survival. Recurrent disease is treated on the basis of site of recurrence and previous therapies. Surgical resection (e.g., pelvic exenteration) is often attempted if the disease is central and not extending to the sidewall, as this offers the best chance of cure (50%). Radiation is another option if recurrent disease is outside a previously irradiated area. Alternatively, chemotherapy can also be used although the optimal regimen remains unclear. Single-agent cisplatin (50 to 70 mg/m^2 IV every 3 weeks) has reported response rates of 20% to 30% and is currently the standard with which other agents/combinations are compared. Five-year survival by stage is as follows: IB, 85% to 90%; IIA, 73%; IIB, 65% to 68%; III, 35% to 44%; and IV, 15%. **Adenocarcinoma of the cervix** is treated in a similar manner as squamous cell carcinoma. **Other histologic variants (small cell: neuroendocrine, carcinoid, oat cell; verrucous carcinoma; sarcoma; lymphoma; and melanoma)** are very rare and are beyond the scope of this text (see Suggested Readings).

5. **Complications.** Surgical complications of radical hysterectomy are prolonged bladder dysfunction (4%), fistula formation (1% to 2%), lymphocyst requiring drainage (2% to 3%), pulmonary embolism (fewer than 1%), and operative mortality (fewer than 1%). Complications of RT can be acute or chronic and vary depending on volume, fractionation, and total dose or irradiation. The normal tissue of the cervix and uterus can tolerate high doses of 20,000 to 30,000 cGy in about 2 weeks. However, ovarian ablation occurs with radiation doses of approximately 25 Gy. Other sensitive pelvic organs include the sigmoid, rectosigmoid, and rectum. Fortunately, precise delivery of radiation to target tissues with intensity-modulated radiation therapy reduces damage to surrounding organs. Nonetheless, acute complications of RT are inflammatory and include cystitis, hematuria, proctitis with tenesmus and diarrhea, as well as enteritis with nausea. Chronic RT complications result from obliterative endarteritis that leads to fibrosis and necrosis of normal tissues. They include, but are not limited to, serious small and large bowel injury (3% to 4%) including bowel obstruction, chronic diarrhea, fecal incontinence, and fistula formation; ureteral or urethral stricture, decreased bladder capacity, hematuria, and urinary fistula formation (2%). Sexual dysfunction is common in up to 60% of women and may include vaginal stenosis, shortening of the vagina, dyspareunia, and decreased orgasm.

6. **Follow-up.** More than one-third of treated patients will have disease recurrence and 80% of them will recur within 2 years of therapy completion. Patients should be seen every 3 months for the first year, every 3 to 4 months for the second year, every 6 months for third to fifth year, and then at 6- to 12-month intervals. Screening CXR, CT, or PET may be useful in evaluating symptomatic or high risk patients. We recommend considering PET at 3, 9, 15, 21 months and then annually for 5 years. During the office visit special attention should be paid to weight loss, abdominal pain, leg pain, and lower extremity edema. Examination should include a complete physical examination including palpation of supraclavicular and inguinal lymph nodes, a bimanual pelvic exam, a Pap test, and rectovaginal exam. The presence of nodularity of the cervix, vagina, or rectum should prompt biopsies.

7. **Current focus.** Multiple chemotherapeutic agents and combinations including cisplatin, carboplatin, liposomal doxorubicin, bevacizumab, topotecan, ifosfamide, and paclitaxel have been investigated for advanced stage, recurrent, or progressive disease, as these patients typically do very poorly. More recently there have been advances using targeted, biologic therapy with bevacizumab. In a four-armed, phase III trial, GOG 240 randomized 452 women with recurrent or metastatic cervical cancer to one

of two chemotherapy regimens alone or combined with 15 mg/kg of bevacizumab. The chemotherapy regiments were (1) cisplatin (50 mg/m^2) plus paclitaxel (135 to 175 mg/m^2); and (2) topotecan (0.75 mg/m^2 days 1 to 3) plus paclitaxel (175 mg/m^2 day 1). At median follow-up of 20.8 months, OS with bevacizumab plus chemotherapy was 17 months versus 13.3 months with chemotherapy alone (HR = 0.71, 95% CI 0.54 to 0.94, p = 0.0035). PFS was 8.2 months for those who received bevacizumab versus 5.9 months for those who received chemotherapy alone (ClinicalTrials.gov identifier: NCT00803062).

III. VULVAR CANCER

A. **Background.** Vulvar cancer is the fourth most common gynecologic malignancy with fewer than 3,000 cases diagnosed annually in the United States. Classically, vulvar cancer has been a disease of elderly women, with peak incidence occurring between ages 65 and 75 years, but there appears to be a bimodal age distribution. There is an increasing incidence of younger patients presenting with early-stage vulvar cancer, which often arises from HPV-related preinvasive disease (e.g., chronic vulvar dystrophies such as lichen sclerosis) and is associated with a history of tobacco use. Although not well-understood, other etiologic factors include environmental/industrial toxins, chronic irritants, and chronic infections. Knowledge of the anatomy of the vulva with special attention to the lymphatic drainage is vital to understanding disease progression.

B. **Presentation.** The vast majority of patients are first seen with complaints of vulvar pruritus or a mass on the vulva, primarily arising from the labia majora. Other common symptoms of vulvar cancer include pain (23%), bleeding (14%), ulceration (14%), dysuria (10%), discharge (8%), and presence of a groin mass (2.5%). Significant delay up to 16 months following onset of symptoms has been reported.

C. **Workup and staging.** Biopsy must be done on all suspicious lesions of the vulva, including lumps, ulcers, pigmented areas, and any existing vulvar lesion that displays changes in elevation, color, surface, or sensation; even if a patient is asymptomatic. There are a wide variety of appearances of vulvar cancers: raised, ulcerative, exophytic, white, red, and pigmented. Application of 4% acetic acid solution or toluidine blue to the vulva can help define the extent of some lesions. Colposcopy is only rarely helpful. Biopsy is performed under local anesthesia using a 3- to 5-mm Keyes punch biopsy to sample the worst-appearing areas. Hemostasis is obtained with direct pressure, silver nitrate, or suture ligature. More than 90% of vulvar cancers are squamous cell carcinomas, and the other cell types (melanoma, extramammary Paget's disease, basal cell carcinoma, adenocarcinoma, verrucous carcinoma, and sarcoma) are all very rare.

D. **Therapy and prognosis.** The trend for surgical management of vulvar cancer has become more conservative over the last decade. Classically, resection included the labiocrural fold bilaterally over the mons veneris and across the posterior fourchette with complete removal of the subcutaneous tissue with coverage by flaps or skin grafts. Current treatment for invasive vulvar cancer is a radical vulvectomy (down to the level of the underlying deep perineal fascia and the pubic periosteum) with bilateral groin node dissection (usually through separate skin incisions). Two exceptions to this recommendation are the following: (1) biopsy results that demonstrate less than 1 mm of invasion, in which case, a radical excision with at least 1 cm margin should be performed. If the final pathology confirms only microinvasion, the groin lymph nodes need not be sampled; and (2) invasive lesions (larger than 1 mm) that are less than 2 cm in diameter and more than 2 cm from the midline may be staged with ipsilateral groin node dissection alone. FIGO staging is summarized in Table 24-9. Surgical resection in patients with pathologically negative groin nodes is curative in more than 90% of patients. More than half of all patients with positive groin nodes will die of their disease. Currently it is recommended that patients with two or more positive groin nodes undergo inguinal and pelvic irradiation after primary surgery.

E. **Complications.** Radical vulvectomy with inguinofemoral lymphadenectomy, although less invasive than prior techniques in the past, is still associated with increased risks of

TABLE 24-9	FIGO Staging of Vulvar Cancer

Stage	Description
0	Carcinoma in situ, intraepithelial carcinoma
I	Tumor is confined to the vulva/perineum
IA	Lesion ≤2 cm in size with stromal invasion ≤1 mm*, no nodal metastasis
IA1	Lesion >2 cm in size with stromal invasion >1 mm, no nodal metastasis
IA2	Measured invasion of stroma >3 mm and ≤5 mm in depth, and ≤7 mm width
II	Tumor of any size with extension to adjacent perineal structures (1/3 lower urethra, 1/3 lower vagina, anus)
III	Tumor of any size with or without extension to adjacent perineal structures (1/3 lower urethra, 1/3 lower vagina, anus) with positive inguinofemoral lymph nodes
IIIA(i)	With 1 lymph node metastasis (≥5 mm), or
IIIA(ii)	1–2 lymph node metastasis(es) (<5 mm)
IIIB(i)	With ≥2 lymph node metastases (≥5 mm), or
IIIB(ii)	≥3 lymph node metastases (<5 mm)
IIIC	With positive nodes with extracapsular spread
IV	Tumor invades other regional (2/3 upper urethra, 2/3 upper vagina), or distant structures
IVAi	Tumor invades upper urethra and/or vaginal mucosa, bladder mucosa, rectal mucosa, or fixed to pelvic bone, or
IVAii	Fixed or ulcerated inguinofemoral lymph nodes

FIGO, International Federation of Gynecology and Obstetrics.
*Depth of invasion is defined as the measurement of the tumor from the epithelial–stromal junction of the adjacent most superficial dermal papilla to the deepest point of invasion.

wound breakdown (15% to 20%), infection, and lymphocyst formation. Fortunately, diligent surgical technique and the use of closed suction drain(s) in the groin sites help reduce the risk of postoperative complications. These drains are typically removed when output is <25 mL per day. Inguinal cellulitis, lower extremity lymphangitis, and lymphedema are later sequelae and are related to the extent of groin therapy (e.g., high risk women include those who undergo superficial and deep lymphadenectomy and groin irradiation).

F. Follow-up. Most recurrences (70% to 80%) occur in the first 2 years after initial surgery. Patients should be examined every 3 months for the first year, every 4 months for the second year, every 6 months for third to fifth year, and then at 6- to 12-month intervals. During this period biopsies should be liberally performed on any suspected lesion(s). Sexual dysfunction and disfiguring body image are common concerns of patients after treatment completion and should be addressed during follow-up visits.

G. Current focus. Chemoradiation in the neoadjuvant setting has potential to produce high rates of surgical respectability without the morbidity and mortality associated with pelvic exenteration. However, significant heterogeneity in the chemotherapy regimens exists. GOG 101 investigated the use of neoadjuvant chemoradiation (4,760 cGy to the primary and lymph nodes, with concurrent cisplatin/5-FU) for patients with locally advanced vulvar carcinoma (*Int JRadiat Oncol Biol Phys* 2000;48:1007). Forty-two of 46 patients (91%) completed the chemoradiation per protocol and of these, 38 patients (83%) had resectable disease. Nineteen (50%) experienced recurrence or progression, and 12 of the 38 patients (32%) who underwent surgery were alive and disease-free with a median follow-up of 78 months. With regards to primary treatment for patients with locally advanced vulvar cancer not amendable to resection, the optimal chemotherapy regimen is under current investigation. Specific agents include 5-FU, mitomycin-C, bleomycin, and cisplatin. GOG 205 was a phase II trial of 58 eligible patients investigating the role of primary chemoradiation using RT 5 days per week in 1.8 Gy fractions to a total dose of 57.6 Gy combined with weekly cisplatin 40 mg/m^2 IV (*Gynecol Oncol* 2012;124:529). Twenty-nine women (64%) achieved a clinical response and of this cohort, 22 (75%) continued to have no evidence of disease after 24 months median follow-up.

IV. VAGINAL CANCER

A. **Background.** Vaginal cancers are very rare, accounting for only 1% to 2% of gynecologic malignancies. Squamous cell carcinomas, the most common primary tumors, are most often located on the anterior wall of the upper third of the vagina and are usually multifocal. The specific etiology is unclear, but as with cervical cancer the presence of HPV16 has been associated with up to two-thirds of all new cases of vaginal cancer. Other risk factors include multiple lifetime sexual partners, early age at coitarche, smoking, DES exposure, and prior cervical dysplasia or cervical or anogenital cancer.

B. **Presentation.** Vaginal bleeding, either spontaneous or after coitus, and vaginal discharge are the most common presenting symptoms. Patients may also present with an abnormal Pap test, pelvic pain, dyspareunia, and/or bowel and bladder complaints. Urinary symptoms are common because often vaginal lesions are close to the vesicle neck resulting in bladder compression at an early stage. However, approximately 5% to 10% of women have no symptoms and the disease is suspected on physical examination.

C. **Workup and staging.** Definitive diagnosis is made by biopsy. A patient with an abnormal Pap test who has previously undergone hysterectomy or in whom evaluation of the cervix showed no disease should undergo colposcopy of the vagina with biopsies. In a study of 269 patients with metastatic vaginal cancer, 84% were from genital sites (the majority cervical and endometrial cancer) and the remaining were from the gastrointestinal tract or breast. Staging of vaginal cancer (Table 24-10) is similar to that of cervix cancer in that it is a clinical staging system. Stage 0 or vaginal intraepithelial neoplasia (VAIN) is a preinvasive disease and is graded in a manner similar to that of CIN, from I to III. Patients with invasive disease should be evaluated with a complete history and physical examination with special attention to supraclavicular and inguinal lymph nodes. CXR and IVP are indicated as part of staging. Location and tumor size will dictate the necessity of cystoscopy and proctosigmoidoscopy to complete staging. Alternatively, one may consider a CT or MRI.

D. **Therapy and prognosis.** Squamous cell carcinoma of the vagina is by far the most common primary vaginal cancer and stage-based treatment is as follows: **Stage 0** (intraepithelial disease) lesions have an unclear malignant potential and usually only VAIN III lesions are treated. Often they are multifocal so the method of treatment should be tailored to

TABLE 24-10	FIGO Staging of Vaginal Cancer

Stage	Characteristics
0	Carcinoma in situ (intraepithelial carcinoma)
I	Carcinoma is limited to the vaginal mucosa
II	Carcinoma has involved the subvaginal tissue, but has not extended into the pelvic wall
III	Carcinoma has extended into the pelvic wall
IV	Carcinoma extension with involvement of the mucosa of the bladder or rectum or extension beyond the true pelvis
IVA	Spread to adjacent organs or direct extension beyond the true pelvis
IVB	Spread to distant organs

FIGO, International Federation of Gynecology and Obstetrics.

the patient's presentation. Simple surgical excision and/or ablation (laser vaporization, cryotherapy) are most often used. However, topical treatments are reasonable alternatives—imiquimod applied three times per week for approximately 8 weeks and topical 5-fluorouracil (5-FU) 5 g intravaginally at nighttime for 5 days repeated every 2 to 3 months. 5-FU is generally not as well-tolerated as a topical imiquimod due to significant irritation and burning. All invasive lesions (**stage I to IV**) can be treated with some form of RT. However, surgical management is an option for lesions 0.5 cm or less, particularly in the upper vagina. Lesions that are thicker than 0.5 cm should undergo radical hysterectomy, upper vaginectomy, and bilateral pelvic lymphadenectomy. For those who have had a prior hysterectomy, pelvic external-beam radiotherapy and interstitial implants are commonly used. Lesions of the lower one-third of the vagina, although staged similarly to upper vaginal lesions, clinically behave more like vulvar carcinomas. Therefore, bilateral inguinal–femoral lymphadenectomy is recommended. Patients may also receive RT tailored to specific lesion(s). Options include brachytherapy alone (tandem and ovoids, intracavitary vaginal cylinder, or interstitial implants) or in conjunction with external-beam radiation to treat pelvic and/or inguinal lymph nodes. **Stage II to IV** lesions are usually treated first with external-beam radiation (5,000 to 6,000 cGy) to treat the pelvic lymph nodes and to shrink the primary tumor, allowing easier application of brachytherapy with interstitial needles. Actuarial disease-free 10-year survival in patients treated with definitive irradiation by stage at our institution is as follows: I, 75%; II, 49%; III, 32%; and IV, 10%. Most study participants received interstitial or intracavitary therapy or both; however, the addition of external-beam irradiation did not significantly improve survival or tumor control. **Clear cell adenocarcinomas, melanomas, rhabdomyosarcomas,** and **endodermal sinus tumors** are rare tumors of the vagina and are beyond the scope of this text—refer to Suggested Readings.

E. **Complications.** Major complications of therapy (primarily radiation) are seen in 10%- to 15% of patients and are directly related to the dose of radiation. Vaginal stenosis, fistulas (large or small bowel, bladder, and ureteral), bowel and ureteral obstruction, and bowel perforation are not uncommon.

F. **Follow-up.** Patients are usually seen every 3 to 6 months for the first 2 years after therapy and then annually. Patient should be evaluated with pelvic examination and Pap test. Vaginal colposcopy and biopsy are indicated for any suspicious lesion(s). As in vulvar cancer, sexual dysfunction and disfiguring body image are common concerns of patients after treatment completion and should be addressed during follow-up visits. Recurrences can be treated successfully with pelvic exenteration.

G. **Current focus.** Due to comparable epidemiologic and histologic findings between carcinoma of the cervix and vagina, the two cancers are often treated in a similar manner. To this end, our institution was interested in studying the utility and effectiveness of PET scan to detect primary tumor and lymph node metastases in patients with vaginal cancer. We performed a prospective registry study of 23 consecutive patients with clinical stage II to IVa. Of the 21 patients with an intact primary tumor, 9 (43%) were visualized by CT versus 100% by whole-body FDG-PET. PET scan was also superior to CT for detecting enlarged groin nodes (4 vs. 3) and both groin and pelvic lymph nodes (2 vs. 1) (*Int J Radiat Oncol Biol Phys* 2005;62:733).

Hodgkin's Lymphoma

Nancy L. Bartlett • Nina D. Wagner-Johnston

I. HODGKIN'S LYMPHOMA

A. Presentation

1. **Subjective.** Classical Hodgkin's lymphoma (HL) usually presents as painless lymphadenopathy in the cervical and/or supraclavicular regions. Isolated subdiaphragmatic lymphadenopathy or organ involvement is rare. Although staging studies reveal mediastinal adenopathy in more than 85% of patients, symptoms of cough, chest pain, dyspnea, and superior vena cava (SVC) syndrome are uncommon, even in patients with bulky mediastinal disease. Systemic symptoms or "B" symptoms, including fevers (temperature greater than 38°C), drenching night sweats, or weight loss (more than 10% of baseline body weight in the preceding 6 months) occur in 30% to 40% of patients with stage III or IV disease, but in fewer than 10% of patients with stage I or II disease. In most series, the presence of B symptoms portends a worse prognosis. Generalized, severe pruritus occurs in approximately 25% of patients with HL, often precedes the diagnosis by months, can be a presenting symptom of both early and advanced-stage disease, and has no known prognostic significance. Alcohol-induced pain in involved lymph nodes is a rare symptom of HL (less than 1%). B symptoms and pruritus usually subside within a few days of initiating therapy. When HL presents in older patients or patients with human immunodeficiency virus (HIV), B symptoms and intra-abdominal and extranodal involvement including lung, bone marrow, liver, or bone are more common. HL should always be considered in the differential diagnosis of fever of unknown origin in an older patient, even without evidence of adenopathy.

   Nodular lymphocyte-predominant Hodgkin's lymphoma (LPHL), which represents less than 5% of cases of HL in the United States and Europe, is often first seen as a solitary cervical, axillary, or inguinal lymph node. In LPHL, the mediastinum is generally spared, and in contrast to the contiguous pattern of lymph node involvement in classic HL, there is no consistent pattern of spread.

2. **Objective.** Although computed tomography (CT) scans and positron emission tomography (PET) scans have replaced the physical examination in staging, thorough examination of all lymph node–bearing areas in patients with HL remains pertinent. Occasionally, small supraclavicular and infraclavicular nodes can be missed on neck and chest CT scans. In addition, chest CT scans do not always include the entire axillae, especially in larger patients. Physiologic uptake in the sternocleidomastoid muscles on PET scan may decrease the sensitivity of this test in the cervical and supraclavicular regions. Identification of all involved nodal areas is especially important in early-stage patients who may receive limited chemotherapy and involved field radiotherapy (IFRT).

B. Workup and staging.
HL is nearly always diagnosed by an excisional lymph node biopsy, although rarely, biopsy of an extranodal site may be the source of diagnostic tissue. Diagnosis requires the presence of Hodgkin's and Reed–Sternberg cells (HRS) within an appropriate cellular background of inflammatory cells. Despite improved diagnostic techniques, excisional biopsies are preferred over core needle biopsies to adequately assess the architecture and the presence of the rare HRS cells. The classification system proposed by the World Health Organization (WHO) classifies HL as either "classical" HL or nodular LPHL. This distinction is essential because LPHL and classical HL have different natural histories, prognoses, and treatments. Immunohistochemical studies accurately distinguish classical HL from LPHL. In classical HL, the large atypical cells generally express CD15 and CD30, whereas other T-cell and B-cell–associated antigens are usually negative. In

contrast, the tumor cells of LPHL are CD20$^+$ (a pan–B-cell antigen), CD45$^+$ (leukocyte common antigen), CD15$^-$, and variably reactive for CD30, an immunophenotype often seen in B-cell NHL. Flow cytometry is not a useful diagnostic test in HL.

Pathologists continue to describe four patterns of classical HL, including nodular sclerosis, mixed cellularity, lymphocyte rich, and lymphocyte depletion. Nodular sclerosis Hodgkin's lymphoma (NSHL) is the most common type (60% to 80%), accounting for most cases of HL in young adults and those with mediastinal involvement. With current therapies, these subtypes have little prognostic significance.

Additional workup after a diagnostic lymph node biopsy includes a history and physical examination, laboratory evaluations, radiographic studies, and in some cases, a bone marrow biopsy. Necessary laboratory tests include a complete blood count (CBC), alkaline phosphatase, calcium, albumin, and erythrocyte sedimentation rate. A significant minority of patients have mild leukocytosis, neutrophilia, lymphopenia, and rarely eosinophilia. HIV testing is recommended. Elevated alkaline phosphatase is common and does not necessarily signify liver or bone involvement. Anemia and decreased albumin are usually seen only in patients with B symptoms and stage III or IV disease.

The Ann Arbor staging system for HL is detailed in Table 25-1. The designation E applies to extranodal involvement, which is limited in extent and contiguous with lymph node disease. Since the inception of the classification system in 1971, subtle modifications have been suggested but never universally adopted. Proper staging requires a whole body PET/CT scan. The mediastinal mass ratio (MMR), defined as the ratio of the maximal transverse diameter of the mediastinal mass to the maximal transverse intrathoracic diameter, is an important prognostic factor and should be calculated in all patients with significant mediastinal adenopathy. An MMR greater than 0.33 by chest radiograph (CXR) or 0.35 by CT portends a worse prognosis and influences treatment recommendations. Traditionally, bilateral bone marrow biopsies were recommended in patients with B symptoms, known stage III or IV disease, or a subdiaphragmatic presentation of stage I or II disease. However, in the age of PET/CT, results of the bone marrow biopsy are unlikely to change the prognosis or treatment strategy and can likely be eliminated as part of the routine workup.

C. **Therapy and prognosis.** The treatment of HL has been a true success story, with approximately 80% of all patients having durable remissions. Current efforts are aimed at minimizing therapy in an effort to avoid both short- and long-term complications. Tailoring therapy based on results of an interim PET/CT scan following one to three cycles of chemotherapy may offer the best approach, yet mature data from randomized trials are not yet available.

1. **Stage I/II classical Hodgkin's lymphoma: low risk.** Early-stage HL is usually considered "favorable" or low risk if there are no B symptoms and no sites of bulky disease, with bulk commonly defined as an MMR greater than 0.33 or a nodal mass greater than 10 cm. With current treatment strategies, nearly 90% of patients with early favorable HL are cured, yet debate continues regarding the best approach to treatment secondary to concerns of late toxicities. Short course chemotherapy, such as with ABVD (Adriamycin, bleomycin, vinblastine, dacarbazine), followed by radiotherapy

---

TABLE 25-1 Ann Arbor Staging System

Stage	Description
Stage I	Involvement of a single lymph node region (I) or a single extralymphatic organ or site (IE)
Stage II	Involvement of two or more lymph node regions on the same side of the diaphragm (II) or localized involvement of an extralymphatic organ or site (IIE)
Stage III	Involvement of lymph node regions on both sides of the diaphragm (III) or localized involvement of an extralymphatic organ or site (IIIE) or spleen (IIIS) or both (IIISE)
Stage IV	Diffuse or disseminated involvement of one or more extralymphatic organs with or without associated lymph node involvement

has been the standard of care for early stage HL adults for the last two decades. In the HD10 trial for early favorable HL, the German Hodgkin Study Group demonstrated no difference in 5-year freedom from treatment failure (FFTF) with two cycles of ABVD followed by 20 Gy IFRT compared with four cycles of ABVD and 30 Gy IFRT (*N Engl J Med* 2010;363:640). Intuitively, less treatment led to less acute toxicity. Longer follow-up is required to determine if the lower radiation dose decreases the known late sequelae of radiation, including second malignancies, cardiovascular disease, pulmonary fibrosis, and hypothyroidism. Of concern, at a median follow-up of 7.5 years, 4.6% of patients in the HD10 trial developed second malignancies, and at early follow-up, there was no difference in the incidence between the 20 and 30 Gy arms. Importantly, eligible patients included **only** those with disease limited to no more than two sites, no extranodal or bulky disease, and ESR <50 if no B symptoms and <30 in the presence of B symptoms. Involved node radiotherapy (INRT) has gradually become accepted as an alternative for IFRT; however, because mediastinal nodes are involved in the majority of patients with HL, most patients undergoing radiation will continue to have at least modest exposure to the heart, lungs, and breasts regardless of efforts to minimize treatment fields.

Omission of radiation altogether may be feasible in carefully selected patients. Chemotherapy alone is particularly appealing in women aged 15 to 30 years, a subgroup particularly susceptible to second breast cancers after mediastinal and axillary radiation; smokers, due to a marked increase risk of lung cancer after mediastinal RT; and patients with a strong family history of cardiovascular disease. Long-term follow-up of a randomized study of ABVD alone versus radiation-based therapy in patients with limited stage HL demonstrated a survival advantage in the chemotherapy alone arm (94% vs. 87%, *p* = 0.04), despite inferior progression-free survival (PFS) (*N Engl J Med* 2012;366:399). While this study utilized an outmoded field and dose of radiation, the finding that chemotherapy was sufficient alone as curative therapy for the majority of patients with favorable disease is still applicable.

A negative early interim PET/CT scan is a strong predictor of prolonged PFS (*Blood* 2006;107:52). The United Kingdom RAPID trial treated clinical stage I/IIA non-bulky HL patients with three cycles of ABVD and randomized PET negative patients to IFRT versus no further treatment (*Blood* 2012;120: abstract. 547). Nearly 75% of patients had a negative PET/CT scan following three cycles of ABVD. The 3-year PFS and OS rates were 93.8% and 97%, respectively, in the 209 PET-negative patients randomized to IFRT, compared with 90.7% and 99.5%, respectively, in the 211 PET-negative patients randomized to no further treatment. These very encouraging results support the use of ABVD alone in patients who achieve an early negative interim PET/CT.

2. **Stage I/II classical Hodgkin's lymphoma: high risk.** The standard treatment for patients with less favorable limited-stage disease, including those with bulky disease, is combined modality therapy. At least 80% of patients are cured with this approach. Standard therapy is four to six cycles of ABVD followed by IFRT. A large cooperative group trial, E2496, for patients with bulky stage I/II HL and good prognosis stage III/IV HL comparing ABVD with the Stanford V regimen plus 36 Gy modified IFRT enrolled 268 patients with stage I/II bulky disease (*J Clin Oncol* 2013;31:684). In the bulky patients, the 5-year PFS and OS rates were 82% and 94%, respectively, with no difference between treatment arms. Randomized trials in early stage bulky HL specifically addressing the role of radiotherapy are not available. In British Columbia, the decision to use CMT is based on the result of an end-of-treatment PET/CT following completion of ABVD. In a retrospective analysis, patients with initial bulky disease and a negative PET after chemotherapy had a 3-year time to progression of 86% without the use of consolidative RT (*J Clin Oncol* 2011;29: 8034). Phase II studies evaluating outcomes of chemotherapy alone in patients with a negative interim PET are ongoing. Outside the context of a clinical trial, combined modality therapy, including ABVD × 4 to 6 cycles plus 30 Gy IFRT/INRT, remains the standard of care,

although for those with a negative interim and end-of-treatment PET, chemotherapy alone is likely adequate in the majority of patients.

3. **Stage III/IV classical HL.** Approximately 60% to 70% of patients with advanced-stage HL can be cured with six cycles of ABVD chemotherapy, the current standard of care. The International Prognostic Factors Project on advanced HL identified seven independent prognostic factors in 1,618 patients with advanced-stage HL (*N Engl J Med* 1998;329:1506). These include serum albumin less than 4 g/dL, hemoglobin less than 10.5 g/dL, male sex, age 45 years or older, stage IV disease, leukocytosis (white blood cells [WBC] greater than 15,000/mm³), and lymphocytopenia (lymphocyte count less than 600/mm³ and/or lymphocyte count less than 8% of the WBC). The International Prognostic Score (IPS) showed that patients at the lowest risk with zero to two high risk features had a 67% to 84% freedom from progression (FFP) at 5 years, whereas those at highest risk with four to seven adverse risk factors had a 42% to 51% FFP. A more recent study evaluating prognosis according to the IPS score among 740 patients treated between 1980 and 2010 showed more favorable outcomes compared with the initial publication, with 5-year PFS rates of 81% for lower risk patients (IPS 0–3) and 65% for high risk patients (IPS 4–7) (*J Clin Oncol* 2012;30:3383). Justifying changes to the initial management based on the IPS score are challenging with these narrower range of outcomes. Early interim PET/CT scans may overcome these challenges and allow us to successfully tailor therapy. In the frequently described multivariate analysis by Gallamini et al., PET results following two cycles of ABVD were prognostically superior to the IPS factors (*J Clin Oncol* 2007;25:3746).

The German Hodgkin's Study Group continues to advocate the more intense regimen of dose-escalated (esc)BEACOPP (bleomycin, etoposide, doxorubicin [Adriamycin], cyclophosphamide, vincristine, procarbazine, and prednisone) for patients with advanced-stage HL (Table 25-2). Ten-year follow-up of the randomized trial comparing COPP/ABVD with escBEACOPP chemotherapy demonstrated FFTF of 64% versus 82% and OS of 75% versus 86%, respectively (*J Clin Oncol* 2009;27:4548–54). Despite these encouraging results, many oncologists are reluctant to recommend escBEACOPP because of toxicity concerns. escBEACOPP results in azoospermia and infertility in the majority of male patients and in premature menopause in the majority of female patients over the age of 30 years. Eight cycles of escBEACOPP were associated with a 20% incidence of grade 3–4 infections and a 3% risk of secondary acute leukemia. However, a randomized trial of six versus eight cycles showed a more

TABLE 25-2 Chemotherapeutic Regimens

ABVD

Doxorubicin	25	mg/m²i.v.	d1, 15
Bleomycin	10	mg/m²i.v.	d1, 15
Vinblastine	6	mg/m²i.v.	d1, 15
Dacarbazine	375	mg/m²i.v.	d1, 15
Cycles are repeated every 28 days			

Escalated BEACOPP

Bleomycin	10	mg/m²i.v.	d8
Etoposide	200	mg/m²i.v.	d1–3
Doxorubicin (Adriamycin)	25	mg/m²i.v.	d1
Cyclophosphamide	1,250	mg/m²i.v.	d1
Vincristine	1.4	mg/m²i.v.	d1 (max, 2 mg)
Procarbazine	100	mg/m²p.o.	d1–7
Prednisone	40	mg/m²p.o.	d1–14
G-CSF	5	mcg/kg s.c.	d8+
Cycles are repeated every 21 days			

G-CSF, granulocyte–colony-stimulating factor.

favorable toxicity profile with fewer cycles, with a lower incidence of leukemia and myelodysplastic syndrome (0.3% vs. 2.8%) (*Lancet* 2012;379:1791). These added toxicities may be acceptable in the highest risk patients if improved overall survival (OS) rates can be confirmed. Ideally, we will be able to tailor therapy more effectively in the future by escalating to more toxic therapy in the small subset of patients with early positive interim PET.

4. **LPHL.** Nodular LPHL is characterized by its indolent nature and favorable prognosis. Nearly 80% of patients present with early stage disease. Ten-year PFS rates of 85% (stage I) and 61% (stage II) and OS rates of 94% (stage I) and 97% (stage II) were described in a single-institution study of over 100 patients treated between 1970 and 2005 (*J Clin Oncol* 2010;28:136). Deaths due to disease are rare with the majority of deaths being potentially treatment-related, primarily cardiac disease and second malignancies. Of note, patients with LPHL are at risk of transformation to diffuse large B-cell lymphoma, especially in the setting of intra-abdominal disease. Most physicians currently recommend either observation following resection or IFRT alone for treatment of early-stage LPHL. Because most patients are first seen with stage I disease in the neck, axilla, or groin, exposure of normal tissues is relatively limited with IFRT. Treatment for the rare patient with stage III to IV disease continues to be chemotherapy usually in combination with rituximab (*Blood* 2013;122:4288). While some advocate the use of standard HL regimens such as ABVD, outstanding results have been reported with R-CHOP chemotherapy.

5. **Recurrent Hodgkin's lymphoma.** All patients younger than 70 years who relapse after chemotherapy or combined modality therapy should be considered for autologous hematopoietic cell transplant (HCT). Initially patients should receive one of several effective salvage regimens for two to four cycles to reduce tumor burden. Non–cross-resistant regimens such as ESHAP (etoposide, methylprednisolone, high-dose cytarabine, cisplatin) and ICE (ifosfamide, carboplatin, etoposide) are associated with response rates of 73% to 88% in relapsed HL. Treatment with GND (gemcitabine, vinorelbine, and liposomal doxorubicin) is a reasonable salvage regimen for non-transplant candidates or those not responding to platinum-based salvage regimens.

High dose chemotherapy with HCT is associated with PFS rates of 40% to 50%. Salvage therapy is most likely to be successful in patients whose initial remission is longer than 12 months, whose relapse is confined to limited sites including no bone marrow or pulmonary involvement at relapse, and who are without constitutional symptoms. The best approach for patients with favorable early-stage disease, treated with chemotherapy alone, who relapse in initial sites of disease must still be determined. Radiation or standard-dose salvage chemotherapy followed by radiation may be adequate in patients with a first remission lasting more than 12 months and relapse limited to the initial site(s) of disease with HCT reserved for second relapse.

Brentuximab vedotin, an anti-CD30 antibody conjugated to a potent microtubule inhibitor, monomethyl auristatin E (MMAE), is approved for patients with relapsed or refractory HL following at least two prior lines of treatment. In a pivotal phase II trial, brentuximab vedotin had an overall response rate of 75%, with a median PFS of 5.6 months (*J Clin Oncol* 2012;30:2183). Among the 34% of patients who achieved a complete response, the median duration of response was 20.5 months. Retreatment with brentuximab vedotin in previously responding patients is an effective option, with a recent report describing a 60% ORR with 30% CR (*J Hematol Oncol* 2014;7:1).

Patients who relapse after treatment with brentuximab vedotin are candidates for investigational drugs. In a recent cohort expansion phase I study of 23 patients with relapsed HL, treatment with a PD-1 blocking antibody, nivolumab, was associated with an ORR of 87% and a PFS of 86% at 24 weeks. 78% of patients had relapsed following treatment with brentuximab vedotin and 78% had relapsed following HCT (*N Engl J* Med 2014; Epub ahead of print). A phase II study of bendamustine reported an ORR of 53% with a median PFS of 5.2 months (*J Clin Oncol* 2013;31:456). Modest activity has been described with novel agents, including panobinostat, lenalidomide, and everolimus. Palliation for months or years is often possible with sequential use of single-agent chemotherapy. Vinblastine, chlorambucil, oral etoposide, CNNU, vinorelbine, and gemcitabine have all shown activity in this setting.

D. Follow-up. Seventy percent of all relapses occur in the first 2 years after therapy, and fewer than 10% occur after 5 years. History and physical examination alone detect 70% to 80% of all recurrences, with at least half of these identified at appointments arranged by the patient for evaluation of symptoms, not at routine follow-up. A common practice is to perform a history and physical examination every 3 to 4 months for the first 2 years, and then every 4 to 6 months for the following 3 years. A routine annual CXR for the first 2 years detects most of the remainder of the asymptomatic recurrences. Additional routine laboratory tests and radiographs rarely detect asymptomatic recurrences. An annual thyroid-stimulating hormone (TSH) test should be performed in all patients treated with mediastinal or neck radiation. CT scans should probably not be performed more often than annually for the first 2 years after therapy, if at all, and only for evaluation of symptoms thereafter. After 5 years, a history and physical examination should be obtained annually to screen for late complications; follow-up with either an oncologist or a primary care physician is appropriate at this time.

Greater emphasis should be placed on patient education, rather than on routine follow-up testing. Patients should be familiar with symptoms and patterns of relapse as well as signs and symptoms of late complications, including thyroid disease, second cancers, and cardiac disease. Education about the need to minimize sun exposure, avoid smoking, and reduce cardiovascular risk factors is essential. Women who received mediastinal or axillary radiation should be encouraged to do breast self-examinations, and annual mammograms should be initiated 7 to 10 years after completion of treatment. An annual breast MRI should be performed in conjunction with an annual mammogram in female patients treated with mediastinal or axillary radiation between the ages of 10 and 30. An annual low dose spiral chest CT should be considered in current or former smokers starting 5 years after treatment with alkylators and 10 years after treatment with supradiaphragmatic radiation. A cardiac stress test should be considered approximately every 5 to 10 years after mediastinal RT to evaluate for coronary artery disease.

E. Background

1. **Epidemiology and risk factors.** Approximately 9,000 cases of HL are diagnosed annually in the United States. HL has a bimodal age distribution in developed countries, with the first peak occurring in the third decade of life and the second peak occurring after the age of 50 years. Men have a slightly higher incidence than women. There is an association between HL and factors that decrease exposure to infectious agents at an early age, including advanced maternal education, early birth order, decreased number of siblings, and living in a single-family residence. A history of infectious mononucleosis increases the risk of HL two- to threefold and suggests Epstein–Barr virus (EBV) as an etiologic agent. Although 30% to 50% of patients with HL have detectable EBV DNA in the HRS cells, direct evidence of a causative role is lacking. There is a slightly increased risk of HL in patients infected with HIV, but not in other conditions associated with chronic immunosuppression. An increased incidence among first-degree relatives, a significant concordance rate among identical, but not fraternal twins, and linkage with certain human leukocyte antigen (HLA) types suggest a genetic predisposition for HL.

2. **Molecular biology.** The amplification and analysis of genes of single HRS cells has provided overwhelming evidence that at least 95% of HL cases represent monoclonal B-cell disorders. Clonal immunoglobulin gene rearrangements are present in the HRS cells of both classical HL and LPHL.

3. **Genetics.** Cytogenetic analysis in lymph nodes involved by HL is limited because of the low number of obtainable mitoses from lymph node suspensions and the inability to attribute abnormalities to the malignant cells. A specific chromosomal marker of HL has not been identified, but a variety of numeric and structural abnormalities have been found in approximately half of the HL cases analyzed. Gene expression profiles demonstrate that variations in the tumor microenvironment correlate with outcome.

SUGGESTED READINGS

Ansell SM, Lesokhin AM, Halwani A, et al. PD-1 blockade with nivolumab in relapsed or refractory Hodgkin's lymphoma. *New Engl J Med* 2014 [Epub ahead of print].

Engert A, Haverkamp H, Kobe C, et al. Reduced-intensity chemotherapy and PET-guided radiotherapy in patients with advanced stage Hodgkin's lymphoma (HD15 trial): a randomized, open-label, phase 3 non-inferiority trial. *Lancet* 2012;379:1791–1799.

Engert A, Plutschow A, Eich HT, et al. Reduced treatment intensity in patients with early-stage Hodgkin's lymphoma. *N Engl J Med* 2010;363:640–652.

Gordon LI, Hong, F, Fisher RI, et al. Randomized phase III trial of ABVD versus Stanford V with or without radiation therapy in locally extensive and advanced-stage Hodgkin lymphoma: an intergroup study coordinated by the Eastern Cooperative Oncology Group (E2496). *J Clin Oncol* 2013;31:684–691.

Hasenclever D, Diehl V. A prognostic score for advanced Hodgkin's disease. *N Engl J Med* 1998;329:1506–1514.

Meyer RM, Gospodarowicz MK, Connors JM, et al. ABVD alone versus radiation-based therapy in limited-stage Hodgkin's lymphoma. *N Engl J Med* 2012;366:399–408.

Younes A, Gopal AK, Smith SE, et al. Results of a pivotal phase II study of brentuximab vedotin for patients with relapsed or refractory Hodgkin's lymphoma. *J Clin Oncol* 2012;30:2183–2189.

26 Non-Hodgkin's Lymphoma

Nina D. Wagner-Johnston

I. Non-Hodgkin's Lymphoma

A. Presentation

1. **Subjective.** Presenting symptoms of non-Hodgkin's lymphoma (NHL) vary substantially depending on the pathologic subtype of NHL and the site(s) of disease. Indolent lymphomas such as follicular lymphoma (FL) or small lymphocytic (SLL) lymphomas usually present with painless peripheral adenopathy or occasionally with abdominal pain, bloating, or back pain related to bulky mesenteric or retroperitoneal adenopathy. Because spontaneous regressions occur in up to 20% of patients with FL, the patient may describe a history of waxing and waning adenopathy. Most patients with indolent lymphoma feel well at presentation, and B symptoms, including fevers, drenching night sweats, and weight loss, are unusual. MALT (mucosa-associated lymphoid tissue) lymphomas and indolent lymphomas occurring in extranodal sites, most commonly the stomach and the lung, usually have mild symptoms referable to the site of involvement. Indolent lymphomas are uncommon before the age of 50 years.

Many aggressive lymphomas, the most common being diffuse large B-cell (DLBCL), also often occur as painless, peripheral adenopathy without other associated symptoms. Fevers, night sweats, or weight loss occur in approximately 20% of patients with advanced-stage disease. Bulky retroperitoneal nodes are common and may be asymptomatic or associated with mild abdominal pain, bloating, or back pain. Mediastinal adenopathy occurs uncommonly, usually among young women with DLBCL with sclerosis, and can present with cough, dyspnea, chest pain, or, rarely, SVC syndrome.

Primary extranodal large cell lymphomas are common, accounting for 15% to 20% of all large cell lymphomas. NHL should remain in the differential diagnosis of a mass in any organ until pathology is confirmed. Approximately half of the extranodal lymphomas occur in the gastrointestinal tract, including the stomach, bowel, tonsils, nasopharynx, and oropharynx. Other sites include bone, testis, thyroid, skin, orbit, salivary glands, sinuses, liver, kidney, lung, and central nervous system (CNS).

The very aggressive lymphomas, lymphoblastic and Burkitt, are rare in the adult population but can occur with acute symptoms and can be life threatening without rapid intervention. In adults, lymphoblastic lymphomas occur most commonly in young men, and are frequently associated with acute respiratory compromise due to bulky mediastinal adenopathy, and pleural or pericardial effusions. Burkitt lymphomas often present with abdominal pain and occasionally bowel obstruction related to bulky abdominal adenopathy and intestinal involvement.

Patients with HIV-associated lymphomas (usually DLBCL or Burkitt subtypes) often have advanced disease, B symptoms, and involvement of liver, bone marrow, or CNS. A unique presentation of HIV-associated lymphomas is primary effusion, or body cavity–based lymphomas, which are characterized by the presence of NHL along serous membranes in the absence of identifiable tumor masses and with ascites or pleural effusions. Primary effusion lymphomas and CNS lymphomas are extremely rare in patients on appropriate antiretroviral therapy.

Less common subtypes of NHL often have a unique clinical presentation. Examples include, but are not limited to, mycosis fungoides, a primary cutaneous T-cell NHL characterized by pruritic patches and plaques; mantle cell lymphoma (MCL), seen most often in older men with marked hepatosplenomegaly; and splenic marginal zone lymphoma seen as isolated splenomegaly.

2. **Objective.** Physical examination with accurate documentation of the size and location of all enlarged lymph nodes, tonsillar enlargement, hepatosplenomegaly, and skin involvement is important at the time of initial diagnosis in patients with NHL. Comparable physical examinations during and after therapy will allow evaluation of ongoing response without the need for frequent scans. Patients with active, indolent lymphomas are often observed without therapy at diagnosis. Regular repeated physical examinations are essential to allow for intervention before significant symptoms develop. A thorough neurologic examination should be performed in all patients with lymphoblastic or Burkitt lymphoma, looking for subtle signs of CNS involvement. Active involvement of the cerebrospinal fluid, meninges, or brain parenchyma requires a more intensive approach to the CNS.

B. **Workup and staging.** An adequate tissue biopsy is critical to the evaluation and treatment of all patients with NHL. The most recent WHO classification includes more than 35 subtypes of NHL, with B-cell neoplasms representing 80% to 90% of cases (Table 26-1). Optimal therapy requires accurate subclassification. Historically, diagnosis and subclassification required an excisional lymph node biopsy or, alternatively, a surgical biopsy of an extranodal site. Although this is still the preferred approach, accurate diagnosis by core needle biopsy is now a realistic possibility in some cases of NHL, for example, SLL, MCL, lymphoblastic lymphoma, and, occasionally, DLBCL. Lymphomas with a unique immunophenotype are those most likely to be diagnosed accurately with limited material. In patients without easily accessible tissue, it is reasonable to start with a radiographically guided core needle biopsy.

Immunohistochemistry (IHC), now routinely performed in most new cases of NHL, is often necessary for accurate subclassification. Common examples include the differentiation of SLL (CD5$^+$, CD23$^+$) and MCL (CD5$^+$, CD23$^-$), the presence of cyclin D1 in MCL, verification of lymphoblastic lymphoma with terminal deoxynucleotidyl transferase (TdT) stains, and identification of peripheral T-cell lymphomas (PTCL) with aberrant expression of one or more of the T-cell markers CD3, CD4, CD5, CD7, and CD8. Even with the aid of IHC, PTCL can be difficult to diagnose because many have a histologic appearance similar to that of a benign, reactive lymph node and do not have a unique immunophenotype. Biopsies on patients in which the clinical history is suggestive of lymphoma but initial histologic review as well as IHC by flow cytometry or on paraffin-embedded tissue sections is nondiagnostic, should be tested for

TABLE 26-1 World Health Organization Classification for NHL

B-cell neoplasms
    Precursor B-cell lymphoblastic leukemia/lymphoma[a]
    Mature B-cell neoplasms
        B-cell chronic lymphocytic leukemia/small lymphocytic lymphoma
        B-cell prolymphocytic leukemia
        Lymphoplasmacytic lymphoma[b]
        Mantle cell lymphoma
        Follicular lymphoma
        Marginal zone B-cell lymphoma of mucosa-associated lymphoid tissue (MALT) type
        Nodal marginal zone lymphoma
        Splenic marginal zone B-cell lymphoma
        Hairy cell leukemia
        Diffuse large B-cell lymphoma[b]
        Subtypes: mediastinal (thymic), intravascular, primary effusion lymphoma
        Burkitt lymphoma
        Plasmacytoma
        Plasma cell myeloma

T-cell neoplasms
    Precursor T-cell lymphoblastic leukemia/lymphoma[a]
    Mature T-cell and NK-cell neoplasms
        T-cell prolymphocytic leukemia
        T-cell large granular lymphocytic leukemia
        NK-cell leukemia
        Extranodal NK/T-cell lymphoma, nasal-type (*angiocentric lymphoma*)
        Mycosis fungoides[b]
        Sézary syndrome
        Angioimmunoblastic T-cell lymphoma
        Peripheral T-cell lymphoma (unspecified)[b]
        Adult T-cell leukemia/lymphoma (HTLV1[+])[b]
        Systemic anaplastic large cell lymphoma (T-and null cell types)[b]
        Primary cutaneous anaplastic large cell lymphoma[b]
        Subcutaneous panniculitis-like T-cell lymphoma
        Enteropathy-type intestinal T-cell lymphoma
        Hepatosplenic γ/δ T-cell lymphoma

NHL, non-Hodgkin's lymphoma; NK, natural killer.
[a]The classification of acute lymphoid leukemias will expand on the classification of precursor B-cell and T-cell malignancies, incorporating both immunophenotypic and genetic features.
[b]Morphologic and/or clinical variants of these diseases are not listed, for the purpose of clarity and ease of presentation.

T-cell receptor and immunoglobulin heavy-chain gene rearrangements. Cases in which the pathologic diagnosis seems inconsistent with the clinical history should be reviewed by an expert hematopathologist.

Additional workup after a diagnostic biopsy includes a history and physical examination with documentation of adenopathy, hepatosplenomegaly, performance status, the presence of B symptoms, laboratory evaluations, radiographic studies, and, in most cases, a bone marrow biopsy. Necessary laboratory tests include a CBC, liver-function tests, calcium, creatinine, and lactate dehydrogenase (LDH). Cytopenias usually signify bone marrow involvement or, less commonly, hypersplenism. LDH is an important prognostic factor in the International Prognostics Index (IPI). If the LDH is elevated, a uric acid level

TABLE 26-2	Ann Arbor Staging System

Stage	Description
Stage I	Involvement of a single lymph node region (I) or a single extralymphatic organ or site (IE)
Stage II	Involvement of two or more lymph node regions on the same side of the diaphragm (II) or localized involvement of an extralymphatic organ or site (IIE)
Stage III	Involvement of lymph node regions on both sides of the diaphragm (III) or localized involvement of an extralymphatic organ or site (IIIE) or spleen (IIIS) or both (IIISE)
Stage IV	Diffuse or disseminated involvement of one or more extralymphatic organs with or without associated lymph node involvement

should be obtained to evaluate for tumor lysis syndrome. Screening for HIV is indicated for patients with aggressive NHL. The Ann Arbor staging system, initially developed for Hodgkin's lymphoma, is also used to stage NHL (Table 26-2). Alternative staging systems have been proposed but never adopted. Proper staging requires CT scans of the chest, abdomen, and pelvis, as well as bilateral bone marrow biopsies. Marrow evaluation is not always necessary in asymptomatic, older patients with indolent lymphomas if a CBC is normal, as the findings are unlikely to alter management of the disease. PET/CT scans have improved the accuracy of initial staging and response assessment, and are routinely incorporated in patients with aggressive subtypes of NHL. The role of PET/CT in indolent lymphomas remains controversial, although it can be useful in patients with equivocal CT findings and in patients who appear to have localized disease at presentation, where finding additional sites of involvement could potentially alter management. PET/CT is also helpful in identifying areas of suspected transformation, and although it should not replace the role of biopsy, it assists with directing the most appropriate site to biopsy. Patients with lymphoblastic or Burkitt lymphoma should have a lumbar puncture. If Waldeyer ring is involved, an upper gastrointestinal (GI) or upper endoscopy should be considered, given the increased incidence of gastric involvement in these patients.

C. **Therapy and prognosis**

1. **Indolent lymphomas.** The Follicular Lymphoma International Prognostic Index (FLIPI) includes five independent poor prognostic factors, including age equal to or greater than 60, stage III or IV, greater than four involved nodal areas, elevated serum LDH, and hemoglobin less than 12 gm/dL (*Blood* 2004;104:1258). The 10-year OS (overall survival) rate for patients with three or more risk factors according to the FLIPI is 35% compared with 70% for patients with none or one high-risk feature. The FLIPI remains prognostic in the rituximab era (*Ann Oncol* 2013;24:441). Despite the marked improvement in recent outcomes for FL, there is still no plateau in the event-free survival curves with the use of chemoimmunotherapy, and "cures" remain to be achieved.

a. **Stages I or II.** Given the improved sensitivity of staging studies including CT scans, PET/CT scans, and the use of flow cytometry to evaluate bone marrow specimens, the diagnosis of limited-stage indolent lymphoma is uncommon. Observation, involved-field radiotherapy (IFRT), single-agent rituximab, a combination of rituximab and chemotherapy, and combined-modality therapy with rituximab plus or minus chemotherapy with IFRT are all options for patients with this unusual presentation. There are no randomized trials comparing these approaches, and treatment decisions should be based on the site and bulk of disease and patients' age, with the more aggressive approaches being preferred for younger patients and those with bulky stage I and stage II disease.

Gastric and other extranodal MALT lymphomas commonly present with early-stage disease. Gastric MALT lymphomas appear to occur as a direct result of antigenic stimulation from Helicobacter pylori infection. Approximately 80% of patients with gastric MALT lymphoma will have complete regression of disease with appropriate therapy for H. pylori, including antibiotics and proton-pump inhibitors. Long-term studies have demonstrated excellent durability of these remissions, with 80% to 90% of patients remaining in continuous histologic remission (*J Clin Oncol* 2005;23:8018; *Gut* 2012;61:507). For the subset of patients with gastric MALT lymphoma who do not respond to or relapse after H. pylori therapy, or are H. pylori negative, results with IFRT are excellent, with one series reporting 10-year freedom from treatment failure and OS of 88% and 70%, respectively (*Ann Oncol* 2013;24:1344). Other isolated extranodal presentations such as salivary gland, thyroid, breast, conjunctiva, or a unifocal skin site are also effectively treated with low-dose IFRT (30 Gy). Transformation of MALT lymphomas to aggressive, large cell lymphomas occurs in a minority of patients, but can be resistant to therapy.

b. **Stage III or IV disease.** Despite many effective, but to date "noncurative" therapies, there has never been any objective evidence that early intervention versus "watchful waiting" improves OS in asymptomatic patients (*Lancet Oncol* 2014;15:424). A subset of patients with indolent lymphomas will have no indications for therapy more than 15 years after diagnosis. Asymptomatic, older patients with low-volume disease may still be best served by close observation until progression. The current standard of care for patients with indolent lymphomas requiring therapy is a combination of rituximab and chemotherapy. The treatment approach has changed recently, following the publication of a randomized trial showing a significant improvement in remission duration and toxicity profile with bendamustine and rituximab (BR) compared with R-CHOP (rituximab, cyclophosphamide, doxorubicin, vincristine, prednisone) (*Lancet* 2013;381:1203). The newly published BRIGHT trial comparing BR to R-CHOP and R-CVP (rituximab, cyclophosphamide, vincristine, prednisone) demonstrated noninferiority of the BR arm compared with the standard chemotherapy arms (ORR 97% vs. 91%) (*Blood* 2014;123:2944). Longer follow-up is necessary for progression-free survival (PFS) and OS comparisons.

Maintenance rituximab following first-line chemoimmunotherapy is frequently adopted on the basis of data demonstrating improved PFS compared with observation (59% vs. 43% at 6 years); however, an OS benefit has yet to be described (*Lancet* 2011;377:42). Previous studies utilized a variety of maintenance schedules including one dose every 3 months for 2 years, four weekly doses every 6 months for 2 years, four weekly doses at 3 and 9 months after completion of chemoimmunotherapy, and one dose every 2 months for 8 months, although these were tested in the relapsed setting. For upfront treatment, the maintenance schedule with the most data is with rituximab administered once every two months for a duration of two years. No convincing data is available to recommend maintenance rituximab beyond 2 years. The toxicities of rituximab are mild and are limited primarily to infusion-related reactions such as fevers, chills, myalgias, transient hypotension, and, rarely, bronchospasm.

An alternative approach for patients with low-volume disease, older patients, and patients with serious comorbid conditions is with single-agent rituximab administered for 4 weekly doses. The role of maintenance rituximab is more controversial following induction rituximab. However, the low toxicity profile as well as the implications for improved quality of life may potentially justify the role of maintenance rituximab following both chemoimmunotherapy and rituximab alone upfront approaches.

c. **Relapsed disease.** Multiple effective options are available for recurrent indolent lymphoma. If the first remission lasted longer than 1 to 2 years, patients often respond to the same regimen given as first-line therapy. However, remission durations are usually shorter with each subsequent treatment. All of the agents described earlier have activity in relapsed disease. Radiation can be given to patients with local, symptomatic disease. Response rates of approximately 80%

have been reported with radioimmunotherapy (RIT) agents such as Zevalin, an anti-CD20 monoclonal antibody conjugated with the radioisotope [^{90}Y]. Despite the early promise of RIT, the approach is underutilized because of concerns about damaging stem cells as well as the risk for developing secondary leukemias.

An exciting treatment for indolent lymphomas is with targeted agents that disrupt the B-cell receptor (BCR) pathway. Idelalisib, an oral phosphatidylinositol 3-kinase (PI3K) delta isoform inhibitor, was recently approved for the treatment of follicular lymphoma and SLL. Several other agents that target the BCR, including inhibitors of BTK (bruton's tyrosine kinase) and SYK (spleen tyrosine kinase), are under investigation. Lenalidomide, an oral agent with unique immunomodulating properties, has significant activity in follicular lymphoma.

Stem cell transplants are another option for relapsed indolent lymphoma. The only randomized trial of autologous transplant versus standard chemotherapy for relapsed indolent lymphoma showed both a PFS and OS advantage to transplant. Treatment-related mortality rates for allogeneic transplants have decreased significantly with the use of reduced intensity conditioning, but serious complications of both acute and chronic graft versus host disease continue to restrict this approach to patients with short remissions or refractory disease following standard approaches. In the era of having novel targeted therapies for indolent NHL, stem cell transplants are less frequently performed, and their use will likely continue to decline.

2. **Aggressive lymphomas.** Large cell, mantle cell, Burkitt, and lymphoblastic lymphomas compose most of the aggressive lymphomas. Peripheral T-cell lymphomas (PTCL) represent a spectrum of distinct subtypes that also usually behave aggressively. PTCL comprise approximately 10% of all the lymphomas. Standard approaches and prognosis vary for these subtypes of lymphoma and are addressed separately.

   a. **Stage I to II large cell lymphoma.** The current standard of care for limited-stage nonbulky large cell lymphoma is three cycles of R-CHOP followed by IFRT. A phase II study of this approach showed 4-year PFS and OS rates of 88% and 92%, respectively (*J Clin Oncol* 2008;26:2944). Long-term follow-up of a previous trial comparing limited chemotherapy plus IFRT to eight cycles of CHOP alone showed no survival advantage to IFRT beyond 9 years because of an excess of late lymphoma relapses in the radiation arm (*J Clin Oncol* 2004;22:3032). These results have resulted in recommendations to consider six cycles of R-CHOP plus or minus IFRT as an alternative approach, especially in older patients and those with other high-risk features such as an elevated LDH.

   Primary mediastinal B cell lymphoma, a unique subtype of large cell lymphoma characteristically affecting young women, has not traditionally responded well to chemotherapy alone. Chemoimmunotherapy is typically followed by consolidative mediastinal radiation. Because of the rarity of this disease, randomized trials are lacking. However, a small phase 2, prospective study of infusional dose-adjusted EPOCH-R (etoposide, prednisone, vincristine, cyclophosphamide, doxorubicin, and rituximab) without radiation demonstrated outstanding results with event-free and OS of 93% and 97%, respectively at a median of 5 years (*N Engl J Med* 2013;368:1408).

   b. **Stage III or IV large cell lymphoma.** The standard of care for advanced-stage DLBCL remains 6 cycles of R-CHOP. Several studies are evaluating the addition of novel agents that have known activity in a particular subtype of DLBCL (germinal center vs. nongerminal center B cell) to R-CHOP. It seems likely that future treatments will vary depending on the cell of origin of DLBCL. Patients with translocations of C-Myc, and particularly patients with "double-hit" lymphomas (dual translocations of C-Myc plus either BCL2 or, less commonly, BCL6) have a significantly worse prognosis. The best treatment for these challenging cases is unknown. Studies are ongoing evaluating the role of dose-adjusted EPOCH-R.

   Prophylactic intrathecal therapy or high-dose methotrexate should be considered for patients with testicular, orbital, epidural, paranasal sinus, or extensive bone marrow involvement with an elevated LDH. These presentations carry an increased risk of CNS relapse, usually meningeal. The best treatment for prophylaxis is unknown, though cross study comparisons of retrospective studies may suggest lower CNS recurrences with high-dose methotrexate (*Cancer* 2010;116:4283). Patients with primary CNS lymphoma should be treated with specialized protocols using high-dose methotrexate, cytarabine, and rituximab with consideration for autologous stem cell transplant (ASCT) consolidation in eligible patients (*J Clin Oncol* 2013;31:3061). Treatment with high-dose methotrexate combined with whole brain radiotherapy (WBRT) increases the incidence of cognitive deficits and is avoided when possible. WBRT as a single modality is mostly reserved for elderly patients who are not eligible for chemotherapy.

The International Prognostic Index (IPI) helps predict prognosis for individual patients with advanced-stage large cell lymphoma. The presence or absence of five independent poor prognostic features (age older than 60 years, stage III or IV disease, more than one extranodal site, performance status greater than or equal to two, and elevated serum LDH) effectively predicts an individual's risk of relapse and death from lymphoma after standard chemotherapy. For patients treated with R-CHOP, 3-year OS rates according to the IPI are approximately 87% for patients with zero to one risk factor, 75% for patients with two risk factors, and 56% to 59% for those with three or more factors (*J Clin Oncol* 2010;28:2373). The nongerminal center B cell (non-GCB), also known as the activated B-cell (ABC), subtype is associated with a worse prognosis compared with GCB. Immunohistochemistry using Hans criteria (CD10, bcl-6, MUM1) as a surrogate for molecular profiling adequately discriminates the subtypes, with 5-year OS rates of 76% for the GCB group compared with 34% for the non-GCB group (*Blood* 2004;103:275). A revised prognostic tool driven by biomarker expression has not been adopted to date.

c. **Burkitt lymphoma.** Burkitt lymphomas have a poor prognosis with standard R-CHOP chemotherapy, and short-duration intensive therapies are indicated. Most current protocols prescribe four to six cycles of chemotherapy including intensive doses of alkylating agents such as cyclophosphamide or ifosfamide, vincristine, anthracyclines, and high-dose methotrexate alternating with high-dose cytarabine and etoposide. Two-year event-free survival rates of 70% to 90% are reported with this approach. CNS prophylaxis with intrathecal methotrexate and cytarabine is an essential component of therapy. Patients with an elevated LDH and bulky disease should be treated with allopurinol or rasburicase and vigorous hydration during initiation of therapy to minimize the risk of tumor lysis.

d. **Lymphoblastic lymphoma.** Treatment for this rare, highly aggressive lymphoma must include intensive combination chemotherapy and CNS prophylaxis. Most centers now use therapies modeled after acute lymphoblastic leukemia (ALL) regimens including induction, consolidation, and maintenance with a total treatment duration of 2 to 3 years. Five-year survival rates with this approach are approximately 60%.

e. **Mantle cell lymphoma.** Mantle cell lymphoma (MCL) often behaves aggressively and is characterized by multiple recurrences, yet in a subset of patients the disease follows a more indolent path. MCL occurs most frequently in men older than 60 years. Intensive approaches, such as with R-hyperCVAD (rituximab, high-dose cyclophosphamide, vincristine, doxorubicin, dexamethasone) alternating with high-dose methotrexate and ara-C, are associated with longer remissions and survivals compared with R-CHOP and R-CVP, but plateaus in PFS have not been demonstrated. Consolidative ASCT in first remission is associated with a 5-year PFS of approximately 60% (*J Clin Oncol* 2009;27:6101). Treatment with the less intensive regimen of bendamustine and rituximab is associated with a median PFS of nearly 3 years. The favorable PFS and OS rates associated with novel nontransplant regimens along with the availability of several active agents in the relapsed setting have challenged the role of transplant. Maintenance rituximab administration has become standard, although its role following rituximab and bendamustine has not been published.

f. **HIV-associated lymphoma.** Treatment approaches have changed with the advent of highly active antiretroviral therapy (HAART). Previously, most clinicians favored low-dose chemotherapy because studies comparing low-dose and standard-dose therapy showed similar response and survival rates and more toxicity with standard-dose therapy. Such practices are no longer followed. Limited evidence suggests that R-EPOCH is the optimal regimen for HIV-associated DLBCL. Randomized data is not available, however CNS prophylaxis should be considered in all patients with HIV-related lymphomas.

g. **Peripheral T-cell lymphoma.** Optimal treatment for PTCL remains unknown. CHOP is associated with an approximately 30% cure rate. Multiple clinical trials are underway evaluating the role of new agents in combination with existing regimens.

h. **Relapsed disease.** Patients younger than 70 to 75 years without significant concurrent illnesses should be considered for high-dose therapy and autologous or allogeneic stem cell transplantation at relapse. Several effective salvage regimens are available as cytoreduction before transplant, including most commonly ICE (ifosfamide, carboplatin, and etoposide), ESHAP (etoposide, methylprednisolone [Solu-Medrol], high-dose cytarabine, cisplatin), or DHAP (dexamethasone, high-dose cytarabine, and cisplatin). Rituximab is typically added to these regimens for patients with B-cell lymphomas. Recent data suggests that R-DHAP is superior to R-ICE in patients with DLBCL of the GCB subtype (*J Clin Oncol* 2011;29:4079). In patients with chemosensitive relapse, the 5-year disease-free survival (DFS) rate after transplant is approximately 50%, whereas in patients with refractory relapse, it is less than 15%. Allogeneic stem cell transplant should be considered for patients with a remission duration of less than 1 year after initial therapy, refractory disease at relapse, and all patients with relapsed Burkitt or lymphoblastic lymphoma.

Treatment options for nontransplant candidates include gemcitabine, oxaliplatin ± rituximab; lenalidomide ± rituximab (especially for non-GCB DLBCL subtype); and bendamustine ± rituximab.

D. **Complications**
1. **Therapy related.** Most first-line therapies for indolent lymphomas are well tolerated, with minimal risk of severe toxicity. Most patients experience moderate to severe infusion-related symptoms, including fevers, chills, dyspnea, and hypotension, during administration of the first dose of rituximab. These side effects are uncommon with subsequent doses. Rituximab has rarely been associated with reactivation of hepatitis B. Concurrent administration of entecavir for patients with positive antibodies is recommended (*J Clin Oncol* 2013;31:2765).

Potential complications of CHOP chemotherapy include hair loss, a moderate risk of fever and neutropenia, minimal nausea and vomiting if serotonin-antagonist antiemetics are used, peripheral neuropathy secondary to vinca alkaloids, cardiomyopathy related to anthracyclines, and, rarely, hemorrhagic cystitis related to cyclophosphamide. The current American Society of Clinical Oncology (ASCO) guidelines recommend prophylactic hematopoietic colony-stimulating factors for patients older than 65 treated with CHOP (*J Clin Oncol* 2006;24:3187). Another clinical scenario that may justify the use of prophylactic growth factors is a patient with extensive marrow involvement and cytopenias at diagnosis.

First-line regimens for Burkitt and lymphoblastic lymphomas, as well as most salvage regimens for relapsed aggressive NHL, have significant toxicities associated with them, most commonly, severe cytopenias and increased risk of life-threatening infection. Prophylactic growth factors should be used with these regimens. Renal insufficiency and mucositis occur frequently with regimens containing high-dose methotrexate. Cerebellar toxicity, somnolence, and, rarely, coma are reported with high-dose cytarabine, particularly in older patients. These regimens should usually be administered in a hospital setting with close monitoring of electrolytes, creatinine, and fluid balance.

Patients with advanced-stage Burkitt or lymphoblastic lymphoma are at significant risk of acute tumor lysis during initiation of therapy. Patients with an elevated LDH or creatinine are at greatest risk. Complications of tumor lysis include hyperkalemia, hyperphosphatemia, hyperuricemia, renal failure, hypocalcemia, and death. Vigorous intravenous hydration (250 to 500 mL/hour) should be given for 2 to 3 days. Bicarbonate should be avoided. While urinary alkalinization improves uric acid excretion, systemic alkalinity increases the chance of hypocalcemia, potentially resulting in tetany and cardiac arrhythmias. Allopurinol or rasburicase should be given before initiation of chemotherapy and in the case of allopurinol continued for 10 to 14 days. If a high urine flow cannot be maintained, urgent hemodialysis may be necessary to treat and prevent life-threatening biochemical abnormalities.

Therapy-related myelodysplastic syndrome (MDS) and secondary acute myelogenous leukemia (AML) are rare, but are the devastating late complications of therapy for NHL. These complications can occur in patients with indolent lymphomas as a consequence of years of intermittent alkylator therapy. There is also an increased risk of MDS/AML after stem cell transplantation with as many as 12% of patients developing this complication, a median of 4 years after transplant. Most have complex karyotypes with deletions in chromosomes 5 and 7. The prognosis is dismal. Radioimmunotherapy drugs such as Zevalin may also be associated with an increased risk of MDS and AML, particularly in heavily pretreated patients.

2. **Disease related.** Most patients with indolent lymphomas are asymptomatic at presentation and have no significant complications of the disease until the terminal stages. Occasionally, lymphedema related to pelvic adenopathy or hydronephrosis related to retroperitoneal adenopathy can require urgent therapy. Both radiotherapy and chemotherapy are effective modalities in this setting.

Patients with aggressive histologies occasionally have serious disease-related complications, particularly those with Burkitt or lymphoblastic lymphoma. Such complications include airway obstruction secondary to paratracheal adenopathy, cardiac tamponade, paraplegia secondary to spinal cord compression, gastrointestinal bleeding, bowel obstruction or perforation, SVC syndrome, ureteral obstruction, cranial neuropathies, or radiculopathies related to meningeal involvement, and very rarely hypercalcemia or uric acid nephropathy. When these complications occur at initial presentation or first relapse, rapid initiation of chemotherapy is imperative. In patients with late-stage or refractory disease, these complications are often fatal, and supportive care is appropriate.

E. **Follow-up.** The goals of follow-up are to provide reassurance to the patient, to detect recurrent or progressive NHL, and to monitor for long-term complications of therapy. Survivorship care plans provide treatment summaries and guidelines and can be useful when care is transitioned to the primary care physician. Anxiety and depression, often related to fear of recurrence, are common in the early period. Individual counseling, support groups, and occasionally short-term use of antidepressants may be needed.

As described earlier, asymptomatic patients with indolent lymphoma are often observed without therapy. Appropriate follow-up for these patients includes a history and physical examination every 3 to 4 months, and a CBC, LDH, and creatinine level once or twice a year. Patients with significant intra-abdominal disease but no peripheral adenopathy may benefit from an annual abdominal and pelvic CT scan. In addition to close monitoring, patients must be educated to report potential symptoms of progression including new or enlarging lymph nodes, abdominal or back pain, bloating, lower extremity edema, or B symptoms. Because of the recurring nature of the disease, most patients with indolent lymphoma need life-long follow-up with an oncologist.

For patients with aggressive lymphomas who achieve remission with initial therapy, recommendations regarding the optimal strategy have recently been revised to reflect the recognition that the vast majority of relapses are not detected by routine scans and that surveillance scans do not equate with earlier detection and a survival advantage. Most of the aggressive NHL recurrences occur in the first 2 years after treatment, and rarely after 5 years. Sites of recurrence include at least one previously involved site in 75% of cases and only new sites in 25% of cases. A reasonable approach for follow-up of these patients includes a history and physical examination every 3 months for 2 years and every 6 months for the next 3 years, with a CBC and LDH at each visit. Scans should probably not be performed more than annually for the first 2 years, and only to evaluate new symptoms during 3 to 5 years. Routine CT scans might not be indicated at all for patients at low risk for recurrence, including those with no high-risk features at diagnosis.

F. Background

1. **Epidemiology and risk factors.** In 2014, it is estimated that were will be 70,800 new cases of NHL. Between 2002 and 2011, the annual incidence rate of NHL increased by 0.5% per year, which represents a decline compared with the preceding 3 decades. Death rates have been declining on average by 2.7% each year from 2001 to 2010. The incidence of NHL is slightly higher in men than women, and increases exponentially with age. Infectious agents, including EBV, HIV, human T-cell leukemia virus (HTLV)-1, H. pylori, hepatitis C, and HHV8, are clearly linked to the pathogenesis of certain subtypes of NHL. Other infectious agents, such as chlamydia psittaci and borrelia burgdorferi, have discrepant associations, demonstrating variability with geographic location. Additional factors associated with a significant increased risk of NHL include autoimmune disorders, most commonly Sjögren syndrome and rheumatoid arthritis, although it is difficult to separate the effects of immunosuppressive drugs used to treat these diseases and the underlying autoimmune disease. Tumor necrosis factor (TNF) inhibitors have been associated with T-cell lymphomas, most commonly hepatosplenic T-cell subtype. Inconsistent associations have been reported with pesticides, hair dyes, certain occupations, smoking, consuming foods high in animal fat, and receiving blood transfusions.

2. **Molecular biology.** Certain lymphomas have hallmark translocations that lead to unregulated expression of genes, resulting in impaired apoptotic signaling and dysregulation of the cell cycle. Most cases of follicular lymphoma contain a t(14;18) chromosomal translocation, resulting in dysregulation of the bcl-2 gene, one of many important genes thought to play a role in apoptosis. Overexpression of bcl-2 appears to inhibit cell death. Extended cell survival may increase the opportunity of cells to acquire additional genetic defects in growth and proliferation genes. Multiple additional translocations and abnormalities of gene expression have been reported in NHL and are beyond the scope of this chapter. Examples of the better-characterized abnormalities include the t(8;14) translocation in most Burkitt's lymphomas, resulting in dysregulation of the c-myc oncogene, and a t(11;14) translocation in most MCLs with dysregulation of bcl-1, and overexpression of cyclin D1.

3. **Pathogenesis.** Lymphomas represent a large collection of unique diseases that exhibit heterogeneity even within a specific subtype at the genotypic, phenotypic, morphologic, and clinical level. Advances in gene expression profiling over the past decade were key in identifying that distinct subtypes of lymphoma resemble their cell of origin. More recent expansion of sequencing technologies have been integral in our improved understanding of the genetic and epigenetic drivers in lymphomagenesis that are ultimately leading to the development of rational targeted approaches. One of the more exciting advances in lymphoma has been the recent approval of agents such as ibrutinib and idelalisib that target key upstream kinases in the B-cell receptor (BCR) pathway that is well understood to be both tonically and chronically activated, leading to tumor viability and resistance.

G. Current focus of research. Examples of ongoing research efforts aimed at improving therapy include the following:

1. Continued evaluation of targeted inhibitors of the B-cell receptor pathway (e.g., BTK, PI3K, SYK).

2. Development of adoptive gene therapy using anti-CD19 chimeric antigen receptor (CAR)-expressing T lymphocytes for patients with B-cell lymphomas.
3. Development of additional monoclonal antibodies directed at targets other than CD20.
4. Validation of new prognostic indices that build on the IPI by adding biologic factors such as the molecular classification of tumors on the basis of gene expression.
5. Clarification of the role of PET/CT in early interim restaging of aggressive NHL to determine whether outcomes improve for high-risk patients when therapy is adapted on the basis of imaging findings.

SUGGESTED READINGS

Campo E, Swerdlow SH, Harris NL, et al. The 2008 WHO classification of lymphoid neoplasms and beyond: evolving concepts and practical applications. *Blood* 2011;117(19):5019–5032.

Flinn IW, van der Jagt R, Kahl BS, et al. Randomized trial of bendamustine-rituximab or R-CHOP/R-CVP in first-line treatment of indolent NHL or MCL: the BRIGHT study. *Blood* 2014;123:2944–2952.

Rummel MJ, Niederle N, Maschmeyer G, et al. Bendamustine plus rituximab versus CHOP plus rituximab as first-line treatment for patients with indolent and mantle-cell lymphomas: an open-label multicenter, randomized, phase 3 non-inferiority trial. *Lancet* 2013;381(9873):1203–1210.

Salles G, Seymour JF, Offner F, et al. Rituximab maintenance for 2 years in patients with high tumour burden follicular lymphoma responding to rituximab plus chemotherapy (PRIMA): a phase 3 randomized controlled trial. *Lancet* 2011;377(9759):42–51.

Acute Leukemias

Armin Ghobadi • Amanda Cashen

I. PRESENTATION

A. Subjective. Acute leukemia often presents with symptoms or signs related to pancytopenia or organ infiltration. Severe neutropenia (absolute neutrophil count [ANC] less than $100/\mu L$) predisposes to fever and infection, especially in the sinuses, perirectal area, skin, lungs, and oropharynx. Thrombocytopenia is associated with purpura, petechiae, gingival bleeding, epistaxis, and retinal hemorrhage. Anemia can cause fatigue, shortness of breath, chest pain, or lightheadedness.

Less common presenting symptoms include lymphadenopathy, splenomegaly, and hepatomegaly, which occur more often with acute lymphoblastic leukemia (ALL) than with acute myeloid leukemia (AML). Five percent to 10% of patients with ALL have involvement of the central nervous system (CNS), causing headache, confusion, and/or focal neurologic deficits. Monocytic subtypes of AML can infiltrate the skin (leukemia cutis) or gingiva, leading to purple, nontender papules or gingival hyperplasia, respectively. Tumors composed of myeloid blasts, known as *granulocytic sarcomas* or *chloromas*, can involve almost any organ and may precede bone marrow involvement by AML.

A syndrome called **leukostasis** occurs in up to 50% of patients with AML and an absolute blast count (white blood cell [WBC] count × percent circulating blasts) exceeding $100,000/\mu L$. Symptoms include respiratory compromise and CNS manifestations such as headache or confusion. Emergency leukapheresis can be lifesaving. Transfusion of packed red cells may increase blood viscosity and should be minimized until leukapheresis can be performed.

B. Objective. Approximately half of patients present with an elevated white count, and most have blasts circulating in the peripheral blood. Thrombocytopenia, anemia, and neutropenia are due to suppression of normal hematopoiesis in the bone marrow. Hyperuricemia, hyperphosphatemia, and hypocalcemia may indicate tumor lysis syndrome (TLS). Elevated lactate dehydrogenase (LDH) is found in most patients with ALL and many with monocytic variants of AML. Spurious laboratory values associated with hyperleukocytosis (WBC more than 100,000/μL) and blast cell metabolism can include falsely prolonged coagulation tests, hypoxemia, and hypoglycemia. Disseminated intravascular coagulation (DIC) is common in acute promyelocytic leukemia (APL) and is associated with microangiopathic hemolytic anemia, thrombocytopenia, hypofibrinogenemia, elevated fibrin split products, and prolongation of the prothrombin time.

The presence of a mediastinal mass on chest radiograph is suggestive of T-cell ALL. Osteopenia or lytic lesions may be seen in up to 50% of patients with ALL.

II. WORKUP AND STAGING. The recommended workup of patients with newly diagnosed acute leukemia is shown in Table 27-1. A thorough history and physical examination is aimed at

TABLE 27-1	Approach to the Newly Diagnosed Patient with Acute Leukemia

History/examination
    Infection: fever; localizing symptoms, especially sinus, mouth, anogenital, skin, and lungs
    Hemorrhage: petechiae, ecchymosis, epistaxis, oral/GI bleeding, visual complaints
            Symptoms of intracranial bleed, including headache and neurologic deficits
    Anemia: exertional dyspnea, CHF, angina, orthostasis, syncope
    CNS leukemia: headache, confusion, neurologic deficits
    Leukostasis: dyspnea, headache, confusion
    Monocytic leukemia: gingival hyperplasia and/or nontender cutaneous nodules
    Other
        Long-standing symptoms suggest preceding myelodysplasia
        Full siblings, allergies, major medical problems
        HIV risk factors, previous hepatitis
        Previous chemotherapy, exposure to benzene
Routine laboratory testing
    Before treatment: blood chemistry, LFT, CBC/manual differential, PT/PTT, FDP, fibrinogen, uric acid, LDH, pregnancy test, HIV, HLA class I/II, urinalysis, type/cross
    During treatment: CBC daily and blood chemistry/LFT twice weekly
Radiographic studies
    Chest radiograph
    MUGA scan
Procedures
    Placement of central venous access
    Lumbar puncture if CNS leukemia is suspected
    Leukapheresis if leukostasis is present
Management of a febrile patient
    Culture blood, urine, suspected sites of infection
    Inspect indwelling line
    Initiate broad-spectrum antibiotics promptly
        Cefepime or ceftazidine or imipenem
        Vancomycin if line infection suspected
        Allergic to β-lactams: ciprofloxacin or levofloxacin and vancomycin
        Clinically septic: add gentamicin
        Oral or possible intra-abdominal infection: add anaerobic coverage

GI, gastrointestinal; CHF, congestive heart failure; CNS, central nervous system; HIV, human immunodeficiency virus; LFT, liver function tests; CBC, complete blood count; PT, prothrombin time; PTT, partial thromboplastin time; FDP, fibrin degradation products; LDH, lactate dehydrogenase; HLA, human leukocyte antigen; MUGA, multiple-gated acquisition.

identifying the duration and severity of symptoms, evidence of extramedullary (including CNS) leukemia, and presence of risk factors like prior exposure to chemotherapeutic agents. Factors that will impact therapeutic decisions include coexisting medical problems, infection with human immunodeficiency virus (HIV) or hepatitis viruses, and presence of full siblings. Comprehensive laboratory testing can uncover organ dysfunction, TLS, DIC, or infection. It is also important to send a peripheral blood specimen for human leukocyte antigen (HLA) typing, as many patients will be future candidates for stem cell transplantation. A multiple-gated acquisition (MUGA) scan or other test of cardiac function is routinely performed before the patient begins anthracycline containing therapy.

Bone marrow aspiration and biopsy and cytogenetic studies including conventional karyotype analysis and fluorescent in situ hybridization (FISH), multicolor flow cytometry and cytochemistry studies are essential for diagnosis and classification of acute leukemias. Molecular studies using reverse transcriptase polymerase chain reaction (RT-PCR) for FMS-like tyrosine kinase 3 (FLT3) internal tandem duplication (FLT3-ITD mutation), nucleophosmin gene (NPM-1) mutation, c-Kit mutation, and CCAAT/enhancer binding protein alpha gene (CEBPA) mutation have prognostic importance and therapeutic implications on postremission therapy choices in AML. Although recently supplanted by the World Health Organization (WHO) classification, the French–American–British (FAB) classification remains a commonly used system for the description of acute leukemias. The FAB classification relies on morphology, cytochemistry, and flow cytometry to define subtypes of AML (M0 through M7) and ALL (L1 through L3). Application of these criteria requires a thorough examination of the peripheral blood and bone marrow aspirate with enumeration of blasts, which are characterized by a high nucleus/cytoplasm ratio with fine nuclear chromatin and one or more nucleoli. The FAB criteria define AML when greater than 30% blasts are present in the bone marrow aspirate; greater than 20% blasts define AML in the WHO classification. There are a few exceptions. For diagnosis of acute myelomonocytic leukemia, myeloblasts and promonocytes together should comprise at least 20% of bone marrow cellularity. Acute erythroid leukemia is another exception in which >50% erythroid precursors are present in the bone marrow and myeloblasts should account for >20% of nonerythroid cells. Additionally, t(8;21), inv(16), t(16;16), and t(15;17) are diagnostic of AML regardless of blast percentage in bone marrow. The diagnosis of ALL requires demonstration of at least 20% lymphoblasts in bone marrow. Cytochemistry can be helpful in the diagnosis of acute leukemia (for instance, myeloid blasts are positive for myeloperoxidase), but now flow cytometry is the primary method for determining the leukemia subtype. Lymphoid cells are identified by the presence of CD10, CD19, and CD20 (B cell) or CD2, CD3, CD4, CD5, and CD8 (T cell). Myeloid markers include CD13, CD33, and CD117/c-Kit; CD14 and CD64 (monocytic markers); glycophorin A (erythroid); and CD41 (megakaryocytic).

Subtypes of AML and ALL as defined by the FAB system are of limited prognostic or therapeutic importance. The WHO classification, on the other hand, incorporates cytogenetic and clinical features of known prognostic significance. In the WHO system, AML subtypes are organized into four categories: AML with recurrent genetic abnormalities, AML with multilineage dysplasia (often associated with a preceding myelodysplastic syndrome [MDS]), therapy-related AML, and AML not otherwise categorized (Table 27-2). Therapy-related AML and AML with multilineage dysplasia have a generally poor prognosis, and patients with these subtypes may be candidates for early allogeneic stem cell transplantation. In the WHO classification, ALL is categorized as precursor B-cell ALL or precursor T-cell ALL. Burkitt's lymphoma/leukemia is grouped with the mature B-cell neoplasms.

It must be emphasized that cytogenetic studies including conventional karyotype and FISH, and molecular studies for FLT3-ITD, NPM1, c-kit, and CEBPA mutations are crucial for the prognosis and treatment of acute leukemia. Therefore, cytogenetic studies and the above-mentioned molecular studies should be obtained on an initial bone marrow and/or peripheral blood sample. Early recognition of APL (FAB-M3, AML with t[15;17]) is particularly important, as these patients are at risk for DIC, and optimal initial treatment includes all-*trans*-retinoic acid (ATRA; see Section III.B.). Advantages and pitfalls of diagnostic tools commonly used in the diagnosis of APL are summarized in Table 27-3.

TABLE 27-2	World Health Organization Classification of Acute Myeloid Leukemia

AML with recurrent genetic abnormalities
t(8;21); (*AML1/ETO*)
inv(16) or t(16;16); (*CBFβ/MYH11*)
APL (AML with t(15;17) and variants)
11q23 (*MLL*) abnormalities

AML with multilineage dysplasia
With a preceding MDS or myeloproliferative disorder
Without a preceding MDS or myeloproliferative disorder

Therapy-related AML and MDS
Related to an alkylating agent
Related to a topoisonerase II inhibitor

AML not otherwise categorized
Minimally differentiated
Without maturation
With maturation
Acute myelomonocytic leukemia
Acute monoblastic and monocytic leukemia
Acute erythroid leukemia
Acute megaloblastic leukemia
Acute basophilic leukemia
Acute panmyelosis with myelofibrosis
Myeloid sarcoma

AML, acute myeloid leukemia; APL, acute promyelocytic leukemia; MDS, myelodysplastic syndrome.

III. THERAPY AND PROGNOSIS. In the absence of antileukemic therapy, the median survival of newly diagnosed patients is 2 to 4 months. Chemotherapy induces responses in most patients with acute leukemia, although for many patients remission is short-lived. The goal of induction chemotherapy is complete remission (CR), which is a prerequisite for cure. CR is defined as normalization of blood counts (ANC more than $1,500/\mu L$, platelet more than $100,000/\mu L$), with bone marrow aspirate/biopsy demonstrating fewer than 5% blasts. Postremission

TABLE 27-3	Advantages and Pitfalls of Diagnostic Tools Commonly Used in the Diagnosis of Acute Promyelocytic Leukemia

Methods	Markers	Time	Advantages	Drawbacks
Morphology	Dysplastic promyelocytes	30 min	Diagnostic >90%	M3 variant difficult
Immunophenotype	CD13$^+$, CD33$^+$, CD9$^+$, HLA-DR$^-$, CD34$^{-/dim}$	2–3 h	Informative for uncertain morphology, detects CD56$^+$ cases	Specificity, 95%
Karyotyping/FISH	t(15, 17)	48 h	Specific for APL	Quality of mitosis, false negatives
RT-PCR/Southern blot	PML/RAR-α	6–12 h	Hallmark of APL	Qualified laboratory

FISH, fluorescence in situ hybridization; APL, acute promyelocytic leukemia; RT-PCR, real time–polymerase chain reaction; PML, promyelocytic leukemia; RAR, retinoic acid receptor.

therapeutic options include additional chemotherapy or stem cell transplantation. Chemotherapy given during CR can include consolidation (intensity similar to that for induction) and maintenance (reduced intensity administered for 18 to 36 months).

A. **AML.** As stated above, the prognosis for patients with AML is largely determined by the leukemia risk group. Based on cytogenetic profiles, AML is classified into three risk groups. Molecular abnormalities including FLT3-ITD, NPM1, c-Kit, and CEBPA mutations have significant prognostic impacts. National Comprehensive Cancer Network (NCCN) guidelines have included these mutations in risk classification of AML (Table 27-4). Translocation between chromosomes 8 and 21 (AML-ETO, t[8;21]), present in some patients with FAB-M2 AML, and inversion 16, present in most patients with FAB-M4Eo, have a favorable prognosis with chemotherapy alone. Unfavorable cytogenetics, found in 30% to 40% of AML patients, include monosomies or deletions of chromosomes 5 and 7 (–5, –7, 5q–, 7q–) and equal to or greater than three chromosomal abnormalities. Half of patients with AML have intermediate-risk cytogenetics, primarily a normal karyotype. In a large series from the Cancer and Leukemia Group B (CALGB), the 5-year survival rate was 55%, 24%, and 5% for patients with favorable, intermediate, and unfavorable cytogenetics, respectively.

An active area of investigation is the identification of molecular prognostic factors that can guide therapeutic decisions in patients with normal cytogenetics. One such abnormality is FLT3-ITD mutation, which is present in 20% to 30% of all AML cases and 30% to 40% of normal karyotype AML (NK-AML). FLT3-ITD mutation is associated with a high WBC and a worse prognosis. For instance, among 224 AML patients with normal cytogenetics, 5-year survival was 20% for patients with an *FLT3* ITD mutation, versus 42% for those with wild type *FLT3*. NPM-1 mutations are found in 30% of all AMLs and 50% of NK-AMLs. Isolated NPM-1 mutation in NK-AML is associated with higher CR rates and improved DFS and OS, resulting in outcomes similar to good-risk AMLs. However, patients with both NPM-1 mutations and FLT3-ITD mutations have outcomes more similar to isolated FLT3-ITD mutations. CEBPA mutations can be found in approximately 10% and 15% of all AML patients and patients with NK-AML respectively. NK-AML with CEBPA mutation has a better remission duration and OS similar to core binding factor AML [CBF-AML, another term for AML with t(8:21) and AML with inv(16)]. Double mutation of CEBPA (mutation of both alleles) is less common (5% of NK-AML). A recent study showed that OS benefit of CEBPA mutation is limited to patients with double mutations. This study showed the 8-year OS rates of 54%, 31%, and 34% in double mutation of CEBPA, single mutated CEBPA, and wild type CEBPA respectively.

TABLE 27-4	AML Risk Status by NCCN	
Risk status	**Cytogenetics**	**Molecular abnormalities**
Better-risk	inv(16) or t(16;16) t(8;21) t(15;17)	Normal cytogenetics with NPM1 mutation in the absence of FLT3-ITD or isolated biallelic CEBPA mutation
Intermediate-risk	Normal cytogenetics +8 alone t(9;11)	t(8;21, inv(16), and t(16;16) with c-KIT mutation
Poor-risk	Complex cytogenetics (>3 clonal chromosomal abnormalities –5, 5q–, –7, 7q– 11q23—non t(9;11) inv(3), t(3;3) t(6;9) t(9;22)	Normal cytogenetics with FLT3-ITD mutation

C-Kit mutation is another molecular abnormality with significant prognostic impact in AML with t(8;21) and AML with inv(16). The main mutation clusters are in exon 17 and exon 8. C-kit mutations are seen in approximately 20% to 30% of patients with CBF-AML. In good-risk CBF-AML, c-kit mutation increases the risk of relapse and decreases OS, especially in patients with t(8;21). According to current NCCN guidelines, CBF-AML with c-kit mutation is considered intermediate-risk AML.

For more than 20 years, standard remission induction chemotherapy for AML has included treatment with cytarabine (cytosine arabinoside, ara-C) and an anthracycline. The most common regimen combines 7 days of continuous infusion cytarabine (100 to 200 mg/m^2/day) with 3 days of daunorubicin or idarubicin (7 + 3; Table 27-5). A bone

TABLE 27-5 Acute Myelogenous Leukemia Chemotherapeutic Regimens

7 and 3 chemotherapeutic regimen for newly diagnosed AML[a]

Ara-C, 100 mg/m^2/day, as a continuous infusion for 7 days

Idarubicin 12 mg/m^2/day or Daunorubicin, 45–90 mg/m^2/day × 3 on days 1, 2, 3 of ara-C

Administration of additional chemotherapy: Perform bone marrow on day 14 of chemotherapy; if cellularity is >20% and blasts are >5%, administer second cycle of chemotherapy (5 and 2): same doses as above with 5 days of ara-C and 2 days of daunorubicin

High-dose ara-C consolidation regimen[b]

Cytosine arabinoside: 3.0 g/m^2 in 500-mL D5W infused i.v. over 3-h period every 12 h twice daily, days 1, 3, 5 (total, six doses)

Before each dose, patients must be evaluated for cerebellar dysfunction; if present, stop drug and do not resume; one way to monitor cerebellar function is to have patients sign name on sheet of paper before each dose; for significant change in signature, physician should evaluate patient before any further therapy is given

To avoid chemical keratitis, administer dexamethasone eye drops, 0.1% 2 drops OU q6h starting 1 h before first dose and continued until 48 h after last dose

APL regimens[c]

ATRA+ATO regimen:

Remission induction: Daily ATO (0.15 mg/kg) IV, plus oral ATRA (45 mg/m^2) until morphologic CR or for a maximum of 60 days

Consolidation therapy: ATO(0.15 mg/kg) IV, 5 days per week, 4 weeks on 4 weeks off, for a total of 4 courses, and ATRA (45 mg/m^2) daily 2 weeks on and 2 weeks off for a total of 7 courses

ATRA+Chemotherapy:

Remission induction: IV idarubicin (12 mg/m^2/day) on days 2, 4, 6, and 8 plus daily oral ATRA (45 mg/m^2) until morphologic CR or for a maximum of 60 days

Consolidation therapy: 3 consolidation courses consisting of idarubicin 5 mg/m^2/day on days 1–4 (first cycle), mitoxantrone 10 mg/m^2/day on days 1–5 (second cycle), and idarubicin 12 mg/m^2 on day 1 (third cycle). Additionally, ATRA 45 mg/m^2/day is given simultaneously with chemotherapy from day 1 to day 15 during each consolidation cycle

Maintenance therapy: 2-year maintenance therapy with oral 6-mercaptopurine 50 mg/m^2/day, intramuscular methotrexate 15 mg/m^2/week alternating with ATRA 45 mg/m^2/day given for 15 days every 3 months

AML, acute myelogenous leukemia; ara-C, cytosine arabinoside.

[a]From Bloomfield CD, James GW, Gottlieb A, et al. Treatment of acute myelocytic leukemia: a study by cancer and leukemia group B. *Blood* 1981;58:1203–1212, and Bob L, Gert JO, Wim van P, et al. High-dose daunorubicin in older patients with acute myeloid leukemia. *N Engl J Med* 2009;361:1235–1248, with permission.

[b]From Mayer RJ, Davis RB, Schiffer CA, et al. Intensive postremission chemotherapy in adults with acute myeloid leukemia. *N Engl J Med* 1994;331:896, with permission.

[c]From Lo-Coco F, Avvisati G, Vignetti M, et al. Retinoic acid and arsenic trioxide for acute promyelocytic leukemia. *N Engl J Med* 2013;369:111–121, with permission.

marrow examination is repeated 14 to 21 days after starting treatment, and patients with bone marrow cellularity 20% or greater and more than 5% blasts are considered to have residual disease. Patients with persistent disease may achieve a remission after a second, usually abbreviated, course of cytarabine and anthracycline $(5 + 2)$. Sixty percent to 70% of patients achieve a CR after standard induction chemotherapy, with neutrophil (ANC more than $500/\mu L$) and platelet (more than $20,000/\mu L$) recovery occurring an average of 21 to 25 days after the start of therapy. Failure to achieve CR with induction chemotherapy can result from resistant leukemia or early death. Therapy-related mortality increases with age, poor performance status, and underlying organ dysfunction and can be as high as 30% to 40% in elderly patients. Resistant leukemia is associated with a preceding hematologic disorder and adverse cytogenetics, both of which are found more commonly in elderly patients.

Patients will invariably relapse if they do not receive additional therapy after achieving CR. In contrast, postremission treatment can result in a cure rate of up to 40%. Commonly used consolidation strategies include high-dose cytarabine (HDAC) or allogeneic stem cell transplantation. HDAC (Table 27-4) can overcome resistance to conventional doses of the drug, producing CR in approximately 40% of patients with resistant leukemia. On this basis, trials of HDAC consolidation for AML in first CR (CR1) were carried out. The value of HDAC consolidation was demonstrated in a CALGB trial, which randomized 596 patients in CR1 to consolidation with four cycles of conventional-dose (100 mg/m²/day × 5 days), intermediate-dose (400 mg/m²/day × 5 days), or high-dose (3.0 g/m², total of six doses over 5 days) cytarabine. Among patients less than or equal to 60 years old, 4-year progression-free survival was 44% for HDAC consolidation versus 24% for conventional-dose cytarabine. Patients older than 60 did poorly regardless of the type of consolidation they received, with fewer than 20% achieving durable remission. The subgroup analysis of this trial underlines the critical role of cytogenetics for predicting the outcome of consolidation therapy for AML. The estimated likelihood of cure among patients with favorable cytogenetics (t[8;21] and inv16) who received HDAC was 84% versus less than 25% for patients with unfavorable cytogenetics.

HDAC can produce significant neurotoxicity, primarily cerebellar dysfunction and, less commonly, somnolence or confusion. Cerebellar function should be assessed before each dose, and the drug should be stopped if there is evidence of neurotoxicity. A sensitive way to assess cerebellar function is to ask the patient to sign his or her name on a signature record before each dose. Another unique toxicity of HDAC is keratitis, which can be prevented by administration of dexamethasone eye drops, 0.1%, two drops to each eye every 6 hours, from the time treatment is started until 48 hours after HDAC ends. Other potential toxicities of HDAC include an erythematous rash, often worse on the palms and soles, and hepatic dysfunction.

Several trials have examined the role of consolidation with allogeneic transplantation for patients younger than 55 to 60 years with AML in CR1. In these studies, transplantation was associated with improved leukemia-free survival compared with chemotherapy. However, the studies did not consistently show improvement in OS, probably because transplantation is associated with higher treatment-related mortality and because some patients who relapse after consolidation chemotherapy can be salvaged with transplantation. These trials also found that cytogenetic risk group was the major determinant of survival, regardless of whether consolidation was with chemotherapy or transplantation.

The available data from clinical trials allow therapeutic recommendations to be made for some groups. Because 60% to 70% of patients with AML and favorable risk achieve 3-year survival with intensive consolidation that includes HDAC, chemotherapy is the treatment of choice for this group. On the other hand, patients with poor risk have a very low disease-free survival with conventional chemotherapy. For these patients, allogeneic transplant in CR1 is the treatment of choice, if a matched sibling or matched unrelated donor (MUD) can be identified. Optimal treatment for patients with intermediate risk is not clear. Consolidative chemotherapy and allogeneic stem cell transplantation are both accepted postremission strategies for intermediate-risk patients.

When patients with AML relapse after conventional chemotherapy, they generally do so within 3 years. The risk of relapse more than 5 years after diagnosis is 5% or less. For patients with relapsed AML and for those who do not achieve CR despite optimal induction chemotherapy, the only treatment option with curative potential is stem cell transplantation. For patients with an HLA-matched donor, allogeneic transplant is the treatment of choice among those younger than 60. Recent results with reduced intensity regimens suggest that, in the absence of major medical problems, older patients can safely undergo allogeneic transplant. However, relapse is common, and only 20% to 30% of those transplanted in second CR (CR2) are cured. Disease status at transplant (CR2 vs. relapse) and the presence or absence of graft-versus-host disease are the most important prognostic factors.

Because outcomes are poor when patients are transplanted with active AML, an attempt is often made to achieve CR before transplant. Salvage chemotherapeutic regimens for relapsed or refractory disease include HDAC ± an anthracycline, etoposide with mitoxantrone, or fludarabine containing regimens. Participation in a clinical trial is strongly recommended.

Gemtuzumab ozogamicin (Mylotarg), a recombinant, humanized anti-CD33 antibody conjugated to the cytotoxic agent calicheamycin, was approved by FDA in the year 2000 for the treatment of relapsed AML in patients 60 years or older. CD33 is present on leukemic blasts in more than 80% of patients with AML and is also expressed by committed hematopoietic progenitors. When the antibody binds to CD33, calicheamycin is internalized, leading to cell death. Gemtuzumab ozogamicin was removed from the market in 2010 in view of safety concerns raised by a randomized trial.

B. APL. APL is a distinct clinical and pathologic subtype of AML, characterized by a reciprocal translocation between the long arms of chromosomes 15 and 17. The breakpoint on chromosome 17 disrupts a gene that encodes a nuclear receptor for retinoic acid (RAR-α), and its translocation, most commonly to chromosome 15, results in a fusion protein, PML-RAR-α. Detection of PML-RAR-α is associated with a good prognosis. Indeed, patients with APL who achieve CR have better long-term survival than do other patients with AML. Given its unique response to specific therapy, rapid and accurate diagnosis is crucial. It is now commonly accepted that molecular evidence of the PML/RAR-α rearrangement is the hallmark of this disease, as it may be found in the absence of t(15,17).

As soon as the diagnosis of APL is entertained, it is critical to identify and manage **APL-associated coagulopathy**. Five percent to 10% of patients with APL die of hemorrhagic complications during induction chemotherapy, and approximately half these deaths occur within the first week of diagnosis. Consequently, monitoring DIC with twice-daily serum fibrinogen levels and aggressive replacement with cryoprecipitate (5 to 10 units for fibrinogen less than 100 mg/dL) is common clinical practice during the first weeks of treatment of APL. Patients may also require liberal transfusion of fresh frozen plasma. If coagulopathy or bleeding is present, the platelet count should be maintained greater than 30 to 50,000/μL.

APL is categorized to three risk groups based on white blood count and platelet count: (1) low risk with WBC $\leq$10,000/μL and platelet count >40,000/μL, (2) intermediate risk with WBC $\leq$10,000/μL and platelet count <40,000/μL, and (3) high risk with WBC >10,000/μL. Outcomes of intermediate-risk and low-risk APL are similar when arsenic trioxide (ATO) is used in consolidation treatment; as a result, APL is mainly categorized to high risk with WBC >10,000/μL, and low/intermediate risk with WBC $\leq$10,000/μL. Treatment of APL has three phases: induction, consolidation, and maintenance. The goal of induction treatment is morphologic CR. Molecular CR (absence of PML/RAR-α in bone marrow by RT-PCR) is the goal of consolidation.

A distinguishing feature of APL is its sensitivity to ATRA. The advantage of including ATRA in the front-line therapy for APL has now been clearly established in several randomized trials, with CR rates ranging from 72% to 95%, and a 3- to 4-year disease-free survival of 62% to 75%. These studies also found that disease-free survival is improved when ATRA is given concurrently with anthracycline-based chemotherapy. ATRA with an anthracycline, often combined with cytarabine, remains the standard of care for patients with high-risk APL.

In some studies, cytarabine was omitted inconsequently from induction and/or consolidation regimens. Given the lack of randomized trials, long-term results of these trials are needed to clarify the role cytarabine plays in the management of APL. A recent randomized phase III trial (APL0406) compared ATRA plus arsenic trioxide (ATO) with ATRA plus idarubicin in low/intermediate-risk APL. The investigational arm received ATRA plus ATO daily until morphologic CR followed by consolidation with ATO 5 days a week for 4 weeks every 8 weeks for 4 courses and ATRA daily for 2 weeks every 4 weeks for 7 courses. The control arm received ATRA plus idarubicin induction followed by consolidation with ATRA plus idarubicin followed by maintenance treatment with ATRA and low-dose chemotherapy. The CR rate was 100% in the ATRA plus ATO arm and 95% in the ATRA plus idarubicin arm. Two-year event-free survival rates were 97% in the ATRA plus ATO arm and 86% in the ATRA plus idarubicin arm, confirming noninferiority and maybe superiority of ATRA plus ATO for induction and consolidation in low-/intermediate-risk APL. On the basis of these results, ATRA plus ATO and ATRA plus idarubicin are both acceptable induction regimens for low-/intermediate-risk patients, but ATRA plus ATO is often preferred for its efficacy and tolerability.

Maintenance is the final phase in APL treatment. Several studies have shown that the addition of maintenance therapy with ATRA and/or chemotherapy after intensive postremission consolidation is associated with improved disease-free and overall survival. However, many questions remain unanswered. There is controversy regarding the benefit of maintenance therapy in APL patients who receive ATO as a part of consolidation and are in molecular CR after consolidation. Additionally, the optimal maintenance regimen is still unknown. In one study, the combination of ATRA ($45 mg/m^2/day$, 15 days every 3 months) with 6-mercaptopurine ($90 mg/m^2/day$, orally) and methotrexate ($15 mg/m^2/$ week, orally) was associated with the lowest relapse rates, especially for APL patients with a high WBC. An approach for the treatment of patients with newly diagnosed APL is summarized in the algorithm in Figure 27-1.

Initial response evaluation to induction treatment should be done by bone marrow aspiration and biopsy upon count recovery (approximately 5 weeks after the start day of induction). Owing to differentiation effects of ATRA, early response evaluation (day 14 bone marrow biopsy) will be misleading. The goal of induction treatment is morphologic CR. Cytogenetic studies are usually normal at this time. PCR for PML/RAR-α is usually positive at this time and is not considered induction failure. Molecular CR (PCR negativity) is the goal of consolidation treatment; therefore, evaluation for molecular CR should be done after at least 2 cycles of consolidation. Patients who have not achieved a molecular remission at the completion of consolidation should receive salvage therapy (discussed in the subsequent text). RT-PCR should be used to monitor for disease relapse, and the emergence of a detectable PML-RARα transcript is reason to consider salvage therapy.

The two most important factors affecting CR rates and survival in patients with APL are age and the WBC at diagnosis. Age younger than 30 and WBC less than 5,000 to 10,000/μL are favorable prognostic factors. In contrast, several other biologic features such as the type of PML-RARα isoform, additional karyotypic abnormalities, and expression of the reciprocal RARα-PML transcript do not appear to influence outcome. Recent data suggest that the expression of CD56 antigen on promyelocytes is associated with an increased risk of relapse.

Although ATRA is usually well tolerated, some patients develop a unique complication called **retinoic acid syndrome** (RAS). RAS occurs usually early after initiation of ATRA (7 to 12 days) and is diagnosed on clinical grounds. It is characterized by unexplained fever (80%), weight gain (50%), respiratory distress (90%), lung infiltrates (80%), pleural (50%) or pericardial effusion (20%), hypotension (10%), and renal failure (40%). RAS is the most serious toxicity of ATRA and is often, but not always, associated with the development of hyperleukocytosis. Its incidence varies from 6% to 25%, and mortality is variable (7% to 27%). The best approach to predict, prevent, or treat this syndrome

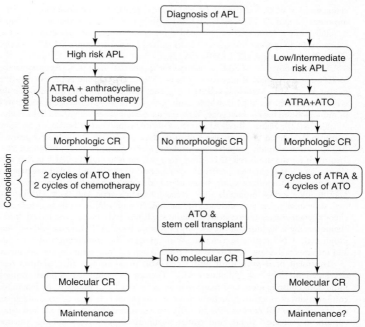

Figure 27-1. Proposed algorithm for patients with newly diagnosed APL (acute promyelocytic leukemia), ATRA, all-*trans*-retinoic acid.

has not been established. Early institution of corticosteroids (dexamethasone, 10 mg i.v. twice daily) simultaneous with cytoreduction (induction chemotherapy or hydroxyurea) is associated with rapid resolution of the syndrome in most patients. Discontinuation of ATRA is common practice after onset of RAS. RAS has not been observed when ATRA was given as maintenance therapy.

Approximately 10% to 25% of patients treated with ATRA-based therapy ultimately relapse. The duration of first CR and the achievement of a second PCR-negative remission after reinduction have been shown to be prognostic determinants. The first choice for salvage therapy is usually ATO. In a U.S. trial, 85% of patients treated with relapsed APL treated with ATO achieved a CR, 91% of whom had a molecular remission. However, most patients will relapse without additional therapy, which may include additional course of ATO, chemotherapy, and/or autologous or allogeneic stem cell transplantation. Toxicities of ATO include QT prolongation, which rarely may lead to torsades de pointes, and APL differentiation syndrome, which is similar to RAS.

Patients with APL who undergo autologous stem cell transplantation while in second remission have a 30% 7-year leukemia-free survival. However, after stratification according to PCR status of the grafted marrow, it appears that patients transplanted with PML-RARα–negative marrow cells are more likely to have prolonged clinical and molecular remissions. In contrast, relapse after autologous transplant is inevitable in patients with persistently positive PCR after reinduction and consolidation therapy. Allogeneic stem cell transplantation may be the preferable treatment modality in this setting.

C. ALL. For ALL, clinically meaningful subtypes are defined by immunophenotype (B-progenitor, B cell, and T cell) as determined by flow cytometry. As for AML, cytogenetics is of critical prognostic and therapeutic value. Translocation between chromosomes 12 and 21 (TEL-AML, t[12;21]), found in 25% of pediatric ALL but rarely in adult ALL, is associated with a good prognosis. Cytogenetics associated with a poor prognosis include abnormalities of 11q23 (mixed lineage leukemia [MLL]) and presence of the Ph chromosome (BCR-ABL, t[9;22]).

Accurate subtyping of ALL is essential for appropriate treatment. Approximately 70% to 75% of patients have B-precursor, 20% to 25% have T-cell, and approximately 5% have mature B-cell ALL. **Mature B-cell ALL** expresses surface-membrane immunoglobulin and is characterized by the t(8;14), which results in fusion of the *myc* oncogene with part of the immunoglobulin heavy-chain gene. Variant translocations involve *myc* and light-chain genes (t[2;8], t[8;22]). Mature B-cell ALL is the leukemic equivalent of Burkitt's lymphoma and is arbitrarily defined by the presence of more than 20% blasts in the bone marrow. B-cell ALL/Burkitt is a rapidly proliferating neoplasm, and treatment is often complicated by TLS. Treatment for mature B-cell ALL differs from that for other types of ALL in that intensive chemotherapy is given over a relatively short period (2 to 8 months) without maintenance chemotherapy. Important components of this therapy include high total doses of cyclophosphamide and/or ifosfamide given in fractions over several days along with HDAC and high-dose methotrexate. Addition of the anti-CD20 monoclonal antibody rituximab to the chemotherapeutic regimen appears to improve CR rate and disease-free survival. Intrathecal chemotherapy is included in the therapy of mature B-cell ALL, because without adequate prophylaxis, CNS relapse is common. With an aggressive combination of chemotherapy and intrathecal therapy, 50% to 70% of patients achieve long-term disease-free survival.

Treatment of **B-progenitor and T-cell ALL** in adults was adapted from regimens developed for high-risk childhood ALL. Therapy is comprised of four components: induction, consolidation, and maintenance, as well as CNS prophylaxis. For induction, combinations of vincristine, prednisone or dexamethasone, L-asparaginase, and an anthracycline result in CR rates of 75% to 90%. Inclusion of cyclophosphamide and cytarabine appears to increase CR rate and remission duration, particularly among patients with T-cell ALL. Standard consolidation therapy includes treatment with several cycles of chemotherapy that include agents used during induction, along with antimetabolites such as 6-mercaptopurine and methotrexate. Several trials have examined the role of intensive consolidation including HDAC and high-dose methotrexate. Patients with Ph+ ALL benefit from the incorporation of a BCR-ABL tyrosine kinase inhibitor (TKI), such as imatinib, into the treatment regimen.

Whereas CNS relapse is very uncommon in AML, in the absence of CNS prophylaxis, the risk of CNS relapse in ALL exceeds 10%; therefore, consolidation therapy has usually included intrathecal chemotherapy and cranial radiation. However, cranial radiation may be associated with long-term neurologic sequelae including impaired cognition. Recent studies indicate that the combination of intrathecal prophylaxis and CNS-penetrating chemotherapy is associated with a risk of CNS relapse similar to that achieved with intrathecal prophylaxis and cranial radiotherapy.

For patients with B-progenitor and T-cell ALL, induction and consolidation usually occupy the first 6 months after diagnosis. Patients then go on to receive maintenance chemotherapy. The most commonly used regimen includes daily oral 6-mercaptopurine, weekly oral methotrexate, a single intravenous dose of vincristine monthly, and 5 days of prednisone/month. Maintenance therapy is continued until 24 to 36 months after diagnosis. With this approach, the likelihood of 5-year disease-free survival is approximately 25% to 50%.

In addition to the importance of cytogenetics in determining the outcome of ALL, presenting white count and age have independent prognostic significance in multivariate models. Another important factor is the rate of clearance of blast cells; patients who achieve CR rapidly are more likely to achieve durable remission. On the basis of data from CALGB, adult B-progenitor and T-cell ALL can be divided into three prognostic groups. Good-risk patients are characterized by all of the following: absence of adverse cytogenetics; age less than 35; presenting WBC less than 30,000/μL; and remission achieved within 4 weeks of diagnosis. These patients have a 50% to 75% likelihood of 3-year disease-free survival with chemotherapy, so that transplant is reserved for relapse. Poor-risk patients are characterized by any of the following: adverse cytogenetics (particularly t[9;22]); for B progenitor, presenting WBC greater than 100,000/μL; more than 4 weeks to achieve CR; and age older than 60. For these patients, 3-year disease-free survival is 0% to 20% with conventional chemotherapy, so that allogeneic transplant is the treatment of choice for patients younger than 60 with histocompatible donors. Older patients may be candidates for allogeneic transplant if they are in good health. Although no randomized trial has been done to evaluate the effect of TKI maintenance after stem cell transplantation for Ph+ ALL, several small studies suggest maintenance TKI results in a better DFS and OS in Ph+ ALL. The remaining intermediate-risk patients represent approximately one-third of all cases of ALL and primarily include patients younger than 60 with B-progenitor ALL. For these patients, chemotherapy is the treatment of choice, because transplantation has not been proven to improve survival.

Most adult patients with ALL will experience disease relapse. Reinduction is most successful if the patient has been in CR for more than 1 year before relapse. Salvage chemotherapeutic regimens can include HDAC, etoposide, or alkylating agents. The ara-guanosine analog nelarabine is active in relapsed T-cell ALL. As for patients with relapsed AML, allogeneic stem cell transplantation is the only potentially curative therapy for patients with relapsed ALL, and eligible patients who achieve a second remission should proceed as quickly as possible to transplantation.

Over the last several years, there have been significant advances in immunotherapy for ALL. The majority of ALLs are pre-B ALL with more than 90%, 80%, and 50% expressing CD19, CD22, and CD20 respectively. Immunotherapy for ALL can be classified to four categories: (1) naked antibody, (2) Bispecific T cell engagers (BiTE), (3) chimeric antigen receptor (CAR)–based T cell therapy, and (4) immunotoxins. Several studies have shown that adding rituximab to induction and consolidation of CD20+ pre-B ALL improve DFS and OS. Rituximab is currently being evaluated in a randomized trial for patients with Philadelphia chromosome negative CD20+ ALL. The investigational agent blinatumomab, a CD19 BiTE (Bispecific T cell Engagers), is one of the most promising new treatments for ALL. It has demonstrated activity in elimination of minimal residual disease and high rate of CRs in patients with relapsed ALL. CD19 CAR (Chimeric Antigen Receptor)–based immunotherapy is another emerging treatment for ALL. Several early phase studies have shown promising results. Several studies using CD19 immunotoxin are in early phase of development.

D. CNS involvement with acute leukemia. Patients with acute leukemia who develop neurologic symptoms or signs should be evaluated with computed tomography (CT) or magnetic resonance imaging (MRI) of the head and, in the absence of a mass lesion, proceed to lumbar puncture. Cerebrospinal fluid (CSF) should be sent for glucose, protein, routine cultures, Gram's stain, cryptococcal antigen, cell count with differential, and cytology. In the absence of contamination with peripheral blood, patients with blasts in the CSF should receive intrathecal chemotherapy, preferably through an Ommaya reservoir. Cranial radiotherapy can also be considered. Intrathecal therapy may include methotrexate, 12 to 15 mg, or cytarabine, 50 to 100 mg. Drugs must be preservative-free and sterile. Cytology and cell count with cytospin differential should be repeated with each intrathecal treatment until blasts have cleared. Intrathecal therapy is given twice weekly until blasts have cleared and then monthly for 6 to 12 months.

The sudden onset of unexplained cranial nerve palsy in a patient with acute leukemia is usually due to CNS leukemia, regardless of whether the CSF shows blasts. Such patients should be treated as described above. Because isolated CNS relapse of leukemia is generally followed soon thereafter by systemic relapse, salvage chemotherapy followed by allogeneic transplant should be considered if patients relapse with CNS involvement.

IV. COMPLICATIONS AND SUPPORTIVE CARE

A. Transfusions. Essentially all adults with acute leukemia will require support with multiple platelet and red cell transfusions. In the absence of bleeding, platelet transfusions can safely be withheld until the platelet count is less than or equal to 10,000/μL. Patients who are bleeding or need a surgical procedure should have their platelet count maintained at greater than 50,000/μL (greater than 100,000/μL for CNS bleeding). Menstruation should be suppressed to reduce uterine blood loss. The threshold for routine transfusion of red blood cells may vary from patient to patient. The policy at Washington University is to transfuse blood to maintain hemoglobin at greater than 8.0 g/dL. However, younger patients may tolerate lower levels, whereas older patients and those who are critically ill may require a higher threshold value for red cell transfusion. Hypofibrinogenemia, usually the result of DIC or treatment with L-asparaginase, should be treated with cryoprecipitate when the fibrinogen decreases to less than 100 mg/dL. All blood products must be irradiated (2,850 cGy), in order to prevent transfusion-related graft-versus-host disease.

Poor response to platelet transfusions may occur when leukocyte contamination of blood products results in alloimmunization. Platelet refractoriness can be reduced by transfusing leukoreduced products and minimizing the number of transfusions a patient receives. Patients with poor increments to platelet transfusions may respond to HLA-matched products. Family members are a potential source of HLA-matched products, although the use of products from related donors may increase the risk of rejecting a subsequent sibling-donor allogeneic stem cell transplant.

An effort should be made to prevent transfusion-related infection with cytomegalovirus (CMV) in any patient who is a potential candidate for allogeneic transplant, as reactivation of CMV after allogeneic transplant can result in life-threatening or fatal disease. To this end, CMV-seronegative patients should receive products that have been collected from seronegative donors. If such products are not available, then the risk of CMV transmission may be reduced by leukoreduction of platelet products. Patients who are CMV seropositive may receive blood products from seropositive or seronegative donors.

B. Infection. Infection is a major cause of death in patients with acute leukemia. These patients are at high risk for infection primarily due to prolonged periods of neutropenia. In addition, indwelling catheters and compromised mucosal barriers (mucositis or enteritis from chemotherapy) provide portals of entry for infectious agents. Because most infections arise from the patient's own microbial flora, rigorous isolation procedures are not necessary. However, good hand washing is always important, and patients should wear a mask when in crowds. Food-borne infection is very uncommon, and it is reasonable to prohibit only consumption of uncooked meat.

Antimicrobial prophylaxis during periods of neutropenia and/or immunosuppression can reduce the incidence of some viral, fungal, and bacterial infections. Acyclovir (400 PO t.i.d. or 125 mg/m^2 i.v. b.i.d.) is recommended for patients with a history of cold sores or herpes simplex seropositivity. Patients with ALL are treated with a long course of steroids and are therefore at risk for *Pneumocystis* pneumonia. They should receive *Pneumocystis* prophylaxis with either trimethoprim/sulfamethoxazole 1 double strength (DS) b.i.d. 2 days/week, dapsone 100 mg daily, or aerosolized pentamidine, 300 mg monthly. During periods of neutropenia or prolonged steroid use, nystatin (15 mL, swish and swallow 5 times a day) or clotrimazole troche (5 times daily) can reduce oral candidiasis. The use of other antibiotics for infection prophylaxis is controversial. Oral fluoroquinolones reduce the risk of infection with gram-negative organisms, but they are associated with an increased risk of gram-positive bacteremia and fluoroquinolone-resistant *Pseudomonas aeruginosa*. Because prophylaxis with systemic antifungals has not been shown to reduce the risk of treatment-related mortality, their routine use during induction chemotherapy is not recommended.

Fever greater than 38.3°C in a neutropenic patient (ANC less than 500/μL) requires prompt evaluation and treatment, as bacterial infections can become rapidly life-threatening. Blood and urine should be cultured, and empiric broad-spectrum antibiotics (cefepime or ceftazidime, 1 g i.v.) should be administered. Vancomycin should be added for the following indications: severe mucositis, evidence of a catheter-related infection, fever equal to or greater than 40°C, hypotension, or known colonization with resistant streptococci or staphylococci. Patients with allergy to β-lactams may receive aztreonam or a fluoroquinolone with vancomycin. Febrile patients with hypotension or respiratory distress should receive at least one dose of an aminoglycoside antibiotic (gentamicin 5 mg/kg i.v.). When fevers and neutropenia persist for more than 3 days and no source of infection has been identified, empiric antifungal coverage can be added (caspofungin 70 mg i.v. loading dose × 1 then 50 mg i.v. qd or fluconazole 400 mg i.v. qd). Febrile patients with newly diagnosed or relapsed acute leukemia should receive empiric broad-spectrum antibiotics whether or not they are neutropenic.

Once antibiotics are begun, they are continued until neutrophil recovery (ANC greater than 500/μL), even if fever resolves. Otherwise, the choice and duration of antimicrobial therapy is dictated by the source of infection. Bacteremia is treated with a 10- to 14-day course of antibiotics. Indwelling catheters should be removed for fungemia, persistent bacteremia, or *Staphylococcus aureus* or *Pseudomonas* bacteremia. Patients with a history of *Aspergillus* or *Mucor* sp. infection should receive prolonged antifungal therapy, especially if profound neutropenia is likely during subsequent courses of chemotherapy.

Typhlitis (neutropenic enterocolitis) is a syndrome of right-sided colonic inflammation in neutropenic patients. It presents with fever, abdominal pain, and tenderness that can mimic appendicitis. The etiology is unclear. Treatment is with broad-spectrum antibiotics, including anaerobic coverage, and nasogastric suction. Surgical intervention is reserved for patients with bowel perforation or suspected bowel necrosis.

C. Growth factors. The use of myeloid growth factors in acute leukemia remains controversial despite multiple randomized trials. Treatment with granulocyte colony-stimulating factor (G-CSF) or granulocyte–macrophage colony-stimulating factor (GM-CSF) after induction chemotherapy shortens the duration of ANC less than 500/μL by 3 to 6 days. The duration of hospitalization and antibiotic use are also shortened by treatment with growth factors. Although the effectiveness of chemotherapy is not compromised by the use of these agents, most evidence indicates that growth factors do not improve the likelihood of CR or long-term survival. Often, growth factors are reserved for older patients or for those with life-threatening infection.

D. Intravenous access. All patients with acute leukemia should have a central venous catheter placed. Temporary catheters, such as the Hohn catheter, are usually chosen because fever, coagulopathy, or poor increments with platelet transfusion represent relative contraindications to placement of a more permanent, tunneled catheter.

E. Tumor lysis syndrome. TLS (see Chapter 35) is a complication of rapid tumor breakdown after chemotherapy. Clinically, it is marked by hyperuricemia, hyperkalemia, hyperphosphatemia, hypocalcemia, and acute oliguric renal failure. Risk factors for TLS include B-cell ALL, WBC greater than 50,000/μL, LDH greater than 1,000 IU/L, renal dysfunction, and elevation of the uric acid or phosphorus before treatment. All patients with newly diagnosed acute leukemia should be vigorously hydrated to maintain urine output at more than 2.5 L/day, and volume status should be closely monitored. If the patient's renal function is normal, allopurinol, 600 mg, is given the day before chemotherapy, followed by 300 mg daily until the WBC is less than 1,000/μL. If the pretreatment uric acid is more than 9 mg/dL, rasburicase can be used in place of allopurinol to reduce the uric acid level rapidly. Patients at high risk for TLS should have electrolytes, calcium, magnesium, and phosphorus monitored two to three times daily for the first 2 to 3 days of induction chemotherapy.

V. FOLLOW-UP. Patients who are in a CR after induction and consolidation therapy require close follow-up. The highest risk of relapse of acute leukemia is within the first 3 years of completion of treatment. During that time, patients should be evaluated with history, physical examination, and complete blood count (CBC) every 2 to 3 months. Bone marrow biopsy should be repeated routinely every 3 to 6 months, or if the blood counts fall or blasts are observed in the peripheral blood. Because patients may have disease relapse at extramedullary sites, suspicious skin or soft tissue lesions should be biopsied to rule out granulocytic sarcoma, and new neurologic deficits should be evaluated by brain imaging and lumbar puncture to rule out CNS leukemia. Molecular monitoring of APL (i.e., RT-PCR for PML-RARα) should be performed every 2 to 3 months for 3 years' postconsolidation for patients at high risk of relapse, particularly those with a presenting WBC of more than 10,000/αL. Relapse of acute leukemia is very uncommon after approximately 5 years, and follow-up can become less frequent after that.

VI. **EPIDEMIOLOGY AND RISK FACTORS.** Approximately 13,000 new cases of acute leukemia are diagnosed in the United States each year. The annual incidence of AML is approximately 3.5 per 100,000 and of ALL is approximately 1.5 per 100,000 persons. Although acute leukemia represents only 5% of all new cancer cases, acute leukemia is the most common cause of cancer death for persons younger than 35 years. ALL has a bimodal age distribution. Most cases occur in childhood, with a peak incidence at approximately age 5 years, and there is a second increase in incidence after 60 years of age. The incidence of AML increases steeply beyond 50 years, and the median age is approximately 65 years.

Fewer than 5% of cases of acute leukemia can be attributed to prior exposure to a leukemogenic agent. Ionizing radiation and benzene are clearly associated with an increased risk of acute AML, with an average latency of approximately 5 years. Two classes of chemotherapeutic agents are associated with an increased risk of acute leukemia (secondary leukemia). Alkylating agents can cause AML approximately 4 to 8 years after exposure. AML that arises in this setting is often associated with a preceding MDS and adverse cytogenetics, particularly abnormalities of chromosomes 5 and 7. Topoisomerase II inhibitors such as etoposide or anthracyclines are associated with AML or mixed lineage leukemia (MLL) with a short (1- to 2-year) latency without a preceding hematologic disorder. The most common cytogenetic abnormalities associated with topoisomerase II inhibitors involve the MLL gene at 11q23. Given the poor prognosis of treatment-related leukemia, allogeneic transplantation in first complete remission (CR) should be considered if a donor is available.

Rare families with a genetic predisposition to acute leukemia have been described, but in the vast majority of cases, there is no clear hereditary risk. However, acute leukemia does occur more frequently in family members than would be expected by chance. Full siblings have an approximately twofold increase in risk, and the concordance rate of infantile leukemias in identical twins has been reported to be as high as 25%. The only infectious agent associated with acute leukemia is human T-lymphocyte leukemia virus (HTLV)-1, which causes T-cell adult leukemia/lymphoma. Congenital disorders that have an increased risk of acute leukemia include Down syndrome, disorders associated with increased chromosomal fragility (Bloom's syndrome and Fanconi's anemia), and those associated with immunodeficiency (X-linked agammaglobulinemia and ataxia telangiectasia).

VII. **FUTURE DIRECTIONS**

A. **Monitoring of minimal residual disease.** After remission induction, most patients with acute leukemia receive several additional courses of aggressive chemotherapy with the goal of eliminating subclinical leukemia. A sensitive and specific technique for detection of minimal residual disease (MRD) could provide important prognostic information, allowing for rational treatment decisions. As discussed earlier, detection of MRD has already an important role in the therapy of APL: detection of the PML-RARα fusion transcript after consolidation therapy identifies patients at high risk for clinical relapse. Monitoring MRD in other AML subtypes is difficult because molecular rearrangements amenable to PCR have been found in a relatively small proportion of patients. Mutlicolor flow cytometry can be used to detect abnormal leukemic immunophenotypes. Monitoring MRD in ALL is facilitated by the presence of clonotypic T cell–receptor gene or immunoglobulin heavy-chain gene rearrangement. Also, BCR-ABL can be followed in patients with Ph+ ALL. However, the role of MRD monitoring and the necessity of obtaining an MRD negative status remain to be defined for AML and ALL.

B. **Identification of molecular prognostic factors.** Although cytogenetics have proved to be extremely valuable for the risk stratification of patients with acute leukemia, there remain a significant proportion of patients who fall into the "intermediate" or indeterminant group. Molecular markers in addition to FLT3-ITD, NPM1, and CEBPA mutations are being sought to distinguish which intermediate-risk patients would benefit from more aggressive therapy such as stem cell transplantation. Mutations in IDH1/IDH2 and DNMT3A can be found in approximately 15% and 30% of NK-AML respectively. The prognostic importance of these mutations requires further studies. Gene expression profiling using microarray technology and whole genome/exome sequencing may better classify patients into risk groups, as well as identify new therapeutic targets.

C. New therapies. Given the high rate of relapsed and resistant disease among adults with acute leukemias, the need for new, effective therapies is significant. Newer drugs for the treatment of relapsed acute leukemia include clofarabine, a purine nucleoside with activity in both AML and ALL and the araguanosine analog nelarabine, which is active in relapsed T-cell ALL. Imatinib and other inhibitors of the BCR-ABL tyrosine kinase have activity in Ph+ ALL and are being investigated as part of upfront therapy or for treatment of relapsed disease. Promising agents for the treatment of AML include the hypomethylating agents azacitidine and decitabine, histone deacetylase inhibitors, farnesyl transferase inhibitors, *FLT3* inhibitors, and the immunomodulatory drug lenalidomide. Many of these new agents are being investigated for the treatment of elderly AML patients, for whom current therapies are particularly toxic and generally ineffective. BiTE- and CAR-based immunotherapy may change the ALL treatment paradigm profoundly.

SUGGESTED READINGS

Advani AS. New immune strategies for the treatment of acute lymphoblastic leukemia: antibodies and chimeric antigen receptors. *Hematology* 2013;2013:131–137.

Burnett AK, Goldstone AH, Stevens RM, et al. Randomised comparison of addition of autologous bone-marrow transplantation to intensive chemotherapy for acute myeloid leukaemia in first remission: results of MRC AML 10 trial. *Lancet* 1998;351(9104):700–708.

Byrd JC, Mrozek K, Dodge RK, et al. Pretreatment cytogenetic abnormalities are predictive of induction success, cumulative incidence of relapse, and overall survival in adult patients with de novo acute myeloid leukemia: results from Cancer and Leukemia Group B (CALGB 8461). *Blood* 2002;100(13):4325–4336.

Fenaux P, Chastang C, Chevret S, et al. A randomized comparison of all transretinoic acid (ATRA) followed by chemotherapy and ATRA plus chemotherapy and the role of maintenance therapy in newly diagnosed acute promyelocytic leukemia. *Blood* 1999;94(4):1192–1200.

Fenaux P, Le Deley M, Castaigne S, et al; European APL 91 Group. Effect of all transretinoic acid in newly diagnosed acute promyelocytic leukemia: results of a multicenter randomized trial. *Blood* 1993;82(11):3241–3249.

Frohling S, Schlenk RF, Breitruck J, et al. Prognostic significance of activating FLT3 mutations in younger adults (16 to 60 years) with acute myeloid leukemia and normal cytogenetics: a study of the AML Study Group. *Blood* 2002;100(13):4372–4380.

Hoelzer D, Thiel E, Loffler H, et al. Prognostic factors in a multicenter study for treatment of acute lymphoblastic leukemia in adults. *Blood* 1988;71(1):123–131.

Jabbour EJ, Estey E, Kantarjian HM. Adult acute myeloid leukemia. *Mayo Clin Proc* 2006;81:247–260.

Jabbour EJ, Faderl S, Kantarjian HM. Adult acute lymphoblastic leukemia. *Mayo Clin Proc* 2005;80:1517–1527.

Jaffe ES, Harris NL, Stein H, et al., eds. *World Health Organization Classification of Tumours: Pathology and Genetics of Tumours of Haematopoietic and Lymphoid Tissues.* Lyon, France: IARC Press, 2001.

Larson R, Dodge R, Burns C, et al. A five-drug remission induction regimen with intensive consolidation for adults with acute lymphoblastic leukemia: cancer and leukemia group B study 8811. *Blood* 1995;85(8):2025–2037.

Larson RA, Boogaerts M, Estey E, et al. Antibody-targeted chemotherapy of older patients with acute myeloid leukemia in first relapse using Mylotarg (gemtuzumab ozogamicin). *Leukemia* 2002;16(9):1627–1636.

Levis M. FLT3 mutations in acute myeloid leukemia: what is the best approach in 2013? *Hematology* 2013;2013:220–226.

Lo-Coco F, Avvisati G, Vignetti M, et al. Retinoic acid and arsenic trioxide for acute promyelocytic leukemia. *N Engl J Med* 2013;369:111–121.

Löwenberg B, Ossenkoppele GJ, van Putten W, et al. High-dose daunorubicin in older patients with acute myeloid leukemia. *N Engl J Med* 2009;361:1235–1248.

Mayer RJ, Davis RB, Schiffer CA, et al. Intensive postremission chemotherapy in adults with acute myeloid leukemia. *N Engl J Med* 1994;331(14):896–903.

Paschka P, Döhner K. Core-binding factor acute myeloid leukemia: can we improve on HiDAC consolidation? *Hematology* 2013;2013:209–219.

Pui CH, Evans WE. Acute lymphoblastic leukemia. *N Engl J Med* 1998;339:605–615.

Rebulla P, Finazzi G, Marangoni F, et al. The threshold for prophylactic platelet transfusions in adults with acute myeloid leukemia. *N Engl J Med* 1997;337(26):1870–1875.

Sanz MA, Tallman MS, Lo-Coco FL. Tricks of the trade for the appropriate management of newly diagnosed acute promyelocytic leukemia. *Blood* 2005;105:3019–3025.

Schiller G. High-risk acute myelogenous leukemia: treatment today . . . and tomorrow. *Hematology* 2013;2013:201–208.

Sievers EL, Larson RA, Stadtmauer EA, et al. Efficacy and safety of gemtuzumab ozogamicin in patients with CD33-positive acute myeloid leukemia in first relapse. *J Clin Oncol* 2001;19(13):3244–3254.

Soignet SL, Frankel SR, Douer D, et al. United states multicenter study of arsenic trioxide in relapsed acute promyelocytic leukemia. *J Clin Oncol* 2001;19(18):3852–3860.

Suciu S, Mandelli F, de Witte T, et al. Allogeneic compared with autologous stem cell transplantation in the treatment of patients younger than 46 years with acute myeloid leukemia (AML) in first complete remission (CR1): an intention-to-treat analysis of the EORTC/GIMEMAAML-10 trial. *Blood* 2003;102(4):1232–1240.

Tallman MS, Gilliland DG, Rowe JM. Drug therapy for acute myeloid leukemia. *Blood* 2005;106:1154–1163.

van Besien K. Allogeneic transplantation for AML and MDS: GVL versus GVHD and disease recurrence. *Hematology* 2013;2013:56–62.

Wetzler M, Dodge RK, Mrozek K, et al. Prospective karyotype analysis in adult acute lymphoblastic leukemia: the cancer and leukemia group B experience. *Blood* 1999;93(11):3983–3993.

Wheatley K, Burnett AK, Goldstone AH, et al. A simple, robust, validated and highly predictive index for the determination of risk-directed therapy in acute myeloid leukemia derived from the MRC AML 10 trial. *Br J Haematol* 1999;107(1):69–79.

28 Chronic Leukemias

Rizwan Romee • Todd A. Fehniger

I. **INTRODUCTION.** Chronic leukemias are malignancies of the myeloid or lymphoid hematopoietic lineages that have historically been characterized as having an indolent course when compared with their acute counterparts. While the indolent nature of these diseases results in a relatively long median survival as compared with other cancers, chronic leukemias have not typically been considered curable, except in some cases following allogeneic hematopoietic cell transplantation (HCT). Here we review clinical features and current treatment approaches to the most common chronic leukemias, chronic myelogenous leukemia (CML) and chronic lymphocytic leukemia (CLL).

CML is the most frequent chronic leukemia of myeloid derivation and is categorized as a clonal myeloproliferative disorder within the World Health Organization (WHO) classification. This disease is characterized by peripheral blood leukocytosis resulting from an expansion of normally differentiated myeloid cells and typically presents incidentally on routine laboratory testing. CML is notable as the first leukemia identified with a causative clonal chromosomal rearrangement, t(9;22), or the Philadelphia chromosome (Ph), which juxtaposes the *ABL* tyrosine kinase next to the break point cluster (*BCR*) region, yielding the BCR-ABL fusion protein. The management of CML has been revolutionized over the past 15 years through targeted inhibition of BCR-ABL by the oral tyrosine kinase inhibitor imatinib mesylate (Gleevec), which has provided the first proof-of-principle for small molecule targeted therapy of cancer. CML therapy continues to rapidly evolve with the advent of new generations of small molecular inhibitors of BCR-ABL, and current challenges include defining the optimal approach to manage CML patients who have developed resistance or are unable to tolerate these agents.

CLL is the most common lymphoid leukemia, and is combined with small lymphocytic lymphoma (SLL) as a mature B-cell neoplasm in the WHO classification. Advances in our understanding of the pathophysiology of CLL have yielded an updated view on the natural history, genomic causes, and important prognostic factors in this disease. Improvements in the initial therapy of CLL include combining chemotherapeutic agents with monoclonal antibodies, and expanded treatment options now exist for patients with disease refractory to purine analogs such as fludarabine, including kinase inhibitors such as idelalisib (PI3Kδ inhibitor) and ibrutinib (BTK inhibitor). Other new agents have preliminary evidence of activity, and the use of immunotherapy appears particularly promising.

II. CHRONIC MYELOGENOUS LEUKEMIA (CML)

A. **Epidemiology.** CML accounts for 14% of all leukemias and 20% of adult leukemias, with an annual incidence of 1.6 cases per 100,000 adults. Since the advent of imatinib, the annual mortality has decreased to 1% to 2%. The median age at presentation is 67, and incidence increases with age. The etiology is unclear; no correlation with monozygotic twins, geography, ethnicity, or economic status has been observed. However, a significantly higher incidence of CML has been noted in survivors of the atomic disasters at Nagasaki and Hiroshima, in radiologists, and in patients treated with radiation to the spine for ankylosing spondylitis.

B. **Pathogenesis.** Historically, CML was the first disease in which a specific chromosomal abnormality was linked to the pathogenesis of the disease: the foreshortened chromosome 22, named the *Philadelphia (Ph) chromosome*. Subsequently, the *BCR-ABL* fusion gene resulting from the common t(9;22) translocation has been noted in 90% to 95% of patients with CML. This fusion of the *BCR* (breakpoint cluster region) serine kinase with the human homologue *ABL1* of the Abelson murine leukemia virus oncogene results in constitutive tyrosine kinase activity of ABL and thereby dysregulated activity of multiple signal-transduction pathways controlling cell proliferation and apoptosis. BCR-ABL may also play a direct role in signals leading to independence from external growth signaling, cell adhesion modulation, and DNA repair. CML patients who truly lack BCR-ABL gene fusion are called atypical CML (aCML) and account for <5% of CML cases. Recently, mutations in G-CSF receptor gene called colony-stimulating factor 3 (CSF3R) were found in 40% of aCML patients and mutations in set binding protein (SETBP1) in 25% of aCML patients. Interestingly, some aCML cases harbor mutations in both of these genes. For this chapter, however, we will focus only on BCR-ABL positive CML.

C. **Clinical and laboratory features.** In most patients, CML is diagnosed incidentally. Symptomatic constellations typically result from concurrent anemia and splenomegaly: fatigue, early satiety, and sensation of abdominal fullness, but may also include weight loss, bleeding, or bruising in advanced disease. Leukocytosis with a myeloid shift is universal. In contrast to cases of acute leukemia, in which an arrest in maturation is the rule, granulocytes at all stages of maturation are observed on the peripheral smear. Anemia and thrombocytosis are common, although basophilia (more than 7%) occurs in only 10% to 15% of patients. Leukocyte alkaline phosphatase (LAP) activity is usually reduced, but can be increased with infections, stress, on achievement of remission, or on progression to blast phase (BP). The diagnosis is confirmed by the detection of the Ph chromosome t(9;22) (q34.1;q11.21). In around 5% of patients, a *BCR-ABL* fusion can be detected without classic Ph chromosomal cytogenetics, and rarely translocations can involve three or more chromosomes. The bone marrow is typically hypercellular and devoid of fat. All stages of myeloid differentiation are present and megakaryocytes may be increased, suggesting that chronic-phase CML is a disease of discordant maturation, where a delay in myeloid maturation results in increased myeloid cell mass.

D. **Natural history.** The natural history of CML is a triphasic process: a chronic phase, an accelerated phase, and a blast phase. Most patients present in chronic phase, characterized by an asymptomatic accumulation of differentiated myeloid cells in the bone marrow, spleen, and peripheral blood. Without therapy, CML patients almost invariably progress from chronic phase to accelerated phase and ultimately into blast phase, though some patients in chronic phase evolve directly into blast phase with no intervening accelerated phase.

In the 2 years after initial diagnosis of CML, 5% to 15% of untreated patients will enter blast crisis. In subsequent years, the annual rate of progression increases to 20% to 25%, with progression commonly occurring between 3 and 6 years after diagnosis.

The definition of accelerated phase CML relies on several clinical and laboratory features and is characterized by increasing arrest of maturation. Current WHO criteria include at least one of the following: 10% to 19% blasts in peripheral blood or bone marrow, equal to or more than 20% peripheral basophils, persistent thrombocytopenia less than 100,000/μL unrelated to therapy, persistent thrombocytosis more than 1000,000/μL and unresponsive to therapy, increasing spleen size and increasing white blood cell (WBC) count unresponsive to therapy, or cytogenetic evidence of clonal evolution. Once either accelerated phase or blast crisis occurs, the success of any therapy declines dramatically.

The current WHO criteria for diagnosis of blast phase (also called blast crisis) include at least one of the following: equal to or higher than 20% blasts in the peripheral blood or bone marrow, large foci or clusters of blasts in the bone marrow biopsy, or extramedullary disease.

Several prognostic models (Sokal score, Hasford, MD Anderson Cancer Center staging system) have been developed to stratify patients into groups with different average survival using variables such as age, spleen size, platelet count, percentage of peripheral blood blast count, hematocrit, cytogenetic clonal evolution, and gender. Although these scoring systems were developed before imatinib, post hoc analysis of the IRIS (International Randomized Study of Interferon vs. STI-571) study provided an initial validation of the Sokal score in this imatinib-treated population. Other predictors of outcome derived from the IRIS study include response to imatinib at 3, 12, and 18 months. EUTOS scoring, which was specifically developed to predict response in CML patients undergoing initial treatment with imatinib, is relatively simple and relies only on spleen size and circulating percentage of basophils. It better predicts complete cytogenetic remission at 18 months after initiation of imatinib therapy, which is an important predictor of outcomes in CML patients. However, it remains to be seen whether EUTOS scoring predicts survival/response in CML patients who are being treated with newer tyrosine kinase inhibitors.

E. Treatment of chronic myeloid leukemia: tyrosine kinase inhibitors

1. Imatinib mesylate (gleevec). Imatinib is a targeted tyrosine kinase inhibitor (TKI), which antagonizes the activity of the *ABL* tyrosine kinase as well as c-Kit, and platelet-derived growth factors α and β. At nanomolar concentrations, imatinib binds to the adenosine triphosphate (ATP)-binding pocket of the BCR-ABL fusion protein while in the inactive conformation, resulting in competitive inhibition. This nearly completely abolishes autophosphorylation of BCR-ABL, inactivates dysregulated downstream signaling through multiple pathways including JAK-STAT, PI3K, RAS, AKT, and ERK, thereby specifically inhibiting the growth of *BCR-ABL* positive bone marrow progenitor cells.

The current practice is to initiate imatinib therapy at a dose of 400 mg once daily, which can be titrated up to 600 mg once daily dose in case of disease progression, lack of hematologic response by 3 months, lack of cytogenetic response after 6 to 12 months, or in case of a loss of previous response at 400 mg dose. In the phase III IRIS trial, an initial dose of 400 mg every day followed by escalation to 400 mg twice daily dosing if needed resulted in 98% complete hematologic response (CHR) and 87% complete cytogenetic response (CCyR) rates at 60 months with an estimated 5-year survival of 90%. However, higher dosing schedules of 600 mg and 800 mg have not been associated with improved survival outcomes.

Side effects of imatinib mesylate are generally mild, but include hematologic suppression (neutropenia, thrombocytopenia, and anemia), constitutional symptoms (diarrhea, edema, and rash) and rare organ damage (transaminitis, hypophosphatemia, and potential cardiotoxicity). These can usually be managed with growth factors or dose reduction, but occasionally require discontinuation, either briefly or permanently.

2. **Imatinib resistance.** Resistance to imatinib has been noted in 2% to 4% of patients annually for the first 3 years of imatinib therapy and may decrease thereafter. Mechanisms proposed include the acquisition of point mutations in the *BCR-ABL* kinase SH1 domain, overexpression of BCR-ABL, activation of BCR-ABL–independent pathways including SRC kinases, increased imatinib efflux through the multidrug resistance (MDR) pump and progressively abnormal cytogenetics. Of these, point mutations in the SH1 kinase domain likely play the most prominent role, and more than 50 distinct mutations have been documented in 42% to 90% of resistant cases. ATP-binding loop (P-loop) and T315I mutations are particularly more common in advanced phase CML patients. Mutations have also been found *de novo* in untreated chronic-phase patients, suggesting they may exist before treatment and are slowly selected out during therapy. As rates of progression decline over time, imatinib therapy is not currently thought to induce new mutations. These mutations act by either decreasing the affinity for imatinib binding in the ATP-binding pocket or shifting the kinetics of BCR-ABL to prefer the active conformation, to which imatinib will not bind.

   Imatinib resistance can be overcome either with increasing doses or a second-generation tyrosine kinase inhibitor. Second-generation tyrosine kinase inhibitors are effective in most of the mutations with the exception of T315I, which imparts a high degree of resistance to all currently available TKI with the exception of ponatinib. Mutational analysis is therefore critical in determining clinical course after resistance is noted.

3. **Second generation tyrosine kinase inhibitors.** Several more potent tyrosine kinase inhibitors have been developed since the initial introduction of imatinib.

   a. **Dasatinib.** Dasatinib is a potent inhibitor of *ABL* tyrosine kinase but also inhibits SRC family kinases, c-KIT, EPHA2, and platelet-derived growth factor receptor β (PDGFRβ). It is active against most of imatinib-resistant mutational forms of ABL1 except for T315I and F317V. First-line therapy for chronic phase CML patients on standard 100 mg daily dose of dasatinib is associated with faster and deeper response rates compared with imatinib. However, so far, no survival advantage has been demonstrated with the use of dasatinib over imatinib as a first-line therapy in chronic phase CML. Dasatinib has also shown excellent response rates as a second-line agent in chronic phase CML patients otherwise intolerant or resistant (except for patients with the above-mentioned mutations) to imatinib. Overall, dasatinib is well tolerated with easily manageable cytopenias and diarrhea. Pleural effusion is a relatively common side effect and tends to be more common in patients with accelerated phase CML, prior cardiac history, hypertension, and those receiving higher doses of dasatinib (70 mg twice a day vs. 100 mg once daily).

   b. **Nilotinib.** Nilotinib is a highly potent inhibitor of ABL tyrosine kinase and also inhibits other tyrosine kinases including c-KIT and PDGFR, but unlike dasatinib, it has no activity against SRC family kinases. Similarly to dasatinib, nilotinib is active against most of the mutations in ABL1 but has no activity against T315I mutation. At a twice daily dose of 300 mg, patients achieve faster and deeper responses compared with imatinib, although without survival improvement. In addition to the common adverse effects including nausea, vomiting, diarrhea, and myelosuppression, nilotinib has also been associated with significant QTc prolongation in some patients, and thus the black box warning in its labeling from FDA. Because of this QTc prolongation, it is important to correct any electrolyte abnormalities prior to its use, and then also to monitor them periodically.

   c. **Bosutinib.** Bosutinib has activity against BCR-ABL and SRC family kinases, but minimal activity against c-KIT and PDGFR. In addition, it has activity against most of the imatinib-resistant mutations except for T315I and V299L. Compared with imatinib, use of bosutinib at a standard daily dose of 500 mg in chronic phase CML patients leads to faster and somewhat deeper responses; however, as with the use of other second-generation TKI's, no survival advantage has been demonstrated. Overall, bosutinib has a favorable toxicity profile with only minimal effect on QTc. Diarrhea is the most common nonhematologic side effect of this medication; the other relatively common nonhematologic side effects are elevation of ALT, increased lipase, hyperglycemia, and electrolyte abnormalities, which are often manageable without needing its discontinuation or dose modification. Currently, bosutinib is approved as a second-line therapy in patients intolerant and/or resistant to prior TKIs (imatinib, dasatinib, and nilotinib).

d. Ponatinib. Ponatinib is a potent orally active tyrosine kinase inhibitor with activity against a wide range of tyrosine kinases including T315I mutant forms of the ABL1 tyrosine kinase. In a phase II using a daily dose of 45mg, patients with chronic phase CML with resistance (including patients with T315I mutations) or intolerance to prior TKI therapy, ponatinib induced a major cytogenetic response rate of 56%, a complete cytogenetic response of 46%, and a major molecular response rate of 34%. Furthermore, the estimated progression-free survival and overall survival at 12 months were 80% and 94%, respectively. Presence of T315I mutations, young age, prior exposure to fewer TKIs, and shorter duration of leukemia were associated with higher response rates. The most common adverse effects reported with the use of ponatinib were thrombocytopenia, neutropenia, rash, abdominal pain, and fluid retention, all relatively easily manageable (*N Engl J Med* 2013;369:1). However serious vascular complications including thromboembolic events (arterial and venous) have been reported in ≥25% of the patients treated with ponatinib, leading to its withdrawal from the market in late 2013. Nevertheless, the drug was reinstated in the spring of 2014 with narrower indications. Ponatinib is currently approved at an oral daily dose of 45 mg for adult CML patients harboring the T315I mutation and for patients where all other TKIs have failed. In addition to thromboembolic events, ponatinib also carries a black box warning for heart failure and liver toxicity. Patients being treated with ponatinib need to be closely monitored for thromboembolic events, and despite lack of evidence for its efficacy, many clinicians now concomitantly use aspirin for the prophylaxis of these thromboembolic events.

4. Initial workup, therapy, and disease monitoring in chronic phase cml. In addition to the routine labs, including CBC with differential and comprehensive metabolic panel, CML patients should undergo bone marrow aspirate and biopsy with conventional cytogenetic analysis (karyotyping) to identify Philadelphia chromosome. In a small minority of patients with variant or cryptic translocations where Philadelphia chromosome is not readily detected by conventional karyotyping, fluorescence in-situ hybridization (FISH) can be used to identify BCR-ABL1 gene fusion in these patients. Peripheral blood (or marrow at diagnosis) quantitative PCR (qPCR) is done at baseline (prior to treatment initiation), then every 3 months to monitor the response once treatment is initiated.

Current recommendations for treatment initiation include either imatinib 400 mg daily, nilotinib 300 mg twice daily, or dasatinib 100 mg daily. Imatinib remains a reasonable first-line agent, although patients with intermediate- or high-risk Sokal or Hasford scores should be considered for either nilotinib or dasatinib. Bosutinib is currently approved for use as a second-line TKI after patients have failed the first line TKI's.

CML patients initiated on TKI therapy are assessed for hematologic, cytogenetic, and molecular responses. Complete hematologic remission (CHR) is defined as normalization of peripheral blood counts (no immature cells, <5% basophils on differential, WBC count <10 × 10^9/L, and platelet count <450 × 10^9/L). CHR also includes absence of palpable splenomegaly on physical exam. Cytogenetic response is defined as complete cytogenetic response (CCyR) by the absence, major by 1% to 35%, minor by 36% to 95%, and no response by >95% Philadelphia chromosome metaphases on bone marrow banding analysis of at least 20 metaphases. Molecular response is defined as major molecular response (MMR) when qPCR for BCR-ABL1 transcripts in the peripheral blood are ≤0.1% on the International Scale (IS), which is equivalent to the ≥3 log reduction from the standardized baseline. Complete molecular remission (CMR) denotes undetectable BCR-ABL1 transcripts by qPCR; however, as the sensitivity of the qPCR has been steadily increasing, it is becoming clear that CMR is a misleading term as very low burden of malignant clone may still be found in patients with otherwise complete CMR, and therefore it has been proposed not to use this term any more.

Increased risk of progression to accelerated and blastic phases has been demonstrated if the initial TKI therapy does not achieve specific clinical goals, which currently include complete hematologic response with normal peripheral counts and *BCR-ABL* transcripts by quantitative polymerase chain reaction (qPCR) of ≤10% (International Scale, IS), and/or ≤35% Ph chromosome-positive bone marrow cells at 3 months, BCR-ABL transcripts by qPCR of ≤1% (IS), and/or 0% Ph chromosome-positive bone marrow at 6 months, BCR-ABL transcripts by qPCR of ≤0.1 (IS) at 12 months after initiation of the TKI therapy. Failure to reach any of these goals warrants close follow-up, change of therapy, and ABL tyrosine kinase domain mutation analysis.

After initiation of therapy, patients should undergo weekly complete blood counts (CBC) with differential until complete hematologic remission. Afterwards, follow-up includes peripheral blood BCR-ABL qPCR with CBCs and chemistries every 3 months for 3 years, and if patient continues to maintain major molecular response, then every 3 to 6 months afterwards. Bone marrow biopsy with cytogenetics is performed at the time of the diagnosis and repeated at 3 and 6 months if qPCR for BCR-ABL transcripts is not available. Bone marrow biopsy with cytogenetics is again performed at 12 months if the patient is still not in MMR and then again at 18 months if the previous marrow at 12 months did not demonstrate a CCyR. Peripheral blood FISH can replace qPCR for BCR-ABL transcripts to monitor disease progression after patients in centers where qPCR is not readily available. Any signs of disease progression such as change in blood counts and/or rising BCR-ABL1 transcripts should be quickly reevaluated with a bone marrow biopsy with cytogenetics as well as mutational analysis of BCR-ABL.

5. **Treatment duration.** Treatment length continues to be defined, but we recommend indefinite tyrosine kinase inhibition. Recent data suggest tyrosine kinase inhibitors are not cytotoxic to early, quiescent BCR-ABL positive precursor cells. Several small recent studies have shown the feasibility of safely discontinuing TKI therapy in patients in MMR and low Sokal risk scores. This is currently an evolving field and at this time discontinuation or TKI drug holidays of TKI therapy should be considered only in the context of a clinical trial.

6. **Conventional chemotherapy.** Until 1980, hydroxyurea and busulfan were the two most effective anti-CML agents. Both offer mild hematologic control associated with myelosuppression but without affecting the uniform transformation to the acute phase of the disease. Subsequently, interferon α used alone or in combination with cytarabine has demonstrated improved response over chemotherapy with major cytogenetic responses in 40% to 50% of patients, with up to 80% of these patients achieving a durable response resulting in a 10-year survival of 75%. However, interferon α therapy is complicated by significant side effects including flu-like symptoms, anorexia, weight loss, depression, autoimmune (AI) disorders, thrombocytopenia, alopecia, rashes, and neuropathies, resulting in discontinuation in approximately a fifth of patients. Given the superior response to tyrosine kinase inhibitors and their relatively benign side effect profile, conventional chemotherapy and interferon have fallen from common use in CML.

F. **Treatment of chronic myelogenous leukemia: transplant options**

1. **Allogeneic hematopoietic cell transplantation.** Allogeneic HCT from either related or unrelated donors remains the only known curative therapy for CML. Transplantation from a matched-sibling donor during the chronic phase is associated with a 10-year survival of 50% to 70%. Results of transplantation from unrelated donors are somewhat less impressive, but are improving with better matching strategies and supportive care. The objective of allogeneic HCT is cure of CML by eradication of the leukemic clone with myeloablative chemoradiotherapy, and restoration of hematopoiesis by transplantation of normal donor-derived stem cells. In addition, the donor-derived

allogeneic immune cells confer an important graft-versus-leukemia (GVL) effect, which acts to prevent recurrence of disease. GVL has been closely associated with the presence of graft versus host disease (GVHD). GVHD does not develop in patients receiving transplants from identical twin donors. These patients have at least twice the risk of relapse of CML compared with transplant recipients from HLA-identical siblings.

The best results occur when patients are transplanted while in chronic phase with 5-year survival in the 50% to 60% range. However long-term survival after allogeneic HCT in accelerated phase is only 20% to 40%, whereas survival after transplants performed in blastic phase further declines to approximately 20%. The highest rates of survival for related and unrelated-donor transplantation in the preimatinib era are documented in patients transplanted within 1 year of their diagnosis where long-term survival in chronic phase approaches the 60% to 70% range.

Use of allogeneic HCT is also limited by histocompatible donor availability as only one-third of patients will have a HLA-matched sibling, and only around 50% of the patients are able to locate a suitable unrelated donor (70% for whites and 15% for African Americans and other minorities in the United States). However, the recent advances in alternate donor allogeneic HCT such as haploidentical and cord blood transplantation have further broadened the availability of the transplant modality to patients who otherwise lack HLA-matched related and unrelated donors. Age older than 50 to 60 years has been found to constitute a significant hurdle for transplant success, especially in the unrelated-donor transplant setting, although this is improved with modified intensity and nonmyeloablative transplant.

Most CML patients transplanted in the chronic phase are cured of their disease, although transplant-related morbidity and mortality remain a significant problem. The cumulative incidence of severe GVHD is approximately 20% to 35% in matched-sibling transplantation and 40% to 55% in recipients of transplants from unrelated donors. Infection is a major cause of nonrelapse mortality in allogeneic transplantation. GVHD and immunosuppression are predisposing factors for infectious complications.

2. **Allogeneic bone marrow transplantation in the TKI era.** The effect of pretransplant tyrosine kinase inhibitor therapy, which will delay transplant and may thereby increase its risks, is still under study. Initial retrospective studies comparing imatinib-treated transplant patients with historical controls show no difference in rates of engraftment and acute or chronic GVHD, suggesting delays due to therapy do not adversely affect the transplant itself. Upfront consideration for allogeneic HCT in the TKI era is suggested for patients who have T315I or other pan-TKI resistant mutations, patients who are intolerant of all currently available TKIs and who present with blast phase.

High-risk patients, who present with cytogenetic changes beyond Ph chromosome, who demonstrate increasing cytogenetic complexity, who do not meet standard goals of therapy at 3, 6, 12, or 18 months, or who have rising qPCR levels of BCR-ABL should be evaluated for human leukocyte antigen (HLA)–matched siblings and potential unrelated donors. Further progressive disease despite appropriate tyrosine kinase inhibition warrants transplant consideration as early as possible.

Relapse following transplant has been successfully treated with both donor lymphocyte infusion and tyrosine kinase inhibition. Mutational analysis of ABL kinase domain may help guide appropriate therapy choice.

G. **Accelerated and blast-phase chronic myelogenous leukemia.** Despite profound advances in the treatment of chronic-phase CML, outcomes of patients with accelerated and blast phase continue to be suboptimal. BRC-ABL mutational analysis should be performed with early consideration for transplant or clinical trial. However, because most patients now developing accelerated phase have been previously treated with imatinib, mutations in and overexpression of BCR-ABL are to be expected. Simple dose escalation of imatinib is rarely sufficient therapy. Patients diagnosed with AP CML are typically treated with second-generation TKIs. Patients with the T315I mutation or intolerant to other

TKIs are treated with ponatinib. Omacetaxine is another option for patients harboring this mutation as it has shown some activity in this setting. Allogeneic HCT is reserved as an option for patients who do not achieve deep response to the TKI therapy.

Blast phase is characterized by cytogenetic evolution in approximately 70% of patients. The most common chromosomal abnormalities are trisomy 8 in 30% to 40% of patients, additional Ph chromosome in 20% to 30%, and isochromosome 17 in 15% to 20%. Corresponding mutations in p53 are also seen in 20% to 30% of patients, amplification of *c-myc* in 20%, and, less commonly, mutations and deletions of *ras*, *Rb*, or *p16*. As with *de novo* acute myelogenous leukemia (AML), complex cytogenetics are associated with decreased response rates and survival.

Treatment of blast-phase CML remains a challenge, and is dictated by hematologic features. Myeloid features are seen in 50% of patients, lymphoid in 25%, and undifferentiated in 25%. Patients with myeloid blast crisis are treated with a second-generation TKI (alone or in combination with AML type of chemotherapy) followed by allogeneic HCT. However, even after allogeneic HCT, the survival continues to be around 20% to 30%.

Patients with lymphoid blast crisis are typically treated with Hyper CVAD or other regimens including vincristine and prednisone plus a TKI. This approach has been shown to induce acceptable response rates with a CHR of around 80% and CCR in the 50% to 60% range. When followed by allogeneic HCT, prolonged survival has been demonstrated in these patients (93 months in one series from MD Anderson Cancer Center).

III. CHRONIC LYMPHOCYTIC LEUKEMIA (CLL)

A. **Epidemiology.** CLL is the most common form of leukemia in adults, accounting for approximately 30% of adult leukemias in the United States. Approximately 16,000 new cases are diagnosed annually, and 4,600 deaths are attributed to CLL each year in the United States. According to the Surveillance, Epidemiology, and End Results (SEER) cancer database, from 2007 to 2011, the median age at presentation was 71 years, and only 14% of patients were less than 60 years old at the time of diagnosis. The age-adjusted incidence for CLL was 6.0 per 100,000 men and 3.1 per 100,000 women per year, with a 2:1 male:female ratio. There are no clear environmental or occupational risk factors that predispose to CLL, and patients who are exposed to radiation do not appear to have an increased frequency of CLL. Interestingly, the incidence of CLL is much lower (10% of that of Western countries) in Asian countries such as China and Japan, which is attributed to genetic rather than environmental factors. CLL (and other malignancies) occur at a higher than predicted frequency among first-degree relatives of patients with CLL (relative risk of approximately 1.5 to 7.5), the highest familial risk of all hematologic malignancies, suggesting a subset of patients have inherited risk factors. Studies of familial cohorts with CLL are ongoing, and the future identification of genes involved in familial CLL may provide insights into the pathogenesis of CLL. Of note, monoclonal B lymphocytosis (MBL) with a CLL phenotype was detected in 3.5% of normal healthy control subjects, and there was a significant increase in the detection of such cells in family members of CLL patients (13.5%). It is now generally accepted that MBL precedes the development of CLL, but only a minority of individuals with MBL eventually develop the disease.

B. **Pathogenesis.** CLL is a clonal lymphoproliferative disorder characterized by the accumulation of neoplastic, functionally incompetent B lymphocytes in the blood, bone marrow, lymph nodes, spleen, or other organs. After encountering antigen, a normal B-cell enters the germinal center and proliferates, where the B-cell receptor genes undergo somatic hypermutation, which allows for B-cell receptor affinity maturation and selection of B-cell clones with high affinity for the antigen. Despite their uniform morphologic appearance and immunophenotype, there appears to be significant heterogeneity in CLL patients with regard to the mutational status of the immunoglobulin (Ig) heavy-chain variable region (IgVH), which usually indicates whether the B cell has experienced somatic hypermutation in the germinal center. In CLL, approximately half of patients have a mutated IgVH (M-IgVH) indicative of a post-germinal center B cell, whereas other patients have an unmutated IgVH (UM-IgVH), a finding that has prognostic significance. The precise normal counterpart(s) of CLL cells during B-cell development has not been definitely identified;

however, the CLL immunophenotype is similar to that of mature, antigen-experienced, activated B cells. Recent gene expression array experiments indicate that both M-IgVH and UM-IgVH CLL cells resemble memory B cells more than any other identified normal B-cell subset. In addition, overexpression of the src tyrosine kinase ZAP-70 in CLL, which is normally expressed in T and natural killer (NK) cells and not B cells, is strongly correlated with UM-IgVH subset. Further advances in defining the relationship between CLL cells and normal B-cell development may yield novel therapeutic targets in CLL.

Unlike many hematologic malignancies, CLL cells do not contain balanced chromosomal translocations, detectable using traditional cytogenetic techniques. However, in fluorescence in situ hybridization (FISH) technology on nondividing cells (i.e., interphase cytogenetics) has identified recurrent chromosomal abnormalities in approximately 80% of CLL cases. The most common cytogenetic abnormalities in CLL are del(13q14), del(11q), trisomy 12, and del(17p), which influence prognosis (Table 28-1). The gene(s) involved in 13q14 deletion have not been definitively identified; however, the retinoblastoma (Rb) gene maps close to this region. Two micro-RNAs (miR-15, miR-16) have been mapped to the 13q locus and are also potential candidates for mediating this locus effect in CLL. Del(11q22-23) encompasses the ataxia telangiectasia mutated (ATM) gene locus, and mutations in the ATM gene have been observed in CLL, suggesting that ATM is the target of this deletion. Similarly, del(17p) encompasses the p53 tumor suppressor gene, and point mutations or deletions of p53 are also present in CLL patients with poor prognosis, suggesting p53 is the target gene in del(17p) CLL patients. The gene(s) important for trisomy 12 effects have not been identified. Approximately 95% of CLLs have increased expression of the antiapoptotic Bcl-2 oncogene, and 70% have expression levels equivalent to follicular lymphoma cells harboring t(14;18). CLL cells utilize other mechanisms to increase Bcl-2 expression, and do not typically contain the classic t(14;18) present in follicular lymphoma. Recent studies using cancer genome sequencing have defined recurrent somatic mutations in CLL patients. These genes affect common pathways including DNA damage and cell-cycle control (ATM, p53), Notch signaling (NOTCH1, FBXW7), RNA splicing (SF3B1, DDX3X), and cytokine/toll like receptor signaling (MYD88 DDX3X, MAPK1). Of these, p53 mutations affect about 10%, NOTCH1 mutations affect about 10%, and SF3B1 mutations affect 10% to 15% of CLL patients, and all confer an independent poor prognosis. Further, substantial clonal heterogeneity exists in CLL patients, and ongoing research is studying how CLL subclonal architecture affects, and is in turn influenced by, anti-CLL therapy.

C. **Clinical presentation, laboratory features, and diagnosis.** Patients with CLL may have a wide range of symptoms, signs, and laboratory abnormalities at the time of initial diagnosis. Many patients are asymptomatic, and a routine CBC reveals a lymphocytosis, whereas fewer patients present with extreme fatigue or B symptoms including fevers,

TABLE 28-1	Cytogenetic Abnormalities in Chronic Lymphocytic Leukemia			
Aberration	**% Patients**	**Prognosis**	**Clinical feature**	**Gene**
13q−	55%	Good	Slower progression Lymphadenopathy	?
11q−	18%	Poor	Rapid progression Shorter PFS with Flu-regimens	ATM
12q+	16%	Intermediate		?
17p−	7%	Poor	Shorter PFS with Flu-regimens	p53

ATM, ataxia telangiectasia mutated; PFS, progression-free survival; Flu, fludarabine; ?, not definitively identified.

night sweats, unintentional weight loss equal to or less than 10% of body weight. Other presentations include painless lymphadenopathy, anemia, thrombocytopenia, and infections. Physical examination findings are normal in 20% to 30% of patients, but may include lymphadenopathy, splenomegaly, and hepatomegaly in approximately half the number of patients. Laboratory findings uniformly include a lymphocytosis (greater than 5,000/μL), and may include anemia, thrombocytopenia, elevated lactose dehydrogenase (LDH) levels, elevated B2M levels, positive Coombs' test, polyclonal increase in γ-globulin levels, or hypogammaglobulinemia. The peripheral blood smear typically shows numerous small, mature appearing lymphocytes with clumped chromatin and no nucleolus, with "smudge" cells present as crush artifacts of fragile CLL cells. Bone marrow biopsy shows infiltration with small lymphocytes in nodular, interstitial, or diffuse pattern. The histopathologic lymph node findings in CLL/SLL consist of diffuse effacement of the nodal architecture by small, mature appearing lymphocytes with a low mitotic rate, and few (less than 10%) large prolymphocytes. Peripheral blood, bone marrow, or lymph node flow cytometry reveals a characteristic immunophenotype (Table 28-2). The essential diagnostic criteria for CLL identified by the CLL international working group (IWG) include an absolute monoclonal B lymphocytosis of more than 5,000/μL with a typical morphology, and commonly, the bone marrow is infiltrated with small lymphocytes accounting for more than 30% of nucleated cells, and a typical immunophenotype (CD5+, CD23+, CD10−, CD19+, CD20^{+dim}, CyclinD1−, CD43±). In addition, the following tests may be useful under certain circumstances: molecular genetic analysis to detect antigen receptor rearrangements, interphase FISH for 17p−, 11q−, 13q−, +12, and determination of CD38 and/or ZAP-70 expression. The differential diagnosis of CLL includes other indolent B-cell lymphomas (mantle cell, follicular, lymphoplasmacytic), hairy cell leukemia, large granular lymphocytic (LGL) leukemia, prolymphocytic leukemia (PLL), and adult T-cell leukemia/lymphoma. Once the diagnosis is made, initial workup should include physical examination, performance status, assessment of B symptoms, CBC with differential count, LDH, comprehensive metabolic panel, and in certain circumstances quantitative Igs, reticulocyte count, direct Coombs' test, computed tomography (CT) scans of the chest/abdomen/pelvis, B2M, and uric acid.

D. Staging and prognosis. The Rai and Binet clinical staging systems were described in the 1970s and provided prognostic information on survival based upon physical examination findings and blood counts (Table 28-3). These clinical staging systems have been extensively validated and are widely used in clinical practice to provide estimates of survival to patients. However, the clinical course of early stage patients is heterogeneous: some patients do not require therapy for many years, whereas others have rapid progression and poor responses to therapy. Further, these staging systems provide little information to help predict the clinical outcome of early stage patients or the response to therapy. Additional laboratory parameters have been identified as markers of tumor burden and independent poor prognostic factors including an elevated LDH, a lymphocyte doubling time of less

TABLE 28-2	Immunophenotypic Features of Malignant Conditions Affecting Mature B Lymphocytes
Disorder	**Common immunophenotype**
CLL	DR+, CD19+, CD20+, CD5+, CD22−, CD23+, CD10−, weak sIg
Prolymphocytic leukemia	DR+, CD19+, CD20+, CD5−, CD22+, CD23−, CD10−, bright sIg
Mantle cell lymphoma	DR+, CD19+, CD20+, CD5+, CD22+, CD23−, CD10−, moderate sIg
Follicular lymphoma	DR+, CD19+, CD20+, CD5−, CD22+, CD23−, CD10+, bright sIg
Hairy cell leukemia	DR+, CD19+, CD20+, CD5−, CD22+, CD23−, CD10−, CD11c+, bright sIg

CLL, chronic lymphocytic leukemia; sIg, surface immunoglobulin.

TABLE 28-3	Chronic Lymphocytic Leukemia Staging Systems		
Staging system	Presentation	Median survival (yr)	Patients (%)
Rai			
0	Lymphocytosis	>10	30
I	LN	9	35
II	Splenomegaly	7	25
III	Anemia	5	7
IV	Thrombocytopenia	5	3
Binet			
A	Lymphocytosis, <3 areas of LN	>10	65
B	Lymphocytosis, >3 areas of LN	7	30
C	Anemia, thrombocytopenia, or both	5	5

LN, lymph node enlargement.

than 12 months, and diffuse bone marrow infiltration pattern. Serum proteins have also been linked to poor prognosis, including elevated levels of thymidine kinase (TK), soluble CD23 (sCD23), and B2-microglobulin (B2M). Notably, patients with an elevated B2M level have a shorter survival, and worse responses to traditional chemotherapy approaches. A summary of prognostic factors in CLL is provided in Table 28-4.

The mutational status of the IgVH locus is an important genetic parameter for prognostication in CLL patients, with the mutated IgVH (M-IgVH) associated with slow progression and long survival, whereas the un-mutated IgVH (UM-IgVH) is associated with an unfavorable course and rapid progression. Surrogate markers of UM-IgVH and poor prognosis include flow cytometry-detected expression of CD38 and ZAP-70 by CLL cells. Recent studies have suggested that more than 20% ZAP-70 expression as assessed by flow cytometry is associated with a median survival of less than 5 years, compared with 10 years in patients with less than 20% expression, and is now widely available. This was superior in predicting outcomes in CLL patients compared with IgVH mutational status testing.

TABLE 28-4	Prognostic Factors in Chronic Lymphocytic Leukemia

Favorable	Unfavorable
Low Rai or Binet clinical stage	High Rai or Binet clinical stage
Lymphocyte doubling time >12 mo	Lymphocyte doubling time <12 mo
Nodular or interstitial BM infiltrate	Diffuse BM infiltrate
Mutated IgVH	Unmutated IgVH
ZAP-70 negative (low)	ZAP-70 positive (high)
CD38 negative	CD38 positive
13q−	17p−/p53 abnormalities, 11q−/ATM abnormalities, +12
	Increased levels of: B2M, LDH, sCD23
	Presence of NOTCH1, SF3B1, TP53, ATM mutations

BM, bone marrow; ATM, ataxia telangiectasia mutated; LDH, lactose dehydrogenase; B2M, beta 2 microglobulin.

Interphase cytogenetics has identified both favorable (13q−) with a longer treatment-free interval and overall survival, and unfavorable (17p−, 11q−) with a short treatment-free interval and overall survival, subsets of CLL (Table 28-2). Consistent with this, subsets of patients with mutations in p53 (17p) or ATM (11q) have a poorer prognosis. When molecular parameters consisting of IgVH mutational status, 17p−, and 11q− were included in a multivariate analysis, the clinical stage was not identified as an independent prognostic factor. Four distinct molecular prognostic groups (17p−, 11q−, UM-IgVH, M-IgVH) have been identified, and have provided a framework for risk-adapted therapeutic strategies. Laboratory testing by interphase cytogenetics for genetic abnormalities of clinical significance in CLL patients is now widely available. Although these advances in genetic and molecular prognostic factors are promising, the decision to treat patients with CLL based upon them requires validation in prospective, randomized clinical trials. More recently, recurrent somatic mutations have been identified in CLL that have been integrated into cytogenetics-based risk scores. For example, a retrospective study of previously untreated CLL patients identified high risk (p53 or BIRC3 abnormalities), intermediate risk (NOTCH1 or SF3B1 mutations and/or 11q deletion), low risk (trisomy 12 or no cytogenetic abnormality), and very low risk (13q− as an isolated abnormality). These findings will require confirmation in prospective clinical trials, and assessment in relapsed/refractory patients.

E. Complications associated with chronic lymphocytic leukemia

1. Richter's transformation. Richter's syndrome (RS), originally described as the development of an aggressive NHL in patients with CLL/SLL, is now commonly used to describe transformation into any aggressive malignancy including diffuse large B-cell lymphoma (DLBCL), or, less commonly, PLL, Hodgkin's lymphoma (HL), lymphoblastic lymphoma, hairy cell leukemia, or aggressive T-cell NHL. RS occurs in 2% to 8% of CLL patients, and results are conflicting on whether purine analog therapy increases the risk for transformation. In about 80% of patients, the malignant clone in RS develops through transformation of the original CLL clone (molecularly related to original CLL), while in about 20% of patients, they arise as an independent neoplasm. This distinction is clinically important, since patients with clonally unrelated RS/DLBLC have a prognosis similar to *de novo* DLBCL and frontline treatment with R-CHOP is adequate. RS is suspected clinically in patients with CLL/SLL that have a rapidly enlarging lymph node group, rapidly progressive splenomegaly or hepatomegaly, elevated LDH and B2M, new B symptoms (fever, night sweats, weight loss), or a sudden decline in performance status. Patients with suspected RS should have a tissue biopsy to confirm the diagnosis. Treatment of clonally related RS usually involves aggressive chemotherapy combinations utilized in NHL (e.g., R-CHOP) with response rates of 5% to 43%, and median survival between 5 and 8 months. For responding patients, an allogeneic SCT in CR1 is preferred, and is typically offered to those patients who respond to initial chemotherapy and who are good transplant candidates with an HLA-matched donor. For patients not responding to R-CHOP, other salvage regimens such as OFAR, RDHAP, or RICE are possibilities. Overall, clonally related RS patients have a poor prognosis, and novel treatment strategies are needed.

2. Autoimmune complications. AI phenomena are common in CLL, occur more frequently in advanced-stage patients and those with UM-IgVH, and include autoimmune hemolytic anemia (AIHA), autoimmune thrombocytopenia (ITP), AI neutropenia, and pure red cell aplasia (PRCA) (Table 28-5). In CLL patients with isolated anemia, laboratory evaluation for hemolysis should be performed, including direct Coombs' (direct anti-globulin) testing, LDH, haptoglobin, indirect bilirubin, and reticulocyte count. It is important to note that these tests may not provide consistent findings of hemolysis in CLL patients, as an elevated LDH may be due to other causes in CLL, and a low reticulocyte count could be due to poor bone marrow responses when infiltrated with CLL. In addition, AI complications may be triggered in CLL patients at the time of treatment with fludarabine. Treatment of AIHA in CLL patients is similar to the steroid approach in non-CLL patients, with a typical course

TABLE 28-5	Complications Associated with Chronic Lymphocytic Leukemia

Complication	Patients affected (%)
Autoimmune	
Hemolytic anemia	10–25
Thrombocytopenia	2
Neutropenia	0.5
Pure red cell aplasia	0.5
Hypogammaglobulinemia	20–60
Infections	
Streptococcus, Staphylococcus sp.	
Haemophilus sp.	
Candida, Aspergillus sp.	
Varicella zoster	
Legionella, Pneumocystis, Listeria sp.	
Toxoplasma sp.	
Disease transformation	
Prolymphocytic leukemia	10
Richter's transformation	3–5
Second cancers (lung, skin, GI)	5–15

GI, gastrointestinal.

of prednisone 1 mg/kg/day until a response is achieved, followed by a prolonged, 2- to 3-month, taper. If the AI complication is not responsive to steroids, other treatments include intravenous immunoglobulin (IVIG), cyclosporine, splenectomy, and rituximab. In addition, treatment of the underlying CLL may improve the AI cytopenias.

3. **Infectious complications.** The immune deficiency associated with CLL is multifactorial, and includes hypogammaglobulinemia, T and NK cell dysfunction, and decreased phagocytic function. Infectious complications are frequent and respond to appropriate antimicrobial therapy. For CLL patients with hypogammaglobulinemia (IgG <500 mg/dL) and recurrent serious infections, treatment with IVIG 400 mg/kg IV every 3 to 4 weeks (goal IgG trough approximately 500 mg/dL) reduces serious bacterial infection rates without clear effects on overall survival. Patients treated with fludarabine or alemtuzumab develop therapy-related T-cell immune defects, and are at a significantly increased risk for cytomegalovirus (CMV) reactivation, pneumocystis, varicella zoster, herpes viruses, listeria, and other opportunistic infections. Prophylaxis against pneumocystis, herpes simplex virus (HSV), and varicella zoster virus (VZV), as well as monitoring for CMV reactivation should be considered when treating CLL patients with these agents.

F. **Decision to initiate treatment.** Treatment of CLL has historically been palliative as chemotherapeutic regimens have not impacted overall survival to date, and therefore the diagnosis of CLL does not mandate the need for therapy. Indications for treatment include (a) eligibility for treatment on a clinical trial, (b) advanced clinical stage (Rai III/IV), (c) AI cytopenias, (d) recurrent infections, (e) B symptoms, (f) threatened compromise of organ function, (g) cytopenias, (h) bulky disease, (i) rapid progression of disease, (j) histologic transformation, or (k) patient preference for immediate treatment. Observation until an indication for treatment arises is not currently thought to impact CLL patients' overall survival or response to therapy when initiated. As therapies for CLL become more effective and strategies to monitor for minimal residual disease develop, this paradigm of initial observation may change in the future.

G. **Initial treatment of chronic lymphocytic leukemia.** The goal of CLL chemotherapy remains palliative; however, these objectives are currently being reevaluated in clinical trials as chemotherapy and monoclonal antibody combinations, kinase inhibitors, and more recently immunotherapy approaches produce high complete remission rates and in some cases elimination of disease based on sensitive molecular and flow cytometric techniques. Accepted first-line therapy options include clinical trials (preferred as standard therapy is not curative), radiation therapy (especially for stage I SLL), alkylating agents (e.g., chlorambucil or cyclophosphamide), purine analogs (fludarabine), or combinations such as fludarabine plus rituximab (FR), fludarabine plus cyclophosphamide plus rituximab (FCR) (see Appendix for treatment regimens). Randomized clinical trials have established higher complete remission rates and PFS intervals for fludarabine over alkylating agents and FC over fludarabine alone; however, no difference in overall survival has been demonstrated. A US intergroup study is comparing upfront FCR, FR, and FR followed by lenalidomide consolidation, and may provide randomized clinical trial data to prioritize these regimens when results are reported. In addition, a European study compared FCR with BR in the upfront setting, and preliminary results suggest equal efficacy and lower toxicity with BR in patients >65 years of age. Treatment duration is clinically aimed at palliating the inciting cause for therapy, and is typically 4 to 8 cycles. Clinical studies suggest a longer duration of remission for patients that achieve a complete remission (CR). Ongoing studies tracking cytogenetic and molecular minimal residual disease are seeking to clarify how MRD impacts relapse, and whether targeting MRD following initial therapy is clinically beneficial. Before initiating treatment, consideration should be given to tumor lysis syndrome prophylaxis, especially in patients with very high lymphocyte counts or bulky disease. In addition, patients treated with purine analogs should receive prophylaxis against pneumocystis and varicella zoster. Moreover, patients treated with anti-CD20 mAbs are at risk for hepatitis B and C reactivation, and testing for these viral infections is recommended prior to starting therapy, and prophylactic entecavir or other appropriate antiviral drug may be indicated. Very rarely, anti-CD20 mAbs may cause progressive multifocal leucoencephalopathy (PML), and this complication should be considered in patients that develop cognitive or neurologic symptoms. We currently utilize FCR as our standard frontline therapy for younger, fit CLL patients, and BR or obinutuzumab/ofatumumab plus chlorambucil for older patients. Patients harboring a 17p deletion or p53 mutation are at considerable risk for not responding or having a very brief remission to standard fludarabine-based therapy, and should be considered for clinical trials. While FCR and FR can induce remissions and represent appropriate therapy for 17p deleted CLL at this time, alternative approaches include alemtuzumab plus rituximab, ibrutinib, idelalisib plus rituximab, high dose methylprednisolone plus rituximab, or obinutuzumab plus chlorambucil. For patients with 11q-deletion, alkylator-based therapy has been shown to improve prognosis. Patients who are younger or have minimal comorbidities may be treated with FCR, BR, PCR, or obinutuzumab plus chlorambucil, while patients aged >70 and comorbidities are better candidates for obinutuzumab or rituximab plus chlorambucil or BR. Clinical research defining the optimal treatment approach for CLL patients continues at a rapid pace, and as new data emerge, these treatment recommendations will also evolve.

H. Treatment of relapsed and relapsed chronic lymphocytic leukemia. Treatment of patients with CLL that have relapsed after at least 1 prior therapy has changed markedly over the past several years. Treatment options now include ibrutinib (Bruton's tyrosine kinase inhibitor), idelalisib (PI3Kγ inhibitor), ofatumumab (2nd generation anti-CD20 mAb) and obinutuzumab (ADCC optimized anti-CD20 mAb), and alemtuzumab (anti-CD52 mAb). Patients who have a long remission after initial therapy with fludarabine–rituximab-based regimens may still be treated in a similar manner as untreated patients, with retreatment with first-line therapies. However, new second-line options provide excellent alternatives with lower incidences of long-term complications and myelosuppression. It remains unclear which second-line therapy is the best initial choice, since this has not been clarified in randomized trials in light of very recent approvals of a number of novel agents. In a randomized study comparing ibrutinib to ofatumumab, the former was associated with a response rate of approximately 70% and a 2-year PFS of 75%. Both PFS and OS were improved compared with ofatumumab (*N Engl J Med* 2014;371:213). Typical adverse prognostic factors such as 17p and 11q deletion did not affect the ORR or PFS. Importantly, ibrutinib can induce an isolate lymphocytosis in CLL patients that occurs in the first weeks of therapy and may persist for weeks to months, that does not signify disease progression. An important uncommon (5%), but poorly understood toxicity of ibrutinib is bleeding events, which do not have a clear mechanistic explanation at this time. Idelalisib represents a PI3K-γ inhibitor with activity in relapsed CLL and is now approved for use in combination with rituximab. In relapsed CLL patients that were not deemed appropriate for cytotoxic agents, idelalisib plus rituximab resulted in an ORR of 81% (0% CR), and improved PFS and OS compared with a rituximab plus placebo control arm (*N Engl J Med* 2014;370:997). Encouragingly, subgroup analysis demonstrated no difference in outcomes in patients with 17p deletion, p53 mutation, or IGVH un-mutated patients. Similar to ibrutinib, a transient lymphocytosis was also observed, which appeared to be dampened by concurrent rituximab therapy. Anti-CD20-mAb options include rituximab, ofatumumab, and obinutuzumab, although combinations with a targeted agent or chemotherapy are commonly utilized. Other treatment strategies for relapsed/refractory CLL patients include retreatment with various combinations of fludarabine, cyclophosphamide, and rituximab, which yield overall response rates of 29% to 59% in this patient population, but also have significant toxicities, especially in older patients previously treated with similar agents. High-dose steroids (e.g., methylprednisolone) in combination with anti-CD20 mAbs, have also provided responses in refractory CLL patients, with response rates up to 77% including patients with p53 or 17p− genetic abnormalities. Alemtuzumab has shown activity in fludarabine-refractory CLL; however, because of its high risk of serious infections, it is reserved for multiply relapsed CLL not responding to other agents, the presence of a 17p deletion, or if the patient transforms to more aggressive prolymphocytic leukemia. Life-threatening infections can occur in patients treated with high dose methylprednisolone or alemtuzumab, and they necessitate routine prophylaxis against infections. While the long-term remission duration with ibrutinib and other novel agents remains unclear, most patients are expected to relapse and require sequential anti-CLL therapy. Clinical trials are also addressing moving novel agents up-front, and combining various agents to optimize rate, depth, and duration of a response.

Myeloablative allogeneic SCT has historically been used in a limited manner in CLL patients, primarily on account of their advanced age. Small single-center and registry studies of selected CLL patients undergoing myeloablative SCT have shown treatment-related mortality rates of 24% to 46%, PFS of 26% to 62%, and overall survival of 31% to 76% at 3 to 10 years of projected follow-up. Recent studies utilizing reduced-intensity or nonmyeloablative allogeneic SCT have shown promising results, with treatment-related mortalities of 15% to 22%, PFS of 52% to 67%, and overall survival of 60% to 80% with a short 2-year projected follow-up. In general, results are superior in younger patients, those with little comorbidity, and those with chemosensitive disease before transplantation. The optimal conditioning regimens, patient age eligible for transplantation, and salvage chemotherapeutic regimens remain under investigation.

Despite the recent FDA drug approvals described above, numerous new drugs are being evaluated in early clinical trials for patients with relapsed and refractory CLL, and enrollment on a clinical trial should be considered routinely for these patients. Lenalidomide is a thalidomide analog with multiple potential mechanisms of action that has shown considerable single-agent clinical activity in multiple hematologic diseases, including multiple myeloma and myelodysplastic syndrome. Two phase II clinical trials have investigated lenalidomide doses of 25 mg daily for days 1 to 21 of a 28-day cycle in relapsed CLL patients, and have shown excellent tolerability and overall response rates of 32% to 65% and a complete response rate of 5% to 9%. Notably, there was a tumor flare reaction noted following treatment that should not be interpreted as rapid disease progression. More recent studies have combined lenalidomide with rituximab with ORR of 66% (12% CR) with similar response rates in patients with 17p deletion, and this combination is an option for relapsed CLL. Flavopiridol is a synthetic flavone with early clinical activity in a single-institution study that demonstrated overall response rates of 43% (many of which were durable for more than 12 months) as well as responses in patients with high-risk genetic features. The most notable toxicity reported was tumor lysis syndrome, which should be monitored for closely when treating CLL patients with this agent. Clinical trials evaluating lenalidomide and flavopiridol alone and with other agents are ongoing.

In summary, depending on patient characteristics, appropriate treatment options for relapsed CLL include clinical trials, ibrutinib, idelalisib, alemtuzumab, ofatumumab, obinutuzumab, combination fludarabine- or bendamustine-based chemotherapeutic regimens, high-dose steroids, lenalidomide, and, in appropriate candidates, allogeneic SCT. Finally, autologous T cells engineered to express an anti-CD19 chimeric antigen receptors (CAR) appear to have preliminary activity in small numbers of refractory CLL patients. Since these T cells have been shown to persist long-term in the patient, this approach provides a potential for long-term anti-CLL immunity without the toxicity of allogeneic HSCT, and will certainly be the focus of future CLL studies. Additional emerging immunotherapy agents under investigation include bispecific T cell engagers (BiTEs) such as blinatumomab, that simultaneously engage tumor cells (via anti-CD19 scFV) and T cells (via anti-CD3 scFv). Immune checkpoint blockade, for example with anti-PD-1/PD-L1/L2 blocking agents, are also being explored.

SUGGESTED READINGS

Chronic Myeloid Leukemia

Baccarani M, Deininger MW, Rosti G, et al. European Leukemia net recommendations for the management of chronic myeloid leukemia: 2013. *Blood* 2013;122:872–884.

Bacigalupo A. Stem cell transplantation for chronic myeloid leukemia (CML): current indications and perspectives. *Curr Cancer Drug Targets.* 2013;13:775–778.

Deininger M, Schleuning M, Greinix H, et al. The effect of prior exposure to imatinib on transplant-related mortality. *Haematologica* 2006;91:452–459.

Druker BJ, Guilhot F, O'Brien SG, et al. Five-year follow-up of patients receiving imatinib for chronic myeloid leukemia. *N Engl J Med* 2006;355:2408–2417.

Melo JV, Ross DM. Minimal residual disease and discontinuation of therapy in chronic myeloid leukemia: can we aim at a cure? *Hematology Am Soc Hematol Educ Program* 2011:136–142.

Osborn M, Hughes T. Managing imatinib resistance in chronic myeloid leukemia. *Curr Opin Hematol* 2010;17:97–103.

Chronic Lymphocytic Leukemia

Brown JR. The treatment of relapsed refractory chronic lymphocytic leukemia. ASH Education Program, Hematology. *Am Soc Hematol Educ Program* 2011:110–118.

Byrd JC, Brown JR, O'Brien S, et al. Ibrutinib versus ofatumumab in previously treated chronic lymphocytic leukemia. *N Engl J Med* 2014;371:213–223.

Byrd JC, Furman RR, Coutre SE, et al. Targeting ibrutinib in relapsed chronic lymphocytic leukemia. *N Engl J Med* 2014;369:32–42.

Byrd JC, Jones JJ, Woyach JA, et al. Entering the era of targeted therapy for CLL: impact on the practicing clinician. *J Clin Oncol* 2014;32:3039–3047.

ESMO Guidelines consensus conference on malignant lymphoma 2011 part 1: DLBCL, FL, and CLL. *Ann Oncol* 2013;24:561–576.

Furman RR, Sharman JP, Coutre SE, et al. Idelalisib and rituximab in relapse chronic lymphocytic leukemia. *N Engl J Med* 2014;370:997–1007.

Gaindano G, Foa R, Dalla-Favera R. Molecular pathogenesis of chronic lymphocytic leukemia. *J Clin Invest* 2012;122:3432–3438.

Hallek M. CLL: 2013 updated on diagnosis, risk stratification and treatment. *Am J Hematol* 2013;88:804–816.

Jones JA, Byrd JC. How will B-cell-receptor-targeted therapies change future CLL therapy? *Blood* 2014;123:1455–1460.

29 Plasma Cell Dyscrasias
Jesse Keller • Ravi Vij

I. MULTIPLE MYELOMA

A. Subjective. Presenting symptoms of multiple myeloma (MM) may include bone pain, fatigue, and recurrent bacterial infections. Lethargy is a common complaint, occurring in up to one-third of patients at diagnosis and usually attributable to ongoing anemia and metabolic derangements. Symptomatic hypercalcemia is common at diagnosis and may occur in approximately 30% of patients. Weight loss may be an accompanying sign in up to 20% of patients. More uncommon events include neuropathy secondary to the mono-clonal paraprotein (M protein), a feature of roughly 5% of newly diagnosed MM patients. Tumor fever is rare, and is a diagnosis of exclusion; febrile MM patients are infected until proven otherwise. One-third of patients have a prior diagnosis of a plasma cell proliferative process preceding the diagnosis of MM.

B. Objective. Physical examination may reveal pallor, bony tenderness, a subcutaneous mass secondary to a plasmacytoma, or focal neurologic signs due to spinal cord compression. Hepatomegaly, splenomegaly, and lymphadenopathy are rare.

C. Workup and staging

1. Laboratory. Anemia is present in three-quarters of patients at diagnosis and is generally normochromic and normocytic. White blood cell (WBC) and platelet counts are usually preserved, although marrow replacement by MM may lead to pancytopenia. Examination of the peripheral smear may reveal rouleaux formation. The erythrocyte sedimentation rate (ESR) is generally elevated in MM. Almost 20% of patients will have a creatinine level of more than 2.0 mg/dL at diagnosis. Hypercalcemia due to extensive bone involvement and hyperuricemia can worsen renal function. Albumin has prognostic significance and is a component of the International Staging System. A serum protein electrophoresis (SPEP) and urinary protein electrophoresis (UPEP) should be performed on patients in whom the diagnosis of MM is suspected. Immunofixation is more sensitive than electrophoresis and is done to confirm the presence and type of a paraprotein (M protein). An M protein is detectable in the serum of more than 90% of patients. The paraprotein is an IgG in approximately half the cases and an IgA in 20% of cases. IgD, IgE, and IgM paraproteins are very rare. IgM paraproteins are almost always associated with Waldenstrom's macroglobulinemia (WM). Free light chains are present in approximately 15% of patients. Kappa (κ) light chains are more common than lambda (λ) by approximately 2:1. Bence–Jones proteinuria occurs when light chains are freely filtered at the glomerulus and are excreted in the urine. The light chain is rarely detected on SPEP, but will be detected on UPEP. If light chains are detected in the urine, a 24-hour urine specimen should be collected to quantify the protein and monitor response to treatment. The serum-free light chain (SFLC) assay now allows for quantification of light chains in the serum in a direct and efficient manner. Nonsecretory myeloma constitutes less than 5% of patients. These patients have no paraprotein detectable on SPEP, UPEP, and immunofixation. However, a majority will have an abnormal SFLC κ:λ ratio.

2. Radiographic imaging. All patients should have a skeletal survey including the skull, spine, pelvis, femurs, and humeri. Almost 80% of patients have at least one abnormality on radiographs with two-thirds of patients having punched-out lytic lesions. Pathologic fractures, vertebral compression fractures, or osteoporosis are each present in one-fourth of patients. Radionuclide bone scans detect osteoblastic response and are therefore less sensitive than plain radiographs in detecting skeletal involvement by MM. Magnetic resonance imaging (MRI) of the spine is more sensitive than plain radiographs in detecting early lesions, and may be considered in patients with negative skeletal surveys or as clinically indicated for suspicious symptoms. Patients thought to have solitary plasmacytomas should undergo MRI imaging to exclude systemic disease. ^{18}F-fluorodeoxyglucose positron emission tomography (FDG PET) is now approved for initial workup and follow-up of patients with MM. It is of particular benefit in those with nonsecretory or oligosecretory disease, an increasing problem in refractory and relapsed patients.

3. **Bone marrow evaluation.** Patients should undergo bone marrow biopsy and aspiration for quantification of bone marrow plasma cells. The malignant plasma cells stain positive for CD138. Monoclonality is established by immunostains that demonstrate κ- or λ-restricted cytoplasmic immunoglobulin staining. Karyotyping is now recommended as a prognostic tool. Conventional cytogenetic analysis in MM is often difficult because of the low-growth fraction and paucity of mitotic cells. However, using a variety of fluorescent in situ hybridization (FISH) probes (del 13q, t[4;14], t[11;14], del 17p, t(14, 16), t(14, 20)) on interphase cells, cytogenetic abnormalities are commonly found in MM. The plasma cell labeling index (PCLI) performed on bone marrow biopsy measures the percentage of MM cells that synthesize DNA; an elevated labeling index implies a more aggressive MM and poor prognosis. Assessment by multiparameter flow cytometry is currently under investigation for the identification of minimal residual disease (MRD). Patients who achieve an MRD negative complete response (CR) may have an improved prognosis as compared with those with persistent disease after treatment.

D. **Diagnosis.** The historic criteria for the diagnosis of MM have been supplanted by the International Myeloma Working Group (IMWG) criteria for the diagnosis of plasma cell dyscrasias (Table 29-1). End-organ damage is the defining feature that separates MM from a monoclonal gammopathy or smoldering myeloma. Revised criteria have recently been published that update the IMWG criteria (Table 29-2). These criteria add several biomarkers as well as radiographic findings as MM defining events.

E. **Staging.** In the past, MM was staged according to the Durie–Salmon staging system. In the modern era, this system has been replaced by the International Staging System (Table 29-3), a simplified system that utilizes only the β-2-microglobulin and albumin.

F. **Treatment.** The initial treatment decision revolves around whether or not a patient is considered a transplant candidate.

1. **Transplant eligible.** High-dose chemotherapy (HDT) with autologous stem cell transplant is considered standard of care for transplant-eligible patients. Response rates (RRs) to HDT approach 90% with approximately half the number of patients achieving CR.

   a. **Induction therapy.** Patients suitable for transplant usually undergo induction therapy with 4 to 6 months of a two- or three-drug regimen including a proteasome inhibitor, immunomodulatory agent (Thalidomide or Lenalidomide), and corticosteroid.

   Three drug regimens such as Bortezomib (bortezomib), Lenalidomide (Revlimid), and Dexamethasone (VRD) or Bortezomib, Cyclophosphamide, and Dexamethasone (VCD) have shown improved efficacy with increased rates of CR when compared with two-drug regimens. Long-term data for an overall survival (OS) benefit with these regimens are still maturing. Since there are only limited data comparing the available regimens, the therapeutic decisions should be made on the basis of patient characteristics and side-effect profiles. Alkylating agents, such as melphalan, should be avoided prior to stem cell collection in transplant-eligible patients as they are toxic to stem cells.

   b. **Stem cell collection and transplant.** Following induction therapy, patients undergo stem cell collection, consolidative HDT, and transplant. Alternatively, patients may undergo harvest and stem cell storage first, and then proceed with additional conventional therapies, postponing transplant until first relapse. Randomized trials have shown equivalent survival with these two approaches. However, quality-of-life analysis and event-free survival favor early transplant. Conditioning for transplant with single-agent melphalan is the standard of care. Although controlled trials

TABLE 29-1   IMWG Classification System

Multiple myeloma	M protein in serum and/or urine
	Bone marrow (clonal) plasma cells ≥10% and/or plasmacytoma
	Related end-organ dysfunction (≥1 of CRAB Criteria)[a,b]
Smoldering myeloma	M protein in serum ≥3.0 g/dL or
	Bone marrow clonal plasma cells ≥10%
	No evidence of related end-organ dysfunction[a]
MGUS	M protein in serum <3.0 g/dL
	Bone marrow clonal plasma cells <10%
	No evidence of other B-cell proliferative disorders
	No evidence of related end-organ dysfunction[a]
Solitary plasmacytoma of bone	No M protein in serum and/or urine[c]
	Single area of bone destruction due to clonal plasma cells
	Bone marrow not consistent with multiple myeloma
	Normal skeletal survey (and MRI of spine and pelvis if done)
	No related organ or tissue impairment (other than solitary bone lesion)[a]
Extramedullary plasmacytoma	No M protein in serum and/or urine[c]
	Extramedullary tumor of clonal plasma cells
	Normal bone marrow
	Normal skeletal survey
	No related organ or tissue impairment[a]

MGUS, monoclonal gammopathy of unknown significance; MRI, magnetic resonance imaging.
[a]CRAB criteria: include hypercalcemia ≥10.5 mg/dL, renal insufficiency with Cr >2 mg/dL, anemia >2 g/dL below lower limit of normal or <10 g/dL, or bone lesions (lytic lesions or osteoporosis).
[b]A variety of other types of end-organ dysfunctions can occasionally occur and lead to a need for therapy. Such dysfunction is sufficient to support a classification of myeloma if proven to be myeloma related.
[c]A small M-component may sometimes be present.

TABLE 29-2   Revised International Myeloma Working Group Classification System

Multiple myeloma	M protein in serum and/or urine
	Bone marrow (clonal) plasma cells cells ≥ 10% and/or plasmacytoma
	Related end-organ dysfunction (≥1 of CRAB Criteria)[a,c]
	Any one or more biomarker of malignancy[b]
Smoldering myeloma	M protein in serum ≥3.0 g/dL or urinary M protein ≥500mg
	Clonal bone marrow plasma cells 10–60%
	Absence of myeloma defining events[b] or amyloidosis

MGUS, monoclonal gammopathy of unknown significance; MRI, magnetic resonance imaging.
[a]CRAB Criteria: includes hypercalcemia ≥11 mg/dL or 1mg/dL > than upper limit of normal, renal insufficiency with CrCl <40mL/min or serum Creatinine >2 mg/dL, anemia >2 g/dL below lower limit of normal or <10 g/dL, or bone lesions (lytic lesions seen on skeletal radiography, CT or PET-CT).
[b]Clonal bone marrow plasma cell percentage ≥ 60%, Involved: uninvolved serum free light chain ratio of ≥100, >1 focal lesions on MRI studies.
[c]A variety of other types of end-organ dysfunctions can occasionally occur and lead to a need for therapy. Such dysfunction is sufficient to support a classification of myeloma if proven to be myeloma related.

of transplant generally excluded patients older than 65 years, improvements in supportive care have allowed the application of high-dose therapy and autologous transplant to patients older than 70. Medicare approves this procedure for patients up to 78 years of age. Toxicities of high-dose therapy include mucositis and infectious complications. The overall transplant-related mortality is 1% to 2%. Repeated HDT and transplant within 6 months ("tandem transplant") may provide a survival benefit in patients who have less than a very good partial response (less than 90% reduction in paraprotein) after their first transplant.

2. **Transplant ineligible.** Newly diagnosed patients ineligible for transplant constitute the majority of cases. The goals of therapy are to gain quick control of disease and limit complications. Numerous regimens exist for management of these patients. Historically, Melphalan and Prednisone (MP) had been the mainstay of therapy. With the advent of novel agents, randomized trials noted superior results for therapies combining MP with newer agents. The addition of Thalidomide (MPT) conferred a survival benefit compared with MP. Likewise, MP plus Lenalidomide (MPR) showed a superior RR and Progression Free Survival (PFS) when compared with MP alone. Bortezomib in combination with MP (VMP) has additionally shown improvements in RRs, time to progression, and OS as compared with MP. While triple-drug Melphalan-based regimens improved results for transplant-ineligible patients, recent data suggest that two-drug novel regimens such as Lenalidomide and Dexamethasone may be as good as triple-drug Melphalan-based therapies.

3. **Maintenance therapy.** In a CALGB study, Lenalidomide maintenance in the post-transplant setting was associated with a benefit in both PFS and OS. In a similar French IFM study, however, the benefit from Lenalidomide maintenance was restricted to PFS. Although Thalidomide has been shown in some studies to have an OS benefit in the posttransplant setting, it is also associated with increased toxicity, particularly with neuropathy and thromboembolism. Likewise, bortezomib maintenance has been shown to confer a PFS and OS benefit when utilized in patients undergoing induction therapy with a bortezomib-based regimen. Even in transplant-ineligible patients, Lenalidomide and Dexamethasone given until progression was associated with an OS advantage compared with fixed duration therapy with MPT.

4. **Relapsed or refractory disease.** Relapse is nearly universal, and refractory disease is frequently encountered in MM patients. Progressive disease (PD) is defined by otherwise unexplained hypercalcemia ($\geq$11.5 mg/dL), new or progressive plasmacytomas, or a predefined absolute rise or 25% increase from best response in a set of markers including the following:
   • Serum M-protein (absolute rise of $\geq$0.5 g/dL)
   • Urine monoclonal protein (absolute rise of 200 mg/24 hours)
   • Percentage of plasma cells in the bone marrow (10% increase if no M-protein)
   • Difference in κ- and λ-FLC studies (must be >10 mg/dL with abnormal K/L ratio)
   There is currently no standard of care for relapsed or refractory disease. For eligible candidates who have not previously undergone stem cell transplant, HDT/autologous stem cell transplant is an option. For those who have previously been transplanted, repeat HDT or further conventional chemotherapy may be tried. If prior response was significant and relapse delayed, repeat trials of previous regimens may be considered. Several agents are approved specifically in the relapsed or refractory setting:
   a. **Carfilzomib.** This is a second-generation proteasome inhibitor approved by the FDA for patients who have been treated with at least two prior therapies, including a proteasome inhibitor and immunomodulatory drug, and have shown progression within 60 days of therapy.
   b. **Pomalidomide.** This is a Thalidomide analog that has demonstrated activity in MM. The combination of Pomalidomide and Dexamethasone is FDA approved for patients who have received at least two prior therapies, including lenalidomide and bortezomib, and whose disease has progressed within 60 days of last treatment.
   c. **Other regimens.** Combinations of conventional chemotherapeutic agents are still utilized frequently after failure of proteasome inhibitor and immunomodulatory

drug therapy. These include a variety of combinations including C-VAD (Cyclophosphamide, Vincristine, Adriamycin, and Dexamethasone), D-CEP (Dexamethasone, cyclophosphamide, etoposide, and cisplatin), DT-PACE (Dexamethasone, Thalidomide, cisplatin, Doxorubicin, cyclophosphamide, and etoposide), and M2 (vincristine, carmustine, cyclophosphamide, and melphalan).

5. **Allogeneic transplant.** Myeloablative allogeneic transplant in MM is associated with a modest rate of potential cure, whereas high upfront treatment-related mortality (TRM) limits its use. Recently, several trials have evaluated tandem autologous transplant compared with autologous transplant followed by nonmyeloablative allogeneic transplant. Although some trials with long-term follow-up have suggested improvement in OS with a tandem autologous and nonmyeloablative allogeneic transplant approach, the majority of trials have not shown a benefit from this strategy, and longer-term follow-up is awaited. Additional trials evaluating the role of autologous transplant followed by allogeneic transplant for relapsed/refractory disease or as initial therapy in high-risk patients are needed.

G. **Adjunct treatments**

1. **Bisphosphonates.** Bisphosphonates inhibit osteoclast-mediated bone resorption and are an integral part of the management of skeletal lesions in MM. They have been shown to decrease skeletal-related events, improve pain control, and limit hypercalcemia. Intravenous pamidronate or zoledronic acid has been approved by the FDA for this indication and is administered on a monthly schedule. Current recommendations suggest 2 years of continued therapy for patients who remain in remission. Bisphosphonates may be continued longer for PD or active bone disease. Key toxicities to monitor include osteonecrosis of the jaw and renal failure. The MRC IX trial revealed an OS advantage for zoledronic acid compared with cladronate independent of the effect on skeletal-related events.

2. **Erythropoietin.** Anemia is a common complication of MM. Erythropoietin decreases transfusion requirements in MM patients, including those with refractory disease.

3. **Radiation.** MM is a radiosensitive tumor. External-beam radiation (RT) can effectively palliate discrete areas of bone pain or areas of mass effect such as spinal cord compression.

4. **Surgery.** Radiographs of long bones done for staging or to evaluate pain may reveal lytic lesions concerning for impending fracture. Orthopedic surgery consultation and prophylactic surgical pinning may prevent some of the morbidity of a fracture. Patients who undergo pinning generally undergo RT to the area postoperatively.

5. **Hemodialysis.** Renal failure may occur early in the course of disease. Renal impairment may be reversible if the MM responds to treatment, and support with hemodialysis is appropriate. The value of plasmapheresis to reduce the paraprotein level in this situation is debatable.

6. **Infection prophylaxis.** MM patients have a deficit in humoral immunity due to decreased levels of normal immunoglobulins. The risk of infection is further increased both by direct marrow suppression from chemotherapy as well as immunosuppression associated with long-term, high-dose corticosteroids. All MM patients should be vaccinated against *Streptococcus pneumonia*. For those undergoing treatment with proteasome inhibitors, Zoster prophylaxis is recommended. Additionally, some patients may benefit from IVIg therapy to supplement chronically low IgG levels.

7. **Venous thromboembolism prophylaxis.** DVT prophylaxis is recommended for patients receiving immunomodulatory drug combinations with high-dose steroids and chemotherapy. Low-dose aspirin is thought to be sufficient for most patients. Patients at high risk for thromboembolism should receive full anticoagulation.

H. **Follow-up.** Close follow-up of serial monoclonal protein levels in the serum and/or urine allows for routine monitoring of disease status. Evaluation of quantitative SFLC should be used as an additional tool to evaluate response in the appropriate patient. In patients who have undergone multiple lines of therapy and have relapsed or refractory disease, malignant plasma cells may de-differentiate and cease secretion of a monoclonal protein or light chain. PET scans may be useful in the follow-up of these patients. Skeletal survey and bone marrow biopsy are usually repeated at the time of suspected disease progression.

I. Natural history

1. **Survival.** Historically, MP was the first regimen to show an OS benefit from a median of 6 months to 3 years. The advent of high-dose therapy with autologous transplant provided additional survival benefit, increasing median OS to 5 years or more. With the advent of bortezomib and the immunomodulatory agents, data support an additional 18 months to 2 years improvement in OS. The recent approval of Pomalidomide and Carfilzomib is expected to further improve on rates of OS. In addition, novel agents in development show promise to extend this benefit even further.

2. **Prognostic factors.** Several factors may be evaluated in the initial workup to assist with prognosis. Serum β-2-microglobulin levels correlate with tumor burden and renal function; elevated levels are an important marker of decreased response to treatment and worse OS. Other poor prognostic factors include high lactate dehydrogenase (LDH), high PCLI, low albumin, plasmablastic features in the bone marrow, and circulating plasma cells. More recently, karyotype has emerged as the most powerful predictor of outcomes. The Mayo Stratification for Myeloma and Risk-adapted Therapy (mSMART) criteria divide patients into standard-, intermediate-, and high-risk groups. The mSMART criteria are detailed below:
   • **High risk.** Del 17p, t(14;16), t(14;20), or high-risk gene expression profiling (GEP)
   • **Intermediate risk.** Del 13 or hypodiploidy, t(4;14), PCLI ≥3%
   • **Standard risk.** All other abnormalities

J. Background

1. **Epidemiology.** Based on SEER data, the incidence of MM is roughly 6 per 100,000/year. It represents 1.3% of all new cancer diagnoses and 1.8% of all cancer deaths. Overall, incidence and prevalence appear to be growing as the population ages and treatment improves. Notably, among African Americans the risk of MM is double that in the white population, and men are more frequently affected than women. It is a disease of the elderly, with the median age at diagnosis being 69 years. The etiology of MM is unknown. Certain environmental factors, such as benzene and radiation exposure, appear to be predisposing.

2. **Pathophysiology.** Cytokines provide autocrine and paracrine growth signals to myeloma cells. IL-6, insulin-like growth factor-1, stromal cell-derived factor-1, and vascular endothelial growth factor have all been shown to be important in myeloma cell survival and growth. The interaction between MM cells and stromal cells involving adhesion molecules such as intercellular adhesion molecule 1 (ICAM-1) and vascular adhesion molecule 1 (VCAM-1) is thought to provide critical survival signals. Clinical symptoms result from the infiltration of end organs by malignant cells, or deposition of excess light chains. Lytic bone lesions, a hallmark of MM, appear to be mediated by increased expression of receptor activator of nuclear factor κB ligand (RANKL) and decreased expression of Osteoprotegrin (OPG). Tumor-derived osteoclast activating factors including increased IL-3, IL-6, and macrophage inflammatory protein-1 α (MIP-1 α) levels, as well as osteoblast inhibition through MM-derived dickkopf-1 (DKK-1) are also thought to play a key role in the development of bony lesions. Osteoblast inhibition and osteoclast activation lead directly to bone breakdown and often result in clinical hypercalcemia associated with MM. Renal dysfunction is usually a result of excess light chains, but heavy chains may be involved. Anemia is a result of bone marrow invasion by malignant cells and subsequent alterations in the marrow microenvironment.

3. **Molecular biology.** The malignant cell in MM is thought to arise from transformation of a postgerminal center plasma cell. The pathogenesis remains unknown, but in almost all cases, initial genetic insults lead to the establishment of a monoclonal gammopathy of undetermined significance (MGUS), a premalignant plasma cell disorder. Most of the karyotypic abnormalities characteristic of multiple myeloma are detectable in patients with MGUS. It is thought that subsequent additional genetic changes in

the plasma cell and alterations in the microenvironment lead to overt MM. Activating mutations of Ras, Myc dysregulation, inactivation of Rb, and loss or mutation of p53 are thought to be critical late events in pathogenesis. Large-scale genomic sequencing has shown an average mutational burden of 35 amino acid changing mutations and 21 chromosomal rearrangements in protein-coding regions. Statistically significant protein-coding region mutations include: *NRAS, KRAS, FAM46C, DIS3, TP53, HLA-A, MAGED1, CCND1, FAM46C, PNRC1,* and *ALOX12B*. Additional mutations are often found in *BRAF*, NF-κB pathway genes, and histone modifying enzymes, including regulators of *HOXA9*.

K. Research frontiers. The number of agents with activity in MM continues to expand. Monoclonal antibodies targeting CS-1 and CD38 are likely to enter the therapeutic armamentarium in the future. Novel oral proteasome inhibitors are being investigated. In addition, a variety of compounds, including signal transduction and cell cycle check point inhibitors, are in clinical trials.

II. OTHER PLASMA CELL DISORDERS

A. Monoclonal gammopathy of undetermined significance. MGUS is defined by the absence of end-organ dysfunction in the setting of a monoclonal protein <3 g/dL and <10% infiltrating plasma cells in the bone marrow. Prevalence varies according to race and age. In a large study of Caucasian patients, the prevalence of MGUS for patients >50 years of age was 3.2%. The African American population and men tend to have higher rates of MGUS. MGUS is often diagnosed incidentally on workup for an increased total serum protein, neuropathy, or in the workup of anemia or renal failure in the setting of other causative factors. MGUS patients should be monitored with SPEP every 6 to 12 months. One percent of patients with MGUS progress to a more clinically significant plasma cell dyscrasia each year. A risk stratification model based on three factors can be used to predict risk of progression over 20 years. These include the following: serum monoclonal protein level ≥1.5 g/dL, non-IgG MGUS, or an abnormal SFLC ratio. The risk of progression for patients with 3, 2, 1, or 0 of these factors is 58%, 37%, 21%, and 5%, respectively.

B. Smoldering myeloma. Smoldering multiple myeloma (SMM) is an intermediate stage between MGUS and MM. It is defined by a monoclonal protein of >3 g/dL and/or BM infiltration of ≥10% plasma cells, in the absence of evidence of end-organ damage. The presence of both defining features in the setting of a FLC ratio outside of the reference range of 0.125 to 8 describes a subset of patients with particularly poor risk for progression to overt MM. At 5 years of follow-up, patients with 3, 2, or 1 of these three features had cumulative risk of progression of 76%, 51%, and 25%, respectively. There is great interest in defining a group of SMM that may benefit from therapy.

C. Plasma cell leukemia. Plasma cell leukemia occurs when high levels of circulating plasma cells are present (greater than 2×10^9/L or greater than 20% in the differential WBC count). The disease is aggressive and survival is worse than MM. In cases arising without an antecedent plasma cell disorder, median survival is 6 to 11 months. When plasma cell leukemia occurs as a late event in a patient with known MM, the median survival is 2 to 6 months. Patients with these disorders usually harbor poor risk cytogenetic abnormalities including p53 deletions at high rates. Aggressive multiagent therapy is employed in treatment for these patients.

D. Solitary plasmacytomas of bone. These patients present with a single bony lesion without signs of systemic disease. An MRI of the spine and pelvis and a PET scan (Table 29-2) should be performed to rule out occult lesions. Radiation provides excellent local control, with 90% of patients free from local recurrence. At this time, there is no evidence that chemotherapy or bisphosphonates during or after radiation provide a benefit to patients with solitary plasmacytoma. Patients with lesions larger than 5 cm have the greatest risk of recurrence after radiotherapy. The median OS is roughly 10 years. Up to 50% to 60% of patients may develop overt MM following radiation therapy.

E. Extramedullary plasmacytomas. Extramedullary plasmacytomas are clonal proliferations of plasma cells that arise outside of the bone marrow (Table 29-1). Lesions occur most frequently in the head and neck, but may occur in virtually any organ. The initial

TABLE 29-3	**International Staging System for Multiple Myeloma**	
	Criteria	**Median survival**
Stage I	β2M <3.5 mg/L and albumin ≥3.5 g/dL	62 months
Stage II	Not I or III[a]	44 months
Stage III	β2M ≥5.5 mg/L	29 months

β2M, β-2-microglobulin.
[a]There are two categories for stage II: serum β-2-microglobulin <3.5 mg/L but serum albumin <3.5 g/dL; or serum β-2-microglobulin 3.5 mg/L to <5.5 mg/L irrespective of the serum albumin level.

workup and evaluation is similar to patients with solitary plasmacytoma, and care must be taken to exclude additional disease. Lesions are sensitive to radiation therapy, and chemotherapy does not provide additional benefit. Five-year OS ranges from 40% to 85%, and 30% to 50% of patients will develop MM at a median of 1.5 to 2.5 years.

III. AMYLOIDOSIS

A. **Subjective.** Patients with AL amyloidosis often present with nonspecific complaints including fatigue, weight loss, and lightheadedness. Orthostasis may be a presenting symptom and can be secondary to several sequelae of amyloidosis, including nephrotic syndrome, intravascular volume depletion, restrictive cardiomyopathy, or autonomic neuropathy. Edema can occur from an amyloid-induced nephrotic syndrome or congestive heart failure. Infiltration of soft tissues can cause capillary fragility and purpuric bruising; periorbital ecchymosis is a classic symptom of AL. Other features include macroglossia, endocrinopathies, neuropathy, and carpal tunnel syndrome.

B. **Objective.** Physical findings in AL vary depending on which organ systems are affected. Examination may reveal macroglossia, periorbital ecchymosis, hepatomegaly, or edema. Nerve involvement can result in sensory, motor, or autonomic deficits. Laboratory evaluation may reveal renal insufficiency or hypoalbuminemia due to nephrotic syndrome. Low voltages in limb leads on electrocardiogram may be noted in roughly 50% of patients. Amyloid cardiomyopathy may appear on echocardiography as hypertrophy with a restrictive filling pattern or with a "sparkling" appearance of the myocardium. Cardiac MRI may reveal a zebra pattern of enhancement within the myocardium.

C. **Workup.** The first step in the workup of AL is to suspect the diagnosis. A clue to the possibility of AL is the discovery of a paraprotein in the serum or urine of the patient. A diagnosis of AL amyloidosis by IMWG criteria requires evidence of a monoclonal plasma cell proliferative disorder in addition to end-organ damage and pathologic confirmation of AL amyloid deposition. In the setting of confirmed tissue amyloid, evidence of an M protein in serum or urine, an abnormal SFLC ratio, or a clonal plasma cell population in the bone marrow is sufficient to complete the diagnosis. The paraprotein may be a complete immunoglobulin, although only the light-chain component contributes to amyloid formation. Only a small quantity (less than 1 g/dL) of paraprotein may be present. SFLC assays can be utilized in patients with a negative serum immunofixation. The λ light chains are three times more commonly associated with AL, presumably because these more often possess amyloidogenic characteristics. Under polarized light, amyloid shows apple-green birefringence when stained with Congo red stain. Immunoperoxidase stains on tissue specimens can differentiate between different types of amyloid. Mass spectroscopy is a more sensitive and specific test when compared with immunohistochemistry and is increasingly used to delineate between types of amyloid. An initial biopsy of abdominal fat is often done in an attempt to make a tissue diagnosis while avoiding biopsy of vital organs. The presence of amyloid is 100% specific, but sensitivity varies and can be less than 75%. A bone marrow biopsy will be positive for amyloid deposition in 60% of cases. In most cases of primary AL, clonal plasma cells represent less than 10% of the marrow. In rare cases, no clonal population may be found, and diagnosis should proceed with caution. MM and

AL sometimes coexist: 20% of patients with AL are found on workup to have myeloma, and in 10% to 15% of patients with MM, AL will eventually develop. Troponin T and N-terminal probrain natriuretic peptide (NT-proBNP) are both powerful predictors of survival in AL patients.

D. Therapy. As with MM, the initial decision in treatment is to determine whether a patient is a candidate for transplantation. As a general rule, transplant-eligible patients should have a low level of Troponin-T and NT-proBNP and limited levels of organ dysfunction.

1. **High-dose therapy/autologous transplant.** Retrospective data support the role of autologous transplantation in amyloidosis, showing significant improvements in OS when compared with traditional chemotherapy. A randomized trial comparing conventional chemotherapy with autologous transplantation showed no improvement in OS. However, the patient population in this study had significant end-organ involvement and a high transplant-related mortality and is thought not to be representative of modern transplant-eligible patients. When transplant is chosen, melphalan-based regimens are standard of care.

2. **Transplant ineligible.** Melphalan and Dexamethasone have been extensively used as therapy for patients who are not transplant candidates. Lately, Bortezomib-containing regimens have shown impressive activity, while immunomodulatory drugs may also have a role in this disease.

3. **Future directions.** Interest lies in the investigation of novel combination therapies as well as new proteasome inhibitors and immunomodulatory agents.

E. Epidemiology and survival. The estimated incidence is 5.1 to 12.8 new cases per million per year. Prognosis depends on the organs affected, with cardiac and hepatic involvement portending worse outcomes. Median survival is approximately 1 to 2 years in untreated patients, but is less than 6 months in patients with cardiac amyloid. However, in those with limited disease, current therapies may offer an OS surpassing 5 years.

F. Pathophysiology. Amyloidosis is a group of syndromes in which symptoms arise from infiltration of tissue with insoluble misfolded proteins. In primary amyloid (AL), the amyloid is composed of paraprotein light chains secreted by monoclonal plasma cells that deposit into tissues in β-pleated sheet conformation. Alternative sources of amyloid protein include chronic inflammation in secondary (AA) amyloid, β-2-microglobulin in hemodialysis-associated amyloidosis, and transthyretin in familial amyloidosis.

IV. WALDENSTRÖM'S MACROGLOBULINEMIA. In the World Health Organization (WHO) classification of non-Hodgkin's lymphoma (NHL), WM is a subset of lymphoplasmacytic lymphoma (LPL), a mature B-cell neoplasm closely related to chronic lymphocytic leukemia/small lymphocytic lymphoma (CLL/SLL).

A. Subjective. Patients may present with nonspecific symptoms such as fevers, night sweats, fatigue, weight loss, and peripheral neuropathy. In up to one-third of patients, monoclonal IgM may lead to the development of the hyperviscosity syndrome (HVS), with a classic triad of symptoms including bruising and bleeding, visual changes, and neuropsychiatric symptoms. Deposits of IgM in end organs may lead to purpuric skin lesions and severe diarrhea with steatorrhea. Mucosal bleeding results from paraprotein-mediated interference with coagulation factors and platelet function. Neuropsychiatric symptoms associated with the HVS include transient ischemic attacks (TIAs), paralysis, seizure, dementia, or coma. Occasionally, the IgM paraprotein may act as a cryoglobulin and cause Raynaud's syndrome and acral cyanosis.

B. Objective. Many patients with WM have no obvious physical findings. On funduscopic examination, patients may have retinal hemorrhages, exudates, or papilledema. Approximately one-third of patients have hepatomegaly, splenomegaly, or lymphadenopathy. IgM can act as an autoantibody against autologous antigens, resulting in autoimmune phenomenon such as demyelinating peripheral neuropathy, cryoglobulinemia, cold agglutinin disease, glomerulonephritis, paraneoplastic pemphigus, or retinitis.

C. Workup and staging. Anemia is the most common laboratory abnormality on initial evaluation. Occasional findings include pseudohyponatremia from elevated protein levels, renal insufficiency, and proteinuria. ESR may be greatly increased or normal.

LDH and β-2-microglobulin are often elevated. Diagnosis is based on the presence of an IgM monoclonal protein, bone marrow involvement of >10% by LPL (small lymphocytes exhibiting plasmacytoid or plasma cell differentiation), and expression of a typical immunophenotype by the bone marrow infiltrate. Immunophenotypic analysis should exclude other lymphoproliferative disorders including CLL/SLL. LPL cells express cytoplasmic immunoglobulin, distinguishing them from CLL/SLL cells, which do not. Other immunophenotypic markers are similar to those of CLL, including expression of CD19 and CD20. Initial assessment should also include measurement of serum viscosity. Symptomatic hyperviscosity usually does not occur until the IgM paraprotein is greater than 3 g/dL and the serum viscosity is more than 5 cp (normal is 1.4 to 1.8 cp), although symptoms can occur at lower levels of paraprotein and lower serum viscosities. The International Prognostic Staging System for WM (IPSSWM) utilizes five adverse features (age >65, Hbg ≤11.5 g/dL, platelet count ≤100,000, β-2-microglobulin > 3mg/L, and serum IgM >70 g/L) to stratify patients into low-, intermediate-, and high-risk groups. Low-risk patients are less than 65 with zero or one risk factor, and have an 87% 5-year survival. Intermediate-risk patients are older than 65 or those with two risk factors. High-risk patients have more than two risk factors. Five-year OS for intermediate- and high-risk patients are 68% and 38%, respectively.

D. Therapy. The goal of treatment is to limit symptoms and prevent end-organ damage. Treatment is directed at reducing serum viscosity and treating the underlying lymphoma. Notably, severe neurologic symptoms or intractable bleeding due to hyperviscosity are an oncologic emergency, requiring urgent plasmapheresis and chemotherapy to reduce circulating IgM levels. Treatment regimens vary, but initial therapy is usually pursued with a Rituximab-based combination. Notably, Rituximab may cause an initial IgM flare, and patients with high IgM levels (>5 g/dL) should be cytoreduced with chemotherapy before Rituximab is added to the regimen. Novel agents such as Bortezomib and Thalidomide in combination with Rituximab and Dexamethasone as initial therapy have produced impressive results. Additional agents with activity include Bendamustine, nucleoside analogs (fludarabine, pentostatin, and cladribine), and alkylator-based regimens. Autologous stem cell transplantation is an option for eligible patients who have relapsed and refractory disease.

E. Epidemiology/natural history. WM is an uncommon disease, occurring in 3.4 per million men and 1.7 per million women per year. Median age at diagnosis is 64. Unlike MM, WM occurs much more often in Caucasians than in African Americans. Median survival varies according to IPSSWM score and ranges from over 10 years in low-risk patients to 44 months in high-risk patients. Patients may eventually develop refractory disease or undergo transformation into a higher-grade neoplasm.

V. POEMS SYNDROME (POLYNEUROPATHY, ORGANOMEGALY, ENDOCRINOPATHY, M PROTEIN, AND SKIN CHANGES).

POEMS syndrome is a rare disorder with variable symptoms. Patients most often present in the fifth to sixth decade of life with stocking-glove numbness, paresthesias, weakness, fatigue, or other nonspecific symptoms. Diagnosis is based on the Mayo clinic criteria, requiring the presence of a monoclonal protein (virtually always κ restricted) and a polyneuropathy, usually peripheral. In addition to these necessary features, diagnosis depends on the presence of at least one major and one minor criterion. Major criteria include Castleman's disease, osteosclerotic bone lesions, and elevated serum VEGF levels (3 to 4 times the upper limit of normal). Minor criteria include organomegaly, endocrinopathy, skin changes, papilledema, thrombocytosis, polycythemia, or volume overload. Osteosclerotic bone lesions are the most common major criteria, occurring in 97% of cases, and diagnosis should proceed cautiously in their absence. Diabetes mellitus and gonadal dysfunction are the most frequent endocrinopathies in POEMS syndrome. Skin changes may include hyperpigmentation, hemangiomas, hair changes, or acrocyanosis. Bone marrow biopsy generally demonstrates less than 5% plasma cells. Radiation may be utilized for the treatment of limited disease, while more widespread involvement usually requires systemic treatment with myeloma-like regimens. Peripheral blood stem cell transplant following high-dose therapy has been successfully used and should be reserved for young patients with extensive disease or rapidly progressive neuropathy. The course of POEMS syndrome is extremely indolent, with median survival of almost 14 years.

VI. LIGHT-CHAIN/HEAVY-CHAIN DEPOSITION DISEASE. Some patients with the clinical features of amyloidosis but without detectable tissue amyloid may have nonamyloid light-chain deposition disease (LCDD). LCDD results from a similar process as AL amyloidosis, but circulating light chains lack the ability to form α-pleated sheets, and thus amyloid is not deposited in end-organ tissues. LCDD tends to present with nephrotic syndrome or renal insufficiency. The mean age of presentation is in the fifties. Unlike AL, φ light chains predominate over κ; LCDD deposits do not take on the amyloid structure or stain with Congo red. Most patients have detectable serum or urinary M protein and may have an associated plasma cell dyscrasia or lymphoproliferative disorder. As with LCDD, patients who have heavy-chain deposition disease (HCDD) have no detectable amyloid, but have evidence of end-organ damage from deposition of monoclonal immunoglobulin heavy chains. Deposits of heavy chains are usually truncated and have no associated light-chain components. Heavy chains most commonly come from IgG and IgA (φ and κ heavy chains). The mean age of presentation is in the fifties. The usual presenting symptoms are renal failure, hypertension, proteinuria, and anemia. The nephrotic syndrome is common. Diagnosis rests on demonstration of heavy chains in end organs. Treatment for both LCDD and HCDD is similar to that described for AL amyloidosis.

VII. HEAVY-CHAIN DISEASE. Rarely, an M protein is found to be a truncated heavy chain with no associated light chain. Three classes of heavy-chain disease are appreciated, based on the class of heavy chain produced—these include alpha (α), gamma (γ), and Mu (μ) heavy chains. The γ- and μ-heavy-chain paraproteins are rare and are usually associated with NHL. α-HCDD is associated with *immunoproliferative small intestinal disease* (IPSID), also called Mediterranean lymphoma. IPSID, now considered to be a mucosa-associated lymphoid tissue (MALT) lymphoma, primarily affects young adults in areas of the Mediterranean, North Africa, and the Middle East who suffer from chronic intestinal diseases and malnutrition. Peripheral adenopathy is rare, but retroperitoneal adenopathy may be palpable as an abdominal mass. Diffuse infiltration of the intestine by lymphocytes or plasma cells results in a thickened, hard, pipelike intestine on endoscopy or imaging. The truncated α-heavy chain M protein associated with IPSID is an abnormal IgA molecule that may be detectable by immunofixation on serum, urine, tissue samples, or jejunal secretions sampled by endoscopy. Electrophoresis is less effective at detecting heavy chains, as they migrate as a smear rather than a discrete band. Biopsy of the intestine or mesenteric nodes is necessary for diagnosis. Patients should be evaluated for intestinal pathogens such as Giardia. Similar to *Helicobacter pylori*–associated gastric MALTomas, early-stage IPSID may respond to antimicrobials directed at any documented intestinal pathogens. More advanced disease may require chemotherapy appropriate for low-grade NHL. IPSID has an indolent course with approximately two-thirds of patients alive at 5 years.

SUGGESTED READINGS

Dispenzieri A. How I treat POEMS syndrome. *Blood* 2012;119(24):5650–5658.

Gatt ME, Palladini G. Light chain amyloidosis 2012: a new era. *Br J Haematol* 2013;160(5):582–598.

Gertz MA. Waldenstrom macroglobulinemia: 2013 update on diagnosis, risk stratification, and management. *Am J Hematol* 2013;88(8):703–711.

Gertz MA. Immunoglobulin light chain amyloidosis: 2013 update on diagnosis, prognosis and treatment. *Am J Hematol* 2013;88(5):416–425.

Giralt S, Koehne G. Allogeneic hematopoietic stem cell transplantation for multiple myeloma: what place, if any? *Curr Hematol Malig Rep* 2013;8(4):284–290.

Landgren O, Kyle RA, Rajkumar SV. From myeloma precursor disease to multiple myeloma: new diagnostic concepts and opportunities for early intervention. *Clin Cancer Res* 2011;17:1243–1252.

Oe Y, Soma J, Sato H, Ito S. Heavy chain deposition disease: an overview. *Clin Exp Nephrol* 2013;17(6):771–778.

Palumbo A, Anderson K. Multiple myeloma. *N Engl J Med* 2011;364(11):1046–1060.

Palumbo A, Mina R. Management of older adults with multiple myeloma. *Blood Rev* 2013;27(3):133–142.

Treon S. How i treat waldenstrom macroglobulinemia. *Blood* 2009;114(12):2375–2385.

30 Sarcoma

Brian A. Van Tine

I. **APPROACH TO THE SARCOMA PATIENT.** Sarcoma patients should be managed by a multidisciplinary team with extensive expertise. As the standard of care for most sarcomas is still clinical trial, access to the latest expertise in sarcoma is vital for this patient population. Second opinions should be considered standard practice for any oncologist that sees less than 10 cases a year and should be considered mandatory for the more rare histologies.

II. **BACKGROUND.** Sarcomas are malignancies of the connective tissue (from the Greek sarx for flesh), including fatty tissue, muscle, blood vessels, and bone. Most of these tissues share a common embryologic origin, arising primarily from tissues derived from the mesoderm. The clinical manifestations of sarcomas depend on the anatomic site of origin. The presenting signs and symptoms vary markedly, from a painless lump to debilitating pain. Because of the large number of neoplasms categorized as a sarcoma, these tumors may be broadly divided into soft-tissue neoplasms (extremity, retroperitoneal, and visceral) and bone sarcomas.

A. **Epidemiology.** Sarcomas comprise 1% of adult malignancies and 7% of pediatric malignancies. In the United States, the incidence of soft-tissue sarcomas is approximately 10,000 cases per year, and the incidence of sarcomas of bone is approximately 3000 cases per year (*CA Cancer J Clin* 2013;63:11). This is likely an underestimation of the total number of cases owing to the lack of a unifying ICD9 code.

B. **Risk factors.** Most cases of sarcoma are sporadic, with no identifiable risk factors. A number of predisposing factors, however, have been recognized.

1. **Radiation.** Sarcomas have been found to originate in or near tissues that have received prior external-beam radiation therapy (RT). These radiation-induced sarcomas generally occur at least 5 years after RT was delivered. Most of these lesions are high grade, and they are typically osteosarcomas, undifferentiated pleomorphic sarcoma (UPS), and angiosarcomas.

2. **Chemical exposure.** Certain chemicals have also been found to lead to the development of sarcomas, including phenoxy herbicides, dioxin, and arsenic. The alkylating chemotherapeutic agents such as cyclophosphamide, melphalan, and nitrosoureas that are used in childhood cancers have also been associated with the development of sarcomas in adulthood.

3. **Genetic conditions.** Several syndromes are associated with sarcomas. Patients with neurofibromatosis type I (mutations in NF1) have a 10% risk of developing a malignant peripheral nerve sheath tumor as adults (*Neuro Oncol* 2013;15:135). Sarcomas occur in patients with Li–Fraumeni syndrome, familial retinoblastoma (osteosarcoma), Gardner's syndrome (desmoids), tuberous sclerosis (rhabdomyosarcoma), and Gorlin's syndrome (rhabdomyosarcoma). Involvement of a genetic councilor is important in the management of patients with these syndromes.

4. **Other risks associated with sarcomas.** Lymphangiosarcomas have been known to develop in a lymphedematous arm after mastectomy (Stewart–Treves syndrome). Kaposi's sarcoma is associated with human herpes virus 8 (HHV8) and human immunodeficiency virus (HIV) disease. Paget's disease of bone is a risk factor for the development of osteosarcoma and fibrosarcoma. Injury is not considered a risk factor for the development of soft-tissue sarcomas.

C. **Molecular biology.** Sarcomas fall into two classes genetically: complex cytogenetic (i.e., osteosarcoma or leiomyosarcoma) and translocation driven. Several cytogenetic abnormalities are characteristic of certain sarcomas. The following is a list of selected tumors and their karyotypic mutations (*J Natl Compr Cancer Netw* 2012;10:951).

1. Peripheral primitive neuroectodermal tumor (PPNET) and Ewing's sarcoma: most commonly, t(11;22) EWS1-FLI
2. Desmoplastic small round cell tumor t(11;22) EWSR1-WT1
3. Alveolar rhabdomyosarcoma t(2;13) or t(1;13) PAX 3 or 7-FOXO1
4. Myxoid/round cell liposarcoma t(12;16) or t(12;22) FUS-DD1T3 or EWSR1-DD1T3
5. Well-differentiated/differentiated liposarcoma amplification of 12q14-15 MDM2 and CDK4
6. Alveolar soft part sarcoma t(X;17) ASPL-TFE3
7. Clear cell sarcoma t(12;22) or t(2;22) EWSR1-ATF1 or EWSR1-CREB1
8. Dermatofibrosarcoma protuberans t(17;22) ColIA1-PDGFRB
9. Low-grade fibromyxoid sarcoma t(7;16) or t(11;16) FUS-CREB2L2 or FUS-CREB3L1
10. Synovial sarcoma t(X;18) SS18-SSX1, 2, or 4.

III. SOFT-TISSUE SARCOMA

A. **Overview.** Soft-tissue sarcomas represent more than 50 different histologies. Pathologic diagnosis is based on the resemblance of these tumors to normal tissues. Despite this diversity, many of the clinical features and treatment decisions are common among the various histologies with some notable exceptions.

B. **History.** The presentation of soft-tissue sarcomas varies according to the site of origin.
   1. **Extremity sarcoma.** Approximately half of all soft-tissue sarcomas arise in the extremities. The majority are first seen as a painless soft-tissue mass. Pain is present in less than one-third of patients at the time of presentation. Patients often report a history of trauma, but in most cases, trauma likely did not cause the mass, but instead brought attention to a mass. Spontaneous hematomas on patients without anticoagulation should be approached with a very high degree of suspicion for malignancy.
   2. **Retroperitoneal sarcomas.** Most patients have an abdominal mass (80%), and approximately half have abdominal pain that is often vague and nonspecific. Weight loss is seen less frequently, with early satiety, nausea, and emesis occurring in fewer than 40% of patients. Neurologic symptoms, particularly paresthesia, occur in up to 30% of patients.
   3. **Visceral sarcomas.** Signs and symptoms relate to the viscus of origin. For example, gastric sarcomas frequently occur with dyspepsia or gastrointestinal bleeding. Rectal bleeding and tenesmus are seen with sarcomas of the rectum. Dysphagia and chest pain are common presenting symptoms of esophageal sarcomas. Painless vaginal bleeding is often seen with uterine leiomyosarcomas.

C. **Physical examination.** The examination of a patient with sarcoma should include an assessment of the size of the mass and its mobility relative to the underlying soft tissues. A site-specific neurovascular examination should also be performed. An assessment of the patient's overall functional status is also important.

D. **Diagnosis and staging.** In addition to a thorough history and physical examination, the evaluation of patients with soft-tissue sarcoma includes a biopsy as well as radiographic imaging.
   1. **Radiographic imaging.** The studies needed for adequate staging vary depending on the site of disease. For soft-tissue masses of the extremities and pelvis, magnetic resonance imaging (MRI) is the imaging modality of choice. MRI allows the differentiation of tumor from surrounding muscle and provides a multiplanar view. For retroperitoneal and visceral sarcomas, however, computed tomography (CT) scans provide the best anatomic definition of the tumor and provide adequate imaging of the liver, the most common site of metastasis for visceral and retroperitoneal sarcomas. Angiography is not usually indicated in the evaluation of sarcomas because MRI accurately delineates vascular involvement. In addition, nuclear medicine bone scanning has poor specificity and sensitivity in detecting bony invasion and is rarely recommended. Positron electron tomography (PET) has not become routine for most

sarcomas, but may be helpful in high-grade sarcomas, angiosarcomas, and gastrointestinal stromal tumors (GISTs).

Since approximately 88% of metastasis from sarcoma of the extremities are in the lungs, chest imaging is necessary. For small, superficial lesions, a preoperative chest radiograph may be sufficient to evaluate for lung metastases, but in patients with high-grade tumors, or tumors larger than 5 cm, a staging CT of the chest should be performed.

2. **Pathology**
   a. **Overview.** The histologic classification of soft-tissue tumors is organized according to the normal tissues they resemble. Unlike carcinomas, sarcomas do not demonstrate in situ changes, nor do they appear to originate from benign soft-tissue tumors (with the exception of malignant peripheral nerve sheath tumors in patients with neurofibromatosis). Clinical behavior is determined more by anatomic site, grade, and size than by a specific histology. Hence, most soft-tissue sarcomas are treated similarly despite different histologies, with the notable exceptions of GIST and rhabdomyosarcoma.

   The histologic grade of a sarcoma is the single best prognostic indicator for the development of recurrent disease. The pathologic features that determine grade include cellularity, differentiation, pleomorphism, necrosis, and a number of mitoses (Table 30-1).

   The three most common histopathologic subtypes are the UPS, liposarcoma, and leiomyosarcoma. It is often possible to correlate a location of a tumor with its histology. For example, most retroperitoneal sarcomas are liposarcomas or leiomyosarcomas.

   b. **Clinical pathologic features of specific tumor types**
      i. **UPS (previously named malignant fibrous histiocytoma)** is a tumor of later adult life with a peak incidence in the seventh decade. It is usually first seen as a painless mass. The most common site of involvement is the lower extremity, but they also occur in the upper extremity and retroperitoneum.
      ii. **Liposarcoma** is primarily a tumor of adults with a peak incidence between ages 50 and 65 years. It may occur anywhere in the body, but most commonly in the thigh or retroperitoneum. Several types of liposarcoma have been recognized, and they have different clinical outcomes. Well-differentiated liposarcoma is usually a nonmetastasizing lesion. Sclerosing liposarcoma also is a low-grade lesion. Myxoid and round cell (or lipoblastic) liposarcomas are low- to intermediate-grade lesions and typically have a t(12;16)(q13-14;p11) translocation. Fibroblastic and pleomorphic liposarcomas are higher-grade lesions and typically more aggressive.
      iii. **Leiomyosarcomas** may arise in any location, but more than half are located in the uterus, retroperitoneum, or intra-abdominal regions.
      iv. **Kaposi's sarcoma** may occur as raised pigmented lesions on the skin. It classically affects elderly Jewish and Italian men and is fairly indolent. It usually

TABLE 30-1	**Guidelines to the Histologic Grading of Sarcomas**
Low-grade sarcomas	High-grade sarcomas
Good differentiation	Poor differentiation
Hypocellular	Hypercellular
Increased stroma	Minimal stroma
Hypovascular	Hypervascular
Minimal necrosis	Much necrosis
<5 Mitoses/high-power field	>5 Mitoses/high-power field

occurs in the lower extremities. An aggressive variant occurs in younger children and is endemic in some areas of Africa. In patients with HIV/ acquired immunodeficiency syndrome (AIDS), a disseminated, aggressive form of this disease may develop.

v. **Angiosarcoma** is an aggressive malignant tumor of the lining of blood vessels. It may arise in any organ, but is most commonly seen in the head and neck region, the breast, the liver, and areas of prior radiation. The skin is frequently involved. Breast angiosarcomas typically occur in young and middle-aged women, often following radiation for breast cancer. Liver angiosarcomas arise in adults previously exposed to thorium dioxide, insecticides, or polyvinyl chloride. Angiosarcomas are also the most common primary malignant tumor of the myocardium.

vi. **Synovial sarcoma** usually occurs in young adults between 15 and 40 years of age. The most common site is the knee. Unlike most soft-tissue sarcomas, these lesions are usually painful.

vii. **Rhabdomyosarcoma** is a malignant tumor of skeletal muscle. Four categories are recognized: pleomorphic, alveolar, embryonal, and botryoid. Pleomorphic rhabdomyosarcoma usually occurs in the extremities of patients older than 30 years. It is highly anaplastic and may be confused with UPS pathologically. Alveolar rhabdomyosarcoma is a highly aggressive tumor that affects adolescents and young adults. Its histology resembles that of lung alveoli. Embryonal rhabdomyosarcoma arises primarily in the head and neck, especially the orbit. It usually affects infants and children, with a peak incidence at age 4. Botryoid rhabdomyosarcoma has been encompassed in the embryonal category. It has a gross appearance of polypoid masses and has a predilection for the genital and urinary tract. It occurs primarily in children at an average age of 7. Rhabdomyosarcomas that arise from dedifferentiated liposarcomas should be treated as liposarcoma.

viii. **GIST** is a sarcoma that can begin anywhere in the gastrointestinal tract but is found most commonly in the stomach (50%) or small bowel (25%). Most GIST tumors have a mutation in c-KIT, resulting in constitutive activation of this receptor.

3. **Staging.** The staging system for soft-tissue sarcomas incorporates histologic grade (G), size of the primary (T), nodal involvement (N), and distant metastasis (M) (Table 30-2). Grade of the tumor is the predominant feature predicting early metastatic recurrence and death. Beyond 2 years of follow-up, the size of the lesion becomes as important as the histologic grade. Recent changes have been made to the staging system with regard to lymph node metastases, as N1 tumors are now considered stage III.

IV. STAGE-DIRECTED APPROACH TO THERAPY

A. Early stage disease (stage I to III)

1. **Extremity soft-tissue sarcomas**

   a. **Surgery.** Surgery is the mainstay of therapy for early-stage soft-tissue sarcomas of the extremities. Over the last 20 years, there has been a gradual shift in the surgical management of extremity soft-tissue sarcomas away from radical ablative surgery, such as amputation and compartment resection, toward limb-sparing surgery. Currently, limb-sparing surgeries are performed in the vast majority of patients.

   When performing a limb-sparing surgery, it is important to obtain adequate margins. In the past, very conservative surgical approaches in which the plane of dissection is immediately adjacent to a pseudocapsule (an area around the tumor that is composed of tumor fimbriae and normal tissue) were associated with a local recurrence rate of 37% to 63%. However, a wide local resection encompassing a rim of normal tissue around the lesion led to improvements in local control, with a local recurrence rate of 30% in the absence of adjuvant therapy. The planned resection should encompass the skin, the subcutaneous tissues, and soft tissue

TABLE 30-2	American Joint Committee on Cancer (AJCC) Staging System for Soft-Tissue Sarcoma

Primary tumor (T)	Regional lymph nodes (N)	Distant metastasis (M)	Grade (G)	Stage
TX: primary tumor cannot be assessed	NX: regional lymph node involvement cannot be assessed	MX: presence of metastasis cannot be assessed	G1: low, well differentiated	Stage I: T1a, bN0M0, G1; T2a, bN0M0, G1
T0: no evidence of primary tumor	N0: no regional lymph nodes metastasis	M0: no distant metastasis	G2: intermediate, moderately well differentiated	Stage II: T1a, bN0M0, G2-3; T2aN0M0, G2-3
T1: tumor is <5 cm in greatest dimension	N1: regional lymph node metastasis	M1: distant metastasis	G3: high; poorly differentiated	Stage III: T2bN0M0, G2-3; any T, N1M0 any grade
T1a: tumor is located above and without invasion of the superficial fascia	—	—	—	Stage IV: any T; any N M1, any G
T1b: tumor is located below and/or with invasion of the superficial fascia	—	—	—	—
T2: Tumor is >5 cm in greatest dimension	—	—	—	—
T2a: tumor is located above and without invasion of the superficial fascia	—	—	—	—
T2b: tumor is located below and/or with invasion of the superficial fascia	—	—	—	—

Adapted from Greene F, Page D, Fleming I, et al. *AJCC Cancer Staging Manual,* 6th ed. New York, NY: Springer-Verlag, 2002, with permission.

adjacent to the tumor, including the previous biopsy site and any associated drain sites. The tumor should be excised with a minimum of a 1-cm margin of normal surrounding tissue.

There is normally no role for regional lymphadenectomy in most adult patients with sarcoma because of the low (2% to 3%) prevalence of lymph node metastases. However, patients with angiosarcoma, embryonal rhabdomyosarcomas, synovial sarcoma, and epithelioid sarcomas have an increased incidence of lymph node involvement and should be examined and imaged for lymphadenopathy.

   b. **Adjuvant radiation therapy.** Wide local excision alone is all that is necessary for small (T1), low-grade, soft-tissue sarcomas of the extremities, with local recurrence rate of less than 10%. Adjuvant RT, however, is required in a number of situations: (a) virtually all high-grade extremity sarcomas, (b) lesions larger than 5 cm (T2), and (c) positive or equivocal surgical margins in patients for whom re-excision is impractical. For T2 extremity soft-tissue sarcomas or any high-grade sarcomas, limb-sparing surgery plus adjuvant radiation to improve local control has become the standard approach. When adjuvant radiation is planned, metal clips should be placed at the margins of resection to facilitate radiation field.

   c. **Adjuvant chemotherapy.** The benefit of adjuvant chemotherapy for most extremity soft-tissue sarcomas is controversial. A formal meta-analysis of individual data from 1,568 patients who participated in 13 trials was performed by the Sarcoma Meta-analysis Collaboration. The analysis demonstrated a significant reduction in the risk of local or distant recurrence in patients who received adjuvant chemotherapy. There was also a decrease in the risk of distant relapse (metastasis) by 30% in treated patients. Overall survival, however, did not meet the criteria for statistical significance between the control group and the adjuvant chemotherapy arm, with a hazard ratio of 0.89 (*Lancet* 1997;350:1647). Most of the randomized trials examined in this meta-analysis were limited by patient numbers, heterogeneous patient and disease characteristics, and varied chemotherapeutic regimens. However, a randomized trial of a homogeneous group of patients with high-grade soft-tissue sarcomas of the extremities and girdle demonstrated a significant survival advantage of five cycles of adjuvant ifosfamide (1.8 g/m^2 days 1 to 5) and epirubicin (60 mg/m^2 days 1 to 2) following definitive local therapy (*J Clin Oncol* 2001;19:1238). In this trial, the chemotherapy arm had an overall median survival of 75 months versus 46 months in the observation arm ($p = 0.03$). An additional trial demonstrated that three cycles of neoadjuvant ifosfamide and epirubicin was equivalent to five cycles of adjuvant therapy (*J Clin Oncol* 2012;30:850). The only exception is with rhabdomyosarcomas, in which neoadjuvant and adjuvant chemotherapy is accepted as standard of care.

   d. **Neoadjuvant radiotherapy.** It may be necessary to administer radiation before definitive resection. This is most commonly performed for tumors that are borderline resectable or for tumors located adjacent to the joint capsule. The typical dose is 50 Gy. Sometimes, a boost is given postoperatively if margins are not adequate. Neoadjuvant radiation, however, is associated with wound healing difficulties. A phase III National Cancer Institute of Canada (NCIC) trial comparing adjuvant (postoperative) and neoadjuvant (preoperative) radiation demonstrated similar local control rates, metastatic outcome, and overall survival rates between the two arms (*Lancet* 2002;359:2235). However, patients receiving preoperative radiation had a significantly higher incidence of wound complications (35% vs. 17%).

   e. **Radiation as definitive therapy.** RT alone in the treatment of unresectable or medically inoperable soft-tissue sarcoma patients yields a 5-year survival rate of 25% to 40% and a local control rate of 30%. Radiation doses, if feasible, should be at least 65 Gy.

   f. **Brachytherapy.** Brachytherapy has also been used in treatment for sarcomas. Iridium 192 is the most commonly used agent. It has comparable local control rates versus adjuvant external-beam RT, although some data suggest a higher rate of wound complications and a delay in healing when the implants are after loaded before the third postoperative day. The advantages of brachytherapy include a decrease in the patient's entire treatment to 10 to 12 days from 10 to 12 weeks, and the advantage that smaller volumes of tissue can be irradiated, which could improve functional results. However, smaller volumes may not be appropriate, depending on the tumor size and grade.

2. **Retroperitoneal sarcomas**
    a. **Surgery.** As with other soft-tissue sarcomas, surgery is the primary treatment of retroperitoneal sarcomas. Tumors that are less than 5 cm in size and not located close to adjacent viscera or critical neurovascular structures are considered resectable. If a tumor has a high clinical suspicion of sarcoma and is resectable, it may not be necessary to perform a preoperative biopsy. One should consider a preoperative biopsy if an incomplete resection is a reasonable possibility to allow neoadjuvant therapy. If a biopsy is performed, it should be a CT-guided core biopsy.

    Unfortunately, only 50% of patients with early stage retroperitoneal sarcomas are able to undergo complete surgical resection. Of the tumors removed, approximately half will develop a local recurrence. Adjuvant therapy, therefore, plays an important role in the management of retroperitoneal sarcomas.

    b. **Adjuvant and neoadjuvant RT.** Adjuvant RT is most frequently recommended for patients with high-grade tumors or positive margins. The radiation is typically started 3 to 8 weeks following surgery to allow wound healing. Two-year local control rates of 70% have been reported with the addition of postoperative RT.

    Neoadjuvant RT is used for patients with retroperitoneal sarcomas. It can be given to patients with marginally resectable tumors and those in whom one would expect to require postoperative radiotherapy. Neoadjuvant RT has a number of advantages over postoperative radiotherapy, including smaller radiation portals and reduction of the extent of the surgical procedure.

    c. **Management of unresectable locally advanced retroperitoneal sarcomas.** Unresectable retroperitoneal sarcomas can be managed in a number of ways. RT can be given for palliation and with the hope that the tumor could be made resectable. Palliative surgery to reduce local symptoms can be performed. Chemotherapy can also be administered.

3. **Visceral sarcomas**
    a. **Overview.** The discovery of the importance of a mutation in the tyrosine kinase c-KIT in GIST has led to a radical change in therapy for this sarcoma. Visceral leiomyosarcomas should be stained for c-KIT to rule out GIST.

    b. **Therapy for visceral sarcomas other than GIST**
        i. **Surgery.** Surgery is the primary treatment of visceral sarcomas.
        ii. **Adjuvant and neoadjuvant radiation.** Adjuvant RT is necessary if the tumor is high grade or if margins are positive. It is usually started 3 to 8 weeks following surgery to allow wound healing. Neoadjuvant radiation can be considered to allow a less radical surgery or make a previously unresectable tumor operable.
        iii. **Management of unresectable locally advanced visceral sarcomas.** Unresectable intra-abdominal sarcomas can be managed in a number of ways. RT can be given for palliation and with the hope that the tumor could be made resectable. Palliative surgery to reduce local symptoms can be performed. Chemotherapy can also be administered.

    c. **Therapy for GIST.** Like other sarcomas, surgery is the primary therapy for non-metastatic GIST tumors. Imatinib is a small-molecule tyrosine kinase inhibitor with significant inhibitory activity against c-KIT. In the initial study, 147 patients with metastatic GIST were treated with either imatinib 400 mg/m^2 or 600 mg/m^2 daily. Partial responses were noted in 54% and stable disease in 28% (*N Engl J Med* 2002;347:472). The initial dose of imatinib is 400 mg daily, which should be continued until the disease progresses. Upon disease progression, treatment options include higher doses of imatinib (600 or 800 mg/day) or the use of sunitinib, another tyrosine kinase inhibitor, which has shown activity in imatinib-resistant GIST. An option for third-line therapy is regorafenib (*Lancet* 2013;381:295).

If a tumor is marginally resectable or the surgery would result in significant morbidity, neoadjuvant therapy with imatinib can be given for 3 to 6 months. Of note, it may take 4 months or more to observe a response to imatinib on CT scan, although changes in FDG-PET imaging can be seen very rapidly (within days).

B. Treatment of local recurrence. Local recurrence of soft-tissue sarcomas should be treated with surgical resection whenever feasible. Adjuvant radiation is often used. For unresectable recurrence of disease, radiation is preferred.

C. Treatment of metastatic soft-tissue sarcomas

1. **Overview.** Metastatic soft-tissue sarcomas can be divided into limited metastasis and extensive metastasis. Limited metastatic disease is defined as resectable metastasis involving one organ system. The prognosis of these two subsets of patients is very different. It is possible (though unlikely) to cure limited metastatic disease, whereas patients with extensive metastatic disease can only be palliated.

2. **Management of limited metastatic disease.** For patients with a limited number of pulmonary metastases, metastasectomy has been performed with some improvement in survival when compared with no surgery. Five-year survival rates range from 23% to 50% if a complete resection is performed (*Ann Thorac Surg* 2011;92:1780). In patients with visceral sarcomas and limited liver metastasis, it is sometimes possible to perform a metastasectomy by surgery, chemoembolization, or radio-frequency ablation.

3. **Management of extensive metastatic disease.** The goal of therapy for patients with metastatic sarcoma is palliation and prolongation of survival. Systemic chemotherapy is the primary modality of treatment. Radiation and surgery may be used with a goal of palliation.

   Numerous chemotherapeutic agents have been used as single agents in soft-tissue sarcomas. Doxorubicin and ifosfamide are among the most active agents. Doxorubicin was the first significantly active agent against soft-tissue sarcomas, with an objective overall response rate of approximately 25%. Continuous infusion of doxorubicin or the use of dexrazoxone decreases the risk of cardiotoxicity and the severity of nausea while maintaining equivalent antitumor activity. Dacarbazine (DTIC) has also been found to have activity in soft-tissue sarcomas, with a response rate of 17%. It is particularly effective in uterine leiomyosarcomas. Ifosfamide has been found to have significant activity in sarcoma, with a response rate of 24% to 38%. On the basis of evidence of an increasing response rate to higher doses of ifosfamide, trials of "high-dose ifosfamide" (with 12 to 14 g/m^2) showed higher tumor response rates (and toxicities) after an ineffective standard dose (5 to 7 g/m^2) of ifosfamide.

   When doxorubicin was combined with DTIC (the AD or ADIC regimen), higher tumor response rates were observed (17% to 40%). To improve the response rate further, several agents were added to the ADIC combination. A combination of [sodium 2-]mercaptoethane sulfonate (MESNA), doxorubicin, ifosfamide, and DTIC (MAID) resulted in a response rate of approximately 47%, with 30% complete responses. Combination chemotherapy has been compared with single-agent doxorubicin in eight randomized phase III trials. Some of them showed superior response rates with combination chemotherapy, but none of the trials found a significant survival advantage. Kaplan–Meier plots of survival are superimposable within each trial and from trial to trial. The MAID regimen is rarely used now in the metastatic setting; instead, either single agent or a combination of doxorubicin and ifosfamide is used.

   Another combination chemotherapeutic regimen that has had activity in soft-tissue sarcomas, in particular, leiomyosarcomas, is gemcitabine and docetaxel, with a response rate of 50% in a phase II trial (*J Clin Oncol* 2007;25:2755). In patients with metastatic angiosarcoma, paclitaxel has shown significant antitumor activity.

V. BONE SARCOMA

A. **Bone sarcomas.** These may be derived from any of the cells in bone, including cartilage (chondrosarcoma), bone (osteosarcoma, parosteal osteogenic sarcoma), notochord (chordoma), or unknown cells of origin (Ewing's sarcoma, malignant giant cell tumor, and adamantinoma).

B. **Presentation.** The clinical presentation of bone sarcomas may suggest the pathologic diagnosis before biopsy.

1. **History.** Localized pain and swelling are the hallmark clinical features of bone sarcomas. The pain is initially insidious but can become unremitting. Occasionally, a pathologic fracture will bring the patient to medical attention. If the tumor arises in the lower extremities, the patient may have a limp. Constitutional symptoms are rare but can be observed in patients with Ewing's sarcoma or patients with metastatic disease. A pertinent history should note how long a lesion has been present and any change in it. Rapid growth or change in a lesion favors a malignant etiology.

   It is also important to inquire about risk factors for development of bone sarcomas. These include any history of RT and chronic bone disease. Paget's disease of bone may give rise to osteosarcoma and giant cell tumors of bone. Sites of chronic osteomyelitis may produce osteosarcomas and squamous cell carcinomas. Fibrous dysplasia may rarely give rise to osteosarcoma. Chondrosarcomas may arise from pre-existing benign enchondroma (solitary or multiple in Ollier's disease), or exostoses (hereditary multiple exostoses).

2. **Physical examination.** Physical examination may reveal a palpable mass. A joint effusion may be observed, and range of motion of the joint may be limited with stiffness or pain. Neurovascular and lymph node examinations are usually normal.

3. **Diagnosis and staging.** Evaluation should include a biopsy and review of appropriate radiographic imaging.

   a. **Radiographic imaging** should include plain films of the lesion and MRI or CT scan. Biplanar radiographs of the affected bone are helpful in determining the specific site of involvement within the bone, the pattern and extent of bony destruction, periosteal changes, and the presence of matrix mineralization within the tumor.

      Osteolytic (bone-destroying) lesions may be seen in metastatic carcinomas, myeloma, and primary bone tumors. Well-defined (geographic) borders of bone destruction may indicate a slower growing or less aggressive lesion, such as a low-grade chondrosarcoma. As the tumor extends beyond the area of lytic destruction, more aggressive growth may be associated with a "moth-eaten" pattern. Rapid, aggressive growth patterns may be associated with cortical destruction, a soft-tissue mass, and a permeative pattern of bone destruction.

      Osteoblastic (bone-forming) lesions may be associated with metastatic disease (e.g., prostate, breast, pancreas, and small-cell cancer of the lung) or osteosarcoma.

      Periosteal reactions may be seen on plain films that give additional clues to the diagnosis. A "sunburst" pattern is associated with classic osteosarcoma. A lamellar or "onion-skin" periosteal reaction is most associated with Ewing's sarcoma. Spiculated periosteal reactions are associated with rapidly growing tumors such as Ewing's sarcoma. A raised periosteal reaction (Codman triangle) may be seen in a number of tumors.

      MRI is the imaging study of choice for the evaluation of most bone sarcomas, allowing for visualization of the relation of the tumor to the neurovascular structures, adjacent joints, and the surrounding soft tissues. MRI can also easily demonstrate the intramedullary extent of the tumor and the presence of skip metastases.

      CT scan of the primary site may be considered in place of MRI to demonstrate cortical destruction more accurately and for the evaluation of pelvic tumors. CT scan of the chest is the preferred imaging of the lungs, which is the most common initial site of metastasis.

Radionuclide technetium Tc99 bone scan imaging is important for assessing extent of tumor within bone at the primary, and the presence of skip metastases or distant bone metastases.

   b. Laboratory features. Anemia or leukocytosis may be present in patients with Ewing's sarcoma. Elevated alkaline phosphatase and lactate dehydrogenase (LDH) levels are observed in patients with osteosarcoma, Ewing's sarcoma, or Paget's disease. An abnormal glucose tolerance test may be seen with chondrosarcoma.

   c. Pathology of bone sarcomas. The classification of bone neoplasms is based on the cell of origin. Primary bone sarcomas can exhibit a phenomenon of dedifferentiation, in which these neoplasms exhibit a dimorphic histologic pattern with low- and high-grade patterns in the tumor. Treatment is dictated by the high-grade lesion.

   i. Osteosarcoma is the most common malignant primary bone tumor, with an annual incidence of three cases per million population. Peaks in incidence occur in adolescents and in the elderly. Most osteosarcomas occur in the metaphyseal region, near the growth plate, of skeletally immature long bones. The distal femur, proximal tibia, and proximal humerus are most common sites.

   ii. Ewing's sarcoma represents 10% to 15% of all primary malignant bone tumors. It is the second most common malignant tumor of bone in childhood and adolescence. The peak incidence is the second decade of life. Ewing's sarcoma tends to occur in the diaphysis of long bones. The most common sites are the femur, followed by the pelvis, and then the skin. Ewing's sarcoma and PPNETs share a common genetic origin, a translocation between chromosomes 11 and 22. When arising in bone, this tumor is recognized as Ewing's sarcoma, and when arising in soft tissue, this sarcoma is recognized as a PPNET. Treatment of these tumors is similar, by using a combination of chemotherapy and local measures (surgery and radiation). Ewing's sarcoma is one of the **small round blue cell tumors**. The differential diagnosis of these tumors includes lymphoma, neuroblastoma, retinoblastoma, and rhabdomyosarcoma.

   iii. Chondrosarcoma is the second most frequent malignant primary bone tumor, representing approximately 20% of all primary bone malignancies. It usually occurs in patients older than 40 years. It can occur in any bone, but the majority occur in the pelvis (30%), femur (20%), and the shoulder girdle (15%).

   iv. Adamantinoma is an indolent, osteolytic tumor that often develops in the upper tibia.

   v. Giant cell tumor of bone, or osteoclastoma, represents approximately 5% of all primary bone tumors. The peak incidence is in the third decade of life, with a female predilection. They are typically epiphyseal–metaphyseal tumors, with the majority in the distal femur and proximal tibia.

   d. Staging of bone sarcomas is shown in Table 30-3. Adverse prognostic indicators include an increased LDH, an increased alkaline phosphatase, and an axial primary. Patients with Ewing's sarcoma should have a bone marrow biopsy as part of staging.

C. Treatment of bone sarcomas

   1. General principles of local therapy. Surgical excision is the mainstay of treatment for patients with low-grade bone sarcomas. For high-grade tumors, multimodality therapy is indicated. As an example, for high-grade osteosarcomas, preoperative multiagent chemotherapy is followed by surgical removal of the tumor and then further adjuvant chemotherapy. It is essential to distinguish high-grade osteosarcoma from a low-grade variant, parosteal osteosarcoma, the latter of which has a lower malignant potential and does not require adjuvant chemotherapy. Occasionally, parosteal osteosarcomas will become dedifferentiated (high grade), and their behavior will resemble that of the classic aggressive osteosarcoma.

TABLE 30-3	American Joint Committee on Cancer (AJCC) Staging System for Bone Sarcoma			
Primary tumor (T)	Regional lymph nodes (N)	Distant metastasis (M)	Grade (G)	Stage
TX: primary tumor cannot be assessed	NX: regional lymph node involvement cannot be assessed	MX: presence of metastasis cannot be assessed	G1: low, well differentiated	Stage IA: T1N0M0, G1,2
T0: no evidence of primary tumor	N0: no regional lymph nodes metastasis	M0: no distant metastasis	G2: intermediate, moderately well differentiated	Stage IB: T2N0 M0, G1,2
T1: tumor ≤8 cm in greatest dimension	N1: regional lymph node metastasis	M1: distant metastasis	G3: high; poorly differentiated	Stage IIA: T1N0M0, G3,G4
T2: tumor is >8 cm in greatest dimension	—	M1a: lung metastasis	G4: undifferentiated (Ewing's sarcoma)	Stage IIB: T2N0M0, G3, G4
T3: discontinuous tumors in the primary bone site	—	M2b: other sites of metastasis		Stage III: T3N0M0, any G
				Stage IVA: any T N0 M1a, any G
				Stage IVB: any T any N M1b, any G; any T N1 any M, any G

Adapted from Greene F, Page D, Fleming I, et al. *AJCC Cancer Staging Manual,* 6th ed. New York, NY: Springer-Verlag, 2002, with permission.

    a. Limb-sparing surgery. The Musculoskeletal Tumor Society and the NCCN recognize wide excision, either by amputation or by a limb-salvage procedure, as the recommended surgical approach for all high-grade bone sarcomas. Currently, 75% to 80% of patients may be treated with a limb-sparing surgery. This type of resection is predicated on complete tumor removal, effective skeletal reconstruction, and adequate soft-tissue coverage. There are three types of limb-sparing procedures.

        i. Osteoarticular resection is an excision of the tumor-bearing bone and the adjacent joint. It is the most common procedure because most bone sarcomas arise in the metaphysic of long bones.

        ii. Intercalary resection is an excision of tumor-bearing bone only.

        iii. Whole bone resection is an excision of the entire bone and adjacent joints. It is used when the tumor extends along or invades the joint. Reconstruction is usually achieved by prosthetic arthroplasty.

2. Osteosarcoma therapy. The 5-year survival for osteosarcoma with surgery alone is less than 20%. This occurs because microscopic dissemination is likely to be present in

80% of patients at the time of diagnosis. The addition of adjuvant chemotherapy has improved survival for high-grade osteosarcoma, permitting long-term survival as high as 80%.

    a. Neoadjuvant and adjuvant chemotherapy. Neoadjuvant chemotherapy began as a strategy to permit limb-sparing surgery, allowing time for creation of custom-made prosthetics. Since its acceptance, other advantages have been recognized with this approach. It permits earlier treatment of occult micrometastatic disease, preventing emergence of resistant clones, and potentially allowing debulking of the primary to improve chances for limb-sparing surgery.

        Chemotherapy drugs active in osteosarcomas include doxorubicin, cisplatin, and high-dose methotrexate with leucovorin rescue. These agents are typically used in combination to improve response, although the optimal combination and duration of therapy remain controversial.

        Histologic response to preoperative therapy is recognized as a significant prognostic factor. Various systems have been developed for grading histologic response to chemotherapy, but greater than 90% necrosis of tumor cells is associated with the best prognosis. If the tumor has been resected to negative margins and had a good histologic response to chemotherapy, the patient continues on chemotherapy for an additional 2 to 12 cycles. If the tumor was fully resected but has less than 90% necrosis, salvage chemotherapy with agents not used in induction is attempted, but the effect of this change in chemotherapy on outcomes is unclear. If the tumor margins are positive, additional local surgery should be attempted.

    b. Radiation therapy. Radiation is not routinely used in the therapy of osteosarcoma, but may prove helpful in patients who refuse definitive resection or palliation of patients with metastatic disease.

    c. Management of metastatic disease. Approximately 10% to 20% of patients with osteosarcoma have evidence of metastatic disease at presentation. Some of these patients may be candidates for surgical resection of pulmonary metastases. For patients with more extensive metastatic disease, chemotherapy is used to provide control of disease and palliation of symptoms.

3. Therapy for Ewing's sarcoma and the related PPNETs use a combined-modality approach.

    a. Treatment of the primary tumor. The optimal treatment for local tumor control is not well defined. Historically, RT has been the mainstay of local therapy, but there has been a recent trend toward surgery. No prospective randomized trials have been performed to compare the two modalities, but retrospective data suggest improvements in local control and survival when surgery is done with a complete resection of the tumor. Patients with unresectable disease or positive margins require RT to improve local control.

    b. Chemotherapy. Before the availability of effective chemotherapeutic agents, fewer than 10% of patients with Ewing's sarcoma survived beyond 5 years, although only 15% to 35% of patients with Ewing's sarcoma/PPNET have evidence of metastatic disease at presentation. This fact suggests that many patients with Ewing's sarcoma had occult microscopic dissemination of the disease at the time of diagnosis. The First Intergroup Ewing's Sarcoma Study demonstrated an improved survival rate for patients receiving systemic therapy with VACA (vincristine, actinomycin D, cyclophosphamide, and doxorubicin). The Second Intergroup Ewing's Sarcoma Study used VACA, but on an intermittent schedule and a higher dose and achieved an improved 5-year survival (73%).

        The addition of alternating cycles of ifosfamide and etoposide to VAC further improved survival in patients with nonmetastatic Ewing's sarcoma and PPNET.

    c. Recurrent metastatic Ewing's sarcoma. Although cure is not a realistic goal, aggressive combination chemotherapy (VAC or IE) and RT can still lead to prolonged progression-free survival.

4. **Therapies for chondrosarcoma.** Chondrosarcomas are a group of tumors that arise from the cartilage matrix and are the third most common bone tumor. There are many subtypes of chondrosarcoma, and not all are treated in a similar manner.
   a. **Treatment of the primary tumor.** As chondrosarcomas are usually slow nonmetastasizing tumors, the majority are treated with surgery alone. **Dedifferentiated chondrosarcoma** should be approached in a similar manner as osteosarcoma, and **mesenchymal chondrosarcoma** should be treated as if it is Ewing's sarcoma.
   b. **Chemotherapy.** As chondrosarcomas are generally slow growing, most chondrosarcomas are resistant to chemotherapy. The standard of care for metastatic chondrosarcoma is clinical trial.

VI. FUTURE DIRECTIONS. In the treatment of sarcomas include the search for more effective chemotherapeutic agents and combinations, and targeted therapies that will exploit the genetic features of these tumors.

SUGGESTED READINGS

Biermann JS, Adkins DR, Agulnik M, et al. Bone cancer. *J Natl Compr Cancer Netw* 2013;11:688–723.

Demetri GD, von Mehren M, Blanke CD, et al. Efficacy and safety of imatinib mesylate in advanced gastrointestinal stromal tumors. *New Eng J Med* 2002;347:472–480.

Demetri GD, Reichardt P, Kang Y-K, et al. Efficacy and safety of regorafenib for advanced gastrointestinal stromal tumours after failure of imatinib and sunitinib (GRID): an international, multicentre, randomised, placebo-controlled, phase 3 trial. *Lancet* 2013;381:295–302.

Gyorki DE, Brennan MF. Management of recurrent retroperitoneal sarcoma. *J Surg Oncol* 2014;109:53–59.

Kolberg M, Holand M, Agesen TH, et al. Survival meta-analyses for >1800 malignant peripheral nerve sheath tumor patients with and without neurofibromatosis type 1. *Neuro Oncol* 2013;15:135–147.

O'Sullivan B, Davis AM, Turcotte R, et al. Preoperative versus postoperative radiotherapy in soft-tissue sarcoma of the limbs: a randomised trial. *Lancet* 2002;359:2235–2241.

von Mehren M, Benjamin RS, Bui MM, et al. Soft tissue sarcoma, version 2.2012: featured updates to the NCCN guidelines. *J Natl Compr Cancer Netw* 2012;10:951–960.

31 Malignant Melanoma and Nonmelanoma Skin Cancer

Lauren S. Levine • David Y. Chen • Lynn A. Cornelius • Gerald P. Linette

I. MALIGNANT MELANOMA
A. Background
1. **Epidemiology.** The Surveillance, Epidemiology, and End Results Program (SEER) data demonstrate a steady rise in the incidence of cutaneous melanoma since 1975 and a continued average of 1.8% year-over-year increase between 2002 and 2011. The American Cancer Society estimates that in 2014, approximately 76,100 cases of melanoma will be diagnosed, and 9,710 individuals will die of melanoma. The lifetime risk of being diagnosed with melanoma in the United States is approximately 1 in 50 for whites, 1 in 1,000 for blacks, and 1 in 200 for Hispanics. Overall, more men account for new cases of melanoma than women (27.7 vs. 16.7 new cases per 100,000).

2. **Risk factors.** There are clear genetic and environmental determinants of melanoma risk. One study found that mutations in the CDKN2A tumor suppressor gene are present in 39% of families with multiple occurrences of melanoma, while another population-based study found that though CDKN2A mutations were associated with greater risk of first degree relatives with melanoma, only one out of 18 families with three or more affected first-degree relatives carried CDKN2A mutations, suggesting other heritable factors. Low penetrance gene variants associated with increased melanoma risk include melanocortin 1 receptor (MC1R), tyrosinase (TYR), cyclin-dependent kinase 4 (CDK4), micropthalmia transcription factor (MITF), BAP1, and others. New genetic risk factors are being described with the proliferation of next-generation sequencing, including a recent study that identified a nongenic polymorphisms affecting the regulatory region in telomerase (TERT) in a family with multiple family members with melanoma. Despite identification of genetic risk factors, the utility of their detection is not established and genetic testing is not a routine practice in the clinical setting.

The most significant environmental exposure that drives melanoma, and non-melanoma skin cancer, risk is ultraviolet (UV) exposure. The WHO has classified UV radiation between 100 and 400 nm as a known carcinogen. UV exposure interacts with genetic risk factors, including fair skin, red hair (MC1R variants), and UV sensitivity syndromes like xeroderma pigmentosum. Fair-skin people are at higher risk of melanoma from UV exposure. Additionally, SEER registry data demonstrate that prior history of melanoma confers 10-fold risk of subsequent melanoma compared to the general population, likely reflecting a confluence of genetic and environmental causes. Other risk factors include increased number of nevi (>50), history of greater than five clinically atypical nevi, large congenital nevi, and history of immune suppression with solid organ transplantation.

B. **Primary cutaneous melanoma**

1. **Diagnosis.** Cutaneous melanomas commonly arise in the absence of a clinically apparent precursor, although in some instances benign nevi are associated with melanoma on histologic examination. Patients may report the appearance of a new skin lesion or change in an existing lesion and will occasionally note associated symptoms such as itching and bleeding. Nonpigmented, or amelanotic, primary lesions comprise approximately 5% of cutaneous melanomas.

   a. **Physical examination.** While evaluating a pigmented skin lesion, the ABCD morphologic criteria are helpful, but not absolute.
      - **Asymmetry.** One half of the lesion does not match the other.
      - **Border irregularity.** The lesion has ragged or notched edges.
      - **Color variegation.** Pigmentation is a heterogeneous mixture of tan, brown, or black. Red, white, or blue discolorations are particularly of concern.
      - **Diameter.** Larger than 6 mm in diameter.
      - **Evolution.** Any change in clinical characteristics of a lesion noted by the patient or physician.

      Particular attention should be given to lesions that are evolving by clinical documentation (i.e., written or photographic records) or by patient report. Together, these sets of criteria are sometimes known as the ABCDE's of melanoma. Lesions with one or more of these attributes should be brought to the attention of a physician, preferably a dermatologist, and evaluated for the possibility of melanoma. Other characteristics such as itching, bleeding, and the presence of ulceration should also prompt a careful evaluation for melanoma. In addition to examination of the lesion in question, a comprehensive skin examination by a dermatologist is critical in evaluating and monitoring patients with multiple or atypical nevi, a history of excessive sun exposure, or a history of melanoma or nonmelanoma skin cancer. Full body examination is essential, including scalp, hands and feet, genitalia, and oral cavity.

   b. **Biopsy.** The differential diagnosis of a pigmented skin lesion includes an atypical nevus, a benign growth such as melanocytic nevus, solar lentigo, seborrheic keratosis, angioma, and other malignant growths such as basal cell carcinoma (BCC) and squamous cell carcinoma (SCC). When melanoma or other malignant lesion is a consideration, a biopsy without delay is required to establish a diagnosis.

- **Excisional biopsy.** Full thickness removal of the entire clinical lesion with 1 to 3 mm margins is optimal for diagnosis and accurate staging by Breslow's depth. Avoiding wider margins facilitates accurate sentinel lymph node mapping if later required.
- **Incisional biopsy.** For large lesions or lesions on special sites like the palms and soles, face, ears, or digits, full thickness incision or punch biopsy of the thickest clinical portion may be appropriate.
- **Deep shave (Saucerization).** Wide sampling is preferred in superficial lesions such as lentigo maligna, where atypical melanocytes may extend beyond the clinically observed lesion. Superficial shave biopsy is not recommended for any lesion suspected to be melanoma.

c. **Histologic reporting and classification.** Breslow's thickness in millimeters, presence or absence of histologic ulceration, dermal mitotic rate per square millimeter, and presence or absence at the lateral or deep margins comprise the bare minimal elements that should be reported with the histologic evaluation of melanoma. Reports may include additional elements encouraged by the American Academy of Dermatology such as the presence or absence of regression, microsatellitosis, tumor infiltrating lymphocytes, lymphovascular invasion, neurotropism, or whether there is vertical growth phase. The pathologist may also report the histologic subtype, which includes superficial spreading melanoma, nodular melanoma, lentigo maligna melanoma, and acral lentiginous melanoma. Superficial spreading melanoma is the most common subtype comprising 75% of all melanomas, while lentigo maligna comprises 10% to 15% and is thought to have an extended radial growth phase. Nodular melanomas are by definition in vertical growth phase. Acral lentiginous melanoma is the least common type and characteristically arises on specialized sites including palmar, plantar, and subungual locations. Aside from the four dominant subtypes, there are rare variants including nevoid melanoma and desmoplastic melanoma. Although histologically distinct, the subtype does not affect staging as it does not influence management or prognosis with the exception of pure desmoplastic melanoma, with which sentinel node biopsy may not be indicated.

d. **Diagnostic dilemmas.** Distinguishing melanoma from benign growths can be challenging, despite thorough clinical exam and adequate sampling of the lesion. Immunohistochemistry may be utilized to highlight cells of melanocytic origin, including S100, MART-1, and HMB-45. These antigens are not specific to melanoma but can highlight the architecture of the lesion as well as aid in the identification of nodal metastases. In certain cases, further testing for chromosomal aberrations and copy number variability with fluorescence in situ hybridization (FISH) or comparative genomic hybridization (CGH) can help distinguish benign from malignant lesions.

Staging. The most commonly used staging system is found in the *AJCC Cancer Staging Manual*, 7th edition. The T stage is defined by the tumor thickness (T1—$\leq$1 mm, T2—1.01 to 2 mm, T3—2.01 to 4 mm and T4—>4 mm). The presence of ulceration defines the b substaging. The N stage is defined by the number of lymph nodes involved (N1—1 lymph node, N2—2 to 3 lymph nodes and N3—4 or more lymph nodes, matted lymph nodes or in-transit metastases). The M stage may be further subdivided into M1 (involvement of skin, subcutaneous tissue, or distant lymph nodes with normal LDH), M2 (lung metastases with normal LDH), and M3 (metastases to other organs or any metastasis with elevated LDH). The melanoma stages are as follows: IA (T1a), IB (T1b or T2a), IIA (T2b or T3a), IIB (T3b or T4a), IIC (T4b), III (N1, N2, or N3), IV (M1). Although many of the staging criteria remained the same, the new staging system reflects the rise in utilization of sentinel lymph node biopsy technique and the attendant increase in detection of micrometastases. Importantly, microstaging now distinguishes mitotic rate less than $1/mm^2$ or $1/mm^2$ or greater as a separate staging criterion in determining T1a from T1b lesions, respectively, in addition to the existing criterion regarding the presence or absence of ulceration. The most important prognostic factors in the staging of melanoma are the thickness of the primary lesion measured in millimeters, the presence of histologic ulceration, the mitotic rate, and regional lymph node involvement. The thickness of the primary melanoma is known as the Breslow thickness and is measured in millimeters from the top of the granular layer in the epidermis to the base of the deepest tumor nest in the dermis. The Breslow thickness cutoffs for primary tumor classification are 1.0, 2.0, and 4.0 mm, while mitotic activity and ulceration modify tumor staging. Tumor staging, in combination with clinical findings, guide the next steps of the staging workup.

   a. Sentinel lymph node biopsy. Stage 0, I, and II melanoma is localized to the skin, while stage III melanoma denotes regional metastasis, which is detected by clinical exam or by sentinel lymph node biopsy. Lymphoscintigraphy and sentinel lymph node biopsy is performed at the time of wide-local excision and offers prognostic value to patients with primary melanoma thicker than 1.0 mm. This is supported by multiple studies and recently reaffirmed in the final analysis of the Multicenter Selective Lymphadenectomy Trial-1 (MSLT-1). Generally, sentinel lymph node biopsy is not recommended for primary melanomas less than 0.75 mm, and there is no general consensus for melanomas between 0.76 and 1.0 mm.

   b. Imaging. Routine imaging is not recommended in stage I or II disease unless used to evaluate specific signs and symptoms. The exception is ultrasonography of a nodal basin for an indeterminate lymph node clinical exam, which can help guide decisions for fine-needle aspiration (FNA) or sentinel biopsy. For stage III disease as determined by sentinel biopsy, clinically positive nodes, or in-transit metastases, baseline contrast-enhanced CT exam is recommended, with or without positron emission tomography with computed tomography (PET-CT) or MRI, based on clinical context. For suspected stage IV disease, in addition to CT of the chest, abdomen, and pelvis, gadolinium-enhanced brain MRI is recommended in the initial staging because of its increased sensitivity for detecting small posterior fossa lesions (<1 cm) compared to head CT. PET-CT is also appropriate for initial staging.

   c. FNA. Suspected regional metastatic disease by clinical exam or imaging should be evaluated histologically by FNA. In the appropriate context, this can be done for suspected stage IV disease except when archival tissue is not available for genetic testing. In this instance, biopsy is preferred over FNA.

   d. Lactate dehydrogenase. Elevated serum level of LDH is an independent predictor of poor outcome in stage IV disease and defines the designation of M1c disease. The two-year survival for normal versus elevated LDH at time of staging is 40% versus 18%, respectively, for stage IV (*J Clin Oncol* 2009;27:6199). For this reason, LDH levels should be evaluated in the initial staging workup of patients with stage IV disease. Monitoring LDH levels in patients with loco-regional disease is not recommended.

C. Treatment of localized disease

   1. Wide local excision. In stage 0, I, and II disease, wide local excision of the primary lesion with appropriate clinical margins provides the greatest chance of local control. Margins of 0.5 to 1.0 cm are recommended for melanoma in situ. A margin of 1.0 cm is adequate for primary melanomas with a Breslow thickness of 1 mm or less, while melanomas between 1.01 and 2.0 mm thickness require a 1 to 2 cm margin. Any melanoma with a Breslow thickness of greater than 2 mm requires a 2.0 cm clinical margin. More aggressive margins than those recommended have not been demonstrated to improve survival. In the case of stage III disease with clinically evident lymph nodes, the same margins apply for optimal local control, while stage III in-transit disease should be completely excised with clear margins if possible.

2. **Nonsurgical therapy.** Although surgical excision is standard of care for in situ melanoma, topical imiquimod may be considered particularly for melanoma in situ or in cases of lentigo maligna when surgical cure is not achievable.

D. **Treatment of advanced melanoma**

1. **Adjuvant therapy.** There is no proven benefit for any adjuvant therapy given to patients with low-risk (stage IA) or intermediate-risk (stage IB, IIA) melanoma. Interferon α 2b (Intron) was granted U.S. Food and Drug Administration (FDA) approval in 1995 for administration to patients with surgically resected stage IIB, IIC, and III (high-risk) melanoma. The approved schedule is 1 year of adjuvant treatment given intravenously for the initial 4 weeks at 20 MU/m^2 each day (Monday to Friday), followed by subcutaneous administration at 10 MU/m^2 for 48 weeks given three days per week. We routinely hydrate patients with 500 mL saline before each i.v. dose of interferon during weeks 1 to 4. Patients are premedicated with acetaminophen 650 mg orally. Three randomized controlled clinical trials have been performed using the FDA-approved schedule and the results of Eastern Cooperative Oncology Group (ECOG) 1684, ECOG 1690, and ECOG 1694 have been published. A recent update of the three trials (*Clin Cancer Res* 2004;10:1670) confirms the durable benefit with improved relapse-free survival (RFS) at a median follow-up of 12.6 months for patients given interferon when compared to the control group.

   Pegylated-interferon α 2b (Sylatron) can be administered as adjuvant therapy to patients with microscopic or macroscopic lymph node involvement with melanoma that has been surgically resected. The greatest risk reductions were observed in patients with ulceration and stage IIb/III-N1. The efficacy of IFN/PEG-IFN is lower in stage III-N2 patients with ulceration and uniformly absent in patients without ulceration. The recommended dose is 6 μg/kg/week subcutaneously for 8 doses, followed by 3 μg/kg/week for up to 5 years (*J Clin Oncol* 2012;30:3810). There is no role for adjuvant cytotoxic chemotherapy or adjuvant high-dose interleukin 2 (IL-2) for treatment of surgically resected melanoma.

   Ipilimumab as adjuvant therapy for high-risk resected stage III patients has been evaluated in two large randomized controlled clinical trials (ECOG 1609 and EORTC 18071). Final RFS data released at ASCO 2014 for EORTC 18071 demonstrated improved median RFS with adjuvant ipilimumab (17.1 months for placebo to 26.1 for ipilimumab (HR 0.75 [CI 0.64 to 0.90], $p = 0.0013$)). Moreover, the 3-year RFS rate of 46.5% in the ipilimumab arm is significantly improved compared with 34.8% in the placebo arm. Data on overall survival (OS) are still not available.

   Targeted agents such as serine/threonine-protein kinase B-Raf (BRAF) inhibitors as single agents or in combination with MEK inhibitors are also currently being evaluated as adjuvant therapy in high-risk surgically resected stage III cutaneous BRAF V600E/K-mutated melanoma. The randomized, placebo-controlled phase III studies are ongoing and no data are currently available.

   a. **Interferon side effects and toxicities.** The side effects and toxicities of interferon are significant and all patients should be counseled before the initiation of therapy (*Oncologist* 2005;10:739). Virtually all patients experience fatigue and many experience fevers, chills, and diaphoresis (70% patients, grade 3 to 4). Myelosuppression, hepatotoxicity, and neurologic symptoms are frequent. Depression can be severe and precautions should be taken with appropriate referral to mental health professionals. The use of selective serotonin reuptake inhibitors (SSRI) is recommended in suitable patients (*N Engl J Med* 2001;344:961). Approximately 50% of patients have treatment delay or dose reduction during the initial 4 weeks of induction therapy. Selection criteria used currently in our practice include patients aged 60 or younger with no other significant medical illness, who understand the risks and benefits of treatment. Excellent guidelines to assist in the management of toxicities and side effects have been published. Finally, there is no role for administration of interferon concurrent with radiation.

2. **Metastatic disease.** Regional and distant lymph nodes, skin, lung, liver, and brain are the most common distant sites of metastases from cutaneous melanoma. Prognosis depends on the sites of metastases with brain and hepatic metastases having the shortest survival followed by lung metastases; nodal and skin metastases have the most favorable prognosis. Patients with regional nodal disease or a single distant site (including brain or lung, particularly with pulmonary disease) should be considered for surgical resection. Complete surgical resection of nodal disease can afford significant long-term survival in many patients. The final analysis of the MSLT-1 data attempted to address whether reflex completion lymphadenectomy in sentinel node positive melanoma patients provided melanoma-specific survival benefit compared to delayed lymphadenectomy. The data for intermediate thickness melanomas suggest survival benefit from reflex lymphadenectomy, though owing to post hoc subgroup analysis these do not provide definitive evidence (*N Engl J Med* 2014;370:599). Despite this controversy, current guidelines support completion lymphadenectomy for sentinel-node-positive nodal basins (*J Clin Oncol* 2012;30:2912). The forthcoming MSLT-2 trial will address whether sentinel-node-positive patients benefit from completion lymphadenectomy or from nodal surveillance with ultrasound.

The treatment of metastatic melanoma has improved substantially since 2011. Advances in immunology as well as molecular oncology provided the foundation for therapeutic strategies that have had a profound effect on patient care. A pivotal discovery in 2002 identified the BRAF V600 mutation as a critical driver mutation that is present in approximmately50% of cutaneous melanoma samples irrespective of geography (*Nature* 2002;417:949). Among patients with BRAF-mutated cutaneous melanoma, the BRAF V600E mutation is detected in 80% to 85% patients and the BRAF V600K detected in approximately10% of cases. It appears that non-V600E genotypes occur more frequently in older (>65 years of age) patients. Rare non-V600E/K (exon 15) mutations are not detected by the FDA-approved companion diagnostic (real-time qPCR) Cobas 4800 BRAF V600 mutation test (Roche/Genentech) and THxID-BRAF mutation test (bioMerieux/GSK). Therefore, in certain cases, DNA sequencing of exon 15 is warranted. An emerging method to detect the BRAF V600E mutation is the implementation of the immunohistochemical (IHC) assay using a monoclonal antibody specific for the V600E-mutated protein. The VE1 monoclonal antibody (specific for BRAF V600E) demonstrates 97% sensitivity and 98% specificity in detecting the V600E mutant protein by IHC assay. It is imperative that BRAF inhibitors are not administered to patients with melanoma that is BRAF wild type (no mutation detected) as there is evidence of a paradoxical activation of the MAPK pathway in various cell lineages, including melanocytes. For selected BRAF wild-type patient groups (e.g., mucosal, acral, and chronic sun-damaged skin), KIT mutation testing is performed.

Since 2011, ipilumumab, vemurafenib, dabrafenib, and trametinib have received regulatory approval for unresectable or metastatic (stage III/IV) melanoma and each single agent has been shown to prolong survival in randomized clinical trials compared to dacarbazine. In addition, the combination of dabrafenib and trametinib was approved in 2014 based on improved response rate and the median duration of response compared to dabrafenib alone. Pembrolizumab was granted accelerated approval in 2014 based upon the tumor response rate (24%) and the durability of response for the treatment of metastatic melanoma following ipilimumab treatment. Nivolumab subsequently received accelerated FDA approval for the same indication shortly thereafter in late 2014 based upon tumor response rate (40%) and one year survival rate (72.9%). Despite the introduction of these novel agents, clinical trial participation remains the best option for most patients. Prior to 2011, dacarbazine and IL-2 were regarded as the standard of care for patients with newly diagnosed metastatic melanoma. High-dose IL-2 is recommended at some specialized centers in the United States as first line therapy based on the observation that 3% to 5% of selected patients can attain a durable complete remission. Dacarbazine and combination cytotoxic regimens such as carboplatin plus paclitaxel are generally reserved for patients that have failed or are not candidates for checkpoint inhibitors or targeted agents such as BRAF inhibitors.

Ipilimumab is an immune-modulatory mAb that promotes T cell activation by blocking the interaction of CTLA-4 with its ligands CD80/CD86 (B7 family). Ipilimumab is a human IgG1 kappa antibody specific for human CTLA-4. Since CTLA-4 is a negative regulator of T cell activation, ipilimumab allows T cell activation and proliferation to continue after antigen stimulation by interfering with a homeostatic checkpoint that normally inhibits T cell growth. Ipilimumab was approved in March 2011 for use in patients with unresectable or metastatic melanoma administered every 3 weeks (at 3 mg/kg i.v. over 90 minutes) times four doses with the initial restaging examination done 2 weeks after the fourth or final dose. The overall response rate is 10% to 15%, with a small subgroup of patients exhibiting disease progression at the initial assessment prior to tumor regression. Ipilimumab has been shown in randomized clinical trials to prolong OS in patients with metastatic melanoma (*New Engl J Med* 2010;363:711). A recent pooled analysis of melanoma patients treated on various clinical trials with ipilimumab confirms a 3-year survival rate of 22%, suggesting a durable long-term benefit in this group. Ipilimumab can cause serious side effects leading to severe, and sometimes fatal, autoimmune reactions resulting in dermatitis, colitis, hepatitis, endocrinopathy, and neuropathy. Additional less common autoimmune toxicities such as nephritis, pneumonitis, meningitis, pericarditis, uveitis, iritis, and hemolytic anemia have been reported. Patients should be evaluated at the start and prior to each ipilimumab dose along with appropriate laboratories (including LFTs and thyroid function tests). Adverse event management guidelines have been issued by the drug manufacturer and should be referred to for specific recommendations and treatment algorithms of specific toxicities. **Permanently discontinue ipilimumab and initiate systemic high-dose corticosteroid therapy for severe immune-mediated reactions.**

Pembrolizumab (Keytruda) is a checkpoint inhibitory mAb that blocks the interaction of PD-1 with its ligands (PD-L1/PD-L2). Pembrolizumab is a humanized IgG4 kappa antibody specific for human PD-1. By binding to the PD-1 receptor and blocking the interaction with the receptor ligands, pembrolizumab releases the PD-1 pathway-mediated inhibition of the T cell response, including the anti-tumor immune response. Results from a randomized dose comparison phase 1 study (2mg/kg versus 10 mg/kg) in melanoma patients who progressed after ipilimumab reports ORR 26% (RECIST v1.1) confirmed by independent central review (Lancet 2014; 384:1109). The most common drug-related adverse events of any grade in the cohort were fatigue, pruritus, and rash. The rate of immune-related serious adverse events is 2%. The FDA approved dose is 2mg/kg intravenously over 30 min every 3 weeks.

Nivolumab (Opdivo) is a checkpoint inhibitory mAb that also blocks the interaction of PD-1 with its ligands (PD-L1/PD-L2). Nivolumab is a fully human IgG4 kappa programmed death 1 (PD-1) immune-checkpoint–inhibitor antibody that selectively blocks the interaction of the PD-1 receptor with its two known programmed death ligands, PD-L1 and PD-L2, disrupting the negative signal that regulates T-cell activation and proliferation. Results from a randomized controlled phase 3 trial in patients with untreated advanced BRAF wild type melanoma reported a 40% ORR with nivolumab compared to 13.9% with dacarbazine (NEJM on line published November 16, 2014). The 1 year survival rate was 73% in the nivolumab group versus 42% in the dacarbazine group (Hazard ratio 0.42, p<0.001). The most common drug-related adverse events of any grade in the nivolumab cohort were fatigue, pruritus, and nausea. The rate of immune-related serious adverse events is ~5%. The FDA approved dose is 3 mg/kg intravenously over 60 min every 2 weeks. Permanent discontinuation of pembrolizumab or nivolumab and initiation of systemic-high dose corticosteroid therapy is advised in the setting of severe immune-mediated adverse events.

Vemurafenib (Zelboraf) is an oral kinase inhibitor for the treatment of patients with unresectable or metastatic BRAF V600E-mutated melanoma. The recommended dose is 960 mg every 12 hours with or without food. Vemurafenib is available as 240 mg tablets. Extensive clinical testing in BRAF V600-mutated melanoma confirms a 50% to 60% response rate, with a median PFS of 6 to 7 months and median

OS 13 to 14 months (*Lancet Oncol* 2014;15:323). Vemurafenib also has clinical activity in patients with the BRAF V600E mutation. The side-effect profile includes warning for cutaneous toxicities such as hypersensitivity reactions (including pruritus, fever, and erythema), photosensitivity, alopecia, rash (including Stevens–Johnson syndrome), and development of invasive SCC as well as keratoacanthoma, skin papilloma, and new primary melanoma. Other known toxicities include arthralgia, myalgia, nausea, fatigue, uveitis, blurred vision, hepatotoxicity with elevated liver function tests, and QT prolongation. Vemurafenib should not be administered concurrently with ipilimumab due to hepatotoxicity. Dermatology assessment is recommended at baseline and every 2 months while taking vemurafenib due to the various cutaneous side effects. Likewise, monitoring ECGs at baseline and at the recommended intervals is recommended to assess for QT prolongation >500 ms.

Dabrafenib (Tafinlar) is an oral kinase inhibitor for the treatment of patients with unresectable or metastatic BRAF V600E/K-mutated melanoma. In January 2014, Dabrafenib in combination with trametinib was approved for the treatment of BRAF V600E/K-mutated melanoma based on response rate and the median duration of response (see below). The recommended dose is 150 mg BID. Dabrafenib is supplied as 50- and 75-mg capsules. Dabrafenib shows similar efficacy compared to vemurafenib with 50% to 60% response rate. The side-effect profile is similar; however, there are several important differences. There is a potential risk of hemolytic anemia in patients with glucose-6-phosphate dehydrogenase (G6PD) deficiency. Pyrexia is more common with dabrafenib. Serious febrile reactions and fever of any severity complicated by hypotension, rigors or chills, dehydration, or renal failure can occur and dabrafenib should be held for fever >101.3 F. Similar to vemurafenib, dermatology assessments for skin checks at baseline and every 2 months are recommended. It should be noted that second (noncutaneous) malignancies such as KRAS-mutated pancreatic adenocarcinoma have been diagnosed in patients taking dabrafenib and are thought to be due to the paradoxical activation of the MAP kinase pathway in RAS-mutated tumors, similar to the experience with vemurafenib-treated patients.

Trametinib (Mekinist) is an oral MEK inhibitor for the treatment of patients with unresectable or metastatic BRAF V600E/K-mutated melanoma. Trametinib as a single agent is not indicated for patients that received prior BRAF inhibitor therapy. At this time, the primary use of trametinib is in combination with dabrafenib for treatment of BRAF V600E/K-mutated melanoma. The recommended dose of trametinib either as a single agent or in combination with dabrafenib is 2 mg daily. Trametinib is supplied as 0.5-, 1-, and 2-mg tablets. Published reports with single-agent trametinib demonstrate a 20% to 25% response rate in patients with BRAF V600E/K-mutated melanoma. Rare toxicities include cardiomyopathy, retinal vein occlusion or retinal detachment, interstitial lung disease, and hyperglycemia. The most common adverse events are rash, diarrhea, and lymphedema.

The combination of a BRAF inhibitor (such as dabrafenib) and a MEK inhibitor (such as trametinib) is the preferred systemic treatment for patients with unresectable or metastatic BRAF V600E/K-mutated melanoma (*NEJM* 2014; 371:1877). The recommended dose is dabrafenib 150 mg BID and trametinib 2 mg daily taken 1 hour before or 2 hour after a meal. Treatment is continued until disease progression or unacceptable toxicity. The most common adverse reactions (>20%) for the combination include pyrexia, chills, fatigue, rash, nausea, vomiting, diarrhea, abdominal pain, peripheral edema, cough, headache, arthralgia, night sweats, decreased appetite, constipation, and myalgia. Major hemorrhagic events such as intracranial or gastrointestinal, venous thromboembolism/pulmonary embolism, and cardiomyopathy occur at higher incidence (5% to 10% incidence) compared to patients receiving dabrafenib alone (none reported) in clinical studies. Left Ventricular Ejection Fraction (LVEF) should be evaluated at baseline and at one month and then every 2 to 3 months for patients receiving the combination (or single-agent trametinib). Frequent dermatology evaluation is recommended to assess cutaneous toxicities and new skin lesions.

3. **Investigational therapies.** Clinical investigation is active for the treatment of metastatic melanoma in two broad areas: new immunotherapy approaches and drug-resistant BRAF V600-mutated tumors. Monoclonal antibodies directed to PD-1 as well as PD-L1 are being studied in patients with metastatic melanoma and the results are encouraging with 30% to 40% response rates reported in ipilimumab-naïve as well as ipilimumab refractory patients. A preliminary signal of activity has been reported for the combination of ipilimumab and nivoloumab, an antiprogrammed cell death (PD1) monoclonal antibody. The development of new inhibitor combinations targeting the MAPK pathway is a priority. Combination therapies with BRAF inhibitor and MEK inhibitor together with checkpoint inhibitor monoclonal antibodies (such as anti-CTLA-4 and anti-PD-1/PD-L1) show promise for BRAF-mutated melanoma and are currently under study in phase 1 trials. Adoptive antigen-specific T cell therapy is being investigated at major academic centers. Clinical trial participation remains the best option since most patients will ultimately develop disease progression, and thus, more effective treatments options are urgently needed.

4. **Brain metastases.** The expected survival of patients with intracranial metastases depends on the number of metastatic lesions as well as the presence of neurological symptoms and performance status. A small percentage (<5%) of patients will develop a Central Nervous System (CNS) only relapse. Patients with greater than 3 intracranial melanoma metastasis and focal neurological deficits have an especially poor prognosis. Despite definitive treatment with corticosteroids and whole-brain radiotherapy in patients with multiple melanoma brain metastases, the median survival is 3 to 4 months. In patients who undergo craniotomy and complete surgical resection of a solitary intracranial metastasis, the median survival is 9 months. Outcomes with stereotactic radiosurgery as definitive treatment for 1 to 2 brain metastases appear equivalent to surgery; however, data from a randomized clinical trial are lacking. Noteworthy is the recent observation that BRAF V600E/K-mutated melanoma in the CNS is sensitive to oral BRAF inhibitors. Both vemurafenib and dabrafenib have been studied in this population when given as single agents. However, caution is advised and the use of BRAF inhibitor with concurrent radiation is not recommended pending formal clinical evaluation. In our experience, it appears safe to administer BRAF inhibitor (with a 10 day window) prior to or after radiotherapy in patients with good performance status; however, additional clinical study in this patient population is warranted.

E. **Follow-up.** Patients with a history of melanoma should be followed closely with detailed dermatologic and lymph node examinations. They should be taught skin self-examination, as they are at increased risk for a second primary melanoma, as well as recurrence of disease. In addition, these patients need to be counseled regarding the daily use of a broad-spectrum sunscreen that blocks both UVA and UVB. Patients should also be taught sun-avoidance strategies such as avoiding the mid-day sun and wearing protective clothing. Patients diagnosed with melanoma of any stage are not eligible to donate blood, tissue, or solid organs.

Patients with stage 0 melanoma should be followed with periodic skin examinations for life. Current recommendations for stage IA to stage IIA with no evidence of disease are to have a history and physical examination (H&P) every 6 to 12 months for the first 5 years, then annual skin examinations for life. Routine imaging is not recommended and should be considered only as the clinical scenario dictates. Stage IIB and greater melanoma with no evidence of disease warrants clinical examinations every 3 to 6 months for the first 2 years after diagnosis, then every 3 to 12 months for 3 years, and then annually. Consider radiographic evaluation with chest radiograph, CT, or PET-CT every 4 to 12 months, as well as a brain MRI every 12 months, to assess for metastatic or recurrent disease. Routine radiologic screening in stage IIB and higher is not recommended if rendered no evidence of disease after 5 years, unless symptoms warrant imaging.

F. **Special considerations**

1. **Melanoma of unknown primary.** Patients may present with metastatic disease without an identifiable primary cutaneous melanoma. Cases of melanoma with unknown

primary represent less than 5% of melanomas overall. Most patients present with subcutaneous disease or localized lymph node metastasis clinically manifesting as lymphadenopathy; however, patients with solitary pulmonary metastasis as well as solitary brain metastasis are frequently found to have metastatic melanoma after pathological examination. In these rare instances, BRAF and KIT mutational analysis should be requested. All patients should have a thorough evaluation including examination of the skin, scalp, perineum, eyes, and mucosal membranes, as melanocytes are also present in the eye (conjunctiva and uvea), gut, inner ear, and nasopharynx. Numerous studies have demonstrated that these patients have the same survival as patients with known primaries according to the stage of disease and should be treated accordingly.

2. **Mucosal melanoma.** Mucosal melanoma is rare and represents less than 1% of all melanomas. Melanomas can occur on any mucosal surface including the nasopharynx, oral mucosa, larynx, vulva, rectum, and anus. These tumors are generally advanced at the time of presentation and, therefore, prognosis is poor. Treatment is wide local excision with negative histologic margins. We recommend molecular testing for BRAF and KIT for mucosal melanoma. Clinical responses to ipilimumab have been reported in patients with advanced mucosal melanoma with an objective response rate of 6.6% and a median OS 6.4 months.

3. **Ocular melanoma.** Ocular melanomas also represent less than 5% of the cases of melanoma. Uveal or choroidal melanomas make up most cases, with conjunctival melanomas occurring less frequently. Specialized ultrasonographic evaluation, together with lesional biopsy, is an important tool in initial diagnosis. Treatment for conjunctival melanoma is complete surgical excision. For localized uveal or choroidal melanomas, there are multiple treatment options and factors such as size of tumor, pathologic diagnosis, and vision in affected eye and contralateral eye, presence of metastasis, patient age, and performance status should be considered. Treatment options include enucleation, radiation, photocoagulation, and thermotherapy. In contrast to conjunctival melanomas, uveal and choroidal melanomas generally metastasize hematogenously to the liver. There is no effective systemic treatment for metastatic ocular melanoma. For patients with liver-dominant metastases, regional therapy should be considered. The MEK inhibitor selumetinib (AZD6244) is currently being evaluated as an investigational agent for metastatic ocular melanoma and preliminary reports confirm single-agent activity (*JAMA* 2014;311:2397). Ipilimumab has also been studied in metastatic ocular melanoma and preliminary reports document minimal clinical activity.

Interestingly, the mutation profile of uveal melanoma is distinct from cutaneous melanoma with >85% uveal melanomas showing a GNAQ/GNA11 mutation (most frequently in codon 209); conversely, BRAF mutations are rare. Conjunctival melanoma can infrequently harbor a BRAF mutation. Most major ocular oncology centers now utilize the DecisionDx-UM gene expression profile test (Castle Biosciences) for primary uveal melanoma. This prognostic test (validated in a multicenter clinical trial) stratifies uveal melanoma into three groups based on the 15 gene classifier (*Ophthalmology* 2012;119:1596). Class 1A patients have a very low risk of metastasis (2% at 5 years), while Class 1B patients have a relatively low risk with 21% developing distant metastasis at 5 years after diagnosis. In contrast, Class 2 patients are at high risk for distant recurrence with 72% developing metastasis at 5 years.

II. SQUAMOUS CELL CARCINOMA OF THE SKIN
A. Background
1. **Epidemiology.** Squamous cell carcinoma (SCC) is the second most common type of skin cancer in the United States. The overwhelming majority of SCCs occur on chronic sun-exposed skin in older individuals. Men are twice as likely to develop SCC, and its incidence is more than 20 times higher in fair-skinned individuals than in patients with pigmented skin. Incidence also increases with latitudes closer to the equator, reflecting the importance of ultraviolet (UV) exposure in the pathogenesis of SCC.

2. **Risk Factors.** The major risk factor for development of SCC is exposure to UV radiation or the sun. Therapeutic sources of UV radiation such as psoralen plus

ultraviolet A (PUVA) greatly increase the risk for SCC as do cosmetic sources of UV radiation—indoor tanning accounts for approximately 72,000 excess cases of SCC each year (*BMJ* 2012;345:e5909). Other risk factors include immunosuppression, especially in the context of solid organ transplant patients, fair skin, exposure to ionizing radiation, infection with certain human papillomavirus subtypes, burn scars, nonhealing ulcers, increased age, and hereditary disorders such as xeroderma pigmentosum or recessive dystrophic epidermolysis bullosa.

B. Diagnosis and Staging. SCC generally presents as an enlarging, erythematous, scaly papule or plaque on sun-exposed skin that is persistent and may bleed and be tender. It is generally thought to exist on a continuum from precursor lesions, known as actinic keratoses, to SCC in situ (Bowen's disease) to invasive SCC. Although SCC may be suspected clinically, a biopsy is necessary to make a definitive diagnosis. Several biopsy techniques are adequate, including shave, punch, incisional, or excisional biopsies. Additionally, a full dermatologic examination and palpation of the draining lymph nodes should be performed. In the absence of evidence of metastatic disease, further workup with imaging and laboratory studies is not necessary. Staging of SCCs in the tumor, node, metastasis (TNM) system has been revised in the seventh edition of the AJCC guidelines to include tumor thickness, as it may have prognostic value. One prospective study of SCC in 615 patients demonstrated no metastases in tumors less than 2.0 mm thick, while the rate increased to 4% in tumors 2.1 to 6.0 mm and 16% in tumors larger than 6.0 mm (*Lancet Oncol* 2008;9:713). However, the existing system tends to cluster poor outcomes to T2 tumors and therefore renders T3 or T4 classifications less meaningful given the rare occurrence of bone metastases. Because of this, an alternative staging scheme has been proposed to better stratify good and poor outcomes.

C. Therapy. Several treatment options exist for the treatment of SCC. In situ or low-risk lesions in non–hair-bearing locations may be treated with curettage and electrodessication. Most lesions are removed surgically with 0.4-cm margins for lesions smaller than 2 cm in size and more than 0.6 cm margins for lesions larger than 2 cm or with ill-defined borders. Such margins provide cure rates of 90% to 95%. Mohs micrographic surgery can be employed for lesions that are at high risk for recurrence and metastasis, for example, SCC on the central face, ears, eyelids, lips, recurrent tumors, SCCs larger than 2 cm, SCCs with aggressive histologic subtypes, SCCs that develop in scars, or SCCs developing in immunocompromised patients. Mohs micrographic surgery involves the use of frozen or permanent sections to evaluate as close to 100% of the surgical margin as possible by evaluating the circumferential and deep margins. Additional therapies for SCCs include cryosurgery, radiation, and, rarely, intralesional chemo- or immunotherapy. Radiation therapy is generally reserved for patients who are poor surgical candidates. Radiation is used as adjunct therapy in patients with metastatic disease and resected high-risk SCCs, including those with extensive perineural invasion. Patients with advanced disease may benefit from platinum-based combination chemotherapy. Cetuximab (Erbitux, BMS/Lilly), the anti-EGF receptor mAb, has been studied in patients with advanced SCC and shows modest clinical activity (*J Clin Oncol* 2011;29:3419). In metastatic disease, multidisciplinary management and clinical trial are recommended.

There has been some attempt to employ chemoprevention in patients with a high risk of developing cutaneous SCC, particularly solid organ transplant patients. These modalities range from the use of topical immunomodulators, such as imiquimod, to topical and oral retinoids and topical 5-fluorouracil (Efudex). The use of these topical agents results in irritation that is typically well tolerated. Oral retinoid therapy, however, may be associated with serum lipid abnormalities that may already be problematic in this patient population. In addition, the discontinuation of oral retinoid may be associated with a rebound in the number of SCCs.

D. Prognosis. The vast majority of SCCs can be cured surgically. However, the incidence of local recurrence is 1% to 10%, depending on the method used and can be approximately 20% for high-risk lesions in high-risk locations such as the ear. The incidence of metastasis from cutaneous SCC is 2% to 6%. When SCCs metastasize, they typically go to the first draining lymph node. Certain SCCs have a more aggressive course and are designated as high-risk. High-risk SCCs carry a metastatic risk greater than 10% and include lesions on the lips and ears, lesions larger than 2 cm, thicker lesions, SCCs in scars, recurrent SCCs, SCCs with perineural invasion, and SCCs in immunosuppressed patients.

E. Follow-up and Prevention. Low-risk SCCs are followed up with full-body skin examinations every 3 to 12 months for the first 2 years, every 6 to 12 months for the next 3 years, and annually thereafter. High-risk SCCs should be followed up with skin and lymph node examinations every 1 to 3 months for the first year, every 2 to 4 months for the next year, then every 4 to 6 months for the next 3 years, then every 6 to 12 months thereafter, according to the 2014 NCCN guidelines. Sun protection and sun avoidance need to be stressed in these patients. In high-risk patients, including solid organ transplant or otherwise immunosuppressed patients, precancerous actinic keratoses should be aggressively treated and threshold for biopsy of suspicious lesions should be low.

III. BASAL CELL CARCINOMA

A. Background

1. **Epidemiology.** Basal cell carcinoma (BCC) is the most common cancer in the United States, with over 2 million new cases each year. It is more common in men than in women, and its incidence is increasing in all age groups (*JAMA* 2005;294:681).

2. **Risk Factors.** Environmental exposure to UV light from the sun or tanning beds confers significant risk for the development of BCC, both of which are preventable exposures. Approximately 98,000 additional cases of BCC are attributable to indoor tanning (*BMJ* 2012;345:e5909). Additionally, a history of immunosuppression, increasing age, exposure to ionizing radiation or arsenic, and a history of prior nonmelanoma skin cancer increase risk. Genetic susceptibility to UV damage from fair skin and hereditary disorders such as xeroderma pigmentosum confer risk for BCC. Rare patients will present with numerous, early-onset basal cell carcinomas as a feature of the nevoid basal cell carcinoma syndrome, or Gorlin syndrome, which is due to mutations in the *PTCH1* gene. Additional syndromes with early-onset BCC include Bazex–Dupré–Christol and Rombo. Patients with multiple or early BCC or extensive family history should be referred for dermatologic evaluation.

B. Diagnosis and Staging. BCC classically presents as a pink, pearly papule with a rolled border and arborizing telangiectasias on sun-exposed skin, although common variants include pigmented, ulcerated, or morpheaform morphology. Patients may report that the lesion bleeds easily, does not heal, or is tender. Although in many instances the diagnosis of BCC is strongly suspected based on clinical appearance, biopsy confirms the diagnosis of BCC and provides valuable information to the treating physician. Metatypical, infiltrative, morpheaform, sclerosing, or micronodular features on histology represent an aggressive growth pattern. Any one of several biopsy techniques is acceptable, including shave, punch, incisional, or excisional biopsies. BCCs rarely metastasize, and further workup, beyond a full skin examination, is generally not necessary.

C. Therapy. BCC is typically treated with destructive or surgical measures. Curettage and electrodessication provides a rapid and effective method to destroy BCCs, with a cure rate more than 90%. Surgical excision of BCCs with at least a 4-mm margin provides a cure rate of approximately 95%. Similar to SCCs, BCCs in high-risk locations, including the "mask areas" of the face and genitals, larger tumors on low-risk areas, tumors with aggressive histology, and recurrent BCCs can be treated with Mohs micrographic surgery. Cryotherapy and radiation therapy are also options for patients with low-risk BCCs who are poor surgical candidates.

For superficial BCC, topical 5-fluorouracil can clear more than 90%, whereas imiquimod has been shown to clear over 80% of such BCCs.

For locally advanced BCC or metastatic BCC, systemic therapy with vismodegib (Erivedge, Genentech) should be considered. Vismodegib is a novel oral small-molecule inhibitor of smoothened homolog (SMO), a downstream target of PTCH1, and has significant clinical activity since most BCCs depend on the activation of the hedgehog

(Hh) pathway. In a multicenter phase 2 clinical trial enrolling patients with either locally advanced BCC ($n = 63$) or metastatic BCC ($n = 33$), treatment with vismodegib demonstrated significant clinical activity, with objective response rates of 43% in locally advanced disease and 30% in metastatic disease (Sekulic A, et al. *NEJM* 2012). The recommended dose is 150 mg daily. The most common adverse reactions (≥10%) were muscle spasms, alopecia, dysgeusia, weight loss, fatigue, nausea, diarrhea, decreased appetite, constipation, arthralgias, vomiting, and ageusia.

D. Prognosis. The prognosis for patients with BCC is excellent. Most patients are cured by the aforementioned modalities. If left untreated, BCCs continue to enlarge and are locally destructive. Metastases occur in less than 0.1% of patients, and common sites are the lymph nodes, lungs, and bones. Although considered incurable, patients with metastatic BCC should be considered for systemic therapy with Hh pathway inhibitor or enrollment in a clinical trial.

E. Follow-up and Prevention. Patients with a history of BCC have a 50% chance of developing a second BCC within 5 years. Therefore, similar to patients with SCC, close follow-up is recommended with full skin examination every 6 to 12 months. Avoidance of precipitating factors such as sun exposure, tanning beds, and ionizing radiation needs to be stressed in these patients.

IV. MERKEL CELL CARCINOMA

A. Background

1. **Epidemiology.** Merkel cell carcinoma (MCC) is an uncommon cutaneous cancer. In the United States, approximately 1,500 cases are diagnosed a year. MCC is more common in fair-skinned, elderly individuals, with a mean age of diagnosis between 74 and 76 years of age and 95% of all cases arising in white patients.

2. **Risk Factors and Pathogenesis.** MCC is thought to arise from the Merkel cell in the basal layers of the epidermis and has both epithelial and neuroendocrine features. The Merkel cell polyomavirus (MCPyV), discovered in 2008, is thought to play an etiologic role in MCC development and is present in 80% to 100% of examined cases, although the Merkel virus can be found on normal skin or in SCCs. Although the pathogenesis is not clear, there are identifiable risk factors for the development of MCC. These include exposure to the sun and man-made sources of UV radiation, immunosuppression, a history of skin cancer, fair skin, and age more than 70.

B. Diagnosis and Staging.

MCC typically presents as an asymptomatic, rapidly growing, pink-to-red, dome-shaped papulonodule on the head and neck or the upper limbs. Tumors are primarily dermal, although around 10% arise in the epidermis. Biopsy and histologic examination is required to make the diagnosis of MCC, while special stains with a profile of CK-20 and neurofilament positive and TTF-1 negative aid in distinguishing MCC from other neuroendocrine tumors such as small cell carcinoma of the lung (*Am J Dermatopathol* 2006;28:99). For equivocal lesions, additional neuroendocrine markers should be considered, including chromogranin A, CD56, and synaptophysin. Patients with lesions suspicious for MCC or those who have a confirmed diagnosis of MCC should have a complete history and physical examination, including a full skin and lymph node examination. The seventh edition of the AJCC staging manual uses 2 and 5 cm as size cutoffs for T1, T2, and T3 lesions. Lesions invading the bone, muscle, fascia, or cartilage are considered T4. Stage I disease includes T1 lesions, while stage II includes T2– to T3 lesions without lymph node involvement (stage IIA/B) or T4 (locally invasive primary, stage IIC). Stage III disease is defined by any T lesion with clinical or pathologically apparent nodal disease or in transit metastases, while stage IV is defined by any distant disease. Patients should also have a staging CT, MRI, or preferably PET-CT, which has a specificity of 90% and sensitivity of 90%, to screen for both regional lymph nodes and distant metastases (*Am J Clin Dermatol* 2013;14:437). PET-CT is particularly useful for evaluation of stage II or stage III disease (tumors larger than 2 cm with no discernable nodal disease). If lymph nodes are negative by clinical examination, it is recommended that patients with stage I or II disease receive a sentinel lymph node biopsy with immunostaining because pathologically negative nodes (stages IA and IIA) confer better outcome than do clinically negative nodes without sentinel biopsy (stages IB and IIB). With clinically positive nodes, fine-needle aspiration should be attempted, and if negative, open biopsy should be considered.

C. **Therapy.** The mainstay of therapy for primary disease is wide local excision with 2-cm margins or Mohs micrographic surgery when 2-cm margins are not feasible. Despite removal with wide margins, the chance of local recurrence is high. It is also important to note that the sentinel lymph node biopsy should be done prior to definitive excision, particularly in the head and neck, where the drainage pattern is complex. Although the NCCN guidelines recommend sentinel lymph node biopsies for staging, their effects on survival remain in question. There is some evidence that a wide local excision, combined with adjuvant radiation therapy, may provide a survival benefit. In one retrospective analysis of 1,187 cases from the SEER database, median survival was prolonged with adjuvant RT versus surgery alone (63 vs. 45 months, $p = 0.03$) (Mojica P, et al. *J Clin Oncol* 2007;25:1043). Patients with recurrent MCC may be treated with a wide local excision, radiation, and chemotherapy if metastatic. Platinum-based chemotherapy with or without etoposide is generally reserved for patients with metastatic disease; however, given the rarity of this tumor, the literature remains sparse regarding systemic therapy for metastatic MCC. For metastatic disease, management by a multidisciplinary management team and enrollment in a clinical trial are recommended.

D. **Prognosis.** The 5-year survival rates for MCC vary by stage, with stage IA offering the best prognosis, around 80%, falling to 60% for stages IB and IIA, then around 50% for stages IIB, IIC, and IIIA. Prognosis is poorest for stage IIIB (25% 5-year survival) and metastatic MCC (stage IV, 20% 5-year survival). These numbers are based on the National Cancer Database outcomes from 1986 to 2000. Outcomes tend to be worse for immunocompromised patients.

E. **Follow-up.** Given the high rates of local recurrence and metastatic disease, patients should be followed up closely with complete physical examination every 3 to 6 months for the first 2 years, including skin and lymph node examinations. The median time to recurrence is 8 months, with 90% of recurrences in the first 24 months. New approaches to disease monitoring are emerging. Patients with positive oncoprotein antibodies at the time of active disease can track recurrence with a serial examination of their oncoprotein titers (*Cancer Res* 2010;70:8388).

SUGGESTED READINGS

Gorantla VC, Kirkwood JM. State of melanoma: an historic overview of a field in transition. *Hematol Oncol Clin North America* 2014;28:415–435.

Eggermont AM, Spatz A, Robert C. Cutaneous melanoma. *Lancet* 2014;383:816–827.

Griewank KG, Scolyer RA, Thompson JF, et al. Genetic alterations and personalized medicine in melanoma: progress and future prospects. *J Natl Cancer Inst* 2014;106:435.

Fecher LA, Agarwala SS, Hodi FS, et al. Ipilimumab and its toxicities: a multidisciplinary approach. *Oncologist* 2013;18:733–743.

Endocrine Malignancies

Jessica L. Hudson • Jeffrey F. Moley

I. THYROID CARCINOMA

A. Definition. Thyroid cancer consists of a group of neoplasms including differentiated (papillary, follicular, Hurthle cell, and follicular variant of papillary); medullary (sporadic and hereditary); poorly differentiated, anaplastic; and lymphoma. The most common site of spread of thyroid cancer is the cervical nodes, with the central nodal compartment affected most often.

B. Epidemiology. In 2013, there were 60,220 new cases of thyroid cancer in US, with a disproportionate number of females and patients under the age of 55. Studies from Asia reveal that thyroid cancer has become the most commonly diagnosed cancer in women. It is estimated that by 2014, thyroid cancer in females will outnumber that in males by 4:1. Despite the rising incidence of thyroid cancer, prognosis remains favorable, reflecting the indolent nature of the disease. The majority of thyroid cancer (90%) is well-differentiated thyroid carcinoma of papillary, follicular, or Hurthle cell pathology. Ten-year survival rates for patients with these subtypes are 93%, 85%, and 76%, respectively.

1. **Differentiated.** Subtypes include papillary, follicular, Hurthle cell, and poorly differentiated. Papillary carcinoma is the most common, accounting for 85%, and commonly metastasizes to the lymph nodes. In contrast, follicular carcinomas are more prone to systemic metastases.

2. **Poorly differentiated.** These tend to be more aggressive, more often are not iodine avid, and have a poorer prognosis.

3. **Anaplastic.** These carcinomas are almost never curable. Management includes surgical excision, if possible, and experimental protocols or palliative radiation. Survival is usually measured in weeks to months.

4. **Medullary thyroid carcinomas (MTC).** These can present as either sporadic tumors (75%) or as part of the multiple endocrine neoplasia syndromes (MEN2A and MEN 2B-25%). Sporadic and hereditary MTCs have similar clinical courses, but sporadic lesions often present later in life with neck masses largely due to lack of screening, almost always have lymph node metastases, and require extensive lymph node dissections. Hereditary MTCs are often detected as a result of familial screening, which allows for earlier detection and performance of preventative thyroidectomy in presymptomatic gene carriers.

   a. **MEN2A and MEN2B.** The hallmark of these syndromes is MTC, which may be bilateral and multifocal. The MEN2A syndrome is characterized by MTC (100% penetrance), hyperparathyroidism (<25% penetrance), pheochromocytoma (<40% penetrance), and Hirschsprung's disease (<3%). The MEN2B syndrome is characterized by MTC (100% penetrance), pheochromocytoma (50% penetrance), megacolon (100% penetrance), and by characteristic facial and skeletal features ("marfanoid habitus"). The MEN2 syndromes are caused by germline gain of function mutations in the RET proto-oncogene. There are strong genotype–phenotype correlations. For example, Hirschsprung's disease is only associated with mutations in codon 609, 611, 618, and 620, while MEN2B is usually associated with codon 918 mutation. Patients with inherited RET proto-oncogene mutations identified by genetic screening should have prophylactic thyroidectomy. Patients with established MTC should be treated with surgery after screening for pheochromocytoma preoperatively. Patients with metastatic MTC are also candidates for therapy with tyrosine kinase inhibitors. Controversy exists over the appropriate age for prophylactic thyroidectomy, extent of lymph node dissection based on calcitonin level, and timing of systemic therapy in metastatic disease.

C. **Presentation**
  1. **Subjective.** Patients with thyroid cancer of any type usually present with a thyroid or nodal mass in the neck, which may be associated with hoarseness, dysphagia, or difficulty breathing.
  2. **Objective.** The physical exam reveals a mass in the thyroid that moves up and down with swallowing, but which may be fixed in position if there is significant local invasion. Cervical lymphadenopathy may be present. Frequently, there is an appreciable hoarse quality to the voice.

D. **Diagnosis.** Generally made by fine-needle aspiration cytology.

E. **Workup**
  1. **Laboratory assessment.** Specific diagnostic labs include thyroid function tests, thyroglobulin, and calcitonin levels. The tumor markers thyroglobulin levels and antithyroglobulin antibodies are used to follow patients after treatment for differentiated thyroid cancer. Following treatment, thyroglobulin is measured either with or without TSH level modulation (achieved either by thyroid hormone withdrawal or administration of recombinant thyroglobulin [Thyrogen™]). Calcitonin levels are followed in patients with MTC, and are used preoperatively to help determine the extent of node dissection, and postoperatively to screen for disease persistence, recurrence, and progression.
  2. **Imaging.** Ultrasound will demonstrate the intrathyroidal tumor mass and adjacent lymph nodes. Computed tomography of the neck, chest, and abdomen may be helpful to distinguish pulmonary and mediastinal disease spread. Features of metastatic nodes in the neck include presence of calcifications; wide but short, rounded lesions; and obliteration of the fatty hilum. The only current recommended role for FDG/PET imaging is in patients with differentiated carcinoma with elevated thyroglobulin levels postoperatively and negative iodine imaging. In medullary carcinoma, computed tomography is highly favored over PET.
  3. **Endoscopy.** Laryngoscopy should be performed on all patients with hoarseness as this may reveal a vocal cord paralysis. If tracheal or esophageal invasion is suspected, bronchoscopy and/or endoscopy is warranted.

F. **Pathology.** Routine light microscopy of the tissue specimen after staining with hematoxylin and eosin may identify the main cytologic subclasses of thyroid cancers. Special stains for calcitonin or immunoglobulin markers may be necessary if medullary carcinoma or lymphoma is suspected. Genetic mutations identified by molecular testing of tissue and aspirates, including BRAF, RAS, PAX8-PPAR gamma, and RET-PTC rearrangements, have been associated with differentiated thyroid cancer, though controversy exists over their utility in guiding surgical therapy.

G. **Treatment.** Surgical resection is usually the treatment modality of choice for thyroid cancer confined to the neck, though the extent of dissection and the adjuvant therapies vary by disease subtype.
  1. **Surgery.** For differentiated thyroid cancer, total thyroidectomy is indicated for tumors >4 cm in diameter or tumors less than 4 cm with risk factors including age >45 years, cervical lymph node metastases, poorly differentiated histology, or extrathyroidal extension. There is controversy regarding whether or not to do prophylactic central lymph node dissection. However, the subcategory of minimally invasive follicular carcinoma generally follows an indolent course and can be treated adequately with lobectomy. For MTC, total thyroidectomy is generally recommended, and preoperative imaging and calcitonin levels should determine the extent of lymph node dissection. For anaplastic thyroid cancers, there is controversy as to whether or not surgery is ever indicated. The role of surgery for lymphoma is usually limited to tissue diagnosis only or in settings of airway compromise.
  2. **Radioactive iodine (RAI).** Thyroid tissue selectively takes up iodine and is the primary location of its use in the body. Therefore, targeted radioactive therapy is possible. RAI is typically recommended for primary tumors >4 cm, gross extrathyroidal extension, or elevated postoperative unstimulated thyroglobulin levels (>5 to 10 ng/mL). RAI may selectively be applied for primary tumors measuring 1 to

4 cm, high-risk histology, lymphovascular invasion, cervical lymph node disease, macroscopic multifocality, or postoperative unstimulated thyroglobulin levels <5 to 10 ng/mL. RAI is not typically indicated for small, intrathyroidal, unifocal lesions, or undetectable postoperative unstimulated thyroglobulin. Additionally, RAI is not indicated in the setting of gross residual disease. Exact timing of adjuvant RAI is institution specific.

3. **External beam radiation therapy.** The role for this therapy in thyroid cancer is limited to tumors of the anaplastic subtype. This can be either adjuvant or palliative in nature.

4. **Hormonal therapy.** Thyroid-stimulating hormone (TSH) is a trophic hormone that stimulates growth of thyroid cancer cells. Maintenance of low TSH levels is usually optimal in these patients. Total suppression by oral supplementation with levothyroxine used to be recommended for all patients; however, recent data suggest that doing so places populations such as the elderly at greater risk of cardiac tachyarrhythmias and bone demineralization. The current guidelines favor a stratified approach. In patients with known residual disease or at high risk for recurrence, TSH levels should be maintained below 0.1 mU/L. In low-risk patients with biochemical evidence but no structural evidence of disease, the TSH should be maintained between 0.1 and 0.5 mU/L. Disease-free patients should have TSH levels near the lower limit of the normal reference range. After several years of being disease free, patients can be maintained within the reference range. Chronic suppression of TSH can lead to deficiencies in calcium and vitamin D.

5. **Systemic therapy.** Conventional chemotherapeutic agents have limited utility in the treatment of metastatic thyroid cancer. However, a role for oral tyrosine kinase inhibitors has clinically been demonstrated in randomized, placebo-controlled trials both in RAI-refractory differentiated thyroid cancer and in locally recurrent but unresectable or metastatic medullary thyroid cancer. Kinase therapy has been shown to be associated with improved progression-free survival but not cure. However, this therapy has significant side effects, the management of which is crucial to therapy compliance. The rate of disease progression is a key variable to determine candidacy for systemic therapy. Treatment should be favored in patients with progressive disease over those with stable or indolent disease. An additional option for systemic therapy is surgical tumor debulking, but there are limited data on this intervention, and the benefit to survival is yet to be determined.

   FDA-approved kinase inhibitors for MTC at the time of this publication include Vandetanib and Cabozantinib. Clinical trials would be ideal for all other subtypes. If no clinical trial is available, one could consider as commercially available kinase inhibitors such as axitinib, pazopanib, sunitinib, or vandetanib.

   Specific to the treatment of anaplastic thyroid carcinoma, the disease often presents with a locally advanced, unresectable tumor. Adjuvant and neoadjuvant chemotherapy is usually employed. This is usually undertaken in the setting of a multidisciplinary team and guided either toward aggressive or palliative care. Current regimens include Doxorubicin, Paclitaxel, Cisplatin, or Paclitaxel plus Carboplatin.

6. **Surveillance and maintenance: patients with differentiated thyroid cancer.** This should be followed with physical exam, TSH and thyroglobulin levels, and antithyroglobulin antibodies at 6 and 12 months postoperatively, then annually until disease free. Periodic neck ultrasounds should be performed. Additional courses of RAI can be considered in select responsive tumors in high-risk patients. Patients with medullary thyroid cancer should have physical exam, calcitonin and CEA levels and ultrasound or CT imaging in patients with elevated serum markers.

II. PARATHYROID CARCINOMA

A. **Definition.** Extremely rare malignant tumor of the parathyroid gland, much less common than benign parathyroid hyperplasia or adenomas.

B. **Epidemiology.** There are fewer than 100 cases per year in the United States. The five-year survival is 90%, whereas 10-year survival is 50%. Recurrence rates of this indolent malignancy are close to 50% even with en bloc resection. Mortality is usually due to the metabolic complications of malignant hyperparathyroidism.

C. **Presentation**

1. **Subjective.** Patients often present with a multitude of symptoms associated with primary hyperparathyroidism, such as nephrolithiasis, osteoporosis, hypertension, mood disturbances, fatigue, muscle weakness, or other subtle symptoms. Patients tend to have severe hyperparathyroidism (serum calcium >15 mg/dL), which may manifest with more severe symptoms or hyperparathyroid crisis.

2. **Objective.** Parathyroid carcinoma is extremely rare, and suspicion is usually raised intraoperatively. Preoperatively, patients may have a palpable neck mass (50%) or symptoms of local invasion, such as hoarseness.

D. **Diagnosis.** Histologic diagnosis at the time of surgery, usually with evidence of vascular or capsular or gross invasion of adjacent structures.

E. **Workup.** Identical to benign disease (serum calcium and parathyroid hormone levels, ultrasound, 99mTc-sestamibi scintigraphy). Patients with persistent elevation of parathyroid hormone levels following surgery should undergo a metastatic workup including whole body imaging by computed tomography, FDG/PET, and/or Sestamibi scan.

F. **Treatment**

1. **Surgical.** Radical en bloc resection with ipsilateral thyroid lobectomy with adjacent lymph nodes.

2. **Systemic therapy.** Very little research, generally poor results.

3. **Surveillance and maintenance.** Patients should be followed with measurement of calcium and parathyroid hormone levels. Imaging should be done in patients with suspected recurrence of persistent disease.

III. ADRENAL TUMORS

A. **Definition.** Benign adrenal tumors are very common, being present in up to 9% of the population. This classification includes adenomas, lipomas, myelolipomas, cysts, and benign pheochromocytomas. Malignant tumors of the adrenal gland include malignant pheochromocytoma, adrenocortical carcinoma (ACC), and metastases. The most common sources of adrenal metastases include lung, renal, melanoma, and thyroid cancer. Tumors arising from the medulla include neuroblastoma and pheochromocytoma. Tumors arising from the cortex are largely nonfunctional and also include aldosteronomas, cortisol-secreting adenomas, and tumors that secrete both cortisol and male hormones, the latter of which is usually malignant, such as ACC. Pediatric patients may develop adrenal neuroblastomas.

B. **Epidemiology.** Incidental adrenal lesions are reportedly found in 1% to 4% of abdominal CTs. Additionally, lesions were found in up to 9% of adult autopsies. In patients with other known malignancies at the time of death, 27% had adrenal metastases. Physicians must weigh the risk of malignancy against the morbidity and cost of additional interventions. Of the histologic diagnoses of adrenal incidentalomas, adenomas account for 55%, metastatic lesions account for 31%, pheochromocytomas and adrenal cancers for 4.3%, hyperplasia for 2%, and lipomas/myelolipoma for 1.4%.

In addition to assessing functionality, the workup for incidentalomas is aimed at detecting ACC. Tumor size is a predictor of likelihood of ACC. The prevalence is roughly 2% for lesions <4 cm, 6% for lesions from 4.1-cm, and 25% for lesions >6 cm. Patients with ACC generally have a very poor prognosis. Long-term survival is related to the tumor stage at the time of diagnosis and the ability to undergo surgical resection by a skilled surgeon. Nevertheless, the five-year survival remains approximately 20% to 25%.

Pheochromocytomas are neuroendocrine tumors of the adrenal gland, arising from the medulla. These tumors can store, synthesize, and secrete catacholamines. Approximately 10% are bilateral, 10% are extra-adrenal, 10% occur in children, 10% are familial (MEN2A, VHL, and NF-1), and 10% are malignant, though the extra-adrenal pheochromocytomas, or paragangliomas, have a higher incidence of malignancy (15% to 35%). A small subset of malignant pheochromocytomas has metastases at the time of initial diagnosis, but a significant number go on to develop metastases after treatment. Unfortunately, even with histologic immunohistochemical evaluation, differentiating between benign and malignant pheochromocytomas in the absence of metastases is challenging. Additional research is needed and long-term follow-up is essential.

C. Presentation

1. **Subjective.** Sixty percent of primary malignant tumors are functional and therefore manifest according to their hormone profile. However, many of these symptoms present on a spectrum and over a prolonged period of time, delaying the diagnosis. Most patients present after an astute clinician has a high degree of suspicion or as an incidental finding from imaging for another reason ("incidentaloma").

2. **Objective.** Rarely is an adrenal tumor identifiable on physical exam; however, the functional overexpression of cortisol, virilization hormones can lead to impressive physical exam findings (i.e., Cushing's syndrome with virilization). In the case of ACC, patients may report abdominal or flank pain or fullness or fevers due to hemorrhage within large lesions.

D. Diagnosis. Usually, a correlation of diagnostic imaging and biochemical testing without preoperative biopsy. Often, the assistance of an endocrinologist is valuable.

E. Workup

1. **Laboratory studies.** The laboratory workup for an adrenal mass is extensive but targeted, aimed at elucidating the functional capacity of the tumor, which affects pre-operative management. Additionally, hormonal markers can be used for postoperative surveillance. Basic screening for hypercortisolism includes either a low-dose dexamethasone suppression test or a 24-hour urine cortisol assessment. For aldosterone, serum potassium and blood pressure are assessed first. If these are abnormal, then plasma renin activity and aldosterone levels are obtained. For pheochromocytomas, screening is accomplished best by plasma metanephrines and plasma normetanephrines.

2. **Imaging.** As stated earlier, many adrenal tumors are found incidentally on computed tomography performed for other indications. Unfortunately, these are often of insufficient quality. The ideal imaging modality is a thin-section, high-resolution CT or MRI of the adrenal gland, ideally with an institution-specific adrenal protocol. CT scanning is usually sufficient in 90% of lesions >1 cm in diameter. MRI is of particular utility when there is clinical concern for pheochromocytoma because of the ability to distinguish between adenomas. ^{131}I-metaiodobenzylguanidine (MIBG) scintigraphy is an additional imaging modality that can be employed to identify both intra- and extra-adrenal pheochromocytomas.

   The appearance of an adrenal lesion on imaging is crucial to the correct diagnosis and therefore warrants review. Regarding specific characteristics, adrenal adenomas tend to be homogeneous and have smooth contours with sharp margins. On noncontrasted CT, the tissue density measures <10 Hounsfield units (HU), while on contrasted CT, it measures <25 HU. On MRI, there is signal dropout on opposed phase chemical shift imaging. Comparatively, ACCs have a nonhomogeneous enhancement pattern with central necrosis, irregular borders, calcifications, sparing of local lymph nodes, and/or invasion into surrounding structures, especially the inferior vena cava. On noncontrasted CT, the tissue densities are >10 HU. ACCs tend to measure >6 cm at the time of diagnosis, though a cutoff of 4 cm for diagnosis is associated with 93% sensitivity and 24% specificity. For pheochromocytoma, CT tissue densities normally range from 40 to 50 HU, and on MRI, the hallmark feature is high signal intensity on T-2-weighted images without signal dropout on opposed phase chemical shift imaging. Extracapsular invasion into adjacent structures is suggestive of malignant pheochromocytoma.

   The role of PET in adrenal cancer is limited to staging for ACC, and in the case of metastatic adrenal lesions, as clinically indicated for the primary malignancy.

3. **Biopsy.** After excluding a pheochromocytoma, it is considered safe to perform a biopsy of an adrenal lesion. Typically, this is performed by image guidance in cases of concern for metastases or lymphoma, if the diagnosis would alter management. Usually, tissue diagnosis is not necessary prior to resection of obviously malignant adrenal masses.

F. Treatment. Any adrenal lesion with concerning characteristics or measuring >4 cm should be considered for surgical resection. Benign but functional lesions are also treated with surgery, but will not be covered. This discussion will focus on malignant pheochromocytoma, ACC, and adrenal metastases.

1. **Surgery.** There is a role for surgery in solitary adrenal metastases, specifically if the patient is symptomatic (i.e., flank pain), there is control of the primary tumor, and the adrenal metastasis is considered fully resectable. There is improved survival in patients after solitary metastasis adrenalectomy due to adenocarcinoma when compared with other pathologic subtypes. There does seem to be improved quality of life when adrenalectomy is performed in symptomatic metastatic disease. While debatable, this can be performed via either an open or a laparoscopic approach.

   For ACC, open adrenalectomy is the preferred operation, aiming for radical en bloc resection of the involved adrenal gland and the surrounding tissues and lymphadenectomy. This could involve the kidney, liver, spleen, and/or inferior vena cava. Avoiding violation of the adrenal capsule reduces the risk of local recurrence. When ACC was not diagnosed preoperatively, retrospective data indicated an increased risk of local recurrence and disease dissemination after undergoing laparoscopic adrenalectomy when compared with open.

   For pheochromocytomas, surgical resection should always be considered, even in the presence of metastatic disease, if only to alleviate symptoms via tumor debulking. Attempts are made to remove local and distant metastatic lesions, which can often be identified preoperatively by MIBG. Specific to hepatic lesions, consideration may need to be given to cryotherapy or transarterial chemoembolization.

2. **Hormonal.** Hormonal therapy for adrenal lesions is targeted at treating or preventing hormone imbalances, rather than targeting the tumors themselves. Nevertheless, it is a crucial component of managing these patients. In the setting of cortisol-producing lesions, all patients should be treated postoperatively with exogenous glucocorticoids for 6 to 18 months to allow the hypothalamic–pituitary–adrenal axis to re-equilibrate. Patients with subclinical or clinical Cushing's disease should also receive preoperative glucocorticoids. With aldosterone excess, supplementation of mineralocorticoids should be considered.

   In the treatment of pheochromocytoma, malignant or otherwise, alpha-adrenergic blockade is necessary 1 to 3 weeks preoperatively in order to prevent intraoperative blood pressure lability. Recent research suggests possible further improvement with the addition of the tyrosine kinase inhibitor metyrosine. If the tumor cannot be fully resected, the alpha-blockade should be continued postoperatively.

3. **Systemic.** For metastatic lesions of the adrenal gland, systemic therapy is guided by the primary tumor guidelines.

   For ACC, a derivative of the insecticide DDT, called mitotane, has been used for adjuvant therapy. It acts to suppress the adrenal cortex directly and therefore has an extensive side-effect profile. It is not yet known whether adjuvant systemic treatment is effective in ACC, and therefore patient selection criteria do not yet exist. At the time of this publication, multiple research trials are ongoing to assess for additive effects of mitotane with more traditional chemotherapeutic agents. Some such combinations include etoposide, doxorubicin, and cisplatin plus mitotane as well as gemcitabine and 5-fluorouracil or capecitabine plus mitotane.

   For inoperable pheochromocytomas, a variety of protocols have been suggested for systemic therapy. Historically, this has included cyclophosphamide, vincristine, and dacarbazine (CVD). More recent approaches have suggested lomustine and 5-fluorouracil for indolent lesions, and etoposide and a platinum-based agent for aggressive lesions.

4. **Radiation.** For treatment of malignant pheochromocytomas, there is a role for neoadjuvant radiation for tumor debulking, palliation, and management of painful bony metastases. In patients who showed radioactive uptake of the noradrenaline analogue MIBG by preoperative imaging, adjuvant administration of radioactive MIBG has been given as a radiopharmaceutical for pheochromocytoma. Most patients experienced symptomatic improvement, which then led to survival benefits proportional to their biochemical response. Since the transition of MIBG from a diagnostic to a therapeutic intervention, and given the poor treatment response to systemic chemotherapy, some suggest that MIBG is the most useful treatment in unresectable pheochromocytomas. Likewise, radiolabeling analogues of somatastatin, such as octreotide,

have been used. Research is still ongoing about the possible combination of these two radiopharmaceutical treatments. Total body radiation dosing limits apply, and the side-effect profile is directly proportional to the dose received.

5. **Surveillance and maintenance.** Patients with adrenal lesions that do not meet the criteria for surgical resection warrant repeat imaging initially 3 and 6 months after diagnosis, then annually. Subsequent hormonal evaluation should be completed every 5 years unless there is a change in the clinical conditions.

SUGGESTED READINGS

Kloos RT, Eng C, Evans DB, et al; American Thyroid Association Guidelines Task. Medullary thyroid cancer: management guidelines of the American Thyroid Association. *Thyroid* 2009;19:565–612.

Beitler AL, Urschel JD, Velagapudi SR, et al. Surgical management of adrenal metastases from lung cancer. *J Surg Oncol* 1998;69:54–57.

Bradley CT, Strong VE. Surgical management of adrenal metastases. *J Surg Oncol* 2014;109(1):31–35.

Dreicer R. Systemic therapy for advanced adrenal cancer. *J Surg Oncol* 2012;106:643–646.

Moley JF. Medullary thyroid carcinoma: management of lymph node metastases. *J Natl Compr Canc Netw* 2010;8:549–556.

Schlumberger M, Bastholt H. Dralle, et al; European Thyroid Association Task. 2012 European thyroid association guidelines for metastatic medullary thyroid cancer. *Eur Thyroid J* 2012;1:5–14.

Schlumberger M, Catargi B, Borget I, et al. Tumeurs de la thyroide refractaires network for the essai stimulation ablation equivalence, strategies of radioiodine ablation in patients with low-risk thyroid cancer. *N Engl J Med* 2012;366:1663–1673.

Tanvetyanon T, Robinson LA, Schell VE, et al. Outcomes of adrenalectomy for isolated synchronous versus metachronous adrenal metastases in non-small-cell lung cancer: a systematic review and pooled analysis. *J Clin Oncol* 2008;26:1142–1147.

Tuttle RM., Ball DW, Byrd RA, et al. National comprehensive cancer, thyroid carcinoma. *J Natl Compr Canc Netw* 2010;8:1228–1274.

Wells SA, Gosnell RF, Gagel RF, et al. Vandetanib for the treatment of patients with locally advanced or metastatic hereditary medullary thyroid cancer. *J Clin Oncol* 2010;28:767–772.

Wells SA, Santoro M, Update: the status of clinical trials with kinase inhibitors in thyroid cancer. *J Clin Endocrinol Metab* 2014;99:1543–1555.

Zheng QY, Zhang GH, Zhang Y, et al. Adrenalectomy may increase survival of patients with adrenal metastases. *Oncol Lett* 2012;3:917–920.

Cancer of Unknown Primary Site

Siddartha Devarakonda • Danielle Carpenter • Daniel Morgensztern

I. **DEFINITION.** Carcinoma of unknown primary (CUP) is defined as a biopsy-proven metastatic malignant tumor whose primary site cannot be identified during pretreatment evaluation that includes a thorough history and physical examination, standard laboratory and radiographic studies, and a detailed histologic investigation.

II. **PRESENTATION**
   A. **Subjective.** Although CUPs comprise a heterogeneous group of tumors with different natural histories, there are still some typical characteristics. Some of the clinical features include a short history of local symptoms related to the metastatic sites (pain, swelling, and cough) and constitutional symptoms (weight loss, fatigue, and fever).

B. Objective. The physical examination is frequently abnormal with findings such as effusions, lymphadenopathy, and hepatomegaly, indicating the site of metastatic involvement. Patients should undergo a thorough examination of the skin to rule out the presence of melanoma or nonmelanoma tumors, breast, rectum, pelvis, and genitals. The most common sites involved are lymph nodes, liver, bone, lungs, and pleura. Most patients present with multiple metastatic sites because of early dissemination and, unlike known primary tumors, the pattern is usually unpredictable.

III. DIAGNOSIS. The diagnosis is made by biopsy. Since several studies may need to be performed, it is important to consult with the pathologist to determine whether the specimen is sufficient, as the commonly used fine-needle aspiration contains limited tissue and does not provide information on tissue architecture.

IV. WORKUP

A. Initial assessment. With the histologically proven diagnosis of malignancy, patients should undergo a limited clinical investigation to identify the primary site and favorable subsets. This evaluation should include a complete history of physical examination including pelvic and rectal examination, complete blood count (CBC), chemistry profile, urinalysis, occult blood stool testing, chest radiography, computer tomography (CT) of the abdomen and pelvis, and symptom-oriented endoscopy. Subsequent diagnostic tests are based on the clinical presentation, gender, and histopathologic findings. Comprehensive and exhaustive radiographic and endoscopic tests should not be performed because even with extensive workup, the primary site becomes evident in less than 25% of the patients. Up to 80% of primaries can be found in autopsy series, most commonly in the lungs and pancreas.

B. Imaging. The initial radiological evaluation may be limited to chest radiograph and CT scans of the chest, abdomen, and pelvis. Chest radiograph is usually performed during the initial evaluation, even in the absence of respiratory symptoms, since a large number of patients will eventually have the diagnosis of lung cancer. Contrast radiographic studies have a low yield and should be reserved for patients with findings related to the organ to be examined. CT scan of the abdomen and pelvis may detect the primary site in approximately one-third of patients. It can also be particularly useful in the detection of occult pancreatic carcinomas. Mammogram is indicated in the diagnostic investigation of all women with CUP, particularly in the cases of adenocarcinoma metastatic to axillary lymph nodes. Breast magnetic resonance imaging (MRI) may be indicated in cases where the suspicion for primary breast remains high despite a negative mammogram. The experience with fluorodeoxyglucose positron emission tomography (FDG-PET) scan in CUP has been limited so far, and larger prospective series are needed before its routine use. Some of the problems associated with the use of PET include the high cost, elevated false-positive rate, and lack of improved survival after the identification of the primary tumor. Nevertheless, PET may be particularly useful in patients with squamous cell carcinoma in the cervical lymph nodes, where it may allow the detection of a primary site in the head and neck area in approximately one-third of the cases, and in patients with single metastatic site, where additional metastases may influence the treatment.

C. Endoscopy. Endoscopy cannot be recommended during the routine workup for patients with CUP in asymptomatic patients. Instead, it should be used according to the clinical presentation. Therefore, ENT endoscopy should be performed in patients with isolated cervical lymph node involvement by squamous cell carcinoma, bronchoscopy in patients with pulmonary symptoms, gastrointestinal endoscopies in patients with abdominal symptoms or occult fecal blood, and proctoscopy or colposcopy in patients with inguinal lymph node involvement.

D. Pathology

1. **Light microscopy.** Routine light microscopy of the tissue specimen after staining with hematoxylin and eosin may identify the five major histologic subtypes of CUP: adenocarcinoma (50% to 60%), poorly differentiated carcinomas or adenocarcinomas (30%), squamous cell carcinomas (5% to 15%), undifferentiated malignant neoplasms (5%), and neuroendocrine carcinomas (1%).

2. **Immunohistochemistry.** Immunohistochemistry (IHC) represents the most widely available specialized technique for the classification of neoplasms and may help identify the tumor lineage by the use of peroxidase-labeled antibodies against specific tissue antigens. Immunoperoxidase (IP) can be used on formalin-fixed specimens, which usually makes repeated biopsy unnecessary and may identify several cell components, resulting in the narrowing of diagnostic possibilities (Table 33-1). IHC can aid in determining whether a poorly differentiated neoplasm is a carcinoma, sarcoma, lymphoma, or melanoma, and if a carcinoma is an adenocarcinoma, squamous cell carcinoma, germ cell tumor, or neuroendocrine carcinoma. Cytokeratins (CKs) are a family of intermediate filaments characteristic of carcinomas. The CK profile may be useful in the identification of the primary tumor site, and the ones most commonly used in patients with CUP are CK7 and CK20. CK7 is more commonly present in tumors of the lung, ovary, endometrium, and breast, and absent in lower gastrointestinal tumors. CK20 is expressed in the gastrointestinal and urothelial cells. Therefore, the CK7/CK20 phenotype can be very useful in narrowing the differential for identification of the primary site, particularly for adenocarcinomas (Table 33-2). Patients with CK7+ and TTF-1 positive are likely to have lung cancer, whereas those with CK7−/CK20+/CDX2+ are likely to have lower gastrointestinal cancer.

3. **Electron microscopy.** Electron microscopy (EM) allows the visualization of the ultrastructural features of the tumors such as cellular organelles, granules, and cell junctions. It may be useful in the identification of neuroendocrine tumors (neurosecretory granules), melanoma (premelanosomes), and poorly differentiated sarcomas. It may also help in differentiating between lymphoma and carcinoma or adenocarcinoma and squamous cell carcinoma, although it does not localize the primary site of the malignancy. Since EM is expensive, time consuming, and not widely available, its use should be reserved for the cases with unclear lineage after light microscopy and IHC.

4. **Tumor markers.** Commonly used serum tumor markers such as CEA, CA 19-9, and CA 125 are of limited value in the diagnosis of patients with CUP. Thyroglobulin may be increased in patients with bone metastases, suggesting an occult thyroid primary. CA 125 may be helpful in women with peritoneal papillary adenocarcinomatosis.

TABLE 33-1	Immunoperoxidase Staining

Tumor type	Immunohistochemistry
Carcinoma	CK, EMA
Lymphoma	CLA (CD45)
Melanoma	S-100, Mart1/MelanA, HMB-45
Sarcoma	Vimentin, desmin, factor VIII antigen (angiosarcoma)
Breast cancer	CK7, EMA, GCDFP-15, mammaglobin, ER, PR,
Germ cell tumor	β-HCG, AFP, PLAP, CK, EMA
Neuroendocrine tumor	Chromogranin, synaptophysin, NSE, CK, EMA, CD56
Prostate cancer	Prostein, PSA, CK, EMA
Thyroid	Thyroglobulin, TTF-1, calcitonin (MTC), CK, EMA
Squamous cell carcinoma	CK 5/6, p63, p40
Urothelial carcinoma	Uroplakin, thrombomodulin
Hepatocellular carcinoma	Hepar1, CD10, CD13
Merkel cell	Chromogranin, synaptophysin

AFP, α-fetoprotein; CK, cytokeratin; CLA, common leukocyte antigen; EMA, epithelial membrane antigen; ER, estrogen receptor; β-HCG, beta-human chorionic gonadotropin; HMB, human melanoma black; MTC, medullary thyroid carcinoma; NSE, neuron-specific enolase; PLAP, placental alkaline phosphatase; PR, progesterone receptor; PSA, prostate-specific antigen; TTF-1, thyroid transcription factor 1.

TABLE 33-2	CK Phenotype

CK phenotype	Tumors
CK7−/CK20−	Head and neck, liver, lung (squamous), prostate, renal
CK7+/CK20−	Biliary tract and pancreas, breast, cervical, endometrial, lung (adenocarcinoma), ovarian (nonmucinous), thyroid
CK7−/CK20+	Colon, Merkel cell carcinoma
CK7+/CK20+	Biliary tract and pancreas, ovarian (mucinous), urothelial

A serum beta-human chorionic gonadotropin (β-HCG) and alpha-fetoprotein (AFP) levels in younger males, and prostate-specific antigen (PSA) in older men should be tested to exclude testicular and prostate cancer, respectively.

5. **Genetics.** Genetic analyses of the biopsy specimen may provide further characterization regarding the origin of the malignancy since a large number of tumors display characteristic cytogenetic abnormalities (Table 33-3).

6. **Expression and micro-RNA profiling.** Molecular profiling including gene expression and micro-RNA can aid in the identification of the primary site of a CUP, as molecular profiles vary across different cancers and are usually comparable to the profiles of their underlying normal tissue of origin. Molecular profiling has the potential to improve outcomes in patients with CUP, especially when the results allow site-specific therapy for favorable tumor types. Studies have demonstrated good agreement between the sites of origin predicted by molecular profiling and suspected primary sites based on clinicopathological findings. These results were, however, shown to be less accurate when IHC suggested two or more sites. While there is little evidence describing the impact of molecular profiling on outcomes in patients with CUP, molecular profiling can be helpful when clinical and pathological workup fails to reveal the primary site.

V. THERAPY AND PROGNOSIS

A. **Favorable subsets.** Following the exclusion of lymphoma and sarcoma by a careful pathologic evaluation, the vast majority of the patients will have the diagnosis of carcinoma. The next step in the investigation is to determine whether they belong to one of the several subsets of CUP patients that require specific treatment approaches that may lead to improved outcomes and possibly cure (Table 33-4).

1. **Women with isolated axillary adenopathy.** Patients with CUP and isolated axillary adenopathy are usually females, and the diagnosis is most likely breast cancer. The

TABLE 33-3	Selected Cytogenetic Abnormalities

Tumor	Abnormality
Lymphomas	
Anaplastic large cell lymphoma	t(2;5)
Burkitt's lymphoma	t(8;14), t(2;8), and t(8;22)
Follicular lymphoma/diffuse large B-cell lymphoma	t(14;18)
Mantle cell lymphoma	t(11;14)
Sarcomas	
Alveolar rhabdomyosarcoma	t(2;13)
Uterine leiomyoma	t(12;14)
Synovial sarcoma	t(X;18)
Germ cell tumors	i(12p)
Retinoblastoma	del(13)
Wilm's tumor	del(11)

TABLE 33-4 Favorable Subsets and Treatment

Subset	Treatment
Women with adenocarcinoma involving only axillary lymph nodes	Treat as stage IIA (T0 N1) or IIIA (T0 N2) breast cancer
Women with papillary serous adenocarcinoma in the peritoneal cavity	Treat for stage III ovarian carcinoma
Men with blastic bone metastases and elevated PSA	Treat for prostate cancer with hormonal therapy
Men with poorly differentiated carcinoma with midline distribution	Treat as extragonadal germ cell tumors
Squamous cell carcinoma of the cervical lymph nodes	Treat as locally advanced head and neck cancer
Isolated inguinal lymphadenopathy by squamous cell carcinoma	Inguinal node dissection with or without adjuvant radiation therapy
Poorly differentiated neuroendocrine carcinoma	Platinum-based chemotherapy
Single metastasis	Local treatment with surgery or radiation therapy

PSA, Prostate-specific antigen.

lymph node specimen should be tested for ER, PR, and HER2/neu. In the case of a negative mammogram, the occult breast primary may be seen on MRI. The primary tumor can be identified after mastectomy in 40% to 80% of cases. Patients with mobile axillary lymph nodes (N1) should be treated as stage IIA breast cancer, whereas patients with fixed nodes (N2) should be treated as stage IIIA disease.

2. **Women with papillary serous adenocarcinoma of the peritoneal cavity.** The presence of ascites and peritoneal adenocarcinoma in women is typical of ovarian carcinoma, although this pattern of spread may also occur in tumors of the lung, breast, and gastrointestinal tract. However, a primary tumor is not found in a large number of these patients. Although the origin of these cells is unknown, histologic features such as papillary configuration or psammoma bodies are typical of ovarian carcinoma. Many of these patients, in whom no ovarian or abdominal primary is obvious on laparotomy, are believed to have primary peritoneal carcinoma. The incidence of primary peritoneal carcinoma is increased in women with a history of ovarian carcinoma and *BRCA1* mutations. Patients in this subgroup should be considered to have stage III ovarian carcinoma and treated with cytoreductive surgery followed by platinum-based chemotherapy.

3. **Men with blastic bone metastases and elevated PSA.** Elderly men with metastatic adenocarcinoma of unknown primary predominantly involving the bones, and those with increased serum PSA or positive PSA staining in the biopsy specimen should be treated for metastatic prostate cancer.

4. **Men with poorly differentiated carcinoma of midline distribution.** Young men with a poorly differentiated neoplasm and predominant midline tumor distribution (mediastinum and retroperitoneum) should be treated as extragonadal germ cell tumors even in the absence of elevated serum levels of AFP or β-HCG. The presence of isochromosome 12p in some tumors allows their classification as germ cell tumors.

5. **Squamous cell carcinoma of the cervical lymph nodes.** Patients with mid or upper cervical lymph nodes are usually middle-aged or elderly, with frequent history of tobacco and alcohol abuse. The main suspicion in these patients is of a primary head and neck tumor, and the workup should involve the complete evaluation of the upper airways. In the absence of an identifiable primary site, patients should be considered to have locally advanced head and neck cancer. Patients with lower cervical lymph or supraclavicular lymph nodes may have lung cancer and should undergo fiberoptic bronchoscopy during the workup, particularly in the case of unrevealing head and

neck examination and nondiagnostic chest imaging. If no primary site is found, the prognosis for this subset of patients is usually poor.

6. **Isolated inguinal lymphadenopathy from squamous cell carcinoma.** Most patients with inguinal lymph nodes have a detectable primary tumor either in the genital or in the anorectal area. Therefore, both the genitalia and the rectum should be evaluated during the initial workup. If the primary cancer cannot be identified, long-term survival may be achieved with inguinal lymphadenectomy with or without adjuvant radiation therapy. Some patients may also benefit from the addition of chemotherapy, either in the neoadjuvant or in the adjuvant settings.

7. **Single metastasis.** In a small number of patients, only a single metastatic lesion is identified despite a complete clinical and radiologic evaluation. Although other metastatic sites may become evident within a short period of time, some patients may achieve prolonged disease-free interval with local therapies such as surgery or radiation therapy. Despite the uncertain role, adjuvant chemotherapy may be considered for patients with good performance status.

8. **Low-grade neuroendocrine carcinoma.** Metastatic carcinoid tumor and islet cell tumors are considered in this subgroup. Treatment includes the use of long-acting octreotide and local therapy when clinically indicated. Cytotoxic agents including streptozocin may be used in selected cases.

B. **Unselected patients.** With the exception of patients in the favorable subsets, most patients with CUP remain relatively resistant to chemotherapy, indicating a very poor prognosis. Although the median survival for patients enrolled into clinical trials ranges between 6 and 10 months, population data from tumor registries report median survivals of 2 to 3 months in unselected patients. A prognostic model proposed by the French study group was based on ECOG (Eastern Cooperative Oncology Group) performance status higher than 1 and abnormal lactate dehydrogenase (LDH). Patients with none, one, or two risk factors had median survivals of 10.8, 6.0, and 2.4 months, respectively (*J Clin Oncol* 2002;20:4679). Patients with good performance status may benefit from chemotherapy. No single chemotherapeutic regimen has emerged as the treatment of choice, and the most commonly used include a combination of platinum and a taxane (Table 33-5). The role for a third agent such as gemcitabine or etoposide remains unclear.

TABLE 33-5	Selected Chemotherapeutic Regimens for Cancer of Unknown Primary Site		
Regimen	**Assessable patients**	**Response rate (%)**	**Median survival (mo)**
PCb[a]	70	39	13
PCbE[b]	66	48	11
PCbG[c]	113	25	9
DCb[d]	40	22	8
DCp[d]	23	26	8
GI[e]	105	18	8.5

Cb, carboplatin; Cp, cisplatin; E, etoposide; D, docetaxel; G, gemcitabine; I, irinotecan; P, paclitaxel.

[a]Briasoulis E, Pavlidis N. Cancer of unknown primary origin. *J Clin Oncol* 2000;18:3101–3117.

[b]Greco FA, Burris HA III, Erland JB, et al. Carcinoma of unknown primary site: long-term follow-up after treatment with paclitaxel, carboplatin, and etoposide. *Cancer* 2000;89:2655–2660.

[c]Greco FA, Burris HA, Litchy S, et al. Gemcitabine, carboplatin, and paclitaxel for patients with carcinoma of unknown primary site: a Minnie Pearl Cancer Research Network study. *J Clin Oncol* 2002;20:1651–1656.

[d]Greco FA, Erland JB, Morrissey LH, et al. Carcinoma of unknown primary site: phase II trials with docetaxel plus cisplatin or carboplatin. *Ann Oncol* 2000;11:211–215.

[e]Hainsworth JD, Spigel DR, Clark BL, et al. Paclitaxel/carboplatin/etoposide versus gemcitabine/irinotecan in the first-line treatment of patients with carcinoma of unknown primary site: a randomized, phase III Sarah Cannon Oncology Research Consortium Trial. *Cancer J* 2010;16:70–75.

VI. BACKGROUND. Metastatic CUP is a common entity, accounting for 2.3% of all cancers reported to the Surveillance, Epidemiology, and End Results (SEER) database between 1973 and 1987. It represents the seventh to eighth most common type of cancer and the fourth commonest cause of death in both men and women. The median age at presentation is approximately 60 years, and it is slightly more prevalent in men.

The characteristic of CUP is the development of metastases before the primary tumor becomes detectable. These tumors are characterized by early dissemination, unpredictable metastatic spread, and very aggressive behavior.

SUGGESTED READINGS

Fizazi K, Greco FA, Pavlidis N, et al. Cancers of unknown primary site: ESMO clinical practice guidelines for diagnosis, treatment and follow-up. *Ann Oncol* 2011;22(Suppl 6):i64.

Culine S, Kramar A, Saghatchian M, et al. Development and validation of a prognostic model to predict the length of survival in patients with carcinoma of an unknown primary site. *J Clin Oncol* 2002;20:4679–4683.

Kamposioras K, Pentheroudakis G, Pavlidis N. Exploring the biology of cancer of unknown primary: breakthroughs and drawbacks. *Eur J Clin Invest* 2013;43:491.

Massard C, Loriot Y, Fizazi K. Carcinomas of an unknown primary origin—diagnosis and treatment. *Nat Rev Clin Oncol* 2011;8:701.

Pavlidis N, Briasoulis E, Hainsworth J, et al. Diagnostic and therapeutic management of cancer of unknown primary. *Eur J Cancer* 2003;39:1990–2005.

Pavlidis N, Fizazi K. Cancer of unknown primary. *Crit Rev Onc Hematol* 2005;54:243–250.

Pavlidis N, Pentheroudakis G. Cancer of unknown primary site. *Lancet* 2012;379:1428–1435.

Rubin BP, Skarin AT, Pisick E, et al. Use of cytokeratins 7 and 20 in determining the origin of metastatic carcinoma of unknown primary, with special emphasis on lung cancer. *Eur J Cancer Prev* 2001;10:77–82.

Van De Wouw AJ, Jansen RLH, Speel EJM, et al. The unknown biology of the unknown primary tumor: a literature review. *Ann Oncol* 2003;14:191–196.

Varadhachary R. Carcinoma of unknown primary: focused evaluation. *J Natl Compr Canc Netw* 2011;9:1406.

34 AIDS-Associated Malignancies

Lee Ratner

GENERAL CARE OF THE PATIENT WITH HIV AND CANCER

I. GENERAL. A malignancy develops in about 20% of patients with human immunodeficiency virus (HIV) during their lifetime, and is often the first clinical evidence of HIV infection. It is also responsible for 28% of AIDS patients' deaths. The most common malignancies in this patient population are non-Hodgkin's lymphoma, Kaposi's sarcoma, and anogenital carcinoma. The incidence of other malignancies is also increased in HIV-infected patients, including Hodgkin's lymphoma (HL), lung cancers, multiple myeloma, testicular tumors, hepatocellular carcinomas (HCCs), and childhood sarcomas. The frequency of non-AIDS–defining cancers has increased significantly over the last 15 years, and has been attributed to expansion of the HIV-infected population and aging. Most of these malignancies are associated with oncogenic viruses, including Epstein–Barr virus (EBV), human herpesvirus-8 (HHV8), and human papilloma viruses (HPV). When CD4 cell counts drop below 200 cell/mL, HIV-infected patients tend to experience greater toxicity with chemotherapy. Dose modifications and dose delays are common in this setting. Often, personalized dose modifications in lower performance status patients may be chosen by treating physicians. Providers need to be cognizant of any drug–drug interactions of highly active antiretroviral therapy (HAART) with antitumor therapies as well as supportive medications. Regular discussion between medical oncologists, infectious disease specialists, and radiation and surgical oncologists are essential. Maximizing nutritional status can assist in minimizing toxicity and accelerating recovery from therapy. Social work assistance is invaluable for these patients, who often have other financial, social, and personality difficulties.

II. **DIAGNOSTIC STUDIES FOR HIV INFECTION** should be considered in patients who are not known to be HIV infected, but who develop a malignancy that occurs at increased frequency with HIV infection. Many patients with HIV infection are unaware of their risk factors or deny their existence. HIV testing is recommended to all individuals presenting with aggressive B-cell lymphomas, Kaposi's sarcoma, or anogenital carcinomas, as well as individuals with any malignancy who have higher than average risk for HIV (i.e., IV drug abusers, homosexuals or bisexuals, individuals with large numbers of sexual partners, and individuals from countries in Africa, southeast Asia, or parts of the Caribbean where HIV is especially prevalent). Appropriate pre- and posttesting counseling services should be available for these individuals. The screening HIV test is an enzyme-linked immunosorbent assay (ELISA), which, if positive, is confirmed by Western blot or plasma HIV RNA assay. The rapid, point-of-care, HIV antibody tests are an acceptable alternative to the ELISA and are in wide use. If HIV is diagnosed concurrently with such a malignancy, additional clinical evaluation of their HIV infection may be indicated. Plasma HIV RNA and CD4 should be determined during the evaluation of HIV-associated malignancies. However, it is important to recognize that chemotherapy can cause wide fluctuations of the CD4 count that may not be an accurate measurement of the immune status.

III. **HAART** will usually be recommended as concurrent therapy for the malignancy, and, in some cases, prophylaxis for opportunistic infections (OIs). Although issues of drug interactions and excessive toxicity must be considered, there is now considerable evidence supporting the concurrent use of HAART in all HIV-1-infected individuals.

A. **HAART regimens** include the use of at least three antiretroviral agents with nucleoside- or nucleotide-reverse transcriptase inhibitors (zidovudine, didanosine; didexoycytidine, stavudine, lamivudine, abacavir, and tenofovir emtricitabine) combined with nonnucleoside-reverse transcriptase inhibitors (nevirapine, delaviridine, efavirenz, rilpivirine, etravirine, and protease inhibitors (PIs); indinavir, ritonavir, nelfinavir, saquinavir,amprenavir, lopinavir plus ritonavir, atazanavir, tipranvir, fosamprenavir, and darunavir), fusion inhibitors (T-20, maraviroc), or integrase inhibitors (raltegravir, dolutegravir, and elvitegravir). Several nucleoside combination pills are available, including Combivir (zidovudine plus lamivudine), Epzicom (lamivudine plus abacavir), Trizivir (zidovudine plus lamivudine plus abacavir), or Truvada (tenofovir plus emtricitabine). A triple nucleoside regimen without a nonnucleoside or PI or integrase inhibitor or entry inhibitor is not appropriate. Combination pills that provide appropriate HAART combinations include Atripla (efavirenz plus tenofovir plus emtricitabine), Complera (rilpivirine plus tenofovir plus emtricitabine), and Stribild (elvitegraivr plus cobicistat plus tenofovir plus emtricitabine).

B. **Benefits of HAART** include a lower incidence of development of HIV-associated malignancies, especially primary CNS lymphoma and Kaposi's sarcoma. Moreover, with HAART the onset of malignancies in individuals is at a higher level of CD4, there is improved tolerance of full-dose chemotherapy, improved response rates and duration of responses, and improved survival during treatment of their malignancy. Pharmacokinetic studies have suggested that metabolism and clearance of several cytotoxic chemotherapeutic agents is not affected by HAART, but caution is still recommended when high doses of chemotherapy are utilized, for example, during stem cell transplantation studies. Several antivirals are inducers and/or inhibitors of cytochrome Cyp3A4, including PIs, elvitegravir (component of Stribild), and, to a lesser extent, nonnucleoside-reverse transcriptase inhibitors. Thus, adverse interactions may occur with targeted chemotherapeutic agents that are also Cyp3A4 inhibitors or inducers (e.g., dasantinib, imatinib, nilotinib, erlotinib, gefitinib, everolimus, sunitinb, sorafenib, and pazopanib).

C. **Specific recommendations for combining HAART with chemotherapy** include avoiding the nucleoside analog zidovudine, in light of excessive neutropenia and anemia. Moreover, the PI atazanavir, which causes hyperbilirubinemia in almost one-third of patients, can also be problematic when anthracyclines or vinca alkaloids are utilized. Some authors have also suggested that HAART regimens, including PIs, may be associated with more myelosuppression when combined with chemotherapy than those lacking PIs, although this remains controversial. Caution is recommended in the use of antiretrovirals associated with neurotoxicity (e.g., didanosine, stavudine, and dideoxycytidine) together with chemotherapy regimens including vinca alkaloids, especially in individuals with pre-existing HIV-associated neuropathy. PIs commonly cause gastrointestinal (GI) toxicities. It should also be recognized that nucleoside inhibitors may cause lactic acidosis, abacavir may cause a multisystem hypersensitivity reaction, emtricitabine occasionally causes hyperpigmentation of the palms and soles, etravirine causes a rash, nevirapine may cause liver toxicity, and efavirenz is frequently associated with central nervous side effects. Atazanavir, ritonavir-boosted lopinavir, and saquinavir are associated with prolongation of the QT interval, as are anthracyclines, arsenic trioxide, dasatinib, lapatinib, nilotinib, sunitinib, and tamoxifen. Therefore, because of the potential for sudden death, these combinations should be avoided. Well-tolerated regimens for a HAART-naïve patient who will receive chemotherapy would be Truvada (300 mg tenofovir plus 200 mg emtricitabine) once daily with Sustiva (600 mg) once daily, or Truvada once daily with raltegravir (400 mg) twice daily. A preferred initial PI-based regimen for a HAART-naive patient is ritonavir (100 mg)-boosted darunvair (800 mg) once daily with Truvada once daily.

D. **Initiation of HAART therapy** should be accompanied by liver function tests; amylase and lipase as baseline values since several antiretrovirals (e.g., didanosine) can cause pancreatitis; an HIV genotype test to identify drug-resistant mutations; fasting glucose and lipid profile since PIs may cause dyslipidemias and glucose intolerance; a serologic tests for syphilis, hepatitis A, B, and C viruses, toxoplasmosis, cytomegalovirus (CMV) assays; glucose-6-phosphate dehydrogenase testing in case dapsone will be needed; cervical Papanicolaou smear, opthalmalogy examination, and anal and cervical screening for HPV if available; and tuberculin skin test, chest radiography, and an electrocardiogram since HIV may be associated with cardiomyopathy. Vaccinations for influenza, hepatitis A and B viruses, and *Streptococcus pneumonia* should also be considered.

E. **Optimal care** of the HIV-infected patient should be done in collaboration with an infectious disease specialist. During active treatment, repeat HIV RNA levels should be assessed, and after completion of therapy, both HIV RNA and CD4 counts should be obtained.

IV. **PROPHYLAXIS FOR OPPORTUNISTIC INFECTIONS (OIs)** is also indicated in individuals with depressed CD4 count. Since chemotherapy can also transiently affect the CD4 count, it has been suggested that OI prophylaxis recommendations be expanded in individuals receiving chemotherapy. Thus, if it is anticipated that the CD4 count will decline below 200/mm,[3] prophylaxis for Pneumocystis jiroveci pneumonia (PCP) is recommended with bactrim thrice weekly, or in allergic patients, dapsone or atovaquone. If the CD4 count is anticipated to decline below 50/mm^3, prophylaxis for *Mycobacterium avium* intracellulare (MAI) is also indicated with weekly azithromycin. In individuals with prior OI, who have a CD4 count above these cut-off values and have discontinued prophylactic antibiotics, resumption of prophylactic antibiotics concurrent with chemotherapy may be indicated. Special attention is also recommended in evaluating possible clinical signs of OI in the HIV-positive patient receiving chemotherapy as follows: (1) any CD4 count: oral and esophageal Candidiasis, Mycobacteria including tuberculosis, bacterial pneumonias, histoplasmosis, or coccidiomycosis, (2) CD4 <100: MAI, Toxoplasma, encephalitis, and (3) CD4 <50: CMV retinitis, pneumonitis, or colitis, or progressive multifocal leukoencephalopathy.

V. **EVALUATION OF ANEMIA IN AN HIV-POSITIVE PATIENT WITH A MALIGNANCY** should consider causes other than chemotherapy or antiretrovirals, and should also include other causes of decreased erythropoiesis including (1) drugs (e.g., trimethoprim-sulfamethoxazole, ganciclovir, and dapsone), (2) nutritional deficiency of iron, folate, or vitamin B12, (3) effects of uncontrolled HIV on bone marrow stromal cells, (4) OIs (e.g., parvovirus, atypical or typical mycobacteria, or histoplasmosis, and (5) preexisting conditions (e.g., sickle cell disease or thalassemia). Alternatively, causes of erythrocyte loss should also be considered, including (1) hemolysis due to thrombotic thrombocytopenic purpura, glucose-6-phosphate dehydrogenase deficiency, autoimmune hemolytic anemia, or drug-induced hemolysis, (2) GI bleeding that may complicate lymphoma, Kaposi sarcoma (KS), or enteric infections due to CMV, Candida, or parasites, or (3) hypersplenism associated with infection, lymphoma, or cirrhosis that may complicate hepatitis B or C virus infections.

VI. **EVALUATION OF NEUTROPENIA IN AN HIV-POSITIVE PATIENT WITH A MALIGNANCY** should consider causes other than chemotherapy or antiretrovirals. These include causes of decreased myelopoiesis from drugs (e.g., ganciclovir, trimethoprim-sulfamethoxazole, pentamidine, rifabutin, and dapsone), nutritional deficiencies (e.g., folate or vitamin B12 deficiency), infections (e.g., uncontrolled HIV, atypical or typical mycobacteria, histoplasma), or bone marrow involvement by the malignancy (e.g., lymphoma, multiple myeloma). Increased loss of neutrophils may occur with autoimmune neutropenia or hypersplenism. Granulocyte colony stimulating factor (G-CSF) has been shown to be safe and effective in HIV-infected patients, although there is controversy about the use of granulocyte–macrophage colony stimulating factor (GM-CSF), which can potentiate HIV replication in macrophages.

VII. **EVALUATION OF THROMBOCYTOPENIA IN AN HIV-POSITIVE PATIENT WITH A MALIGNANCY** should consider causes other than chemotherapy or antiretrovirals. Causes of decreased thrombopoiesis include (1) drugs (e.g., trimethoprim-sulfamethoxazole, pyrimethamine, ganciclovir, fluconazole, and clarithromycin), (2) nutritional deficiency (e.g., folate or vitamin B12), (3) infection (e.g., uncontrolled HIV, mycobacteria, histoplasma, or Bartonella henselae), or (4) bone marrow involvement by lymphoma. Causes of decreased platelet survival include (1) immune thrombocytopenic purpura from HIV infection or autoimmune conditions, (2) thrombotic thrombocytopenic purpura, or (3) hypersplenism.

ACQUIRED IMMUNODEFICIENCY SYNDROME-ASSOCIATED DIFFUSE LARGE B-CELL LYMPHOMAS (DLBCL)

I. **CLINICAL PRESENTATION**

A. **Non-Hodgkin's lymphomas (NHL)** are 100- to 200-fold more frequent in HIV-positive individuals than the general population, and occur in 5% to 10% of HIV-infected individuals. HIV-DLBCL accounts for about 5% of all DLBCL cases in the United States. AIDS-associated lymphomas are generally aggressive B-cell malignancies that present at an advanced stage with extranodal involvement in more than two-thirds of individuals.

B. **Pertinent history** should include performance status, duration of HIV infection, treatment of OIs, and current antiretroviral regimen.

C. **B symptoms,** such as fever, night sweats, and weight loss in excess of 10% of the normal body weight, are very common, but should be attributed to AIDS-associated lymphoma only after the exclusion of OIs. Extreme fatigue from anemia caused by bone marrow involvement may be seen.

D. **Lymph node enlargement** may be asymptomatic or associated with pain or obstructive symptoms. This should be differentiated from persistent generalized lymphadenopathy (PGL) due to HIV replication or other AIDS-related OIs. Splenomegaly is commonly present, and may be related to the cause of lymphadenopathy.

E. **GI involvement** causing anorexia, nausea, vomiting, hemorrhage, change in bowel habits, or obstruction occurs in 10% to 25% of patients. Jaundice and abdominal discomfort may be due to lymphomatous hepatic or pancreatic involvement.

F. **CNS or meningeal involvement** resulting in seizures, altered mental status, and neurological defects occurs in 10% to 30% of patients. Other causes of neurological defects in this patient population should also be considered, such as HIV-associated encephalopathy.

G. **Pleural or pericardial effusions** may cause dyspnea and chest discomfort.

H. **The physical examination** should include careful examination and measurements of enlarged lymph nodes, spleen, and liver. Pulmonary and cardiac examinations may reveal pleural or pericardial effusions. A thorough neurological examination should be done to determine the presence of meningismus or focal neurological defects.

II. DIAGNOSTIC WORKUP AND STAGING

A. **Pathology.** Definitive diagnosis of AIDS-associated NHL is made with the identification of lymphoma in lymph node biopsies or other tissues (bone marrow, cerebrospinal fluid (CSF), pleural fluid, and liver), in an HIV-infected individual. DLBCL is characterized by large noncleaved cells that usually express cell surface pan-B-cell marker, CD20, and lymphocyte common antigen, CD45, but not CD3. The transcription factor Bcl-6 is expressed in the centroblastic subtype but not the immunoblastic subtype. In contrast, the immunoblastic subtype is typically characterized by CD138 expression as well as EBV latent membrane protein-1 (LMP-1). Centroblastic DLBCL is thought to arise in the germinal center (GC), whereas immunoblastic DLBCL is a post-GC lymphoma. GC B-cell-like type DLBCL is considered when CD10 is expressed in >30% of the malignant tumor cells, or if cells are CD10−, BCL6+, and IRF4/MUM1−. All others are considered to be activated B-cell-like type or non-GC types. Cytogenetics or FISH should be performed for MYC translocations, since these variants have a poor outcome with CHOP therapy.

B. **Laboratory tests.** Complete blood counts may reveal anemia, leukopenia, or thrombocytopenia, even if there is no marrow involvement. Serum chemistries may show abnormalities in liver function tests, elevated lactate dehydrogenase (LDH), calcium, or uric acid. Electrolytes and creatinine should also be monitored during therapy.

C. **Radiology/procedures**

1. **Computed tomography (CT) scan** of the chest, abdomen, and pelvis with a CT or an MRI scan of the brain is necessary for the staging of AIDS-related NHL. Special attention should be given to mesenteric adenopathy, a site not usually affected in PGL.

2. **PET** scans are helpful in distinguishing adenopathy due to lymphoma that generally shows significant uptake of fluorodeoxyglucose (FDG) from that associated with PGL or OIs, which show less intense FDG uptake. Alternatively, gallium scanning may be useful for this purpose. PET or gallium scans are useful to detect residual disease after therapy, and to distinguish fibrosis from refractory tumor.

3. **Bone marrow aspiration and biopsies** reveal bone marrow involvement in approximately 20% of patients, and may be associated with increased risk of CSF involvement.

4. **Lumbar puncture** should be performed and CSF sent for cytological examination. Cell count and protein may be normal or elevated, whereas glucose may be low. Analysis of CSF by flow cytometry or for EBV DNA by polymerase chain reaction (PCR) may predict lymphomatous meningitis.

D. **The Ann Arbor staging** for NHL also is used for AIDS-related NHL. Prognostic factors correlating with poor survival in patients with AIDS-related NHL include stage IV disease, Karnofsky performance status less than 70%, CD4 count less than 100/mm^3, elevated LDH, and history of OIs before lymphoma diagnosis.

III. THERAPY

A. **m-BACOD** (methotrexate, bleomycin, doxorubicin, vincristne, and dexamethasone) was used in AIDS-DLBCL patients in the pre-HAART era. Given in a low-dose regimen, this resulted in 41% complete remissions and median survival of 35 weeks, whereas standard dose m-BACOD with GM-CSF resulted in 52% complete remissions with a median survival of 31 weeks and more grade 3 toxicity (70% vs. 51%). Since the demonstration in the HIV-negative population that m-BACOD was similar in efficacy to CHOP, the m-BACOD regimen has not been routinely utilized in AIDS-DLBCL.

B. **CHOP** (cyclophosphamide, doxorubicin, vincristine, prednisone) given at the same doses as in the HIV-negative patient population together with HAART and G-CSF is feasible and effective (*J Clin Oncol* 2001;19:2171). In a nonrandomized study, this therapy resulted in a complete response (CR) rate of 30% when given in low doses, and 48% when full doses were provided. The chemotherapy had no adverse effect on HAART activity. Moreover, HAART with a PI, indinavir, had no effect on doxorubicin clearance and only a 1.5-fold reduction in cyclophosphamide clearance, which did not translate into excessive neutropenia.

C. **R-CHOP** was not significantly more effective than CHOP in AIDS-NHL (CR rates of 58% and 47%, respectively) in one study, but was significantly more toxic (14% and 2% serious treatment-related toxicities). The increase in mortality with R-CHOP compared with CHOP, in this randomized study, was primarily due to infectious deaths, particularly in individuals with CD4 lymphocyte counts <50/mm³. However, subsequent trials using prophylactic quinolone antibiotics for individuals with <100 CD4 cells/mm³ obviated this complication. Moreover, a meta-analysis of trials using various different forms of chemotherapy with or without rituximab found a reduced risk of lymphoma recurrence and death from any cause with the addition of rituximab to combination chemotherapy (*Blood* 2013;122:3251).

D. **CDOP** (cyclophosphamide, liposomal doxorubicin, vincristine, and prednisone) in combination with rituximab resulted in a 47% CR rate in a study of 40 patients.

E. **The infusional dose-adjusted (DA) EPOCH regimen** (etoposide, prednisone, vincristine, cyclophosphamide, and doxorubicin) with growth factor support resulted in complete remission in 74% of 39 patients, with 60% disease-free survival at 53 months. In this trial, antiretrovirals were withheld during chemotherapy, and after reinstitution of HAART, CD4 cells recovered by 12 months and viral load decreased below baseline by 3 months. Important features of this regimen are that it utilizes 5 days of oral prednisone (60 mg/m²/day), a 4-day infusion of etoposide (50 mg/m²/day), vincristine (0.4 mg/m²/day up to 2 mg total), and doxorubicin (10 mg/m²/day), and day 5 cyclophosphamide, followed by G-CSF or Neulasta. Cycle 1 cyclophosphamide dose is 375 mg/m² for patients with CD4 <100 and 750 mg/m² for patients with CD4 ≥100. In subsequent cycles, the cyclophosphamide dose is increased by 187 mg/m² each cycle up to a maximum of 750 mg/m² if grade 3 or 4 neutropenia or thrombocytopenia has not occurred, and decreased by 187 mg/m² each cycle if one of these complications has occurred. Thus, monitoring of the CBC at days 8, 10, and 12 of each cycle is necessary for guiding subsequent therapy. Concurrent use of rituximab plus EPOCH resulted in a 73% CR in one study, and 5-year progression-free (PFS) and overall survivals (OS) of 84% and 68%, respectively, in another study.

F. **Short-course EPOCH-RR regimen** includes rituximab given on days 1 and 5 of each cycle. To determine the number of cycles of therapy, all patients undergo restaging with CT and FDG-PET after the second treatment cycle, and each cycle until achieving CR or no further tumor shrinkage. The criteria for stopping therapy after a minimum of 3 cycles of therapy is that there is less than 25% reduction in bidimensional tumor products compared with the previous interim CT scan and the standardized uptake values on FDG-PET have decreased at least 50% compared with the pretreatment FDG-PET. With 5 years of follow-up, PFS and OS were 84% and 68%, respectively, and 79% of patients only required 3 treatment cycles.

G. **CDE** (cyclophosphamide, doxorubicin, and etoposide) is an alternative infusional regimen that has resulted in CR rates of 46% to 86%, but grade 3 or 4 neutropenia and thrombocytopenia in 75% and 55% of participants, respectively.

H. **ACVBP** (doxorubicin, cyclophosphamide, vindesine, bleomycin, and prednisolone) is an alternative intensive regimen used primarily in Europe. In one study, the 5-year OS was 51% for good-risk patients.

I. Indications for **CNS prophylaxis** in AIDS-DLBCL are not well defined. Bone marrow involvement has been suggested as increasing the likelihood of CNS relapse, as well as paraspinal, paranasal, epidural, testicular, or widespread systemic involvement. When CNS prophylaxis is provided, the usual recommendation is 4 weekly treatments of either intrathecal cytarabine (50 mg) or methotrexate (12 mg).

J. **Lymphomatous meningitis** should be treated with intrathecal cytarabine or methotrexate 2 to 3 times weekly via Omaya reservoir until the CSF is clear of malignant cells, then weekly for 4 weeks, and then monthly. The duration of therapy remains poorly defined, but is often given for 6 to 12 months. Alternatively, liposomal cytarabine (Depocyt) can be given with a 5-day course of decadron 4 mg bid with each treatment, on weeks 1 and 3 for induction, on weeks 5, 7, 9, and 13 for consolidation, and weeks 17, 21, 25, and

29 for maintenance. In patients failing to respond to intraventricular chemotherapy, CSF flow studies can be performed after instilling radioisotope to identify possible blockade.

K. **Radiotherapy** may be given as palliation to bulky, rapidly enlarging, organ compressing, or CNS lesions or as consolidation to patients with localized lymphoma after chemotherapy.

L. **Duration of first-line therapy** for AIDS-DLBCL should be 3 to 8 cycles, unless there is severe toxicity or lymphoma progression. This should include 1 to 2 cycles after obtaining a CR. For patients with stage I disease and good prognostic characteristics, 3 cycles of therapy followed by involved field radiation is appropriate therapy.

M. **Salvage chemotherapy** regimens for AIDS-associated lymphomas are not highly effective (response rates of 10% to 25%) with most patients relapsing within months, as in the HIV-negative population. This includes the use of rituximab with etoposide and high-dose cytosine arabinoside and cisplatin (ESHAP), mitoguazone, or a combination of etoposide, mitoxantrone, and prednimustine. The use of rituximab with ifosfamide, carboplatin, and etoposide (R-ICE) is a reasonable choice for a salvage regimen, but trials in AIDS patients have not yet been reported. There is little reported experience with dexamethasone, cisplatin, cytarabine (DHAP), mesna, ifosfamide, mitoxantrone, etoposide (MINE), or carmustine, etoposide, cytarabine, melphalan (miniBEAM) regimens in this patient population.

N. **Autologous stem cell transplantation** has also been utilized for refractory or relapsed AIDS-associated lymphomas, particularly in the HAART era. In individuals with a good performance status, lacking severe immune compromise, stem cell collections were successful in 80% to 100% of cases, and graft failure was rare. Long-term survivors have been reported from such studies, but the number of patients in each series remains low. In one study of 68 patients from 20 institutions, including 16 patients in first CR and 44 patients in CR more than 1, partial remission, or chemotherapy-sensitive relapse, and 8 patients with chemotherapy-resistant disease, nonrelapse mortality was 30% at 24 months. Only anecdotal reports have appeared thus far for the use of allogeneic transplants in HIV-infected individuals.

IV. COMPLICATIONS

A. **Complications of disease.** Rapidly enlarging tumors may compromise airways and other vital organs. Significant hepatic dysfunction, hypercalcemia, and CNS relapse may occur. OIs and other AIDS-related illnesses are causes for morbidity and mortality in patients with AIDS-NHL; thus, PCP and mycobacterial prophyalxis should be continued during active lymphoma therapy, if indicated.

B. **Complications of therapy**
   1. **Lymphocytotoxic chemotherapy** may cause depletion of CD4 and total lymphocyte counts, increasing the risk of severe myelosuppression and infections. Potential interactions with chemotherapy and HAART may produce substantial and unexpected toxicity that may require dose delay or reduction, possibly compromising optimal antilymphoma therapy.
   2. **Intrathecal chemotherapy** may cause chemical arachnoiditis that is relatively acute, subacute neurological deficits occurring within days to weeks, or chronic encephalopathy occurring over weeks to months.
   3. **Cardiomyopathy** may occur after the use of doxorubicin, particularly in individuals receiving cumulative doses of more than 550 mg/m^2, but may occur at lower cumulative doses in individuals who received chest radiotherapy, or have other cardiac disorders, such as HIV-associated cardiomyopathy.
   4. **Virus reactivation** is a potential complication of rituximab-based therapies, particularly HBV, HCV, and JCV. Monitoring HBV and HCV levels during therapy is indicated in individuals with chronic persistent infections. Antiviral therapy is recommended for high-risk HBV-positive patients.

V. FOLLOW-UP.
During treatment, intervening history, physical examination, CBC, chemistries, and LDH should be obtained prior to the initiation of each cycle of therapy, and as clinically indicated. With DA-EPOCH-R, more frequent measurements of CBC are required to guide the dose level for the subsequent cycle. After completion of therapy, for patients in complete

remission, follow-up visits and laboratory studies are required every 1 to 3 months for 1 year, every 2 to 4 months during the second year, and then every 3 to 6 months. CT scans are usually performed every 3 to 6 months for 2 years. It is important to remember that these patients are at risk for relapse of their AIDS-NHL or development of a second AIDS-NHL.

VI. BACKGROUND

A. **EBV infection** occurs in nearly 50% of AIDS-associated DLBCL. In these cases, latency type 3 antigens are expressed, including EBV nuclear antigens 1 and 2 (EBNA-1 and 2), latent proteins (LP) 3A and 3C, as well as latent membrane protein-1 (LMP-1). Immunohistochemical stains for LMP-1 or in situ hybridization for EBV-associated RNAs (EBERs) are often used to identify EBV in pathological samples.

B. **Chronic antigen induction** of polyclonal B-cell expansion and cytokine deregulation (especially interleukins 6 and 10) during HIV infection may also contribute to transformation.

VII. CURRENT FOCUS OF RESEARCH.

Current studies of AIDS-DLBCL are evaluating (1) the combination of vorinostat with DA-EPOCH-R chemotherapy for first-line therapy, (2) the safety and efficacy of antiviral and antitumor activity of bortezomib combined with R-ICE in subjects with relapsed or refractory disease, and (3) the safety and activity of DA-EPOCH therapy with or without rituximab in c-Myc positive diffuse large B-cell lymphoma. Future trials will (1) compare CHOP with oral chemotherapy with concomitant antiretroviral therapy in patients with HIV-associated lymphoma in sub-Saharan Africa, and (2) evaluate ibrutinib in patients with relapsed or refractory B-cell NHL or in first-line therapy in combination with chemotherapy. There is also considerable interest in examining the effects of allogenic stem cell transplantation with or without CCR5-depleted cells on HIV reservoirs.

ACQUIRED IMMUNODEFICIENCY SYNDROME-ASSOCIATED BURKITT-LIKE LYMPHOMAS

I. **CLINICAL PRESENTATION.** Burkitt-like lymphoma (BL) accounts for 15% to 40% of AIDS-NHL cases. AIDS-BL accounts for about 20% of all BL cases in the United States. The clinical presentations of AIDS-BL patients are similar to those of HIV-negative patients in terms of histology, disease stage, and proportion with bone marrow and CNS involvement.

II. **DIAGNOSTIC WORKUP AND STAGING.** The pathology of AIDS-BL is characterized by a population of small noncleaved lymphocytes, typically exhibiting a "starry-sky" appearance and a cohesive growth pattern, but atypical variants are noted with medium-sized cells with plasmacytoid differentiation or with nuclear pleomorphism. The tumor cells are generally CD10+ and CD20+ and usually express proliferation antigen Ki67 on almost 100% of malignant cells, transcription factor Bcl-6, and, uncommonly, antiapoptosis protein Bcl-2. These tumors are classified as high-grade lymphomas. Molecular diagnostic or cytogenetic studies can be used to confirm the presence of the 8;14 translocation or the variant location 2;8 or 8;22, all of which involve a translocation of myc with an immunoglobulin locus.

III. **THERAPY**

A. **CHOP** therapy was used for AIDS-associated BL, prior to the development of HAART, and responses were similar to those of AIDS-associated DLBCL. However, with HAART therapy, AIDS-BL may have a worse prognosis than AIDS-DLBCL when treated in the same fashion, suggesting a need for more aggressive therapy in this setting.

B. **R-hyper-CVAD** is a regimen of hyperfractionated cyclophosphamide, vincristine, doxorubicin, dexamethasone, and rituximab given in alternating cycles with high doses of both cytosine arabinoside and methotrexate, followed by leucovorin for a total of 8 cycles. Antibiotic prophylaxis is provided with a quinolone, fluconazole, and valganciclovir, together with standard prophylactic regimens for PCP, MAI, and CMV, where indicated. In a single-center study, 9 of 11 patients achieved CRe, and 1 patient PR. Grade 3 or 4 myelosuppression occurred in all patients, and fever or infection during 35% of chemotherapy cycles. Six of seven patients given HAART concurrently with chemotherapy remained in CR for a median of 29 months.

C. **R-CODOX-M/IVAC** (cyclophosphamide, doxorubicin, high-dose methotrexate/ifosfamide, etoposide, and high-dose cytarabine) was used for the treatment of 14 HIV-positive patients, of whom 63% had CRs, with a 2-year disease-free survival of 60%.

Grade 3 or 4 toxicities included anemia (100%), neutropenia (88%), thrombocytopenia (75%), mucositis (75%), neutropenic fever (63%), sepsis (38%), neuropathy (38%), and nephrotoxicity (24%). In a study of 34 AIDS-BL patients with R-CODOX-M/IVAC, 1-year overall survival was 83%.

D. DA-EPOCH-R was utilized in 30 subjects with BL, including 13 individuals with AIDS-BL who received 3 to 6 cycles of therapy, including 1 cycle after obtaining complete remission, resulting in PFS and OS in 12 of these 13 subjects at a median of 36 months of follow-up (*New Engl J Med* 2013;369:1915). This regimen is generally better tolerated than R-Hyper-CVAD or R-CODOX-M/IVAC.

E. Prophylactic intrathecal chemotherapy with methotrexate or cytosine arabinoside should be given to all AIDS-BL patients, generally 4 to 6 weekly doses of therapy in patients who do not have positive CSF cytology.

IV. COMPLICATIONS. The risks of myelosuppression, tumor lysis syndrome, and neurotoxicity are higher for AIDS-BL patients given more intensive therapies, such as R-Hyper-CVAD or R-CODOX-M/IVAC, than for AIDS-DLBCL patients given R-CHOP.

V. FOLLOW-UP is as described for AIDS-DLBCL patients.

VI. BACKGROUND. AIDS-BL is associated with EBV infection in 80% of cases. However, the pattern of latency differs from that of AIDS-DLBCL, with expression of EBNA-1 but not LMP1 or EBNA2. As in BL not associated with HIV, translocations between immunoglobulin genes and myc are uniformly present. Mutational inactivation of tumor suppressor protein p53 is also prevalent.

VII. CURRENT FOCUS OF RESEARCH. A confirmatory study of the results with DA-EPOCH-R for AIDS-BL is planned.

ACQUIRED IMMUNODEFICIENCY SYNDROME-ASSOCIATED PRIMARY CENTRAL NERVOUS SYSTEM LYMPHOMAS

I. CLINICAL PRESENTATION. Primary central nervous system lymphoma (PCNSL) usually presents in severely immunocompromised individuals with CD4 counts less than $50/mm^3$. AIDS-PCNSL accounts for about 13% of all PCNSL cases in the United States. Thus, with widespread use of HAART, the incidence of AIDS-associated PCNSL has declined significantly. Typical presentations are with confusion, memory loss, lethargy, or focal neurological signs. Patients may also present with seizures, headaches, memory loss, or dementia.

II. DIAGNOSTIC WORKUP AND STAGING

A. Differential diagnosis includes systemic lymphomas with CNS involvement, toxoplasmosis, HIV encephalopathy, progressive multifocal leukoencephalopathy, and other infections associated with viral, fungal, or mycobacterial infections. Some investigators have suggested that in patients with serological evidence of prior toxoplasma exposure, a 14-day course of antitoxoplasmosis therapy may be indicated to assess response. However, given the other diagnostic modalities available, this approach is rarely utilized now, and the delay in therapy resulting from this approach is potentially risky.

B. Diagnostic workup should include chest, abdomen, and pelvis CT scans in order to exclude systemic lymphoma. Body PET scans may be indicated as well in selected cases. If these scans are negative, it is unclear whether or not bone marrow biopsy is needed, since the yield of positive results in this setting may be very low. Patients should undergo slit-lamp ophthalmologic exam to exclude concurrent intraocular lymphoma.

C. Brain MRI or CT scan typically shows multifocal disease. However, lesions are typically larger and fewer than those associated with *Toxoplasma* encephalitis. Lesions may be ring enhancing and are often associated with edema and shift of normal brain structures, and may be found at any location in the brain.

D. Brain PET or single-photon emission computer tomography (SPECT) is helpful in distinguishing PCNSL from other HIV-associated brain lesions, such as toxoplasmosis, which exhibit less uptake of FDG.

E. Brain biopsy is the gold standard for diagnosis, but tumor location and other factors may preclude this procedure. CT-guided stereotactic brain biopsies can produce diagnostic rates with acceptable morbidity, comparable to that of open brain biopsy.

F. CSF EBV PCR is a sensitive (80%) and specific (99%) test for AIDS-associated PCNSL, since EBV infection is uniformly associated with this condition. For patients with positive CSF EBV PCR and PET or SPECT scans showing intense uptake in the brain lesion, biopsy may be obviated. **Pathology** is typically a diffuse large B-cell lymphoma, usually of the immunoblastic subtype, with angiocentric distribution.

III. THERAPY for PCNSL should also include HAART, which significantly improves survival.

A. Whole brain radiotherapy alone was used in the pre-HAART era, since the median survival of patients presenting with PCNSL was only 1 to 3 months as a result of OIs. Typically, 4,000 cGy is used in fractions of 267 cGy each. Cranial irradiation alone results in a 53% rate of tumor regression and slightly improved survival compared with untreated individuals. Because of the multifocal nature of AIDS-PCNSL, radiation should be directed to the whole brain and meningeal fields to the level of the second cervical vertebra without spinal irradiation. In patients with poor performance status, who are severely immune compromised, and/or patients with multidrug-resistant HIV infection, this may be the most appropriate therapy. Autopsy studies showed that patients who did not receive radiotherapy died of lymphoma progression, whereas those that did receive radiotherapy died of OIs.

B. High-dose methotrexate (2.5 to 3.5 g/m^2 every 14 days) with leucovorin rescue was reported to produce a CR of 50%, a median OS of 10 months, and improved quality of life. For patients with a good performance status, who are not severely immunocompromised and are responding to HAART therapy, a chemotherapy regimen including high-dose methotrexate may be appropriate, followed by cranial irradiation, as in the HIV-negative PCSNL population. However, recent studies have questioned the need for cranial irradiation in those individuals who achieve complete remission with chemotherapy. High-dose methotrexate therapy requires careful monitoring of methotrexate levels and adjustment of leucovorin doses if delayed methotrexate clearance is found. Methotrexate should not be used in individuals with a third space fluid collection.

C. High-dose cytosine arabinoside added to high-dose methotrexate has been reported in a small randomized phase 2 trial to improve response rates in HIV-negative PCNSL, although there were higher rates of myelosuppression and neutropenic infections.

D. Steroids are used to limit edema, but the impact on survival is unclear.

E. Rituximab has been reported to play a role in CNS lymphomas not associated with AIDS, when given systemically, but there are only anecdotal reports of its use for AIDS-PCNSL. Intrathecal rituximab remains investigational.

F. Other agents (e.g., temozolomide, topotecan, procarbazine, vincristine, and ifosfamide) and stem cell transplantation remain to be evaluated in AIDS-associated PCNSL.

IV. COMPLICATIONS

A. Complications of PCNSL include ocular lymphoma that may involve the vitreous, uvea, or retina, and is usually bilateral. Bilateral ocular irradiation, or high-dose cytarabine or methotrexate, which penetrate the vitreous, may be given. Leptomeningeal lymphoma can be treated with intrathecal methotrexate or cytarabine via Ommaya reservoir.

B. Complications of therapy of AIDS-associated PCNSL are coincident OIs and neurological toxicity from whole brain radiotherapy.

V. FOLLOW-UP should be performed monthly in the first year after completion of therapy, with MRI brain scans performed every 3 months and less often thereafter.

VI. BACKGROUND. AIDS-PCNSL occurs in 2% to 11% of HIV-infected patients, representing a 3,600-fold higher incidence of this disease, compared with that of the general population. Latent EBV-infected cells develop into malignant clones in the relatively immunoprivileged CNS, secondary to decreased immunosurveillance resulting from HIV-related T-cell depletion.

ACQUIRED IMMUNODEFICIENCY SYNDROME-ASSOCIATED PRIMARY EFFUSION LYMPHOMAS

I. CLINICAL PRESENTATION

A. Primary effusion lymphomas (PELs) account for 1% to 5% of HIV-NHL. PEL presents 200-fold less commonly in HIV-negative patients, including elderly individuals or organ transplant recipients. In the HIV-positive patients, these lymphomas are uniformly associated with HHV8.

B. **Classical presentations** of PEL are ascites, pleural effusion, or pericardial effusions without infiltrative growth patterns or tumor masses. Some cases of PEL extend into tissues underlying serous cavities, including the nodes, omentum, mediastinum, and lung. Other cases of HHV8-positive solid lymphomas are extracavitary variants of PEL.

C. **PEL occurs primarily in homosexual men** and late stages of HIV infection (mean CD4 count 98/mm³). In one study, 64% of patients had previous manifestations of AIDS. PEL commonly occurs in patients with previous manifestations of HHV-8 infection, such as Kaposi's sarcoma or Castleman's disease.

II. DIAGNOSTIC WORKUP AND STAGING

A. **Diagnostic thoracentesis, pericardiocentesis, or paracentesis** is usually required to diagnose patient with PEL.

B. **PEL is classified as a stage IV NHL.**

C. **Pathology** of PEL usually demonstrates plasma cell differentiation as shown by expression of CD138 or syndecan-1. The cells typically express leukocyte common antigen, CD45, EMA, and activation antigens, HLA-DR, CD23, CD25, CD30, CD38, CD70, and CD77. However, they are usually negative for T- and B-cell markers, including CD20, although clonal immunoglobulin gene rearrangements are present. Although the large, pleomorphic malignant cells may resemble Reed–Sternberg (RS) cells, they are CD15 negative.

III. THERAPY

A. **CHOP** therapy was generally ineffective in the pre-HAART era (*Nador Blood* 1996;88:645). However, now that HAART is available, the CHOP regimen is an appropriate choice of therapy for these patients, if they have adequate performance and immune status. Rituximab is not recommended for use in these lymphomas, which are typically CD20 negative. There are also anecdotal reports of use of other combination chemotherapy regimens for PEL, as described for DLBCL. Other regimens, such as DA-EPOCH, may be effective for PEL.

B. **HAART alone** has been reported to be effective for AIDS-PEL, according to anecdotal reports.

C. **Major prognostic** factors for response are good performance status and preexisting use of HAART therapy. In a study using a variety of treatment regimens, of which CHOP was the most common, OS was greater than 3 years in 32% of patients.

IV. BACKGROUND. AIDS-associated PELs are uniformly associated with HHV8 infection and frequent coinfection with EBV. It is unclear why PEL arises in body cavities, but there is evidence that viral Bcl-2 is activated by hypoxia, which may contribute to lymphoma development.

ACQUIRED IMMUNODEFICIENCY SYNDROME-ASSOCIATED HODGKIN'S LYMPHOMAS

I. CLINICAL PRESENTATION. HL is 10- to 25-fold increased in incidence in the HIV-positive population compared with the HIV-negative population.

A. **At diagnosis,** 74% to 92% of HIV-HL patients present with advanced disease, with frequent extranodal involvement, including the bone marrow, liver, and spleen, but mediastinal involvement is uncommon. Moreover, 70% to 96% of patients have B symptoms. Bone marrow involvement is present in 40% to 50% of patients, and is the first indicator of disease in 20% of cases. In contrast to the HIV-negative population, noncontiguous nodal spread of lymphoma is common, for example, liver without splenic involvement or lung without mediastinal node involvement.

B. **Median CD4** count at presentation is in the range of 275 to 300/mm³.

II. DIAGNOSTIC WORKUP AND STAGING

A. **Lymph node enlargement** may be due to HIV or HL, and PET scans may be helpful in distinguishing the etiology. Other coincident causes of lymph node enlargement should also be excluded, such as mycobacterial or cytomegalovirus infection or NHL.

B. **Pathology** shows the mixed cellularity subtype as the most common variant in HIV-infected individuals, as well as an increased frequency of the lymphocyte-depleted subtype compared with HIV-negative HL. LMP-1 is expressed in almost all cases in the RS cells. RS cells are typically CD15+CD30+CD45−.

C. **Staging evaluation** is as described by AIDS-DLBCL except that brain MRI/CT scans and lumbar puncture may be omitted unless there are neurological symptoms. Pulmonary function tests should be performed prior to the use of bleomycin.

III. THERAPY

A. **Full-dose chemotherapy regimens** are recommended, combined with HAART and G-CSF. However, it should be recognized that G-CSFs increase the likelihood of bleomycin pulmonary toxicity, and thus the fewest possible doses of CSFs should be utilized.

B. **ABVD** (doxorubicin, bleomycin, vinblastine, and dacarbazine) given with G-CSF support is the most commonly used regimen, given at the same doses as in the HIV-negative population. In the pre-HAART era, this regimen resulted in a CR of 42%. In the post-HAART era, CR rates of 87% and 91% have been reported in separate studies. Recent studies show that HIV infection does not adversely affect the overall survival or event-free survival for individuals with HL treated with ABVD (*J Clin Oncol* 2012;30:4056).

C. **EBVP** (epirubicin, bleomycin, vinblastine, and prednisone) resulted in a CR rate of 74%, with grade 3 or 4 leukopenia in 32% of patients.

D. **The Stanford V regimen** (doxorubicin, vinblastine, mechlorethamine, etoposide, vincristine, bleomycin, and prednisone) resulted in a complete remission rate of 81%, 3-year overall survival of 51%, and disease-free survival of 68%. This regimen maintains or increases the dose intensity of individual drugs, but reduces the cumulative doses of bleomycin and doxorubicin compared with ABVD, and may reduce the incidence of pulmonary or cardiac dysfunction.

E. The **BEACOPP** regimen (cyclophosphamide, doxorubicin, etoposide, procarbazine, prednisone, bleomycin, and vincristine) resulted in CR in all 12 treated patients and 83% 2-year survival, but grade 3 or 4 leukopenia in 75% of cases.

F. **Risk-adapted therapy** was utilized in a study of HIV-associated HL. Subjects with early-stage favorable disease received 2 to 4 cycles of ABVD plus involved field radiation, whereas patients with early-stage unfavorable disease received 4 cycles of BEACOPP or a combination of 4 cycles of ABVD, followed by involved radiotherapy if disease was >5 cm or residual disease >2 cm. Patients with advanced disease received 8 cycles of BEACOPP. CRs occurred in 96% of subjects, and 2-year progression-free survival was 92%, and 2-year OS was 91%.

G. **Salvage** therapy studies have not been reported in AIDS patients. However, patients relapsing more than 12 months after obtaining an initial complete remission may be candidates for treatment with one of the first-line regimens described earlier. Patients relapsing in a shorter period of time may be candidates for similar salvage approaches as described for AIDS-DLBCL patients. The role of brentuximab in salvage therapy remains to be defined in HIV-associated HL.

IV. COMPLICATIONS of the disease or treatment are as described for AIDS-DLBCL with the addition of possible pulmonary fibrosis resulting from use of bleomycin. This complication, characterized by acute pneumonitis with fever, congestion, cough, and dyspnea, occurs most commonly after doses of more than 200 to 400 U/m^2, but may occur at lower doses when chest radiotherapy is also utilized.

V. FOLLOW-UP should be as described for AIDS-associated diffuse large B-cell lymphomas.

VI. BACKGROUND. EBV has been identified in 80% to 100% of HIV-HL cases compared with about 50% in the HIV-negative population. The RS cells of HL from HIV-negative patients are generally derived from GC B cells, whereas those of HIV-HL patients are derived from post-GC B cells.

VII. CURRENT FOCUS OF RESEARCH. Current research is focusing on the possible substitution of brentuximab for bleomycin in the ABVD regimen, given the excellent response rate of

brentuximab in relapsed HIV-negative HL, but significant pulmonary toxicity when bleomycin and brentuximab are used concurrently. Other research is examining the use of stem cell transplantation, either autologous or allogeneic, in the treatment of HIV-HL, as well as therapeutic strategies targeting EBV infection.

ACQUIRED IMMUNODEFICIENCY SYNDROME-ASSOCIATED ANAL CARCINOMAS

I. CLINICAL PRESENTATION

A. HIV-infected individuals have a 30- to 120-fold higher rate of anal carcinoma than HIV-negative individuals. These squamous cell carcinomas result from high-risk HPV infections. These malignancies are not clearly associated with immune suppression, occur in individuals with a wide range of CD4 counts, and are not considered AIDS-defining illnesses. The incidence of anal cancers appears to have increased since the introduction of HAART, although clinical features and overall survival have not changed.

B. **The most common clinical presentations** are pain or bleeding. However, larger tumors may interfere with anal sphincter function and lead to incontinence.

C. **Clinical examination** will identify a mass, and the size and position within the anal canal or anal margin should be documented. Rectal examination may detect enlarged perirectal lymph nodes.

D. **Proctosigmoidoscopy** should be done in all of these patients.

E. **A thorough gynecological examination** should be done in women, especially if the tumor is situated in the anterior anal canal or if the perineum is involved. Evidence of vaginal mucosal involvement suggests that rectovaginal fistula might develop during treatment. If pelvic examination cannot be performed due to pain, this examination should be done under anesthesia.

II. DIAGNOSTIC WORKUP AND STAGING

A. **Screening strategies** for anal or cervical dysplasia are based on CD4 count and the local expertise.

B. **Pathology** shows that distal anal tumors tend to be keratinized, whereas more proximal tumors are nonkeratinized and referred to as cloacogenic or basaloid. However, the clinical behavior of both types of tumors is similar.

C. **Differential diagnosis** includes other rare tumors arising in the anal canal that need to be distinguished from squamous cell carcinoma including adenocarcinomas of the anal ducts or glands, melanomas, clear cell sarcomas, and neuroendocrine tumors.

D. **Staging** evaluations should include endoanal ultrasonography, CT, MRI, or PET.

E. **Prognosis** depends on sex, tumor stage, nodal status, and response to chemoradiation. Patients with well-differentiated tumors have a more favorable outcome than those with poorly differentiated cancers.

III. THERAPY is generally with concurrent chemotherapy with radiotherapy.

A. **Chemotherapy options** may include fluorouracil and mitomycin, as in the HIV-negative patient population, fluorouracil alone, or fluorouracil with cisplatin. Local control rates are 80% to 90% for tumors less than 4 cm, and 70% to 85% for larger tumors. The addition of mitomycin to fluorouracil improves local control and disease-free survival. HIV-infected patients with CD4 counts greater than $200/mm^3$ generally tolerate therapy similar to that of the HIV-negative patient population, although the rate of local skin/ mucous membrane toxicity and bone marrow suppression may be higher in HIV-positive than in HIV-negative individuals. Individuals with CD4 counts less than $200/mm^3$ may tolerate chemotherapy less well, and consideration should be given for withholding or reducing the dose of mitomycin.

B. **Recurrent or residual disease** is associated with substantial morbidity, associated with poor wound healing and wound infections or sinuses. Salvage therapy for recurrent local disease in selected cases may include inguinofemoral lymph node dissection, pelvic exenteration, or additional radiotherapy if the region has not received the maximum tolerated doses.

C. **Distant metastatic disease** is managed with palliative intent, and active chemotherapy agents include cisplatin and fluorouracil. Resection of isolated metastases in the liver or lung may be considered in select cases.

IV. COMPLICATIONS. Late complications of chemoradiotherapy occur in 3% to 16% of patients after 3 to 10 years, and include necrosis of the anus, especially with more than 60 Gy external radiotherapy or after interstitial implants. Other complications include neurogenic bladder, urethral stenosis, small bowel damage, cytopenia, intractable diarrhea, and radiation-induced sarcoma. These complications are more common in patients with CD4$<$200/mm^3 (*J Clin Oncol* 2008;26:2550).

V. FOLLOW-UP of treated patients involves digital rectal examination and proctoscopy every 2 months for 1 year, every 3 months in the second year, and then every 6 months thereafter. If persistent thickening is present after 3 months, follow-up CT or MRI exams and/or biopsies may be indicated.

VI. BACKGROUND. Anogenital squamous cell carcinomas are uniformly associated with HPV infection, particularly high-risk strains 16, 18, 31, and 35. The HPV E6 protein binds tumor suppressor protein p53 and promotes its degradation, abrogating its cell cycle arrest and apoptosis functions. The HPV E7 protein binds retinoblastoma family proteins, p105, p107, and p130, and promotes cell cycle transition into the S phase.

VII. CURRENT FOCUS OF RESEARCH is examining the efficacy of vaccines in preventing acquisition of high-risk HPV strains. Moreover, vaccines expressing epitopes of HPV E6 or E7 are also being examined as therapeutic vaccines. The use of infrared coagulation for treatment of high-grade squamous intraepitheal neoplasia of the anal canal is also being studied. In addition, the role of cidofovir against HPV for high-grade perianal dysplasia will be investigated.

ACQUIRED IMMUNODEFICIENCY SYNDROME-ASSOCIATED KS
I. CLINICAL PRESENTATION

A. **KS** occurs 500- to 10,000-fold more commonly in HIV-positive individuals than in the general population. Although occurring more commonly in patients with $<$200 CD4 lymphocytes/mm^3, the CD4 count at presentation can be quite variable, and KS may be the first manifestation of AIDS.

B. **Clinical presentation** depends on the site and degree of KS involvement. Manifestations of disease may range from asymptomatic innocuous cutaneous macules to life-threatening visceral lesions. The clinical course of KS is also highly variable, with rapid increase in the number and size of lesions in some patients over the course of weeks to months, or indolent lesions gradually shrinking over years.

C. **Pertinent history** should include a description of all areas of initial KS involvement, lesion duration and rates of progression, oral lesions, GI and pulmonary lesions, presence of KS-associated edema, and other KS-associated symptoms, AIDS-defining illnesses, other sexually transmitted diseases, OIs, and past and current antiretroviral treatment.

D. **Physical examination** includes evaluation of performance status, complete evaluation of the skin, oral cavity, and lymph nodes, with assessment of the chest, abdomen, and neurological assessment, and genital and rectal examinations. **Baseline measurements** of at least five indicator lesions, description of whether lesions are flat or raised, and determination of the number of lesions per area (i.e., left leg, torso, head, and neck) are necessary for later assessment of rate of progression and response to therapy. Photographs or drawings of sites of KS involvement are helpful for follow-up evaluations.

1. **Cutaneous manifestations.** Typically, KS presents with pigmented skin lesions, from a few millimeters to several centimeters in size, that may be flat or raised, with a pink to purple or brown color. These lesions tend to be painless and nonpruritic, although bleeding and superficial infection or cellulitis may occur. Visceral KS can occur without skin manifestations.

a. **Facial KS** typically involves the nasal, periorbital, or conjunctival areas. These may be cosmetically unappealing and cause anxiety and social stigmatization.

   b. **Oral KS** occurs in 30% of patients, and often involves the hard and soft palates, and occasionally the gums, tongue, tonsils, and pharynx. The lesions may be macular, nodular, or exophytic, causing dysphagia, odynophagia, or speech difficulties.
   c. **Genital KS** is characterized by irregular erythematous patches on the foreskin or shaft of the penis.
   d. **KS of the feet** may cause pain and ambulation difficulties.
   e. **Lymphedema** may occur because of dermal and lymphatic involvement of KS, resulting in a nonpitting, sometimes woodlike edema of the lower extremities and genitals, sometimes disproportionally more severe than the degree of KS involvement. Skin breakdown may cause weeping, ulceration, and subsequent superimposed bacterial infections.
   2. **Nodal KS** may present with painless lymph node enlargement, caused by focal or total replacement with KS. This should be differentiated from lymphoma, mycobacterial, or HIV lymphadenitis.
   3. **Visceral manifestations** most often affect the lungs and GI tract.
   a. **Pulmonary KS** affects 40% of KS patients and is usually associated with dyspnea without fever, cough, or hemoptysis. This may be progressive, debilitating, and rapidly fatal if left untreated.
   b. **GI KS** occurs anywhere in the GI tract in 40% of patients at diagnosis, and is generally asymptomatic, although bleeding, obstruction, or enteropathy can occur.
   c. **Other visceral organs**, such as spleen, bone marrow, liver, heart, and pericardium, may be involved with KS. However, CNS involvement with KS is highly unusual.

II. DIAGNOSTIC WORKUP AND STAGING

   A. **Diagnosis of KS** should be confirmed in all patients by biopsy on at least one occasion. **Differential diagnosis** of pigmented skin lesions in HIV-infected patients includes ecchymosis, nevi, melanoma, Bartonella henselae-associated skin lesions, and dermatofibromas.
   B. **Clinical Evaluations**
   1. **Evaluation of cutaneous disease** includes counting the number of lesions if <50, or the number of lesions on a single portion of the body, measurement of biperpendicular diameters of five lesions, description of the color of the lesions, and whether they are raised or flat, whether there is tumor-associated edema, and photographic documentation of the lesions.
   2. **Evaluation of mucosal lesions** should include description of the size of the lesions and their site of involvement.
   3. **Evaluation of visceral disease** should be directed primarily at assessing pulmonary and GI tract lesions. Patients should have a baseline and at least annual chest radiograph, or, if indicated, chest CT. If GI bleeding, vomiting, pain, or other abdominal symptoms are present, upper or lower endoscopy should be strongly considered.
   C. **Pathology.** The diagnosis of KS is made by biopsy and histological examination of cutaneous lesions, enlarged lymph nodes, or visceral tissues. Typical pathology shows a proliferation of spindle cells that may express endothelial markers such as PECAM-1 (CD31), CD34, LYVE1, podoplanin (D2-40), and FLI1 and KS herpes virus (KSHV, HHV8) markers such as LANA, mixed with endothelial cells, fibroblasts, inflammatory cells, and extravasated erythrocytes. Similar histological findings are present in non-AIDS–related KS.
   D. **Radiology and endoscopic procedures**
   1. A baseline **chest radiograph** is done for all patients with KS to exclude pulmonary KS and other cardiopulmonary disorders associated with HIV infection. Localized or diffuse interstitial reticulonodular infiltrates with mediastinal prominence may be seen in patients with pulmonary KS, and should be differentiated from lymphoma or PCP and other typical (i.e., bacterial) and atypical pneumonias (i.e., mycobacterial, CMV, or histoplasma pneumonias). KS may also present with alveolar infiltrates, pleural effusion, or isolated pulmonary nodules. KS lesions are generally thallium or PET positive and gallium negative, in contrast to pulmonary infections.
   2. **Bronchoscopy** may reveal endobronchial erythematous KS-like lesions even with radiologically normal studies. Because transbronchial biopsies have poor histologic

yield, a presumptive diagnosis of pulmonary KS can be made on the basis of dyspnea without fever, chest radiograph, and bronchoscopic findings after exclusion of other disease processes.

E. Staging of KS utilizes the AIDS Clinical Trials Group (ACTG) classification system, which characterizes patients as good risk or poor risk, on the basis of their tumor burden (T), immune function (I), and presence of systemic illness (S). T0 denotes good-risk KS confined to skin and/or lymph nodes and/or minimal oral disease, whereas T1 poor-risk lesions are associated with symptomatic lymphedema, tumor ulceration, extensive oral disease, and/or visceral involvement. Immune function is categorized according to whether the CD4 count is $<$ or $\geq 150/mm^3$. S0 is defined as no history of OIs, B symptoms, other HIV-related illness, and Karnofsky score of at least 70%. Good-risk KS patients are T0I0S0.

F. Prognosis in the HAART era is largely determined by the T and S stages, whereas in the era of HAART use, CD4 count does not have a significant impact on survival. The 3-year OS is 88% for individuals with T0S0, 81% for T0S1 patients, 80% for T1S0 patients, and 53% for T1S1 patients.

G. Morbidity from KS is associated with painful lesions in the mouth or on the soles of the feet, lymphedema, symptoms associated with visceral KS, or psychological disturbances resulting from the cosmetic effects of KS lesions.

H. Mortality from KS is associated primarily with pulmonary KS and less commonly with hemorrhage from GI lesions.

III. THERAPY

A. Patients with good-risk or asymptomatic and stable poor-risk KS may be offered local or systemic therapy.

1. **Local therapies** include electron beam radiotherapy, topical 9-cis retinoic acid (Panretin Gel), intralesional injections or iontophoresis of vinblastine (0.1 mL of 0.1 mg/mL) or 3% sodium tetradecyl sulfate (0.1 to 0.3 mL), cryotherapy, laser coagulation therapy, or surgical excision. Despite the effectiveness of these procedures, there are several possible complications. Radiotherapy may result in chronic residual lymphedema, postirradiation telangiectasias, woody skin changes, and reappearance of KS after treatment. It is more toxic for mucosal than skin lesions. Panretin gel can cause local inflammation and lightening of the skin, resulting in inadequate cosmetic results. Photodynamic therapies can result in moderate pain and photosensitivity for a number of weeks after treatment. Intralesional injections cause necrosis or sclerosis of mucocutaneous lesions, which may be quite painful. Cryotherapy can result in hypopigmented areas, particularly troublesome for dark-skinned individuals. Surgical excision is not optimal for large lesions due to reappearance of KS at the margins.

2. **HAART therapy alone** produces a response rate of about 80% in patients with T0 lesions, but responses are unusual in patients with T1 lesions. This approach is more likely to be effective in patients naïve to HAART who have previously poorly controlled HIV, and who will be compliant with subsequent use of HAART. The time to response is 3 to 9 months. PI-based and nonnucleoside reverse transcriptase inhibitor-based HAART regimens have been verified to be similarly effective. It should be noted that progressive KS may also develop in patients who have recently initiated HAART, attributed to an immune reconstitution syndrome.

3. **Thalidomide** has been reported to produce responses in 30% to 50% of patients, at doses of 100 to 1,000 mg/day (200 mg/day is the usual maximal tolerated dose), but is complicated by fatigue, constipation, neuropathy, xerostomia, neutropenia, orthostatic hypotension, risk of birth defects, and, less commonly, hyper- or hypoglycemia, hypothyroidism, tremor, elevated serum transaminases, or thrombosis. The use of other thalidomide analogs, such as lenalidomide and pomalidomide, is currently under investigation.

4. **Interferon-α** produces responses in about 30% of patients, when used in high doses, >20 mU/m^2 three times per week, but fewer responses at lower doses when used alone, although responses at low doses are improved when combined with PIs.

Interferon-α can result in neutropenia, flulike symptoms, and depression. The use of pegylated interferon for KS has not been reported.

B. Patients with poor-risk symptomatic visceral KS or rapidly progressive KS should be treated with HAART combined with chemotherapy or investigational agents. Pharmacological doses of systemic corticosteroids should be avoided, since this can cause marked acceleration of KS.

1. **Liposomal anthracyclines** are the most appropriate initial therapy, and either liposomal doxorubicin (Doxil, 20 mg/m^2 IV every 2 to 3 weeks) or daunorubicin (DaunoXome, 40 mg/m^2 IV every 2 to 3 weeks) results in response rates of 25% to 90%. Grade 3 or 4 adverse effects include myelosuppresion (36%), nausea and vomiting (15%), anemia (10%), and hand-foot syndrome. The incidence of extravasation injury, mucositis, nausea, alopecia, and cardiomyopathy with liposomal anthracyclines is lower than that with nonliposomal anthracyclines.

2. **Paclitaxel** 100 mg/m^2 q 2 to 3 weeks is generally considered the most effective and best-tolerated second-line agent, although some oncologists recommend it as first-line therapy for life-threatening KS. Response rates of 59% to 71% have been reported, with a median duration of response of more than 10 months. Myelosuppresion (grade 3 or 4 in 35%), alopecia, neuropathy, and hypersensitivity reaction are the major toxicities. Liposomal paclitaxel (xyotax) and abraxane have not been studied in AIDS-KS.

3. **Oral etoposide** may be useful as a third-line agent, given at a dose of 50 mg/day for 7 days of each 14-day cycle. In a trial of 36 patients, the response rate was 36%, with a median duration of response of 25 weeks. This therapy was complicated by grade 3 or 4 neutropenia in 36% of patients.

4. **Vinorelbine** has a 43% response rate in patients with one or more prior systemic therapies for KS, but is associated with myelosuppression.

5. **Alternative chemotherapy regimens** that may be considered include bleomycin, docetaxel, or a combination of doxorubicin, bleomycin, and vincristine.

6. **Duration of therapy** depends on individual patients. Generally, chemotherapy is given until a plateau in the response has been achieved, and then doses of therapy can be discontinued or given less frequently. Chronic chemotherapy can be associated with limiting cumulative treatment-related toxicities.

IV. COMPLICATIONS

A. Complications of AIDS-KS. Although visceral KS, especially GI and pulmonary KS, may prove fatal, AIDS-related immunosuppression and OIs remain the major cause of morbidity and mortality in patients with KS. Superimposed bacterial, fungal, and parasitic infections in ulcerated, weeping lesions are not uncommon. Severe dyspnea from pulmonary KS and hemorrhage from GI involvment of KS also may be seen.

B. Complication of therapy. The use of HAART with systemic anti-KS therapy, such as paclitaxel, may potentially cause profound toxicity in some patients with AIDS-KS. The metabolism of paclitaxel, docetaxel, and anti-HIV PIs involves cytochrome P450 3A4 isoform.

V. FOLLOW-UP.
The frequency of follow-up may vary from every 2 weeks to every 6 months, depending on the stage of disease, rate of disease progression or regression, and the type of therapy. During follow-up visits, *indicator lesions* should be measured, the number of KS lesions in indicator regions should be counted, and the character of the lesions described. Repeat photographs and follow-up chest radiographs should be performed as clinically indicated.

VI. BACKGROUND

A. KS develops in HIV-negative individuals, including older men primarily of Eastern European, Mediterranean, and/or Jewish descent, individuals undergoing immunosuppression (e.g., associated with bone marrow or organ transplantation), and young males in equatorial Africa, as well as in HIV-infected individuals. AIDS-associated KS occurs in individuals who are homosexual or bisexual and very rarely, if at all, in other HIV risk groups. The incidence of AIDS-KS has decreased significantly with the use of HAART in the United States. However, in other parts of the world with limited access to HAART, KS incidence continues to increase.

B. **Pathogenesis of KS** is thought to involve expression by the spindle cells of cytokines such as interleukin-6, basic fibroblast growth factor, vascular endothelial growth factor (VEGF), matrix metalloproteinases, tumor necrosis factor-α, oncostatin-M, platelet-derived growth factor, and interferon-γ.

C. **HHV8,** also designated KSHV, is thought to be the etiologic agent of this disorder, with primarily latently infected cells contributing to the development of this disorder. A small proportion of cells with lytic HHV8 replication may also contribute to disease pathogenesis. HHV8 is present in AIDS-KS, as well as KS developing in HIV-negative populations. Several viral genes implicated in the pathogenesis of KS include those encoding homologs of antiapoptosis proteins Bcl-2 and an inhibitor of Fas-mediated apoptosis, interleukin-6, cyclin D, interferon-regulatory factors, chemokines, and G protein-coupled receptors. Serologic tests for HHV8 are not yet routinely available. The median time for KS development in HHV8-positive, HIV-1-infected individuals is estimated to be about 10 years. HHV8 is thought to be transmitted sexually, although concentrations of virus in semen appear to be very low. Blood-borne transmission is thought to occur, but inefficiently. Mother-to-child transmission also occurs, which is primarily through saliva.

VII. CURRENT FOCUS OF RESEARCH

A. **Antiangiogenic agents** have been extensively studied in AIDS-associated KS. This includes thalidomide, as well as several agents studied in phase I and II trials, including fumagillin analog TNP-470, a VEGF receptor inhibitor SU5416, antiangiogenic dipeptide IM862, bevacizumab, lenalidomide, and ephrin and Notch pathway inhibitors. The matrix metalloproteinase inhibitor, COL-3, a tetracycline analog, resulted in a 44% response rate for a median duration of more than 25 weeks in a cohort of 17 patients. This therapy was complicated by headache, photosensitivity, or rash. An inhibitor of collagen synthesis, halofuginone, is also undergoing clinical study in AIDS-KS. Interleukin 12 has also been shown to be a potent inhibitor of angiogenesis, perhaps through induction of inducible protein 10, and clinical trials are underway with this agent. An antisense oligonucleotide to VEGF mRNA will also be studied in AIDS-KS. There is also evidence that antiretroviral PIs may function as angiogenesis inhibitors.

B. **Inhibitors of growth factor receptor signaling** were studied, including imatinib, as an inhibitor of platelet-derived growth factor and c-kit receptors. In a trial of 10 individuals given 600 mg/day, 5 exhibited a PR, but grade 3 or 4 diarrhea, depression, or neutropenia occurred in 8 patients. Other studies are based on the mediators of signaling pathways, including phosphatidyl inositol 3-kinase, serine-threonine kinase Akt, extracellular receptor kinase Erk, nuclear factor kappa B, target of rapamycin (TOR), and cyclin D.

C. **Cell-differentiating retinoids** have also been used systemically in AIDS-KS patients. Oral 9-cis-retinoic acid (alitretinoin or Panretin) resulted in a 37% response rate, but almost half of the patients discontinued treatment because of headache or skin toxicity. Hypertriglyceridemia and subclinical pancreatitis have also been reported with retinoids, including alitretinoin. There are no reports of the use of bexarotene for AIDS-KS.

D. **Anti-HHV8** therapy with cidofovir or foscarnet has been reported in anecdotal or retrospective studies. For example, time to KS progression was prolonged in patients treated with foscarnet compared with patients treated with ganciclovir (211 days vs. 22 days). Histone deacetylase inhibitors, such as butyrate and valproic acid, and nuclear factor kappa B inhibitors (e.g., bortezomib), which have been shown to induce lytic gene expression of HHV8, are being evaluated in clinical trials.

OTHER ACQUIRED IMMUNODEFICIENCY SYNDROME-ASSOCIATED MALIGNANCIES

Although a number of other malignancies may be more frequent among HIV-positive than among HIV-negative individuals, treatment approaches are generally similar, especially if virus load is well controlled and CD4 is not profoundly depressed.

I. HCC is about fivefold more common in HIV-positive individuals than in the general population, primarily because of a higher rate of persistent hepatitis B and C virus infection. However, higher rates of alcohol abuse, nonalcoholic steatohepatitis, and diabetes may contribute to HCC development in HIV-positive individuals. Screening for active HBV and HCV infection is recommended for all HIV-positive individuals. Hepatitis B vaccine should be provided to all individuals who are not immune to HBV. Antiviral treatment is recommended for individuals with persistent infection and evidence of liver disease. Screening for HCC in patients with cirrhosis is recommended every 6 months with ultrasound. Treatment of HCC in HIV-positive patients, with transplantation, TACE, or sorafenib (depending upon the stage), is similar to that in HIV-negative individuals. However, outcomes of transplantation for HCC may be worse in HIV-positive individuals, in terms of HCV and HCC recurrence.

II. LUNG CANCERS occur 2.5- to 5-fold more commonly in HIV-positive individuals than in the general population, and are the most frequently diagnosed non-AIDS–defining malignancy in this population. Lung cancer risk is unrelated to level of HIV-induced immunosuppression.

III. LIP CANCERS occur 3.1-fold more commonly in HIV-infected patients than in the general population. Some of these cancers may be HPV related.

IV. CERVICAL CANCERS occur threefold more commonly in HIV-infected women than in the general population. Pap smears are recommended at the time HIV is diagnosed, and repeated at least once within 6 months if normal. If the initial or follow-up Pap smear shows severe inflammation, a repeat study should be performed in 3 months. If a Pap smear shows squamous intraepithelial lesions or atypical squamous cells of undetermined significance, colposcopic examination and, if indicated, biopsies should be performed. High-risk HPV infections are found more commonly in sexually active HIV-infected women than in women not infected with HIV. When cervical cancer presents in an HIV-infected woman with CD4$<$500/mm,^{3} it appears at a younger age and with more advanced disease, and it is associated with a worse outcome than in women without HIV infection. The incidence and therapeutic response of cervical cancer, however, appears unchanged by HAART therapy. The use of radiation therapy combined with chemotherapy may also be less well tolerated in HIV-infected women than in women lacking HIV. As for HIV-negative patients, early-stage, nonbulky cervical tumors respond well to surgical intervention, and for more advanced tumors, the standard of care is concomitant chemoradiotherapy with cisplatin.

V. PENILE CANCER occurs 3.9-fold more commonly in HIV-positive individuals than in the general population.

VI. OTHER. Higher rates of testicular seminomas, multiple myeloma, multicentric Castlemans's disease, nonmelanotic and melanotic skin cancer, prostate carcinoma, brain tumors, leukemia have also been described in HIV-infected individuals than in the general population.

SUGGESTED READINGS

Ammari ZA, Mollberg NM, Abdelhady K, et al. Diagnosis and management of primary effusion lymphoma in the immunocompetent and immunosuppressed hosts. *Thoracic Cardiovasc Surg* 2013;61:343–349.

Antman K, Chang Y. Kaposi's sarcoma. *N Engl J Med* 2000;342:1027–1038.

Barta SK, Xue X, Wang D, et al. Treatment factors affecting outcomes in HIV-associated non-Hodgkin lymphomas: a pooled analysis of 1546 patients. *Blood* 2013;122:3251–3262.

Clark MA, Hartley A, Geh JI. Cancer of the anal canal. *Lancet Oncol* 2004;5:149–157.

Dunelavy K, Pittaluga S, Shovin M, et al. Low-intensity therapy in adults with Burkitt's lymphoma. *New Engl J Med* 2013;369:1915–1925.

Dunleavy K, Wilson WH. How I treat HIV-associated lymphoma. *Blood* 2012;119:3245–3255.

Kaplan LD. Management of HIV-associated Hodgkin lymphoma: how far we have come. *J Clin Oncol* 2012;30:4056–4058.

Martis N, Mounier N. Hodgkin lymphoma in patients with HIV infection: a review. *Curr Hematol Malig Rep* 2012;7:228–234.

Oehler-Janne C, Huguet F, Provencher S, et al. HIV-specific differences in outcome of squamous cell carcinoma of the anal canal: a multicentric cohort study of HIV-positive patients receiving highly active antiretroviral therapy. *J Clin Oncol* 2008;26:2550–2557.

Pria AD, Hayward K, Bower M. Do we still need chemotherapy for AIDS associated Kaposi's sarcoma? *Expert Rev Anticancer Ther* 2013;13:203–209.

Ratner L, Lee J, Tang S, et al. Chemotherapy for human immunodeficiency virus-associated non-Hodgkin's lymphoma in combination with highly active antiretroviral therapy. *J Clin Oncol* 2001;19:2171–2178.

Rudek MA, Flexner C, Ambinder RF. Use of antineoplastic agents in patients with cancer who have HIV/AIDS. *Lancet Oncol* 2011;12:905–912.

Spano J-P, Costagliola D, Katlama N. AIDS-related malignancies: state of the art and therapeutic challenges. *J Clin Oncol* 2008;26:4834–4842.

Yarchoan R, Tosato G, Little RF. AIDS-related malignancies—the influence of antiviral therapy on pathogenesis and management. *Nat Clin Pract* 2005;2:406–415.

35 Care of the Older Adult with Cancer

Tanya M. Wildes

I. **INTRODUCTION.** Cancer is a disease of aging; the incidence of most malignancies increases with age. Over half of cancer diagnoses and nearly 70% of cancer deaths occur in patients over the age of 65. With the aging of the population, the number of older adults with cancer will increase by 67% by 2030. There are significant differences in cancer-specific death rates between older and younger individuals. These age-related disparities likely differ in cause among different malignancies, but contributory factors include differences in screening, more advanced stage at presentation, differences in biology of disease across the age spectrum, and less aggressive treatment in older adults.

   A. **Knowledge gaps in treatment of older adults with cancer.** Contributing to differences in treatment between older and younger adults are the increased vulnerability of older adults to toxicity of therapy and the underrepresentation of older adults in clinical trials. Older adults are less likely to be enrolled in clinical trials owing to restrictive exclusion criteria based on organ function or comorbidities. In addition, clinicians are less likely to propose participation in a clinical trial, though, if asked, older adults are as likely as younger adults to agree to participate. This under-representation of older adults in clinical trials has resulted in substantial gaps in our knowledge about the safety and efficacy of cancer therapies when applied to older adults. With the growth in the number of older adults with cancer, thankfully, increasing attention is now being directed to the need to increase our knowledge base on treating older adults with cancer.

II. **BIOLOGY OF CANCER IN OLDER ADULTS.** There is a commonly held perception that, overall, cancer in older adults is less aggressive than in younger adults. Breast cancer is one example of this, being more likely to be hormone-receptor positive. Overall, however, most cancers do not exhibit substantial age-related differences in biology. In some cases, older age is actually associated with more aggressive, treatment-resistant biology, as in acute myeloid leukemia and diffuse large B-cell lymphoma. Thus, in older adults, treatment decisions are largely not driven by biology of disease, but rather by the patient's individual health status.

III. **COMPREHENSIVE GERIATRIC ASSESSMENT.** Increasing chronologic age is associated with an increasing prevalence of comorbidities and functional or cognitive impairment. A comprehensive geriatric assessment (CGA) is a multidimensional assessment of geriatric domains (Table 35-1). While the screening tools used are often referred to as "CGA," in geriatrics, CGA refers to the multidisciplinary assessment, interpretation of screening tools, and recommended tailored interventions.

TABLE 35-1	Domains of a CGA

Domain	Commonly used scales/measures
Comorbidities	• Charlson comorbidity index • Cumulative illness rating scale—geriatrics • Adult comorbidity evaluation-27 (ACE-27) • Hematopoietic cell transplantation comorbidity index (HCT-CI)
Physical performance	• Timed up and go • Short physical performance battery

Functional status	• Activities of daily living
	  • Bathing
	  • Continence
	  • Dressing
	  • Toileting
	  • Transferring
	  • Feeding
	• Instrumental activities of daily living
	  • Using telephone
	  • Getting to places out of walking distance
	  • Shopping for groceries
	  • Preparing meals
	  • Doing housework
	  • Doing laundry
	  • Taking medications
	  • Managing finances
	• Performance status

Cognition	• Short Blessed test • Montreal cognitive assessment (MOCA) (http://www.mocatest.org) • Mini-mental status examination
Depression	• Geriatric depression scale (GDS) • Patient-health questionnaire-9 (PHQ-9)
Polypharmacy and inappropriate medications	• Beers criteria for potentially inappropriate medications in the elderly • STOPP/START criteria

Geriatric syndromes are extremely common in older adults with cancer, and are inadequately described in a routine oncology assessment. Coexisting medical conditions are present in more than 80% of cancer patients over the age of 80. Functional decline or disability refers to the greater need for assistance with daily activities owing to physical or cognitive decline. Cognitive impairment is also common among older adults with cancer, with 15% to 25% in the outpatient setting, and 40% to 50% in the inpatient setting screening positive.

Furthermore, evaluating only performance status significantly underestimates the level of impairment in an older individual. Comorbidities and functional status are entirely independent. Among older adults with cancer who had an Eastern Cooperative Oncology Group performance status (ECOG PS) of 0–1, 10% were dependent in one or more activities of daily living (ADLs), nearly 40% were dependent in one or more instrumental activities of daily living (IADLs), nearly 30% were cognitively impaired, and 30% were depressed. Thus, PS is an inadequate measure of the heterogeneous health statuses of older adults.

IV. TREATMENT OF CANCER IN OLDER ADULTS

A. Surgery. Surgical management of cancers does not differ between older and younger patients overall. Studies that appropriately control for confounders (such as comorbidities, advanced cancer stage, and functional impairment) demonstrate similar outcomes in older and younger patients undergoing cancer surgery. That said, some older adults are at greater risk for postoperative complications. In the Preoperative Assessment of Cancer in the Elderly (PACE) study, dependence in IADLs, self-reported fatigue, and an Eastern Cooperative Oncology Group performance status (PS) of two or more were associated with increased risk of complications of surgery (*Crit Rev Onc Hem* 2008;65:156). Similarly, dependence in ADLs, IADLs, and poor PS were associated with longer length of stay. Age was not associated with increased 30-day mortality, though male gender, advanced cancer stage, and extent of surgery were. Thus, age alone should not be a primary consideration in decisions regarding cancer surgery; decisions are better made in the context of evaluation of the patient's individual functional status.

B. Radiation. Similarly, age alone is generally not a primary consideration in decision making regarding radiation therapy (RT) for cancer. Some studies have demonstrated greater acute functional decline during chemotherapy in older adults undergoing RT, but similar longer-term outcomes in patients undergoing curative-intent RT. Thus, among patients being treated with curative intent, the initial toxicity may be warranted given the longer-term outcomes. Conversely, among older adults treated with palliative intent, the risk of toxicity and functional decline must be balanced with the potential benefit of therapy. Among patients with glioblastoma, older age is associated with greater toxicity and cognitive impairment related to radiation with concurrent temozolomide. Little is known about predictors of toxicity of RT in older adults with cancer. In a small study of older adults with rectal cancer, comorbidities were associated with greater risk of acute toxicity. The role for evaluation with geriatric assessment in older adults undergoing RT remains to be examined.

C. Systemic therapy. Age-related physiologic changes may increase the risk of toxicity of chemotherapy among older adults; these include reduced gastrointestinal motility, decreased splanchnic blood flow, changes in body composition resulting in altered volume of distribution, decreased hepatic blood flow, polypharmacy and drug interactions, and declining renal function (*J Clin Oncol* 2007;25:1832).

   1. Chemotherapy. A comprehensive discussion of age-related differences in toxicity of individual chemotherapeutic agents is beyond the scope of this chapter. However, some important themes merit discussion.

   a. Hematologic toxicity. Older adults are at greater risk for myelosuppression than younger adults, particularly with the exposure to the alkylating agents, due to age-related decreases in hematopoietic stem cell reserve.

   b. Mucositis. Older adults are at greater for mucositis with fluoropyrimidines, the liposomal anthracyclines, and high-dose melphalan, likely due to decreased ability to respond to mucosal damage.

   c. Dose adjustments for renal insufficiency. Renal function declines with age. Serum creatinine levels alone are an inadequate reflection of renal function, which is better estimated with an equation, such as the Cockcroft–Gault or Modification of Diet in Renal Disease (MDRD) equation, or measured with a 24-hour urine collection. Many chemotherapeutic agents have not been thoroughly studied in patients with renal insufficiency.

   2. Targeted agents. A large number of targeted agents have been brought from the bench to clinical trial and into the clinics in the past 15 years. The underenrollment of older adults in clinical trials has resulted in a paucity of data on most of these targeted agents in older adults, particularly older adults with comorbidities. A number of agents, including erlotinib, sorafenib, bevacizumab, imatinib, bortezomib, and lenalidomide, have been shown to have greater toxicity in older adults (*Crit Rev Onc Hematol* 2011;78:227). In other cases, subgroup analyses of patients fit enough to participate in clinical trials may demonstrate similar efficacy and toxicity, only to be found to have increased toxicity and decreased effectiveness when applied in "real-world" settings, among patients with comorbidities and functional impairment. Caution must be used in using targeted agents in older adults.

V. PREDICTING TOXICITY OF CHEMOTHERAPY IN OLDER ADULTS. With the increased vulnerability to toxicity and lack of data on treating older adults with cancer, clinicians are left to

TABLE 35-2	Interventions for Geriatric Syndromes
Domain	**Intervention**
Comorbidities	Comanagement with primary care physician
Functional decline	Physical therapy consult
	Occupational therapy consult
Falls	Physical therapy consult
	Occupational therapy consult for home-safety evaluation
	Screen for neuropathy
	Medication review
Nutritional risk	Consultation with dietitian
	Social work consult for resource assistance (meals-on-wheels, cancer foundation support for nutritional supplements)
Polypharmacy and inappropriate medications	Medication reconciliation and review
	Home-health nursing for medication setup
	Consultation with pharmacist
Lack of social support	Consultation with social worker

make decisions by combining clinical trial data and clinical judgment. Several instruments are being evaluated to aid in risk stratification and decision making for older adults considering chemotherapy. In the Cancer and Aging Research Group study, over 500 patients underwent CGA prior to initiation of chemotherapy. Factors including age $\geq$73 years, anemia, renal insufficiency, recent falls, hearing impairment, limited ability to walk 1 block, decreased social activities, and requiring assistance with medications predicted greater risk of grade 3 to 5 toxicity of chemotherapy (*J Clin Oncol* 2011;29:3457). In the Chemotherapy Risk Assessment for High Age Patients (CRASH) trial, diastolic blood pressure, dependence in IADLs, elevated LDH, and the intensity of chemotherapy were associated with hematologic toxicity of chemotherapy, while ECOG PS, cognitive impairment, nutritional compromise, and intensity of chemotherapy were associated with nonhematologic toxicity (*Cancer* 2012;118:3377).

VI. PRACTICAL GUIDE TO ADDRESSING GERIATRIC SYNDROMES IN OLDER ADULTS WITH CANCER. Table 35-2 lists some potential interventions for geriatric syndromes identified in older adults.

VII. SURVIVORSHIP IN OLDER ADULTS. With the coming increase in the number of older adults with cancer, there will be a consequent increase in the number of older adult cancer survivors. Older adult cancer survivors are at greater risk for developing geriatric syndromes. In a study of over 12,000 older adults, cancer survivors were more likely to report hearing impairment, incontinence, depression, falls, and osteoporosis. Even after completion of cancer therapy, older adults will remain increasingly vulnerable and will require attention to long-term effects of their cancer therapy.

VIII. SUMMARY. The population is aging, and with the increased incidence of cancer with age, the number of older adults with cancer will increase significantly over the coming years. Older adults may be at increased risk for chemotherapy toxicity, but tools to better predict toxicity are being validated. CGA is a tool that holds promise to aid in individualizing cancer treatment for older adults.

SUGGESTED READINGS

Audisio RA, Pope D, Ramesh HS, et al. Shall we operate? Preoperative assessment in elderly cancer patients (PACE) can help: a SIOG surgical task force prospective study. *Crit Rev Oncol Hematol* 2008;65:156–163.

Exterman M, Boler I, Reich RR, et al. Predicting the risk of chemotherapy toxicity in older patients: the chemotherapy risk assessment scale for high-age patients (CRASH) score. *Cancer* 2012;118:3377–3786.

Gonsalves W, Ganti AK. Targeted anti-cancer therapy in the elderly. *Crit Rev Oncol Hematol* 2011;78:227–242.

Hurria A, Togawa K, Mohile SG, et al. Predicting chemotherapy toxicity in older adults with cancer: a prospective multicenter study. *J Clin Oncol* 2011;29:3457–3465.

Lichtman SM, Wildiers H, Chatelut E, et al; International Society of Geriatric Oncology Chemotherapy Taskforce. International Society of Geriatric Oncology Chemotherapy Taskforce: evaluation of chemotherapy in older patients—an analysis of the medical literature. J Clin Oncol 2007;25:1832–1843.

Cancer and Thrombosis

Kristen Sanfilippo • Tzu-Fei Wang

I. **INTRODUCTION.** Cancer patients have a 5- to 7-fold increased risk of developing venous thromboemboli (VTE) compared with noncancer patients (*JAMA* 2005;293:715), with cancer-associated VTE accounting for 20% to 30% of all VTEs (*J Thromb Haemost* 2007;5:692). Patients with cancer-associated VTE had decreased survival compared with their thrombosis-free counterparts matched by cancer type and stage. When treated with anticoagulation, cancer patients have higher rates of major bleeding events compared with patients with VTE without cancer (*Blood* 2002;100:3484).

II. **PATHOPHYSIOLOGY AND RISK FACTORS.** A clearer understanding of the complex pathophysiology of cancer-associated thrombosis is beginning to emerge. In response to cancer-induced inflammatory cytokines, tissue factor (TF) or cancer procoagulants are aberrantly expressed on the surface of cancer cells, monocytes, and endothelial cells, promoting a hypercoagulable state, angiogenesis, and tumor metastasis. Secondly, decreased patient activity due to the disease or therapy leads to increased venous stasis. In addition, vascular injury from surgery, chemotherapy, radiation, and central venous catheters (CVCs) are major risk factors for VTE, completing Vichow's triad. Thus, cancer is a heterogeneous disease, with varying VTE risk based on cancer subtype and stage, patient-associated factors, and cancer-specific therapy.

A. **Type of cancer.** A higher VTE risk has been noted in biologically aggressive malignancies with early metastatic potential and short overall survivals. Cancers associated with the highest risk of VTE include lung, pancreas, brain, ovary, and hematologic malignancies (myeloma, lymphoma, leukemia) (*JAMA* 2005;293:715).

B. **Stage of cancer.** As expected, more advanced stage is associated with higher risk (*JAMA* 2005;293:715).

C. **Timing related to cancer diagnosis.** Patients are at highest risk for VTE in the time period immediately following cancer diagnosis. This is hypothesized to be due to the presence of the largest disease burden; in addition, this period correlates with initiation of therapy (i.e., chemotherapy/surgery). In a study by Blom et al., VTE risk was highest in the 3 months after diagnosis (53-fold risk) and decreased over time (*JAMA* 2005;293:715).

D. **Patient-associated risk factors.** These are similar to those in noncancer patients and include age, race, obesity, presence of medical comorbidities, surgery, history of VTE, presence of hereditary thrombophilia, and leukocytosis and/or thrombocytosis.

E. **Cancer treatment.** Recent surgery is a well-documented risk factor for VTE in both cancer and noncancer patients. Pathophysiology is attributed to direct vascular damage, prolonged immobility, and presence of an inflammatory state. It should be assumed that all patients receiving chemotherapy or hormonal therapy are at increased risk of VTE. Plausible mechanisms for this prothrombotic state include decreased activity of physiologic anticoagulants, release of procoagulants from apoptotic cancer cells, and drug-induced injury to endothelial cells. Some of the specific therapies that have been associated with increased risk of VTE in randomized, prospective trials include cisplatin therapy, hormonal therapy, antiangiogenic agents, erythrocyte-stimulating agents (ESAs), and immunomodulatory agents (i.e., lenalidomide and thalidomide).

The knowledge of these potential risk factors for VTE in cancer patients can guide clinicians to identify patients with increased risk of VTE.

Several risk prediction models have been generated to identify cancer patients at greatest risk of developing VTE. The 2013 American Society of Clinical Oncology (ASCO) VTE guidelines recommend the use of the model proposed by Khorana et al., given that it has been validated in a large population of cancer patients (*Blood* 2008;111:4902). The model was generated using a cohort of 4,066 ambulatory cancer patients initiated on chemotherapy. Several important risk factors for VTE were identified in multivariate analysis, including site of cancer, prechemotherapy platelet and leukocyte counts, hemoglobin or use of red cell growth factors, and body mass index (BMI). Each risk factor was assigned a corresponding score in the point system. Patients were then divided into three groups: high risk (≥ 3 points), intermediate risk (1 to 2 points), and low risk (0 points), with VTE rates of 6.7%, 2%, and 0.3%, respectively, over a 2.5-month period. While the clinical utility of such models remains poorly defined beyond patient education, incorporation of these tools in the future will allow identification of patients at highest risk of VTE and potential consideration for thromboprophylaxis.

III. **VENOUS THROMBOSES AND OCCULT CANCER.** About 20% to 30% of all newly diagnosed VTE are cancer associated. The majority of these cases will present with thrombosis following diagnosis of an established malignancy. However, a significant percentage of patients with seemingly idiopathic VTE will subsequently be diagnosed with cancer. This association has raised the question of the clinical benefit of cancer screening in patients who present with idiopathic VTE.

In a landmark study by Prandoni et al. (*N Engl J Med* 1992;327:1128), 260 consecutive outpatients with objectively diagnosed deep vein thrombosis (DVT) were followed for 2 years. Development of cancer in patients was compared between the idiopathic ($n = 153$) and secondary DVT ($n = 107$) groups. History, physical, and routine laboratory testing were performed at VTE diagnosis in each group, identifying 3.3% ($n = 5$) of patients in the idiopathic (2 lung cancers, 1 multiple myeloma, 1 chronic lymphocytic leukemia, and 1 osteosarcoma) compared to no patients in the secondary DVT group with an underlying malignancy. During the 2-year follow-up in the remaining patients, symptomatic malignancies were diagnosed in 11 of 145 patients (7.6%) with idiopathic DVT compared to 2 of 105 patients (1.9%) with secondary DVT. The majority of malignancies (77%) were diagnosed in the first 12 months of follow-up, with all cases diagnosed by 18 months. A similar association between occult malignancy and idiopathic VTE is further supported by findings from retrospective studies using hospital discharge administrative databases.

Given the association, oncologists may be asked to evaluate patients with idiopathic VTE for occult cancer. Limited prospective data are available for guidance. In the SOMIT trial, 233 patients with newly diagnosed, idiopathic VTE were randomized to receive cancer screening (abdominal/pelvic ultrasound or computed tomography [CT], endoscopy, colonoscopy, hemoccult testing, sputum cytology, serum tumor markers, mammogram, and pelvic exam with cytology for women and prostate ultrasonography for men) or routine follow-up (*J Thromb Haemost* 2004;2:884). At baseline, all patients underwent history, physical, and routine laboratory tests, during which 32 cancers were diagnosed (14%). An additional 13 of 99 patients (13%) in the screening group were diagnosed with cancer based on the additional procedures. During the 2-year follow-up, one cancer was diagnosed in the screening arm compared to 10 cases in 102 patients in the control arm, with no significant difference in mortality between the arms (2% vs. 3.9%, respectively). However, the study was closed early due to poor accrual, failing to meet a target enrollment of 1,000 patients. A cost-effective analysis of the trial concluded that abdominal/pelvic CT was the most cost-effective test, and tumor markers were associated with high false-positive rates generating additional unnecessary testing.

In a second, large prospective cohort study (*J Thromb Haemost* 2004;2:876), the impact of cancer screening was also assessed in new, idiopathic VTE. In this trial, 864 patients were initially evaluated with history, physical (including rectal), breast and pelvic exam in women, routine laboratory tests (in addition to erythrocyte sedimentation rate and serum protein electrophoresis), and chest X-ray (CXR), at which time a total of 34 cancers were detected, the majority of which were limited in stage (61%). Patients who did not have a cancer diagnosed in step 1 (*n* = 830) underwent a "limited" workup consisted of an abdominal/pelvic ultrasound, Carcinoembryonic antigen (CEA), and Prostate-specific antigen (PSA) in men and CA-125 in women, revealing an additional 13 cancers. The remaining patients (*n* = 817) were followed for 12 months for the occurrence of cancer. During the 12-month follow-up, 14 additional malignancies were diagnosed, of which 14% were limited stage for a total of 61 malignancies. The results of this study suggest that in adults with idiopathic VTE, more than 50% of underlying occult malignancies can be detected with a limited initial evaluation, followed by age/sex appropriate cancer screening. Patients diagnosed at the time of presentation tend to be diagnosed with earlier stage cancers compared with those diagnosed during follow-up. Despite diagnosis at early stage, data have not yet indicated a proven survival benefit for cancer screening in patients with idiopathic VTE.

In summary, 20% to 30% of all newly diagnosed idiopathic VTEs are cancer associated. While a significant proportion of cancers are known at the time of VTE diagnosis, the majority of the remaining cases will be established between presentation and the following 12 months. Aggressive screening for occult cancers in asymptomatic patients with idiopathic VTEs has not been associated with improvement in survival and is thus not recommended. However, limited evaluation with history, physical, routine labs, and age/gender appropriate cancer screening is a reasonable strategy.

IV. **PREVENTION OF VTE IN PATIENTS WITH CANCER.** Cancer patients have a sevenfold increased risk of VTE compared to persons without cancer, with risk highest in the first 3 months after cancer diagnosis (53-fold increased risk) (*JAMA* 2005;293:715). One of the main reasons for this high risk of VTE is due to surgical, chemotherapy, and hormonal interventions, and can be reduced by employing prevention strategies.

A. **Prophylaxis against VTE in patients with cancer in the perioperative setting.** The incidence of VTE after cancer surgery may be as high as 50% without prophylaxis. Although mechanical prophylaxis can reduce postoperative VTE by approximately 50%, it is inferior to anticoagulant prophylaxis.

Prospective studies comparing prophylactically dosed low molecular weight heparin (LMWH) versus unfractionated heparin (UFH) for 7 to 10 days postoperatively in cancer patients have consistently shown equivalent efficacy and safety with VTE rates of approximately 15% and major bleeding incidents of approximately 4%. These findings formed the basis for recommendations that cancer patients should receive postoperative VTE prophylaxis for 7 to 10 days following major surgery.

There are compelling data to support extended DVT prophylaxis beyond 10 days following some types of cancer surgery (i.e., abdominal and pelvic). In the ENOXACAN II study, patients were randomized to receive prophylactic enoxaparin for 6 to 10 (routine prophylaxis) versus 25 to 31 days (extended prophylaxis) after curative open surgery for abdominal or pelvic malignancies (*N Engl J Med* 2002;346:975). The incidence of DVT was significantly different: 12% for routine and 4% for extended prophylaxis, while bleeding complications were comparable (3.6% and 4.7% respectively). On the basis of this, the 2012 American College of Chest Physicians (ACCP) guidelines recommend extended DVT prophylaxis with LMWH for patients undergoing abdominal/pelvic open surgery for cancer (*Chest* 2012;141:e227S).

There is limited consensus on prophylactic regimens following minor or less invasive surgeries. Patients undergoing laparoscopic colorectal, urologic, and gynecologic cancer surgeries have documented increased risk for VTE complications. Thus, 7 to 10 days of postoperative DVT prophylaxis with UFH or LMWH is reasonable until future studies determine the ideal prophylaxis schedule for this population.

Lastly, patients who undergo surgery for central nervous system neoplasms have one of the highest rates of postoperative VTE and lowest tolerance for bleeding complications. Several prospective randomized trials have validated the safety and efficacy of VTE prophylaxis with UFH and LMWH starting approximately 24 hours after surgery (*Br J Haematol* 2004;128:291–302). These findings are supported in the ACCP guidelines recommending pharmacologic prophylaxis following craniotomy in cancer patients (*Chest* 2012;141:e227S).

B. Prophylaxis against VTE in hospitalized cancer patients. All hospitalized oncology patients admitted for management of acute medical conditions or cancer therapy should be considered for mechanical or pharmacologic VTE prophylaxis. Unfortunately, there is a lack of data supporting these recommendations that are primarily based on studies in general hospitalized, acutely ill medical patients. Several prospective, randomized VTE prevention studies have confirmed the efficacy and safety of LMWH and UFH prophylaxis in acutely ill medical patients; however, cancer patients have comprised only 5% to 14% of these populations. A subset analysis of cancer patients in the MEDENOX (*N Engl J Med* 1999;341:793) study detected a 50% reduction in VTE risk in patients receiving enoxaparin versus placebo.

On the basis of the available data, the 2012 ACCP guidelines recommend UFH or LMWH for VTE prophylaxis in hospitalized cancer patients (*Chest* 2012;141:e227S). Temporary risk factors for bleeding complications, including invasive procedures or thrombocytopenia, may require interruption of anticoagulant prophylaxis. Substitution of mechanical devices until the bleeding risk is resolved should be pursued, and should not lead to complete avoidance of UFH or LMWH. Ambulation should also be conscientiously encouraged during hospitalization.

C. Prophylaxis in ambulatory cancer patients. Given the high risk of developing VTE in cancer patients, numerous investigators have assessed the efficacy of thromboprophylaxis. One smaller trial randomized patients with metastatic breast cancer receiving chemotherapy to warfarin 1 mg/day for 6 weeks followed by dose adjustment to an international normalized ratio (INR) target of 1.3 to 1.9 versus placebo showed an 85% reduction of symptomatic VTE in the treatment arm (incidence 0.16%/month vs. 0.7%/month, respectively) without a significant increase in bleeding (*Lancet* 1994;343:886). Two larger trials, the PROTECHT trial and the SAVE-ONCO trial, also showed a risk reduction in the incidence of VTE with thromboprophylaxis (*N Engl J Med* 2012;366:601) (*Lancet Oncol* 2009;10:943). In the PROTECHT trial, 1,166 patients with metastatic or locally advanced cancer were randomized in a 2:1 manner to prophylaxis with nadroparin versus placebo, starting on day 1 of chemotherapy to a maximum of 4 months. Patients receiving nadroparin had a significant reduction in the risk of VTE with an incidence of 1.4% compared to 2.9% in the placebo arm. The SAVE-ONCO trial was the largest of the three trials, randomizing 3,212 patients with metastatic or locally advanced cancer to prophylaxis with semuloparin versus placebo, starting on day 1 of chemotherapy to a maximum of 4 months. The primary outcome was development of any VTE or VTE-related death, and the study revealed a 64% risk reduction in patients receiving semuloparin (HR 0.36; 95% CI 0.21 to 0.60).

Despite the efficacy and safety of primary VTE prophylaxis in the cancer population, routine primary VTE prophylaxis with anticoagulants during chemotherapy is not currently recommend. This is likely in part due to the overall low occurrence of VTE in the available studies, and the concern of increased risk of bleeding in cancer patients receiving chemotherapy. However, guidelines do recommend consideration of LMWH prophylaxis on a case-by-case basis in selected cancer patients with highest risk of VTE, accompanied by a thorough risk–benefit description. Additionally, patients with multiple myeloma receiving thalidomide- or lenalidomide-based therapy and/or dexamethasone have been documented to have an exceedingly high risk of VTE. Therefore, the guidelines do recommend pharmacologic prophylaxis with either aspirin 81 mg or prophylactic dose of LMWH in this unique population.

V. CVC AND THROMBOSIS. Percutaneous inserted CVCs and port-a-caths provide reliable venous access for blood collection, as well as administration of chemotherapy, medications, and blood components to cancer patients. However, it is associated with several complications, one of which is thrombosis (including occluded catheter lumen, external catheter fibrin sheath, and partial or occlusive venous thrombus). The reported frequencies of symptomatic upper extremity DVT associated with CVC in cancer patients not using prophylactic anticoagulants decreased from approximately 38% (*Ann Intern Med* 1990;112:423) in the 1990s to around 4% in more recent years (*J Clin Oncol* 2005;23:4057), most likely reflecting refinements in catheter materials and insertion techniques. Although earlier randomized control trials (RCTs) have demonstrated a significant reduction in venography-confirmed upper extremity DVTs with either warfarin 1.0 mg/day or dalteparin 2,500 IU/day, further RCTs have failed to show a significant reduction of asymptomatic or symptomatic CVC-associated DVTs with warfarin 1.0 mg/day, enoxaparin 40 mg/day, or dalteparin 5,000 IU/day compared with placebo. On the basis of the results of these contemporary studies, the 2012 ACCP guidelines do not recommend routine anticoagulant DVT prophylaxis for cancer patients with CVCs. Patients with hematologic malignancies treated with intensive chemotherapeutic regimens appear to have a 2- to 4-fold higher risk of CVC-associated symptomatic DVTs compared to patients receiving outpatient chemotherapy for solid tumors. However, studies evaluating the risks and benefits of DVT prophylaxis in the population with hematologic malignancies have not been published, and routine anticoagulation is not recommended. Although several cohort studies have shown an increased relative risk of CVC-associated DVT in cancer patients who are also heterozygous for factor V Leiden or prothrombin gene G20210A mutation, routine screening for these inherited thrombophilia risk factors in cancer patients without a VTE history is not recommended.

Optimal treatment for symptomatic CVC-associated DVTs is controversial. While the risk of symptomatic pulmonary embolism (PE) appears to be low, it remains a potentially fatal complication. Because of the lack of high-quality evidence, expert opinions have been used to guide routine practices. It is now thought that catheters can remain in place as long as it is still needed, functional, and with no other compelling reason for removal such as infections. Catheter should be removed whenever it is not needed or not functional. It is recommended to continue anticoagulation as long as the catheter is present, until 3 months after removal of the catheter, unless if bleeding risk is unacceptable. Current studies are underway to investigate whether shorter duration of anticoagulation (4 to 6 weeks) is appropriate after catheter removal.

VI. DIAGNOSIS AND TREATMENT OF VTE IN CANCER PATIENTS

    A. Diagnosis of VTE. Although the combination of a low clinical assessment score and a negative quantitative D-dimer result has been validated for ruling out VTE in patients with a low risk of thrombosis, this strategy should be used with great caution in cancer patients suspected of VTE. In cancer patients, a higher underlying prevalence of VTE may produce an unacceptably high false-negative rate and low negative predictive value using the same decision rule. In addition, D-dimer is typically elevated in cancer patients in the absence of an underlying VTE, producing a high false-positive rate and a low positive predictive value for the detection of VTE. A clinical suspicion for VTE in cancer patients requires sensitive imaging studies, guided by the presenting signs and symptoms, to assess for VTE. The noninvasive imaging techniques, including lower extremity duplex ultrasonography, spiral chest CT, and ventilation–perfusion scan, are likely to have similar sensitivities and specificities for the detection of DVT and PE in cancer patients as have been reported in patients without underlying malignancies.

        CVC-associated upper extremity DVTs tend to be more centrally located, and ultrasonographic techniques have consistently been shown to have suboptimal sensitivities (ranging from 56% to 94%) with specificities of 100%. Therefore, although a positive upper extremity duplex color ultrasonographic study confirms a suspected CVC-associated DVT, a negative study in the setting of high suspicion requires more sensitive imaging techniques such as venography, CT, or magnetic resonance imaging to rule out a thrombus.

B. Therapy of VTE in patients with cancer

1. **Special issues in patients with cancer.** Three important issues related to treatment of cancer-associated VTE are the safety, type, and duration of anticoagulation therapy. The only absolute contraindication to therapeutic anticoagulation is active bleeding that cannot be rapidly and reliably controlled. However, the bleeding risk can be difficult to predict in a quantitative manner for each individual patient. Treatment of VTEs in patients with primary and metastatic brain tumors is particularly challenging, due to the potentially devastating complications of intracranial hemorrhage associated with anticoagulation therapy, the high risk of recurrent VTE, and the inadequacy of high-quality evidence to guide management. Therapeutic anticoagulation is considered by some oncologists and neurosurgeons to be an absolute contraindication in patients with highly vascular brain metastases or recent craniotomies. For patients in whom the benefit of anticoagulation therapy is judged to outweigh the risk, one approach involves cautious initiation of continuous infusion of UFH, and, if tolerated, to switch to other long-term anticoagulation therapy such as LMWH.

   Thrombocytopenia, either cancer related or secondary to chemotherapy, complicates anticoagulation therapy. While data to define an evidence-based, safe, minimal platelet count are not available, expert opinions and anecdotal clinical experiences support the safety of therapeutic anticoagulation when the platelet count is >50,000/μL. When the platelet count drops below this level, lower intensity or interruption of chronic anticoagulation should be considered.

2. **Role of inferior vena cava (IVC) filters.** IVC filters are used to prevent development of a PE in patients with acute, lower extremity DVT when anticoagulation cannot be safely administered. Placement of an IVC filter is an option in cancer patients with acute lower extremity DVT and unacceptable bleeding risk or active bleeding. However, IVC filters are thrombogenic, and over time increase the risk of lower extremity DVT. Therefore, a retrievable filter should be used whenever possible, with reinitiation of anticoagulation and removal of the filter once the risk of acute bleeding has resolved.

3. **Role of thrombolytic therapy.** Indications for thrombolytic therapy in cancer patients with VTE are limited due to the increased risk of bleeding, especially in patients with brain tumors. Use should be considered for a PE causing severe hemodynamic instability, a DVT causing arterial insufficiency due to severe venous congestion, clinically significant extension of a thrombus despite therapeutic anticoagulation, and an occluded CVC that must be kept patent.

4. **Initial treatment of VTE.** Options for initial anticoagulation in cancer patients include continuous UFH, LMWH, and fondaparinux. The traditional approach was initial anticoagulation with UFH, using activated partial thromboplastin time (aPTT) for therapeutic monitoring, and concurrent warfarin until two therapeutic INRs (2 to 3) were obtained ≥24 hours apart, at which time UFH was stopped. Subgroup analyses of cancer patients initially treated with LMWH versus UFH for acute VTE showed similar efficacy for VTE recurrence. However, LMWH is now the preferred initial anticoagulant in cancer patients due to the ease of administration, ability to use in the outpatient setting, elimination of need for therapeutic monitoring, and lower risk of heparin-induced thrombocytopenia (HIT). In a study comparing twice-daily (1 mg/kg) versus once-daily (1.5 mg/kg) dosing of enoxaparin for acute VTE, the cancer patient subgroup had a nonsignificant higher VTE recurrence rate with once-daily dosing (12.2%) compared with twice-daily dosing (6.4%) (*Ann Intern Med* 2001;134:191). Limited data exist on the use of fondaparinux in cancer patients. Limitations include its long half-life (17 to 21 hours), 100% renal clearance, and inability to reverse. However, small studies have shown the safety of fondaparinux in patients with HIT. In summary, LMWH is the recommended treatment of choice for initial management of acute VTE in patients with cancer. UFH should be considered in patients with severe renal insufficiency (CrCl [creatinine

clearance] <30 mL/minute), while fondaparinux can be considered for patients with active or a history of HIT.

5. **Long-term anticoagulation for VTE in patients with cancer.** While oral vitamin K antagonists (VKA) are the standard for treatment and secondary prevention of VTE in noncancer patients, they pose several dilemmas in cancer patients. Cancer patients have more thrombotic recurrences (fourfold higher) and bleeding complications (twofold higher) than patients without malignancies during long-term VKA therapy. It translates into cumulative recurrent VTE and bleeding incidences of 20% and 12%, respectively, after 1 year of anticoagulation therapy (*Blood* 2002;100:3484). Additionally, VKAs require frequent therapeutic monitoring, have a slow onset and offset of action, depend on adequate gastric absorption, and have numerous food and medication interactions.

Several prospective, randomized, open-label studies have shown that LMWH is superior to VKAs in long-term management of VTE in cancer patients. The largest of these trials, the CLOT trial, randomized cancer patients to VKA versus dalteparin (LMWH) for 6 months following diagnosis of a first symptomatic VTE (*N Engl J Med* 2003;349:146). Patients receiving LMWH had a 52% reduction in VTE recurrence and no significant difference in major bleeding compared to those receiving VKA. A meta-analysis supported these findings when combing the results of eight prospective, randomized trials, reporting an overall 53% reduction in risk of recurrent VTE with LMWH compared to VKA (HR 0.47; 95% CI 0.32 to 0.71) (*Cochrane Database Syst Rev* 2008:CD006650). The same meta-analysis found no difference in rates of bleeding or overall mortality between the two groups.

Based on the aforementioned evidence, the 2012 ACCP, 2013 ASCO, and the National Comprehensive Cancer Network, all recommend chronic anticoagulation with LMWH when possible for treatment of DVT or PE in cancer patients.

Novel oral anticoagulants (NOACs) such as rivaroxaban (Xarelto), dabigatran (Pradaxa), and apixaban (Eliquis) were approved for VTE and stroke prevention and VTE treatment in recent years. Among them, rivaroxaban is the only FDA-approved NOAC for VTE treatment in the general population currently. NOACs are attractive options in the cancer population, with their oral formulation, no need of monitoring, and less interactions with drug and diet. However, in all pivotal phase III trials leading to drug approval, cancer patients only constituted a small proportion of the enrollees. In addition, NOACs have not had head-to-head comparison with LMWH as the treatment of VTE, the superior and standard therapy for cancer patients. Given the lack of high-quality data, at the current time, major guidelines including ACCP, ASCO, and NCCN all recommend against routine use of NOAC for the treatment of VTE in the cancer population, and advocate further dedicated studies.

6. **Duration of anticoagulation in cancer patients with VTE.** The duration of anticoagulation in cancer patients must be individualized. In general, if cancer treatment leads to cure or durable remission, 3 to 6 months is appropriate. In the setting of ongoing active malignancy, the risk of recurrence is much higher, and consideration of long-term anticoagulation is appropriate and often used.

7. **Treatment of incidental VTE.** Incidental VTEs (VTE found incidentally on imaging studies without symptoms) are common in the cancer population, given the baseline high risk of thrombosis and the frequency of imaging studies for cancer staging. Several retrospective studies showed that 35% to 50% of DVTs and PEs were incidentally discovered in cancer patients. The need of treatment for incidental VTEs has been questioned, given the lack of symptoms. However, many studies have revealed that rates of VTE recurrence, bleeding, and mortality are similar in cancer patients with incidental VTE compared to those with symptomatic VTE. Therefore, expert consensus recommends the same treatment for incidental VTE as compared with symptomatic VTE.

8. **Thrombosis despite anticoagulation.** Cancer patients commonly have recurrent VTE despite anticoagulation. Approximately 10% to 17% of cancer patients on warfarin and 6% to 9% on LMWH will have recurrent VTE (*N Engl J Med* 2003;349:146). There is no standard therapy for patients with recurrent VTE despite anticoagulation, since no high-quality evidence is available. In this setting, it is important to first confirm compliance and rule out HIT. In the case of true failure of therapeutic anticoagulation, various treatment strategies have been employed, including switching anticoagulation from warfarin to LMWH (if the patient were to be on warfarin at the time of VTE recurrence), switching to a different type of LMWH (if the patient were to be on LMWH at the time of VTE recurrence), increasing the dose of LMWH, placement of IVC filter, addition of antiplatelet agents such as aspirin, or a combination of these methods. Studies are needed for optimal management of this group of challenging patients.

SUGGESTED READINGS

Agnelli G, George DJ, Kakkar AK, et al. Semuloparin for thromboprophylaxis in patients receiving chemotherapy for cancer. *N Engl J Med* 2012;366:601–609.

Agnelli G, Gussoni G, Bianchini C, et al. Nadroparin for the prevention of thromboembolic events in ambulatory patients with metastatic or locally advanced solid cancer receiving chemotherapy: a randomised, placebo-controlled, double-blind study. *Lancet Oncol* 2009;10:943–949.

Blom JW, Doggen CJ, Osanto S, et al. Malignancies, prothrombotic mutations, and the risk of venous thrombosis. *JAMA* 2005;293:715–722.

den Exter PL, Hooijer J, Dekkers OM, et al. Risk of recurrent venous thromboembolism and mortality in patients with cancer incidentally diagnosed with pulmonary embolism: a comparison with symptomatic patients. *J Clin Oncol* 2011;29:2405–2409.

Falanga A. Thrombophilia in cancer: semin thrombosis. *Hemostasis* 2005;31:104–110.

Geerts WH, Pineo GF, Heit JA, et al. Prevention of venous thromboembolism: the Seventh ACCP Conference on Antithrombotic and Thrombolytic Therapy. *Chest* 2004;126:338S–400S.

Khorana AA, Kuderer NM, Culakova E, et al. Development and validation of a predictive model for chemotherapy-associated thrombosis. *Blood* 2008;111:4902–4907.

Lee AY, Levine MN, Baker RI, et al. Low-molecular-weight heparin versus a coumarin for the prevention of recurrent venous thromboembolism in patients with cancer. *N Engl J Med* 2003;349:146–153.

Lee AY. Management of thrombosis in cancer: primary prevention and secondary prophylaxis. *Br J Haematol* 2004;128:291–302.

Lyman GH, Khorana AA, Kuderer NM, et al. Venous thromboembolism prophylaxis and treatment in patients with cancer: American Society of Clinical Oncology clinical practice guideline update. *J Clin Oncol* 2013;31:2189–2204.

Piccioli A, Lensing AW, Prins MH, et al. Extensive screening for occult malignant disease in idiopathic venous thromboembolism: a prospective randomized clinical trial. *Journal of thrombosis and haemostasis. JTH* 2004;2:884–889.

Prandoni P, Lensing AW, Buller HR, et al. Deep-vein thrombosis and the incidence of subsequent symptomatic cancer. *N Engl J Med* 1992;327:1128–1133.

Prandoni P, Lensing AW, Piccioli A, et al. Recurrent venous thromboembolism and bleeding complications during anticoagulant treatment in patients with cancer and venous thrombosis. *Blood* 2002;100:3484–3488.

37 Growth Factor Support in Oncology

Melissa Rooney • Janelle Mann

I. **INTRODUCTION.** Myelosuppression is one of the most common dose-limiting toxicities of cytotoxic agents. An understanding of hematopoiesis and the roles of growth factors can significantly improve complications of treatment. Hematopoiesis is the process of production multiplication and specialization of blood cells in the bone marrow. The proliferation and differentiation of the pluripotent stem cell to the myeloid and the lymphoid progenitors and the further differentiation of those to the mature circulating blood cells involve complex interaction of the stem cells, bone marrow stromal cells, and cytokines. The cytokines also activate the mature hematopoietic cells. Hematopoietic growth factors' action and effect on cell lines are still not fully understood; however, some identified growth factors and potential therapeutic options are described later.

II. **MYELOID GROWTH FACTORS**

A. **Granulocyte colony-stimulating factor (G-CSF)**

1. **Endogenous G-CSF.** G-CSF is a glycoprotein secreted by monocytes, fibroblasts, and endothelial cells. It targets G-CSF receptors on myeloid precursor cells in the bone marrow, promotes the maturation of the granulocyte colony-forming unit to the polymorphonuclear leukocyte, and enhances neutrophil function.

2. **Recombinant preparations (rHuG-CSF).** Filgrastim (Neupogen and Granix) and pegfilgrastim (Neulasta) are the two currently available formulations of recombinant G-CSF in the United States. Filgrastim and pegfilgrastim function through the same mechanism of action promoting neutrophil proliferation, differentiation, and activation. Filgrastim has a half-life of 3.5 hours. Pegfilgrastim, which is a covalent conjugate of filgrastim and monomethoxypolyethylene glycol, has a prolonged half-life of 15 to 80 hours.

3. **Recommended dose.** The recommended dose of filgrastim is 5 μg/kg administered subcutaneously daily until an absolute neutrophil count (ANC) of 10,000/mm³ has been reached following a chemotherapy-induced nadir. When filgrastim is used following high-dose chemotherapy with autologous stem cell rescue, a higher dose of filgrastim of 10 μg/kg daily is recommended. When used in this setting, filgrastim should be continued until an ANC of 1,000/mm³ is reached on three consecutive days. The dose of filgrastim should then be reduced to 5 μg/kg subcutaneously daily until ANC remains >1,000/mm³ for three consecutive days at which therapy can be discontinued. When filgrastim is utilized in stem cell mobilization and collection prior to stem cell transplantation, filgrastim is administered at a dose of 10 μg/kg daily 4 days prior to apheresis and continued until the stem cell collection is complete. Of note, filgrastim should not be administered within 24 hours from the administration of cytotoxic chemotherapy because of the potential cellular toxicities to rapidly dividing myeloid cells. Filgrastim administration should also be avoided in patients receiving concurrent chemotherapy with radiation to the chest.

   Pegfilgrastim is administered at a dose of 6 mg given subcutaneously, one time 24 to 72 hours following the administration of chemotherapy, and at least 14 days prior to the initiation of subsequent doses of chemotherapy. The safety and efficacy of pegfilgrastim in the setting of concurrent chemotherapy and radiation have not been established. Pegfilgrastim is not currently indicated for stem cell mobilization (*J Clin Oncol* 2006;24:4451).

   Filgrastim and pegfilgrastim doses do not need to be adjusted for renal or hepatic function.

4. **Adverse effects.** The most common adverse reactions associated with the use of recombinant G-CSF include bone pain, fever, and injection-site reactions. Rare adverse reactions including splenic rupture, adult respiratory distress syndrome (ARDS), and alveolar hemorrhage have also been reported. In patients with sickle cell anemia, the use of recombinant G-CSF has been associated with severe and potentially fatal sickle cell crisis (*Blood* 2001;97:3998). Allergic reactions of varying severity are also described with the use of recombinant G-CSF.

B. **Granulocyte–macrophage colony-stimulating factor (GM-CSF)**
1. **Endogenous GM-CSF.** GM-CSF is a protein that stimulates stem cell precursors to produce all types of white blood cells including neutrophils, lymphocytes, eosinophils, basophils, and monocytes. GM-CSF also enhances neutrophil and monocyte/macrophage function.
2. **Recombinant granulocyte–macrophage colony-stimulating factor (rHuGM-CSF).** Sargramostim (Leukine) is the only rHuGM-CSF formulation available in the United States. Administration of rHuGM-CSF results in increased production, differentiation, and activation of neutrophils, eosinophils, monocytes, and macrophages. When administered subcutaneously, sargramostim has a half-life of 2.7 hours.
3. **Recommended dose.** The recommended dose of sargramostim is 250 $\mu g/m^2$/day for all indicated treatment settings. Subcutaneous and intravenous dosing are available; however, subcutaneous dosing is the preferred route of administration. Sargramostim is indicated following induction chemotherapy for AML in adults ≥55 years old, engraftment failure or delay following bone marrow transplant, myeloid reconstitution following autologous or allogeneic bone marrow transplant, and stem cell mobilization. In the setting of primary prophylaxis of neutropenia in patients receiving chemotherapy, GM-CSF is administered off label, 24 to 72 hours after chemotherapy, and is discontinued once the ANC has recovered to 10,000/mm^3 or the ANC is more than 1,500/mm^3 for 3 days. GM-CSF is contraindicated 24 hours preceding and following chemotherapy and radiation therapy. Hepatic and renal function should be monitored closely during the administration of sargramostim.
4. **Adverse effects.** The most common adverse effects associated with sargramostim include fever, headaches, diarrhea, bone pain, myalgias, arthralgias, and injection-site reactions. Fluid retention manifested by edema, capillary leak syndrome, pleural effusion, and pericardial effusion have also been reported. Sargramostim is contraindicated in patients with myeloid blast counts exceeding 10% in the peripheral blood or bone marrow. Allergic reactions to sargramostim are uncommon, but severe anaphylactic reactions have been described. Sargramostim is contraindicated in patients with previous reactions to GM-CSF, other products derived from yeast, or any of the other ingredients used to make sargramostim. In addition, a rare constellation of symptoms consisting of respiratory distress, hypoxia, hypotension, flushing, and tachycardia may be seen following the first dose of sargramostim. The "first dose" reaction is treated with supportive care and does not typically recur with subsequent doses.

C. **Clinical applications of myeloid growth factors.** The current recommendations for the use of colony-stimulating factors are based on the 2005 American Society of Clinical Oncology (ASCO) clinical practice guidelines (*J Clin Oncol* 2006;24:3187).
1. **Primary prophylaxis.** An initial risk assessment for chemotherapy-induced neutropenic fever should be performed prior to the first cycle of chemotherapy. When performing a thorough risk assessment, factors including the patient's underlying disease, planned chemotherapeutic drug regimen, treatment intent, and individual patient risk factors must be considered. Primary prophylaxis is recommended for chemotherapeutic regimens with a high risk (>20%) of inducing neutropenic fevers. A list of chemotherapeutic drug regimens associated with a >20% risk of neutropenic fevers are conveniently located in the NCCN guidelines on growth factor support. All dose-dense regimens require the use of growth factor support. In addition to considering the chemotherapeutic regimen, certain patient factors are known to predispose

individuals to a higher rate of neutropenic fevers and include older age (>65 years old), poor performance status, poor nutritional status, prior chemotherapy or radiation, and comorbid conditions (renal dysfunction, liver dysfunction, recent infection, and recent surgery). In patients with high-risk features, primary prophylaxis may be considered in chemotherapeutic regimens with a risk of febrile neutropenia of less than 20%. Lastly, the treatment intent must be considered as growth factor support may avoid treatment delays in curative settings.

2. **Secondary prophylaxis.** For patients who experience a neutropenic complication from an earlier cycle of chemotherapy (for which primary prophylaxis was not administered), secondary prophylaxis with CSFs is recommended in situations in which dose reduction or delay may compromise disease-free survival, overall survival, or treatment outcomes.

3. **Afebrile neutropenia.** CSFs should not routinely be administered for afebrile patients with neutropenia.

4. **Febrile neutropenia.** The routine use of CSFs as an adjunct to antibiotic therapy in the setting of neutropenic fever is not currently recommended. The 2005 ASCO guidelines support the use of CSFs in patients with neutropenic fevers who are at high risk for infection-related complications (prolonged and profound neutropenia, age >65 years old, uncontrolled primary disease, pneumonia, hypotension, multiorgan dysfunction, invasive fungal infection, or development of fever during hospitalization). Additionally, the recently updated Infectious Disease Society of America (IDSA) guidelines from 2010 also do not recommend the routine use of CSFs as an adjunct to antibiotic therapy in neutropenic fever (*Clin Infect Dis* 2011;427).

5. **Dose-dense/dose-intense regimens.** Dose-dense/dose-intense regimens have been shown to increase disease-free and overall survival in the treatment of node-positive breast cancer, small cell lung cancer, and non-Hodgkin's lymphoma. In those situations, it is appropriate to use CSFs to maintain the use of dose-dense/dose-intense chemotherapy regimen (*J Clin Oncol* 2006;24:3187).

6. **Bone marrow transplant.** CSFs are routinely used in conjunction with chemotherapy to mobilize peripheral stem cells. CSFs are recommended following autologous stem cell transplant, but not allogeneic stem cell transplant.

7. **Acute myeloid leukemia (AML).** The administration of CSFs following induction chemotherapy for AML can decrease the duration of neutropenia when begun shortly after chemotherapy; however, studies have not consistently shown a positive impact on the duration of hospitalization and incidence of severe infections. CSFs following induction chemotherapy in AML are considered reasonable, and may have the most benefit in patients over the age of 55 years old. In the setting of consolidative therapy for AML, CSFs are recommended following chemotherapy, as CSFs have convincingly been shown to decrease the incidence of infection and decrease hospitalization rates. There is also a more pronounced shortening of the duration of neutropenia following consolidative chemotherapy when compared with induction chemotherapy. There are currently no data surrounding the use of pegylated CSFs in patients with myeloid leukemias, and so their use in this setting is not recommended at this time. The use of CSFs for priming of leukemia cells is also not recommended.

8. **Acute lymphoid leukemia (ALL).** CSFs are recommended following the completion of induction or first postremission course of therapy as this has been shown to shorten the duration of neutropenia (<1,000/mm^3) by approximately one week. Although G-CSF has been shown to shorten the duration of neutropenia, the data have not been consistent relating to G-CSFs' effect on the duration of hospitalization, incidence of febrile neutropenia, or incidence of severe infections. G-CSF can be given concurrently with corticosteroids/antimetabolite therapies as the combination of drug therapies does not appear to prolong myelosuppression induced by chemotherapy.

9. **Myelodysplastic syndromes.** CSFs can increase ANC; however, there is no data supporting long-term continuous use. Intermittent administration may be considered in the subset of patients with severe neutropenia and recurrent infection.

10. **Concomitant chemoradiotherapy.** CSFs should be avoided in patients receiving concurrent chemotherapy and radiation therapy, especially involving the mediastinum. CSF use can be considered in patients receiving radiation therapy alone, if prolonged treatment delays secondary to neutropenia are expected.

III. ERYTHROID GROWTH FACTORS

A. Erythropoietin (EPO)

1. **Endogenous EPO.** EPO is a glycoprotein hormone that regulates red blood cell production by stimulating erythroid colony-forming units to proliferate and maturate, which is essential for erythroid cell maturation. Healthy individuals require 5 to 30 mU/mL of EPO to maintain a normal hemoglobin and hematocrit. Under normal circumstances, EPO increases in the setting of hypoxia or anemia. In patients receiving chemotherapy, inappropriately low and high concentrations of EPO can occur.

2. **Recombinant erythropoietin (rHuEPO).** Currently there are two preparations of recombinant EPO, erythropoiesis-stimulating agents (ESAs) available in the United States, epoetin alfa (Epogen and Procrit) and the hyperglycosylated recombinant EPO, darbepoetin alfa (Aranesp). ESAs exert their effect on erythroid progenitors, leading to induction, proliferation, and differentiation. This results in an increase in reticulocyte counts, followed by a rise in hematocrit and hemoglobin levels. Epoetin alfa has a half-life of approximately 16 to 67 hours when given subcutaneously compared with darbepoetin alfa that has a half-life of 24 to 144 hours for cancer patients.

3. **Recommended dose.** It is imperative to appropriately select patients for the use of ESA therapy given increased risks associated with the use of these products. On the basis of the 2010 ASCO/ASH guidelines and the FDA guidelines for ESA use, ESAs are recommended as a treatment option for chemotherapy-induced anemia and patients with an hgb≤10 g/dL (ASCO/ASH guidelines). In patients with a declining hemoglobin, ≤12 g/dL but ≥10 g/dL, initiation of ESA therapy should be determined by clinical circumstances. Patients must be enrolled in the FDA risk evaluation mitigation (REMS) program, APPRAISE, prior to initiating therapy.

The recommended starting dose of epoetin is 150 U/kg subcutaneously three times weekly for 4 weeks, with a possible increase in dose level to 300 U/kg three times weekly for an additional 4 to 8 weeks in those who do not respond to the initial dose. An alternative weekly dosing regimen (40,000 U/week) based on common clinical practice may be considered, although this is supported by lower level evidence. Dose escalation to 60,000 U/week may also be considered in patients who do not respond to the initial dose. Darbepoetin alfa is also approved for the management of chemotherapy-induced anemia. The recommended starting dose for darbepoetin alfa is 2.25 µg/kg subcutaneously weekly or 500 µg subcutaneously once every 3 weeks. In the setting of inadequate response in hemoglobin (≤/= 1 g/dL increase and below 10 g/dL after initial 6 weeks), the dose should be increased to 4.5 µg/kg weekly. For the every 3-week regimen, there is no current recommendation to increase the dose.

If the rate of hemoglobin increase is more than 1 g/dL in a 2-week period or hemoglobin reaches a level sufficient to avoid red blood cell transfusions, the dose of epoetin should be decreased by 25% and the dose of darbepoetin should be decreased by 40%.

If the rise in hemoglobin is less than 1 g/dL at 8 weeks of treatment, the ESA should be discontinued, and an evaluation for iron deficiency and tumor progression should be considered.

The dose of EPO should be withheld if hemoglobin exceeds a level sufficient to avoid red blood cell transfusion or =12 g/dL, and therapy can be restarted when the hemoglobin falls to 10 g/dL. When restarting epoetin alfa, reduce the previous dose by 25% and resume treatment with darbepoetin alfa with a 40% dose reduction.

4. **Clinical indications.** In patients with nonmyeloid malignancies, EPO is indicated for the treatment of anemia due to the effect of concomitantly administered chemotherapy. EPO therapy should be discontinued once chemotherapy is stopped, regardless of hemoglobin. The role of ESAs in anemia due to myelodysplastic syndrome is under debate, and ESAs are not currently FDA approved for these indications.

5. **Adverse effects.** Common adverse effects with EPO therapy include edema, high blood pressure, fever, headache, insomnia, rash, nausea, vomiting, injection-site reaction, arthralgia, myalgias, fatigue, cough, and dyspnea. Less commonly reported but potential adverse effects include chest pain, arrhythmia, diarrhea, seizure, and thromboembolic events. A rare but serious adverse event is antibody-mediated pure red cell aplasia (PRCA) leading to severe anemia. Patients who develop a loss of response to ESAs should be evaluated for PRCA, and these drugs should be discontinued. Additionally, iron deficiency is common during ESA administration, which is a result of the consumption of available iron stores and decline in transfusion rate.

In 2007, the FDA required ESA therapy labeling changes to include a new black box warning. The black box warning indicates that ESAs can increase the risk of thromboembolic events, serious cardiovascular events, and death when administered to patients with a goal hemoglobin greater than 12 g/dL. Several studies have shown shortened time to tumor progression, specifically in patients with advanced breast, cervical, head and neck, lymphoid, and nonsmall cell lung cancer in patients receiving ESA therapy with a target hemoglobin $\geq$10 g/dL. (*J Clin Oncol* 2010:4996) Additionally, ESA therapy is no longer indicated for patients receiving myelosuppressive chemotherapy with curative intent owing to increased risk of thromboembolic events.

As a requirement of the REMS program, access to these medications is restricted. Healthcare providers and hospitals must be enrolled in the ESA APPRISE Oncology Program to prescribe or dispense ESAs to patients with cancer.

IV. PLATELET AND MEGAKARYOCYTIC GROWTH FACTORS

A. **Thrombopoietin (TPO)**

1. **Endogenous TPO.** TPO stimulates growth and maturation of megakaryocyte-erythroid progenitor cells into mature megakaryocytes. Normally 10^{11} platelets are produced daily, with platelets having a lifespan of 8 to 9 days in circulation. TPO is produced in the liver primarily and is regulated through the TPO receptors available for binding on platelets (*Transfusion* 2002;42:321). In the setting of thrombocytopenia, TPO levels are high due to decreased production. Intermittent platelet transfusions in the thrombocytopenic patient may actually blunt the TPO response (*N Engl J Med* 1998;339:746).

2. **TPO receptor agonist.** The initial thrombopoietic agents were recombinant and pegylated human megakaryocyte growth factor. Although initially promising, development of antibodies against endogenous TPO resulted in refractory thrombocytopenia. Romiplostim (NPlate) and eltrombopag (Promacta) are synthetic second-generation platelet-stimulating agents that are currently FDA approved for the treatment of chronic idiopathic thrombocytopenia purpura (ITP), but may have a potential role for chemotherapy-induced thrombocytopenia. Second-generation agents are still under research and safety concerns still exist with these agents, including risk of thrombosis, rebound thrombocytopenia, and formation of bone marrow reticulin (*Curr Opin Oncol* 2008;20:690).

B. **Oprelvekin (neumega).** Interleukin (IL)-11 is a thrombopoietic growth factor that directly stimulates the proliferation of hematopoietic stem cells at various steps in the hematopoiesis process including the megakaryocyte progenitor cells, which induces megakaryocyte maturation resulting in increased platelet production. Oprelvekin, recombinant IL-11, was the first cytokine to reach the market with the indication of prevention of chemotherapy-induced thrombocytopenia. Early clinical trials in cancer patients have shown increased steady-state platelet counts and to reduce the risk of thrombocytopenia from chemotherapy (*J Clin Oncol* 1997;15:3368). The dose is 50 µg/kg/day, given subcutaneously starting 24 hours after chemotherapy, until the postnadir platelet count is greater than 50,000/µL or 48 hours before beginning the next cycle of chemotherapy. Dose adjustments are recommended in patients with impaired renal function, CrCl </= 30 mL/min. The most common side effects associated with oprelvekin treatment include peripheral edema, dyspnea, tachycardia, atrial arrhythmia, papilledema, and conjunctival redness. Reversible dilutional anemia may occur within 3–5 days of starting therapy owing to increased plasma volume, and this resolves over one week following discontinuation. Allergic or hypersensitivity reactions have been reported, and if they develop therapy should be discontinued permanently.

V. FUTURE DIRECTIONS. A better understanding of stem cell trafficking is essential to the development of newer agents that will potentiate the effects of the currently available CSFs. Newer EPO and TPO agonists are currently in development. Efforts are being made to develop oral, longer acting agents that could possibly be incorporated into the treatment of chemotherapy-induced anemia and thrombocytopenia.

SUGGESTED READINGS

Freifeld AG, Bow EJ, Sepkowitz KA, et al. Clinical practice guideline for the use of antimicrobial agents in neutropenic patients with cancer: 2010 Update by the Infectious Diseases Society of America. *Clin Infect Dis* 2011;52:427–431.

Levy B, Arnason JE, Bussel JB. The use of second-generation thrombopoietic agents for chemotherapy-induced thrombocytopenia. *Curr Opin Oncol* 2008;20:690–696.

Rizzo JD, Brouwers M, Hurley P, et al. American Soceity of Clinical Oncology/American Society of Hematology Clinical Practice Guideline Update on the Use of Epoetin and Darbepoetin in Adult Patients with Cancer. *J Clin Oncol* 2010;28:4996–5010.

Smith TJ, Khatcheressian J, et al. Update of Recommendations for the Use of White Blood Cell Growth Factors: An Evidence-Based Clinical Practice Guidelines. *J Clin Oncol* 2006;24:3187–3205.

38 Oncologic Emergencies
Manik Amin

I. METABOLIC EMERGENCIES

A. Hypercalcemia

1. **Pathophysiology.** Most common cancers associated with hypercalcemia are breast cancer, lung cancer, and multiple myeloma. Patients with hypercalcemia of malignancy often have poor prognosis. Hypercalcemia of malignancy results from three main mechanisms: (1) secretion of a PTHrP, (2) local osteolytic activity, and (3) abnormal production of 1,25-dihydroxyvitamin D (Calcitrol). Humoral secretion of PTHrP accounts for more than 70% of patients with hypercalcemia of malignancy and is seen in a variety of cancers such as squamous cell cancer (e.g., of head and neck, esophagus, cervix, or lung), renal cancer, ovarian cancer, endometrial cancer, non-Hodgkin's lymphoma, and breast cancer. Malignant hypercalcemia due to osteolytic activity is seen in approximately 20% of patients with hypercalcemia of malignancy and is mediated by osteoclasts and is a complex interplay between RANKL/RANK interaction/activation and cytokine production. It usually develops in patients with extensive skeletal metastases (e.g., breast cancer, lung cancer, prostate cancer, or multiple myeloma). In Hodgkin's lymphoma and few non-Hodgkin's lymphoma, malignant lymphocytes secrete the active form of vitamin D, 1, 25-dihydroxyvitamin D, resulting in increased osteoclastic bone resorption and intestinal absorption of calcium resulting in hypercalcemia.

2. **Signs and symptoms.** Patients with mild hypercalcemia, with calcium levels less than 12 mg/dL, are usually asymptomatic or may have nonspecific symptoms such as constipation and fatigue. Symptoms generally develop at serum calcium levels greater than 12 mg/dL and depend upon the acute rise in serum calcium concentration. Serum calcium levels between 12 and 14 mg/dL developing over few months may be well tolerated by patients, whereas a sudden increase in the serum calcium levels may manifest with altered mental status. Patients with severe hypercalcemia

of more than 14 mg/dL usually present with nausea, vomiting, anorexia, abdominal pain, constipation, muscle weakness altered mental status, coma, and seizures. Patients usually develop renal dysfunction with dehydration, elevated creatinine, polyuria (from decreased concentrating ability in distal tubules), and polydipsia. Chronic hypercalcemia (from nonmalignant cause) may present as nephrogenic diabetes insipidus and nephrolithiasis. Long-standing hypercalcemia can also result in demineralization and frequent fractures of the long bones. Acute hypercalcemia, on the other hand, can cause myocardial damage leading to conduction abnormalities such as ventricular or supraventricular arrhythmias. Physical examination may reveal altered mental status, distended abdomen from ileus, and signs of dehydration. In the absence of prompt recognition and treatment, hypercalcemia can progress to renal failure, coma, and death.

3. **Workup.** The normal range for total serum calcium is 8.6 to 10.3 mg/dL (2.15 to 2.57 mM). About half the amount of the circulating calcium is bound by albumin, and the remaining unbound ionized calcium (normal range, 4.5 to 5.1 mg/dL) is responsible for the biologic functions. Since a low or high albumin level may result in an inaccurate ionized calcium level, the effective total calcium should be calculated with following formula: corrected Ca (mg/dL) = measured Ca (mg/dL) − albumin (g/dL) + 4.

In patients with hypercalcemia without malignancy, other causes of hypercalcemia should be considered such as primary hyperparathyroidism, thyrotoxicosis, adrenal insufficiency, 1, 25$(OH)^2$ vitamin D toxicity (through ingestion or granulomatous conversion), and inherited disorders of calcium metabolism. Patients with elevated PTH rather than PTHrpP are more likely to have primary hyperparathyroidism than malignant hypercalcemia. But if both Parathyroid hormone (PTH) and Parathyroid hormone-related protein (PTHrP) concentrations are high, then coexisting primary hyperparathyroidism along with hypercalcemia of malignancy are likely.

4. **Treatment.** The treatment of hypercalcemia depends on the serum calcium level and the symptoms. Asymptomatic or mildly symptomatic patients (calcium <12 mg/dL) may not require immediate treatment, whereas symptomatic patients or calcium >14 mg/dL irrespective of symptoms require aggressive treatment. The main goals of treatment are lowering the serum calcium and treatment of underlying disease. The treatment of severe hypercalcemia involves simultaneous administration of isotonic saline, calcitonin, and bisphosphonate (Table 38-1).

   a. **Volume expansion.** Patients should be rehydrated with isotonic saline at an initial rate of 200 to 300 mL/hour up to 2 to 3 L and then adjusted to maintain the urine output at 100 to 150 mL/hour. Saline infusion should be stopped in patients who develop fluid overload due to impaired renal function or heart failure and loop diuretics should be used. Loop diuretics not only reduce the volume load but also decrease calcium reabsorption in the loop of Henle. Potassium and magnesium should be carefully monitored and replaced as needed. Hypophosphatemia is common in hypercalcemia but should not be reple unless symptomatic, because an increase in the calcium × phosphorus product to 70 or more can cause precipitation of calcium salts in the kidney and other soft tissues.

   b. **Calcitonin.** Calcitonin decreases the serum calcium concentration by increasing renal calcium excretion and by decreasing bone resorption by osteoclasts. Salmon calcitonin (4 to 8 IU/kg) is usually administered intramuscularly or subcutaneously every 12 hours, with a dose increase to 6 to 8 IU/kg every 6 hours if needed. Nasal calcitonin is not efficacious in the treatment of hypercalcemia. Calcitonin works rapidly and usually decreases the serum calcium concentration by 1 to 2 mg/dL within 4 to 6 hours of administration. It is safe, nontoxic, and rapidly acting, but efficacy is limited to the first 48 hours, owing to the development of tachyphylaxis by receptor downregulation and hence may be used to manage severe hypercalcemia (serum calcium >14 mg/dL) before bisphosphonates reach full effect.

   c. **Intravenous bisphosphonates.** The bisphosphonates are nonhydrolyzable analogs of inorganic pyrophosphate, which adsorb to the surface of bone hydroxyapatite and inhibit calcium reabsorption by reducing the activity of the osteoclasts.

TABLE 38-1	Treatment of Hypercalcemia		
Hypercalcemia grade	**Treatment**	**Dose**	**Comment**
Mild hypercalcemia (calcium <12 mg/dL) Moderate hypercalcemia (calcium 12–14 mg/dL)	a. No immediate treatment required b. Avoid things that would increase calcium levels such as high calcium diet, prolonged inactivity, thiazide diuretics, etc. c. Maintain hydration with 6–8 glasses of water every day d. Treat the cause		If sudden rise in the calcium level is noted with altered mental changes, treat like severe hypercalcemia
Severe hypercalcemia (calcium >14 mg/dL)	Isotonic normal saline	Initial rate of 200–300 mL/h	Required for volume expansion
	Calcitonin	4 IU/kg	Can be repeated in 6–12 h
	Bisphosphonates-Zoledronic acid, Pamidronate	4 mg IV over 14 min 60–90 mg over 2 h	
	Loop diuretics	Dosing varies depending upon the requirement	Advised to use loop diuretics with concurrent renal failure or heart failure
	Glucocorticoids	Prednisone 20–40 mg a day	Usually used in patients with lymphoma, leukemia, or chronic granulomatous disease
	Dialysis	Frequency will vary depending upon the requirement	Recommended for severe hypercalcemia with acute mental status changes with end organ damage such as severe acute renal failure, heart failure, etc.

These drugs have become the agents of choice for malignancy-associated hypercalcemia, and can successfully control serum calcium in 80% to 90% of patients. They are more potent, but their maximum effects occur in 2 to 4 days and hence are given with isotonic saline and calcitonin. Current bisphosphonates of choice are intravenous pamidronate and zolendronic acid (ZA). ZA is a third-generation bisphosphonate and is administered at a dose of 4 mg i.v. over 15 minutes, whereas pamidronate can be used as either 60 or 90 mg over 24 hours. Other bisphosphonate as effective as pamidronate is Ibandronate given at the dose of 2 mg IV over 2 hours. The side effects of bisphosphonates are flulike symptoms (fever, arthralgia, fatigue, and bone pain), hypocalcaemia, hypophosphatemia, nephrotic syndrome, uveitis, and osteonecrosis of jaw. Clodronate and etidronate are first-generation bisphosphonates and are weak inhibitors of bone resorption and not very commonly used. Oral bisphosphonates have not been shown to be as effective and are not recommended.

d. Other agents. Corticosteroids may be effective in controlling hypercalcemia due to sarcoidosis or other granulomatous diseases. A dose of 20 to 40 mg/day prednisone orally or its equivalent can be given to control hypercalcemia from excess ingestion of vitamin D or endogenous production of calcitrol. In patients with malignancies producing 1,25dihydroxyvitamin D such as myeloma or lymphomas, IV steroids can be used alone or in combination with bisphosphonates before definitive therapy of the underlying malignancy. Steroids are not effective in the treatment of hypercalcemia in patients with solid tumors. Hemodialysis is usually reserved for severe cases of hypercalcemia not responding to recommended treatments. Several new inhibitors of bone resorption such as osteoprotegerin (an antagonist of RANKL receptor), monoclonal antibodies directed against RANKL, monoclonal antibodies neutralizing PTHrP, and 22-oxacalcitriol are being studied currently.

B. Tumor lysis syndrome

1. Pathophysiology. The tumor lysis syndrome (TLS) results from excessive tumor breakdown either spontaneously or during therapy, leading to sudden and large amount of potassium, phosphates, and nucleic acids into systemic circulation. Catabolism of nucleic acid to uric acid causes hyperuricemia and other variety of metabolic abnormalities such as hyperkalemia, hyperphosphatemia, secondary hypocalcaemia, and acute kidney injury. The TLS occurs most frequently in patients with tumors having high growth rate and substantial systemic tumor burden that are very sensitive to chemotherapy and radiotherapy such as leukemia's (ALL) and high-grade lymphomas (Burkitts). TLS is rarely encountered in patients with epithelial malignancies.

2. Signs and symptoms. The onset of TLS can be before the initiation of cytotoxic therapy, but is often within 12 to 72 hours after administration of cytotoxic therapy and/or radiation therapy (RT). A high level of suspicion is required because TLS symptoms can be very nonspecific and symptoms are often a result of associated electrolyte imbalances. The patients may present with nausea, vomiting, diarrhea, anorexia, congestive heart failure, cardiac arrhythmias, seizures, tetany, syncope, and possibly sudden death, often due to cardiac arrest.

The most worrisome metabolic consequences of TLS are hyperkalemia, hypercalcemia, and renal failure. Acute renal failure results from precipitation of phosphate and uric acid in the renal tubules causing renal vasoconstriction decreased renal blood flow and acute kidney injury, which creates a vicious cycle, thereby resulting in further deterioration of renal function. Patients with baseline elevated levels of uric acid, phosphorus, and lactate dehydrogenase (LDH) before treatment may be at risk for TLS.

3. Classification of TLS. *Laboratory TLS* (LTLS) is defined as the presence of two or more of the following laboratory parameters within three days before or seven days after cytotoxic chemotherapy: (a) uric acid ≥8 mg/dL or 25% increase from baseline; (b) potassium ≥6.0 mEq/L or 25% increase from baseline; (c) phosphate level ≥4.5 mg/dL or 25% increase from baseline; and (d) calcium ≤7 mg/dL or 25% decrease from baseline. *Clinical TLS* (CTLS) is defined as the presence of laboratory TLS plus at least one clinical complication such as renal failure and/or cardiac arrhythmias and/or seizures and/or sudden death (*Br J Haematol* 2004;127:3).

4. **Management.** Management of TLS involves treatment of the underlying electrolyte abnormalities along with coexisting renal failure or cardiac arrhythmias. The best approach to managing TLS is prevention. Tumor- and patient-related factors are used to calculate the risk of TLS in individual patients. High-risk patients are pretreated with isotonic saline to maintain high urine output (80 to 100 mL per hour) and are recommended to give at least single dose of Rasburicase and should also be pretreated for at least 2 days with allopurinol (600 mg/day). Uric acid levels are closely monitored and dose of Rasburicase may be repeated for persistent hyperuricemia. The dose of allopurinol should be decreased for preexisting renal insufficiency.

   a. Intermediate-risk patient are also pretreated with isotonic saline to maintain high urine output and pretreatment allopurinol if the baseline uric acid levels are <8 mg/dL. If the uric acid levels are ≥8 mg/dL, Rasburicase should also be given.

   b. For low-risk patients, a wait-and-watch approach is used with hydration and close monitoring.

   c. Furosemide may be given to maintain urine output and also to decrease the hyperkalemia. Urine alkalinization with either one ampoule of $NaHCO^3$ in 0.5 N saline or two to three ampoules in D5W may be needed to maintain the urine solutes (calcium, uric acid, and oxalates) in ionic form and thereby prevent crystallization and also to help correct metabolic acidosis accompanying TLS. Blood chemistries (electrolytes, creatinine, phosphorus, calcium, and LDH) need to be checked in patients at risk every 8 to 12 hours during the first 2 to 3 days of treatment.

   d. Hyperkalemia may develop rapidly, and patients at risk should have serum electrolytes checked at least every 12 hours, and more frequently if TLS develops. Mild hyperkalemia (5.5 to 6.0 mEq/L) may be treated with sodium polystyrene sulfonate (Kayexalate resin) and hydration. More severe hyperkalemia (greater than 6 mEq/L or with electrocardiogram [EKG] changes) may be treated immediately with 50 mL of 50% glucose solution with 15 U of regular insulin, i.v. piggyback over an hour. Indications for hemodialysis include volume overload, serum uric acid greater than 10 mg/dL, or rapidly increasing phosphorus levels and uncontrolled hyperkalemia. Renal failure caused by TLS is usually reversible, and even patients requiring hemodialysis often regain normal kidney function as the TLS subsides.

C. **Syndrome of inappropriate antidiuretic hormone (SIADH)**

   1. **Pathophysiology.** SIADH is a syndrome of excessive inappropriate secretion of ADH resulting in water retention and hyponatremia. Excessive secretion of ADH causes increased urine osmolality and increased sodium loss, resulting in concentrated urine. Small-cell lung cancer (SCLC) is the most common cancer causing SIADH, with over 15% patients with SCLC developing SIADH at some point during the course of the illness. Head and neck cancers, olfactory neuroblastomas, and extrapulmonary small-cell carcinomas are some less common causes of SIADH.

   2. **Signs and symptoms.** Patients initially present with headache and fatigue and if left uncorrected may rapidly progress to confusion, seizure, coma, and death. A low plasma osmolality with elevated urine osmolality (more than 100 mosmol/kg), urine sodium more than 40 mEq/L, low blood urea nitrogen (BUN) 10 mg/dL, serum uric acid level <4 mg/dL, FE_{Na} >1%, and normal acid–base and serum potassium levels are all suggestive of SIADH.

   3. **Management.** The treatment of SIADH varies with the severity of hyponatremia and presence of symptoms. Fluid restriction is the initial step of management for patients

with mild-to-moderate SIADH. In patients with acute (less than 48 hours) and severe symptomatic hyponatremia, an urgent intervention with 100 mL of hypertonic saline is given as bolus and can be repeated 1 to 2 times at 10 min interval depending upon the persistent of neurological symptoms. This treatment should raise the serum Na concentration by approximately 1.5 to 2.0 mEq/L. For patients with serum sodium <120 mEq/L and less severe symptoms (more than 48 hours), the goal of correction is to increase serum sodium 1 mEq/L per hour for 3 to 4 hours. When the serum Na levels reach 120 mEq/L, then the 3% saline should be stopped and fluid restriction instituted. For patients with no symptoms or mild symptoms, initial treatment with fluid restriction with oral salt tablets is recommended (Table 38-2).

a. Maintenance therapy in previously symptomatic patients is to maintain fluid restriction to less than 800 mL/day with monitoring of serum sodium levels to >130 mEq/L (Table 38-3).

b. For chronic SIADH, treatment options include demeclocycline (300 to 600 mg daily) and vasopressin receptor antagonists such as tolvaptan (15 to 60 mg oral daily) or conivaptan (20 to 40 mg intravenously daily) (*J Endocrinol Metab* 2013;98:1321).

TABLE 38-2 | **Treatment of Symptomatic and Asymptomatic Hyponatremia from SIADH**

Severity of Hyponatremia	Symptoms	Treatment	Comment
Serum sodium <120 mEq/L (Hyponatremia developing within 48 hours)	Very severe symptoms (acute altered mentation, seizures, comatose patients)	• Hypertonic saline 100 ml bolus of 3% saline • If urine osmolality is excessively high, loop diuretics may be required to increase urinary water excretion	a. Can be repeated 1–2 times depending upon the symptoms b. Measure serum sodium levels every 2–3 hours and watch for rapid correction since it can cause a complication of osmotic demyelination c. Watch for urine osmolality
Serum sodium <120 mEq/L (Hyponatremia developing within more than 48 hours)	Less severe symptoms (forgetfulness, lethargy, confusion etc.)	Hypertonic saline slow infusion. Bolus is usually not required	Be cautious not to overcorrect the hyponatremia. Goal is rise in serum sodium of <10 mEq/L in 24 h
Serum sodium 120–129 mEq/L	asymptomatic	Treat the underlying cause	
Chronic moderate Hyponatremia		Fluid restriction Oral salt tablets Demeclocyclin and vasopressin receptor antagonist	Less than 800 ml/day 9 gm per day in three divided doses Used as deemed appropriate

TABLE 38-3	Maintenance Treatment in SIADH	
Treatment	**Dose**	**Comment**
Fluid restriction	Intake less than 800 mL/d	Do not restrict fluids in patients with SIADH from subarachnoid hemorrhage
Oral salt	9 g/d in three divided doses	May need to increase the dose to increase urine volume
Loop diuretics	Furosemide-20 mg PO twice daily	This may be needed to increase urinary water excretion
		Watch closely for hypokalemia and hypovolemia from diuretics

II. NEUROLOGIC EMERGENCIES

A. Epidural spinal cord compression

1. **Pathophysiology.** Spinal cord compression is a common complication of cancers most commonly due to metastasis to the spinal column, causing pain and possibly irreversible loss of neurologic function involving the thoracic spine (65%), the lumbosacral spine (25%), and the cervical spine (10%). Intramedullary, intradural, or leptomeningeal metastases are rarely encountered. Patients with neurologic impairment secondary to cord compression have a markedly reduced quality of life and a significantly shortened overall survival. Spinal cord compression is seen most commonly in patients with following underlying cancers: lung, breast cancer, multiple myeloma, Hodgkin's and non-Hodgkin's lymphoma, and prostate cancer. The main mechanism involved is the tumor invading the epidural space causing compression of thecal sac. The direct extension of the soft tissue epidural disease can compromise epidural venous plexus causing vasogenic edema, inflammation with release of serotonin and prostaglandins, and eventually infarction of the spinal cord. Other less common causes of cord compression include metastases to the posterior vertebral elements, benign and malignant tumors primary to the spine, vascular malformations, and infections. It is critical to begin therapy as soon as possible.

2. **Signs and symptoms.** The symptoms of cord compression may begin abruptly or progress gradually. Back pain is the most common symptom in almost all patients with spinal cord compression. New onset of back pain in a patient at risk mandates a careful neurologic examination. The pain may be localized to the back or may radiate either unilaterally or bilaterally in the distribution of spinal roots. Back pain may be exacerbated by flexion of the back, Valsalva maneuver, and coughing. Unlike back pain resulting from degenerative disc disease, the back pain due to spinal cord compression is not relieved by recumbent position but may be exacerbated. Majority of patients may present with motor weakness symmetric in both lower extremities and depending upon the level of the lesion may present with either typical pyramidal symptoms (lesion at or above conus medullaris) or weakness of extensors of upper extremities (lesion above thoracic spine). Sensory findings are overall less common, but ascending numbness and paresthesias along the dermatome of the corresponding spinal roots may be seen.

   Other symptoms such as bowel and bladder dysfunction (sphincter disturbances, urinary/fecal incontinence, or retention) and gait ataxia occur late in the course of cord compression but are serious symptoms and need urgent attention since associated with poor prognosis. Acute, severe cord compression can cause spinal shock, with hyporeflexia and flaccid paralysis of all regions below the lesion.

3. **Workup.** The workup involves detailed clinical neurologic examination and preferably a magnetic resonance imaging (MRI) for all patients with suspected cord compression. MRI is the modality of choice when available since it can provide a detailed evaluation of spinal cord and extent of disease with involvement of bone and soft tissue. Myelography combined with contrast computed tomography (CT) is recommended if MRI cannot be performed. It is important to image the entire spine, as some patients may have more than one region of compression. Plain films and bone scans have a limited role since they do not provide anatomical information regarding epidural space and thecal sac. If the nature of the compressing mass is uncertain, surgical or image-guided biopsy for tissue diagnosis may be required. When cord compression is the initial presentation of cancer, further staging evaluation may reveal more accessible lesions such as a lymph node for biopsy and subsequent diagnosis.

4. **Management.** Spinal cord compression requires prompt recognition because delay in treatment may result in permanent neurologic damage and poor outcome. Pretreatment neurological status is the most important prognostic indicator of post-treatment outcome. Immediate treatment of cord compression includes corticosteroids administration, surgery, and RT with external beam radiation therapy (EBRT).

Corticosteroids decrease the edema associated with cord compression and improve neurologic symptoms transiently. We recommend a 10-mg loading dose of Dexamethasone IV or PO followed by 4 mg every 6 hours. Dexamethasone should be tapered off over a few weeks. Spinal cord stability should be assessed. Traditional indications for surgical intervention include the need for a tissue diagnosis, resection of "radioresistant" tumors and tumors primarily treated by surgery (such as sarcomas), and cord compression in a previously irradiated spine. A very rapid onset of symptoms suggests the possibility of vertebral burst fracture causing bony impingement on the cord and hence is an indication for urgent surgical intervention. Patients with extensive bony destruction by tumor and vertebral instability may be at risk for further compression fracture and symptom recurrence after completing X-ray therapy (XRT); these patients should be considered for vertebral stabilization with vertebroplasty and kyphoplasty.

EBRT is the treatment of choice and should begin as soon as the diagnosis is confirmed. Standard radiation doses range from 2,500 to 4,000 cGy delivered in 10 to 20 fractions. Surgical patients usually require 7 to 10 days for wound healing before beginning radiation. In select groups of patients, the addition of decompressive surgery to RT improved neurologic outcomes as compared with radiotherapy alone (*Lancet* 2005;366(9486):643). Systemic therapy using hormonal and/or chemotherapeutic agents should be considered when appropriate (e.g., in patients with lymphoma).

Symptomatic treatment is considered with pain medications, appropriate ambulatory restrictions, anticoagulation if no other contraindications (no anticoagulation if surgery planned), and symptom management from sphincter dysfunction (urinary/bowel retention vs. incontinence).

III. HEMATOLOGIC EMERGENCIES
A. Leukostasis
1. **Pathophysiology.** Leukastasis is a syndrome commonly seen in acute leukemia's and comprises of hyperleukocytosis (WBC >50,000 to 100,000/μL) with respiratory distress, abnormal chest radiograph (CXR), confusion, and CNS bleeding. If not treated, leukostasis has very poor prognosis with a high mortality rate. High and rapidly increasing blast counts are characteristic of leukostasis with classic pathologic finding of occlusive intravascular aggregates of blasts blocking the circulation in multiple organs, especially the lungs and brain.
2. **Signs and symptoms.** Leukostasis is a clinical diagnosis. Patients may present with respiratory symptoms of dyspnea, hypoxia, fever, etc. Pulse oximetry assesses the O_2 saturation more accurately than arterial blood gas (ABG) analysis since WBC in the blood sample consume oxygen and spuriously lower the PO_2 of the specimen if not

processed in a timely manner. Chest X-ray may show diffuse alveolar or interstitial infiltrate. Fever may be from inflammation or concomitant infection and broad-spectrum antibiotics are recommended. CNS involvement may present with head-aches, dizziness, vision changes, confusion, gait abnormality, and even coma. These patients have a high risk of intracranial hemorrhage after starting chemotherapy even in the absence of disseminated intravascular coagulation (DIC) or thrombocytopenia. Less commonly, impairment of other end organs with leukastasis may present as heart failure, myocardial infarction, renal failure, bowel infarction, priapism, etc. Symptoms may be fulminant, leading to death in a matter of days or even hours.

3. **Management.** Leukastasis is treated with prompt cytoreduction treatment in conjunc-tion with leukapheresis with the goal of rapidly decreasing WBC count. Cytoreduction with induction chemotherapy should be initiated whenever possible, especially in acute leukemia, but if induction chemotherapy is delayed, cytoreduction with hydroxyurea is attempted. Hydroxyurea given at 50 to 100 mg/kg/day usually reduces the WBC by 50% in 24 to 48 hours and is continued until WBC is <50,000/μL. Patients who receive leukapheresis have a lower incidence of intracerebral bleeds after starting chemotherapy and also decrease the incidence of TLS. Leukapheresis should be considered in all patients with a leukemic blasts count greater than 100,000/dL. Leukapheresis is not recommended if acute promyelocytic leukemia (APL) is suspected since it may worsen the coagulopathy associated with leukemia. Red blood cell transfu-sion should be avoided since it can worsen the symptoms associated with leukastasis. Thrombocytopenia and coagulation factors need to be corrected to minimize the risk of CNS bleeding. Patients with signs of sepsis need to have blood drawn for culture and treated empirically with broad-spectrum antibiotics. The underlying malignancy needs to be treated appropriately. Low-dose cranial irradiation may be considered in patients with very severe CNS symptoms.

IV. CARDIAC EMERGENCIES
A. Cardiac tamponade
1. **Pathophysiology.** Cardiac tamponade is an accumulation of pericardial fluid under pressure causing abnormal compression of all cardiac chambers and impaired cardiac filling and subsequently hemodynamic compromise. This can be acute, subacute, or chronic. Some of the causes of moderate-to-large pericardial effusions leading to tamponade are idiopathic, malignancy, uremia, iatrogenic, acute myocardial infarc-tion, collagen vascular diseases, hypothyroidism, etc. Overall 10% of patients dying of cancer are found to have pericardial involvement at autopsy. Thoracic malignancies are the most common cause of malignant pericardial effusion and tamponade.

2. **Signs and symptoms.** Presenting symptoms may vary depending upon the acuteness of tamponade. Patients with acute tamponade present with chest pain and dyspnea, whereas patients with subacute or chronic tamponade may present with fatigue, cough, chest pain, and edema. Hypotension is a common feature due to the decline in cardiac output. Severe hypotension and pulseless electrical activity are the final con-sequences of untreated tamponade. More often cardiac tamponade manifests in a less dramatic way with increased filling pressures and decreased cardiac output. Features of right-heart failure, such as peripheral edema, hypotension, and elevated jugular venous pressure (JVP), may be seen. Pulsus paradoxus (a decrease in systolic blood pressure of 10 mmHg or more on inspiration) is classically associated with pericardial effusion. Often a pericardial rub may be heard due to associated inflammatory pericarditis. Acute cardiac tamponade presenting with signs of right heart failure must be differen-tiated from a right-sided acute myocardial infarction and an aortic dissection.

3. **Workup.** The clinical diagnosis of cardiac tamponade is usually confirmed by the physical findings supplemented by electrocardiography (EKG), CXR, and echocardiog-raphy (ECHO). The EKG shows sinus tachycardia with low voltage. The characteristic findings on EKG in patients with pericardial effusion include electrical alternans (beat-to-beat alteration in QRS complex) as the heart swings within the pericardial fluid.

Electrical alternans has a low sensitivity but high specificity. CXR may reveal an enlarged cardiac silhouette (water-bottle heart) with clear lung fields. At least 200 mL of fluid must accumulate before the cardiac silhouette is enlarged on chest X-ray, and hence this is often absent in acute tamponade. ECHO shows moderate-to-large effusion and swinging of the heart within the effusion and diastolic collapse of the right atrium and right ventricle. Collapse of the right atrium occurs when the extrinsic compression by the effusion overcomes venous pressure and prevents right heart filling. Right atrial collapse for more than one-third of the cardiac cycle is highly sensitive and specific for cardiac tamponade. Examination of pericardial fluid is often required in cancer patients to ascertain the diagnosis of malignant effusion and to rule out other causes. In malignant pericardial effusion, cytology will be positive in only 65% to 85% of cases. A positive cytology may be predictive of a poorer outcome in patients with neoplastic pericardial disease. Pericardial biopsy is the gold standard for establishing definitive diagnosis.

4. **Management.** Asymptomatic patients with mild effusion do not require treatment unless the etiology is unclear. Symptomatic patients, however, require intervention. Definitive treatment of tamponade involves removal or drainage of pericardial fluid and relieving intrapericardial pressure. Pericardial fluid can be drained percutaneously by pericardiocentesis with echocardiographic guidance or surgical pericardiectomy. Pericardiocentesis is usually safely done in most of the patients; however, it is relatively contraindicated in severe pulmonary hypertension and severe coagulopathy. Pericardiocentesis is done after local anesthesia; the needle is inserted to the right of the xiphoid and advanced toward the tip of the left scapula, with constant aspiration during the procedure. A large syringe or a catheter with a stopcock should be available to allow removal of 50 to 60 mL of fluid. This results in rapid improvement in symptoms. Despite marked improvement in the symptoms, reaccumulation of fluid occurs in as many as 60% of patients. In this situation, a surgical pericardial window will usually prevent repeat accumulation. Balloon pericardiotomy is an alternative to surgical creation of a pericardial window. In this procedure an uninflated balloon catheter is placed in the pericardial space using a subxiphoid approach under guidance. The balloon is then inflated and pulled out of pericardium to create a "window," thereby allowing drainage of fluid into the pleural or peritoneal space. This technique has shown a decrease in the reaccumulation in 80% to 100% of cases. This approach may be a reasonable alternative to surgery in patients with malignant tamponade, especially in those who are poor surgical candidates.

B. **Superior vena cava syndrome**

1. **Pathophysiology and mechanism.** Superior vena cava (SVC) syndrome results from the obstruction of blood flow in the SVC caused by invasion or external compression of the SVC by a pathologic process involving right lung, lymph nodes, and mediastinal structures. When the blood flow in SVC is obstructed, venous collaterals are formed as alternate pathways to venous return. Thoracic malignancies such as lung cancer (SCLC more often than non-SCLC), non-Hodgkin's lymphoma- DLBCL, lymphoblastic lymphoma, and primary mediastinal B cell lymphoma are common cause of SVC syndrome. Other nonmalignant causes of SVC syndrome are compression of the SVC from indwelling central venous devices that result in SVC thrombosis, aortic aneurysms, and fibrosing mediastinitis.

2. **Signs and symptoms.** Dyspnea is common. Patients with SVC syndrome commonly complain of dyspnea, swelling of the face, neck, upper extremities, and pain (chest pain or headaches). Symptoms may develop rapidly or gradually and may vary in severity by position. Bending forward or lying flat may worsen symptoms as a result of increased venous pressure proximal to the obstruction. Even in the presence of severe symptoms, patients are rarely critically ill as a result of SVC syndrome alone. Dilated neck veins are usually present along with collateral veins that develop as a result of long-standing occlusion.

3. **Workup.** The CXR may show mediastinal widening and pleural effusion. Contrast-enhanced CT is extremely helpful in detecting the location and extent of venous blockage and presence of collateral venous drainage. It also provides very useful

information regarding the adjacent structures, including the presence or absence of compressive mass lesions, and is useful in planning subsequent biopsy or therapeutic intervention. MRI may be useful for patients who are unable to undergo a contrast CT. A histologic diagnosis is essential in the management of SVC syndrome, as specific treatment may be influenced by the tumor type. Patients without a tissue diagnosis or in whom the diagnosis is uncertain should undergo surgical or percutaneous biopsy of an accessible site. Sputum cytology, pleural fluid cytology, and biopsy of enlarged thoracic lymph nodes may be diagnostic in most cases. Bronchoscopy, mediastinoscopy, or thoracotomy may be required if the diagnosis is in doubt. Bone marrow biopsy may provide a diagnosis in suspected NHL or SCLC.

4. **Treatment.** Relief of symptoms and treatment of the underlying disease is the mainstay in the treatment of SVC syndrome. Accurate histologic diagnosis of the underlying etiology is essential prior to initiation of therapy. Malignancy-associated SVC syndrome has poor prognosis.

Malignant SVC was considered an emergency in the past, requiring emergent RT to relieve obstructive symptoms, but nowadays emergent RT is no longer considered necessary treatment unless patients present with severe symptoms including respiratory stridor due to airway obstruction and laryngeal edema or comatose patients presenting with cerebral edema in whom RT and intraluminal stent placement is considered an emergent treatment option.

Prebiopsy empirical treatment may obscure the histologic diagnosis and make further management of the underlying disease complicated. For patients with SCLC, NHL, and germ cell tumors, initial chemotherapy is the treatment of choice for symptomatic patients. In limited SCLC and some NHLs, the addition of RT to chemotherapy decreases the local recurrence rate. Endovascular therapy (i.e., intraluminal stenting) may be considered in some patients with severe symptoms and in patients with underlying malignancy not responsive to chemotherapy or radiation.

The role of steroids in managing SVC syndrome is not proven and hence not recommended except in steroid responsive malignancies such as lymphomas. If SVC thrombus is present, systemic anticoagulation should be considered.

SVC obstruction resulting from indwelling central venous catheters and pacemakers can be managed effectively by thrombolytic therapy (unless contraindicated). Anticoagulation is recommended as long as the central catheter is in place and can be discontinued in 3 months if the catheter is removed.

SUGGESTED READINGS

Ahmann FR. A reassessment of the clinical implications of the superior vena cava syndrome. *J Clin Oncol* 1984;2:961–969.

Arrambide K, Toto RD. Tumor lysis syndrome. *Semin Nephrol* 1993;13:273–280.

Body JJ, Bartl R, Burckhardt P, et al. Current use of bisphosphonates in oncology. *J Clin Oncol* 1998;16:3890–3899.

Cairo MS, Bishop M. Tumor lysis syndrome: new therapeutic strategies and classification. *Br J Haematol* 2004;127: 3–11.

Dempke W, Firusian N. Treatment of malignant pericardial effusion with ^{32}P-colloid. *Br J Cancer* 1999;80:1955–1957.

List AF, Hainsworth JD, Davis BW, et al. The syndrome of inappropriate secretion of antidiuretic hormone (SIADH) in small-cell lung cancer. *J Clin Oncol* 1986;4:1191–1198.

Loblaw DA, Laperriere NJ. Emergency treatment of malignant extradural spinal cord compression: an evidence based guideline. *J Clin Oncol* 1998;16:1613–1624.

Mundy GR, Guise TA. Hypercalcemia of malignancy. *Am J Med* 1997;103:134–145.

Peri A. Clinical review: the use of vaptans in clinical endocrinology. *J Clin Endocrinol Metab* 2013;98:1321–1332.

Shepherd FA. Malignant pericardial effusion. *Curr Opin Oncol* 1997;9:170–174.

Silverman P, Distelhorst CW. Metabolic emergencies in clinical oncology. *Semin Oncol* 1989;16:504–515.

Spinazze S, Caraceni A, Schrijvers D. Epidural spinal cord compression. *Crit Rev Oncol Hematol* 2005;56:397–406.

Spinazze S, Schrijvers D. Metabolic emergencies. *Crit Rev Oncol Hematol* 2006;58:79–89.

Spodick DH. Acute cardiac tamponade. *N Engl J Med* 2003;349:684.

Stewart AF. Hypercalcemia associated with cancer. *N Engl J Med* 2005;352:373–379.

Tanigawa N, Sawada S, Mishima K, et al. Clinical outcome of stenting in superior vena cava syndrome associated with malignant tumors. *Acta Radiol* 1998;39:669–674.

Wilson LD, Detterbeck FC, Yahalom J. Superior vena cava syndrome with malignant causes. *N Engl J Med* 2007;356:1862–1869

Wuthner JU, Kohler G, Behringer D, et al. Leukostasis followed by hemorrhage complicating the initiation of chemotherapy in patients with acute myeloid leukemia and hyperleukocytosis. *Cancer* 1999;85:368–374.

Transfusion Medicine

Ronald Jackups • George Despotis

I. **RED BLOOD CELLS (RBCs).** The therapeutic goal of a blood transfusion is to increase oxygen delivery according to the physiologic need of the recipient. It is difficult to determine an appropriate transfusion threshold, however, because the benefits of blood are hard to define and measure. In a multi-institutional Canadian study, 418 critical care patients were to receive red cell transfusions when the hemoglobin (Hgb) level decreased to less than 7 g/dL, with Hgb maintenance in the range of 7 to 9 g/dL, and 420 patients were to receive transfusions when the Hgb was less than 10 g/dL, with Hgb levels maintained in the range of 10 to 12 g/dL. There was a trend in reduced 30-day mortality rate in the patients randomized to the conservative Hgb threshold (18.7% vs. 23.3%; $p = 0.11$), indicating that a transfusion threshold as low as 7 g/dL is as safe as a higher transfusion threshold of 10 g/dL in critical care patients without active end-organ ischemia (*N Engl J Med* 1999;340:409). These findings of tolerance of lower hemoglobin levels were also replicated recently in additional trials. An important confounding factor in the efficacy of red cell transfusions involves the variable capacity of red cell units to enhance or provide tissue oxygenation based on 2,3-diphosphoglycerate (DPG) levels, which vary with the age of the red cell units. Clearly, more data are needed to characterize how these red cell storage changes impact on the clinical efficacy of red cells transfusion on tissue oxygenation.

Data on morbidity also are unclear. Silent perioperative myocardial ischemia has been observed in patients undergoing noncardiac as well as cardiac surgery. Hemoglobin levels in the range of 6 to 10 g/dL as well as clinical signs or indicators of end-organ ischemia other than [Hgb] may identify patients who may benefit from blood transfusion. Accordingly, elderly patients undergoing elective, noncardiac surgery have been shown to be at risk for intraoperative or postoperative myocardial ischemia with hematocrits less than 28%, particularly in the presence of tachycardia. This finding was also recently confirmed in the study involving the postoperative period after orthopedic surgery. In this study, transfusion was more commonly triggered by the development of symptoms (e.g., threefold increase in bleeding, twofold increase in angina, 10-fold increase in congestive heart failure, and two-and-a-half-fold increase in the development of hemodynamic instability) in the patient cohort whose Hgb trigger was set at 8 g/dL (*N Engl J Med* 2011;365:2453). Therefore, in the absence of a physiologic need such as end-organ ischemia in a stable, nonbleeding patient, correction of anemia may not be indicated and may, in fact, predispose patients to adverse outcomes. However, when clinicians implement lower transfusion thresholds, the implementation of a proactive surveillance program should be considered to detect important symptoms of organ ischemia of dysfunction.

Guidelines for blood transfusion have been issued by several organizations including a National Institutes of Health consensus conference on perioperative transfusion of red cells, the American College of Physicians, the American Society of Anesthesiologists, AABB (formerly known as American Association of Blood Banks), and the Canadian Medical Association. These guidelines consistently recommend that blood should not be transfused on a prophylactic basis and suggest that in patients who are not critically ill, a Hgb level of 6 to 8 g/dL is well tolerated and acceptable. Adherence to these guidelines has raised questions about whether transfusion is now underused. A Hgb level of 8 g/dL seems an appropriate threshold for transfusion in surgical patients with no risk factors for critical or target (end-organ) ischemia, whereas a higher threshold may be more appropriate for patients who are considered at higher risk or, more importantly, patients who develop symptoms consistent with organ ischemia. However, prophylactic transfusion of blood cannot be endorsed, particularly because studies have found an association between transfusion and less favorable outcomes in critically ill patients. It is unlikely that one specific hemoglobin value can be used as a universal threshold for transfusion.

II. TRANSFUSION THERAPY

A. General considerations. The transfusion of blood or blood components has inherent risks, summarized in Table 39-1. Informed consent (a clear explanation of relative benefits, risks, and alternatives regarding the transfusion to the patient) is mandatory, and is accompanied in many institutions by a consent form that documents the conversation and patient acceptance. In the elective transfusion setting, alternatives to blood transfusion have previously included autologous or directed (from a donor known to and selected by the patient) blood. However, recent evidence indicates that this approach may not be as safe in part related to the fact that these represent first time donations (*Transfusion* 2013;53:1250). Another important measure for any blood management program includes, when feasible, the evaluation of patients with respect to uncovering treatable anemias (e.g., iron, folate, B_{12}, and erythropoietin) before initiating blood transfusion.

Risks, side effects, and indications of blood and blood products are available in the Circular of Information for Blood and Blood Products, issued jointly by the American Red Cross, America's Blood Centers, and the AABB and approved by the US Food and Drug Administration (FDA), and can be obtained from hospital transfusion services.

TABLE 39-1	Risks with Blood Transfusion
Risk factor	**Frequency/unit transfused**
Infection	
Hepatitis A	1/1,000,000
Hepatitis B	1:2,652,580
Hepatitis C	1:3,315,729
HIV	1:1,461,888
HTLV	1/2,678,836
Parvovirus	1/10,000
Bacterial contamination	
Platelets	1/12,000
Red cells	1/500,000
Acute hemolytic reaction	1/250,000 to 1/1,000,000
Delayed hemolytic reaction	1/1,000
TRALI	1:138,000

[a]Kaufman RM, Djulbegovic B, Gernsheimer T,et al. Platelet transfusion: a clinical practice guideline from the AABB [Epub ahead of print]. *Ann Intern Med* 2014. http://www.ncbi.nlm.nih.gov/pubmed/25383671.

Administration of blood must be preceded by confirmation that two unique identifiers (such as name and hospital number or social security number) match between the patient and the blood-unit label, immediately before initiating infusion of the blood unit. The blood must be infused through a dedicated intravenous line with no other concurrent drugs or fluids, except 0.9% NaCl (normal saline) except when approved for use by the FDA. Signs should be recorded immediately before transfusion and within 5 to 10 minutes after starting; some institutions require the patient to be also carefully monitored, and at regular intervals (e.g., hourly or more frequently as predicated by the patient's condition) thereafter. Each blood unit should be administered within 4 hours. A standard macroaggregate filter (170 to 260 μm) is used to prevent infusion of fibrin, cell clumps, and debris.

An order for blood type and screen involves testing the patient's RBCs blood type for the A, B, and D (Rh) antigens, whereas the antibody screen involves testing the serum/plasma for the presence of alloantibody against other (minor) RBC antigens. The frequency of detecting such alloantibodies varies between patient populations (e.g., 0.2% of healthy donors, vs. 1% to 1.5% in the general population vs. up to 8.4% of patients who receive blood) and is related to previous exposure from pregnancy or transfusion. A crossmatch order leads to in vitro testing of the patient's serum against donor RBCs to confirm compatibility between the blood unit selected and the patient.

B. Complications of transfusion

1. **The Transfusion Medicine Service** typically provides clinicians with a list of distinct diagnostic criteria (e.g., cardiopulmonary or allergic symptoms along with signs of hemodynamic, respiratory, and/or febrile reactions) with respect to early identification of transfusion reactions to alert medical personnel regarding potential problems with the transfusion. These criteria include a temperature elevation of greater than 1°C; the appearance of symptoms (e.g., shortness of breath, nausea/vomiting, pruritus, pain at infusion site, back pain, and palpitations); or signs (changes in vital signs, rash, hives, edema, or stridor) indicating a change in the patient's clinical status. When a transfusion reaction is considered, the transfusion must be stopped immediately, and a physician is notified to assess the patient's status. The transfusion is terminated if there is a significant change in the patient's clinical status during the transfusion. At that time, the blood bag, patient blood samples, and urine are sent to the blood bank, where patient and blood-unit identification are reverified; direct antigen test, blood group confirmation, and potential repeat antibody screen testing are repeated; serum and urine are inspected for signs of hemolysis; and the residual contents of the blood bag may be cultured. The patient's blood should be drawn for blood culture if fever or blood pressure changes occurred during the transfusion.

2. **Nonhemolytic febrile-associated transfusion reactions (NHFTRs)** are characterized by fever (i.e., at least a one degree rise in temperature), which may or may not be associated with other signs and symptoms. These types of reactions used to occur in 0.5% to 2% of RBC transfusions and in 8% to 30% of platelet transfusions in the era prior to use of leukoreduced blood. Within certain populations such as multiparous women and frequently (or chronically) transfused patients, the prevalence can be higher. These reactions are generally mild and occur during the latter part of the transfusion. The potential mechanisms involve either recipient antibodies against donor leukocyte antigens and/or soluble cytokines (interleukins and tumor necrosis factor) contained within the blood component, or both. Symptoms are treated with acetaminophen (650 mg) for fever, and occasionally, rigors and chills may require meperidine (25 to 50 mg i.v.). Although these reactions are typically mild and self-limiting, if the rise in temperature is related to infusion of blood component contaminated with bacteria, there may be a more profound presentation with high fevers and hemodynamic instability related to sepsis (refer to infectious complications of transfusion).

3. **Nonhemolytic allergic transfusion reactions (NHATR)** are invariably accompanied by pruritus, rash, or hives consistent with urticaria and on occasion, histamine release results in more significant and on occasion life-threatening perturbations such as severe bronchospasm, angioedema involving swelling of supraglottic structures (e.g., glossal,

epiglottis, and other pharyngeal structures), or substantial hemodynamic compromise such as severe hypotension with reflex tachycardia or, on occasion, myocardial depression. While mild allergic reactions occur in 0.5% to 2% of RBC transfusions and in 8% to 30% of platelet transfusions, severe reactions occur at a much lower frequency (0.3% to 0.01% of transfusions) and are typically related to allergy to one or more unidentified donor plasma proteins. Therapy depends on the severity of signs and symptoms and includes either continued monitoring or with progressive symptoms beyond a rash, antihistamine therapy involving both an anti-H1 antagonist diphenhydramine (25 to 75 mg), p.o. or i.v. when the patient is NPO, and an anti-H2 blocker such as ranitidine (50 mg) or pepcid (20 mg). For more severe reactions, SQ or IV epinephrine and glucocorticoids should be considered for severe allergic reactions involving hemodynamic perturbations while inhaled beta agonist therapy to abate either bronchospasm (e.g., albuterol) or stridor (e.g., racemic epinephrine). The transfusion may be continued at the discretion of the physician, particularly in patients with prolonged transfusions with mild dermatologic reactions. Some patients may benefit from prophylactic treatment with antihistamine agents shortly before transfusion, to prevent or attenuate reactions. Bedside leukodepletion filters are infrequently utilized (i.e., >90% of blood is leukoreduced prior to storage) for patients with a history of two or more febrile reactions but prevent only 50% of reactions, because they affect only those due to antibodies against leukocytes. However, severe hypotension can occur in susceptible patients (e.g., patients on angiotensin-converting enzyme [ACE] inhibitors) and is secondary to the hemodynamic effects of bradykinin, which is released due to the filtration process and by sustained blood levels as related to reduced clearance (i.e., as related to the use of ACE inhibitors). The clinical manifestations include vital sign instability, particularly, hypotension. Bedside leukodepletion filters should therefore be avoided in patients with cardiovascular compromise and in those treated with ACE inhibitors.

Severe anaphylactic reactions have been observed (i.e., generally with the first or second transfusion) in patients with immunoglobulin A (IgA) deficiency who have no detectable IgA levels and who have developed anti-IgA antibodies and receive blood products (all of which contain IgA). If IgA deficiency is considered, both IgA levels (i.e., with a method that can detect levels as low as 0.05 mg/dL as highlighted by Vassallo RR) and anti-IgA antibody testing should be pursued. Patients with suspected IgA deficiency should receive washed cellular blood components until the diagnosis is confirmed, at which time, components from IgA deficient donors may be potentially procured from the American Red Cross if available.

4. **Acute hemolytic transfusion reactions are caused** by preformed antibodies (IgM or IgG antibodies against A or B antigens, or complement-fixing IgG antibodies against minor RBC antigens, such as Kidd) in the patient and are characterized by complement-mediated intravascular hemolysis subsequent to initiation of the transfusion. Hypotension, fever, nausea/vomiting, and back and/or chest pain may develop, along with hemoglobinuria, renal failure, and disseminated intravascular coagulation (DIC). If such a reaction is suspected, the transfusion should be immediately terminated. Treatment includes resuscitative measures, support of the cardiovascular system with intravascular volume and vasopressor therapy, and preservation of renal function with i.v. hydration, along with alkalinization of urine (i.v. sodium bicarbonate therapy) and administration of hemostatic blood components in the setting of bleeding and laboratory evidence of hemostatic factor deficiency secondary to DIC.

5. **Delayed hemolytic transfusion reactions (DHTRs)** are usually detected 7 to 21 days after RBC transfusion. They are related to a primary or anamnestic IgG response on exposure to minor RBC antigens, the latter seen particularly in patients previously exposed to such antigens through pregnancy or previous blood transfusion. Clinical manifestations may include an unexplained and perhaps severe (i.e., dependent on the number of incompatible units transfused) posttransfusion anemia, icterus, or jaundice (due to accelerated intravascular RBC destruction), a failure to increase Hgb (1 g/dL/U)

levels after RBC transfusion, or most commonly in asymptomatic patients through serologic evidence (i.e., the appearance of a new alloantibody on antibody screen before subsequent transfusion). Occasionally, the reactions can be clinically severe, with renal impairment and even reported deaths (Table 39-2). Treatment in these cases is the same as for acute reactions. Patients should be informed that they have an allergy (e.g., antibody to non-ABO antigens) to prevent subsequent DHTRs since many of these antibodies (50%) fade within 3 to 6 months and therefore lead to negative antibody screens obtained at the same or another institution.

6. **Transfusion-related acute lung injury (TRALI)** is an underrecognized and serious reaction to transfusion often due to an antihuman leukocyte antigen (HLA) or anti-neutrophil (HNA) antibody from a donor (usually a multiparous woman) that reacts to the corresponding antigen on recipient leukocytes. Alternatively, transfusion of accumulated lipids or cytokines in the plasma of stored blood products has also been implicated as a cause of TRALI, especially when related to transfusion of platelet units. In addition, there is substantial evidence to suggest that TRALI represents a two-hit mechanism and that the patient's underlying condition (e.g., sepsis, systemic inflammatory response, major surgical intervention) predisposes patients to an exaggerated response to the primary trigger (e.g., anti-HLA/HNA antibodies, biologically active lipids or cytokines, etc.) that leads to an increase in adverse consequences. This has been recently supported in the cardiac surgery environment; Vlaar et al. demonstrated a 2.4% incidence of TRALI in 668 patients undergoing cardiac surgery. In this cardiac surgical series, TRALI was associated with substantial (i.e., fourfold and twofold) increase in ICU and hospital lengths of stay, doubling of ventilation intervals and a fourfold higher mortality. In addition, TRALI was only associated with anti-HLA antibodies using multivariate statistical methodology. TRALI is now the leading cause of transfusion-related mortality in the United States, exceeding the number of deaths due to transfusion of ABO-incompatible or bacterially contaminated units. Most studies have indicated that plasma is associated with roughly 50% of TRALI cases, whereas apheresis or whole blood platelets are the next most common precipitant, and packed red cells and cryoprecipitate are rare causes of TRALI. Other publications, however, have indicated the highest incidence with platelets (1:400 platelet units), but this has not been uniformly reported. Clinical manifestations of TRALI include fever, hypotension, tachycardia, and noncardiogenic pulmonary edema that can lead to profound hypoxemia and respiratory distress necessitating intubation and mechanical ventilatory support in 70% of patients. Chest radiographs demonstrate a noncardiogenic pattern of bilateral infiltrates without cardiomegaly consistent with acute respiratory distress

---

TABLE 39-2   Indications for Leukocyte-Reduced Blood Components

Established indications
  Prevention of recurrent nonhemolytic febrile transfusion reactions to RBC transfusions
  Prevention or delay of alloimmunization to leukocyte antigens in select patients who are
    candidates for transplantation or transfusion on a long-term basis
Indications under review
  Prevention of the platelet-refractory state caused by alloimmunization
  Prevention of recurrent febrile reactions during platelet transfusions
  Prevention of cytomegalovirus transmission by cellular blood components
Not indicated for
  Prevention of transfusion-associated graft-versus-host disease
  Prevention of TRALI due to the passive administration of antileukocyte antibody
  Patients who are expected to have only limited transfusion exposure
  Acellular blood components (fresh frozen plasma, cryoprecipitate)

syndrome. Typically, signs and symptoms of TRALI occur within 2 hours of receipt of the blood product, but can occur up to 6 hours following transfusion. Treatment is supportive, and while more than 70% of patients require mechanical ventilation, most patients are extubated within 24 to 72 hours.

In patients who meet the clinical criteria for TRALI, confirmation first requires the identification of potentially involved blood products and their respective donors. Other banked blood products from the donor(s) suspected in a TRALI case must be quarantined during evaluation. To implicate a donor in a case of TRALI, the presence of an anti-HLA or antineutrophil antibody with specificity to an antigen expressed by the recipient is required. Implicated donors are typically permanently deferred from further donation.

To date, measures to prevent TRALI have focused on the identification and deferral of donors at high risk to form anti-HLA or antineutrophil antibodies. The United Kingdom adopted a policy to manufacture and import male donor plasma only, whereas centers in Spain screen previously pregnant donors for anti-HLA antibodies and, if positive, do not manufacture plasma products from these donors. Data from the SHOT UK Surveillance program (i.e., years 1996 to 2006) involving 206 cases of TRALI demonstrated a substantial (i.e., 80%) decline in the incidence of TRALI after implementation of exclusive use of male donor plasma in the United Kingdom in 2003. Accordingly, in 2007, the American Red Cross has also adopted the use of plasma from only male donors as well. However, this risk still persists with the use of AB plasma; despite the fact that AB plasma represents 4% of all plasma transfused, 50% of the TRALI cases were observed with AB plasma from female donors who had HLA or HNA antibodies (*Transfusion* 2013;53:1442). This has led to preferential utilization of non-AB plasma in an attempt to mitigate this risk. In multiparous donors from the United States, the incidence of anti-HLA antibodies is approximately 25% and, therefore, policies to exclude high-risk donors can potentially adversely affect the supply of blood products, especially platelets. It is currently unclear which preventative measures such as anti-HLA/HNA testing versus use of platelet additive solution for platelets will be implemented to definitively decrease the incidence of TRALI from platelet derived from female donors.

7. **Volume overload** with symptoms and signs of congestive heart failure can be seen in patients with cardiopulmonary compromise, particularly in elderly patients with substantial anemia who already have expanded plasma volume, patients with substantial renal dysfunction, or patients who have received excess fluids prior to transfusion. Diuretic therapy should be used prophylactically in such patients to minimize this complication. The distinction between volume overload and TRALI can be difficult. Recently, a small study involving 19 patients suspected to have transfusion-associated circulatory overload (TACO) found beta natriuretic peptide (BNP) to be 81% sensitive and 89% specific in the diagnosis of volume overload following a transfusion. Therefore, along with essential clinical data, BNP may be a helpful marker to distinguish TACO from TRALI, although future studies are needed validate this approach.

8. **Transfusion-associated graft-versus-host disease (GVHD)** is a syndrome in which donor lymphocytes that share an HLA haplotype with the patient's lymphocytes successfully engraft and attack the host (patient) with clinical manifestations of rash, pancytopenia, and liver and gastrointestinal damage (diarrhea). This appears to be unique to immunocompromised patients such as solid organ or bone marrow transplantation patients, and patients with certain malignancies (Hodgkin's disease, non-Hodgkin's lymphoma, leukemia, and multiple myeloma), particularly in those undergoing intensive chemotherapy (e.g., fludarabine or myeloablative therapy). Interestingly, a patient with human immunodeficiency virus (HIV) infection has not yet been reported to have this complication, probably because of the suppressive effect of HIV infection on donor lymphocytes. Mortality is in excess of 80% and is usually secondary to bone marrow failure. This complication can be prevented by irradiation of blood products

for patients at risk. On the basis of the pathogenesis, directed blood transfusions from any blood relative of the transfusion recipient also must be irradiated.

9. **Posttransfusion purpura (PTP)** is a rare complication, which is manifested by a profound immune-mediated thrombocytopenia that is observed 7 to 10 days after blood transfusion. Platelet alloantibodies within the recipient initiate the destruction of allogeneic platelets and are thought to trigger a complement-mediated consumption of the patient's own platelets. Most commonly, recipients lack human platelet antigen (HPA)-1a, which is present in approximately 99% of whites. Although controversial, additional platelet transfusions with HPA-1a–positive units may increase complement generation, so further transfusions are often withheld unless an HPA-1–negative donor is identified. The treatment for PTP is intravenous IgG (IVIG), and if this fails, plasma exchange may be initiated to eliminate the antibody after 4 to 5 procedures.

C. **Infections**

1. **Human immunodeficiency virus infection.** Since the recognition that HIV infection is transmissible by blood, major advances in blood safety have been made. With the implementation of nucleic acid testing (NAT) for direct detection of viral (HIV and hepatitis C) contamination, the window period (time from infection to detectability by testing) is 11 days for HIV and 8 to 10 days for hepatitis C. Following the institution of NAT testing, the estimated risk for HIV and hepatitis C transmission is 1:1.5 × 10^6 and 1:1.2 × 10^6, respectively. In contrast, the risk of hepatitis B approximates 1:293,000. *The risk of fatality from acute hemolytic transfusion reaction (usually due to ABO incompatibility secondary to patient or blood-unit misidentification) approximates 1:1.5 × 10^6, which approximates the estimated death risk from viral transmission.* Nevertheless, prudent utilization of transfusion support is important because blood is a scarce resource and because of possible, unknown future blood risks.

2. **West nile virus (WNV).** Queens, New York, was the epicenter of a WNV epidemic in 1999, which thereafter spread to numerous states throughout the country. The first of the cases of transfusion-transmitted WNV was reported in 2002, when 23 transfusion recipients who developed symptoms of a viral illness within 4 weeks of transfusion and then had laboratory confirmation of WNV. The cases were linked to 16 donors who were viremic at the time of collection (*N Engl J Med* 2003;349:1236). NAT testing of blood donors was started in 2003, and data from the American Red Cross reported 540 positive donations in 2003 and 2004. It is not clear whether NAT testing for WNV in blood donors will need to continue as the number of WNV cases throughout the country has declined since 2002.

3. **Cytomegalovirus (CMV) infection.** CMV infection has been a substantial cause of morbidity and mortality for immunocompromised oncology patients. Patients who receive allogeneic bone marrow/stem cell transplantation are at risk because of cytotoxic preparative regimens, immunosuppressive therapy (cyclosporine and corticosteroid), and/or GVHD. Up to 60% of this patient population will experience CMV infection, with half of them developing CMV disease. Even with the use of CMV-negative blood products, CMV seroconversion has been reported in 1% to 4% of CMV-negative donor–recipient transplantation patients.

   CMV infection and CMV disease are much less common in patients undergoing conventional chemotherapy or autologous bone marrow/stem cell transplantation, and are not thought to be a significant clinical problem.

   A randomized, controlled clinical trial in allogeneic bone marrow transplantation patients compared the value of CMV-seronegative blood products with unscreened blood products that were subjected to bedside leukofiltration. Four (1.3%) of 252 patients in the CMV-seronegative cohort developed CMV infection, with no CMV disease or fatalities; 6 (2.4%) of 250 patients in the leukoreduced cohort developed CMV disease, of whom 5 died. A much larger study would have to be performed to eliminate a type II statistical error with the insignificant rise in CMV infection of 40%. The filtered cohort had an increased probability of developing CMV disease by day 100 (2.4% vs. none; $p = 0.03$). Even when the investigators eliminated CMV infections that occurred within 21 days of transplantation, two cases of fatal CMV disease occurred in the filtered arm as compared with none in the leukoreduced arm. The conclusion by the authors of this study that leukoreduced blood products are "CMV safe" remains controversial. In a consensus conference held by the Canadian Blood Service, 7 of 10 panelists concluded that patients considered at risk for CMV disease should receive CMV-seronegative products, even when blood components are leukoreduced.

4. **Bacterial contamination.** The risk of platelet-related sepsis is estimated to be 1:12,000 for apheresis platelets but is greater with transfusions of pooled platelet concentrates from multiple donors (e.g., 1:2,000 after receiving six concentrates). Transfusion-related sepsis was the second leading cause of transfusion-associated fatalities from 1990 to 1998. In descending order, the organisms most commonly implicated in fatalities (as reported to the FDA) are *Staphylococcus aureus*, *Klebsiella pneumoniae*, *Serratia marcescens*, and *Staphylococcus epidermidis*. Platelets are prone to bacterial contamination because they are stored at 20°C to 24°C (room temperature). There is an increasing risk of bacterial overgrowth with time and, consequently, the shelf life of platelets is limited to 5 days. However, with new procedures, this may be extended to 7 days. In 2004, AABB implemented standards that require blood banks to perform bacterial testing of platelets. The bacterial testing systems are inoculated 24 hours after collection (to allow for bacterial growth) and then incubate for an additional 24 hours. Approximately 1:2,000 platelet units are found to be bacterially contaminated and often bacteria are detected after the 24-hour incubation and subsequent transfusion. Late positive tests likely indicate a reduced bacterial load and a smaller risk of sepsis. When platelets are released from bacterial testing, only 3 days remain of the 5-day shelf life, which challenges blood banks to maintain an adequate platelet inventory without substantial wastage. The use of rapid culture technology has been shown to reduce the transfusion of bacterially contaminated components (i.e., especially platelets with Gram-negative organisms), and this has also been accompanied by diminishing rates of septic reactions via hemovigilance programs. However, ongoing reports of culture negative products leading to either septic reactions or being associated with positive outdate cultures underscore persistent limitations in this technique. Recently, the FDA has approved a bacterial testing system that prolongs the shelf life of platelets to 7 days, which is currently being utilized in some centers.

Another method to reduce the risk of transfusion-associated sepsis is photochemical treatment of platelet products. Photochemical treatments utilize ultraviolet (UV) light and psoralen to inactivate a broad range of Gram-negative and -positive organisms, as well as viruses. Treatment of platelet concentrates with amotosalen (a synthetic psoralen) and UVA light will result in a >4.5-log reduction in bacterial pathogens. Two randomized, controlled trials have evaluated the safety and efficacy of platelet concentrates treated with psoralen and UVA and both concluded that platelet products treated with photochemical inactivation were as efficacious as conventional platelets in achieving hemostasis with a comparable safety profile. Further studies are needed to better elucidate the role of pathogen inactivation in platelet products to reduce transfusion-associated sepsis and the risk reduction, if any, these methods provide in addition to the AABB-mandated bacterial cultures. In addition, Benjamin et al. have demonstrated that diversion pouches in conjunction with bacterial culture at the time of collection can minimize the rate of bacterial contamination of donated blood.

The clinical presentation of bacterially contaminated platelet infection can range from mild fever (which may be indistinguishable from febrile, nonhemolytic transfusion reactions) to acute sepsis, hypotension, and death. Sepsis caused by transfusion of contaminated platelets is underrecognized in part because the organisms found in platelet contamination are frequently the same as those implicated in "catheter" or "line" sepsis. The overall mortality rate of identified platelet-associated sepsis is 26%.

In the clinical setting, any patient in whom fever develops within 6 hours of platelet infusion should be evaluated for possible bacterial contamination of the component, and initiation of empiric antibiotic therapy should be considered. Because of their storage at room temperature, platelets are more prone to bacterial infection than are other blood products. FATRs occur in only 0.5% of red cell transfusions; of these, 18% and 8% of patients experience a second and third Febrile Transfusion Reaction (FTR),, respectively. Approximately 18% of platelet transfusions are associated with FTR, although the prevalence of platelet-associated FTR can be as high as 30% in frequently transfused populations such as oncology patients. Reactions characterized as severe occur in only 2% of platelet transfusions, and bedside leukofiltration has not been found to reduce the overall prevalence of FTR. Risks of transfusion-transmitted diseases are the same as those for red cells and are summarized in Table 39-1.

D. Plasma therapy. Plasma therapy should be administered to patients who have abnormal prothrombin time (PT) or partial thromboplastin time (PTT) assays in the setting of correction with a mixing study and clinically significant hemorrhage. The most common setting is in patients with liver disease who have multiple coagulation deficiencies, along with ongoing consumption due to impaired reticuloendothelial system (RES) clearance of substances activating the coagulation system. Another setting is in vitamin K deficiency. Vitamin K is derived from dietary sources and from intestinal bacteria, so that deficiency is caused by either poor dietary intake and/or with concomitant antibiotic therapy (e.g., intubated or cachectic patients treated with prolonged and multiple antibiotic therapy). Patients who have had Coumadin overdose or who are sensitive to this agent can also have markedly elevated international normalized ratio (INR) values. Parenteral vitamin K (5 to 10 mg s.q. or i.v. daily) administration should be considered in both patients with liver disease (impaired enterohepatic circulation of bile salts leading to deficiency of vitamin K and the vitamin K–dependent coagulation factors II, VII, IX, and X) and patients with Coumadin overdose. For patients with life-threatening hemorrhage, 15 mL/kg of plasma will increase factor levels by 20% to 30%, but there are limitations with plasma related to time required to obtain and administer the units as well as the propensity for fluid overload in susceptible patients (e.g., patients with poor myocardial function or patients who require larger doses). Recent guidelines have highlighted the potential usefulness (Grade 2c recommendation) of three and four factor concentrates that can be used to immediately reverse the effects of warfarin with minimal requirements for volume; the newer factor concentrates may also attenuate thrombotic risk since they also contain substantial quantities of protein C and S.

E. Platelet transfusions

1. Platelet-transfusion practices

a. Threshold for transfusion. Several studies have evaluated prophylactic platelet-transfusion practices and thresholds for patients who are thrombocytopenic due to myelosuppressive therapy. One study found that most patients undergoing stem cell transplantation were transfused prophylactically with platelets when their platelet counts were between 10×10^9/L and 20×10^9/L, indicating that a threshold of 20×10^9/L was most common. Only 9% of hemorrhagic events reported in this study occurred when platelet counts were less than 10×10^9/L.

Two prospective, randomized studies evaluated the relative merits of platelet-transfusion thresholds of 10×10^9/L versus 20×10^9/L for leukemia patients undergoing chemotherapy. One found that the lower transfusion threshold was associated with 22% fewer platelet transfusions. No differences between the two patient cohorts were seen with respect to hemorrhagic complications, number of red cell transfusions, duration of hospital stay, or mortality. In a second study, a platelet threshold of 10×10^9/L was safe and effective when compared with a threshold of 20×10^9/L. Two (1.9%) of the 105 patients in this study died of hemorrhagic complications; each patient had a platelet count greater than 30×10^9/L at the time of death. However, these studies were not adequately powered to detect a difference in fairly infrequent but catastrophic complications (e.g., subarachnoid bleeds). Nevertheless, it seems that other patient-related factors (i.e., qualitative platelet abnormalities, von Willebrand disease, or other hemostatic system defects) may play a role with respect to bleeding complications in the setting of thrombocytopenia.

b. Platelet dose. Standards of the AABB require that 75% of single-donor platelet (SDP) or apheresis products contain more than 3×10^{11} platelets and that 75% of platelet concentrates (i.e., six pack is equivalent to a SDP) contain more than 5.5×10^{10} platelets. However, there is a broad range of platelet doses in several clinical trials, indicating that there is no consensus for a standardized platelet-transfusion dose.

High-dose platelet therapy was investigated in a clinical trial that randomized patients with hematologic malignancies to prophylactic platelet transfusions with standard, high, and very high platelet doses (4.6×10^{11}, 6.5×10^{11}, and 8.9×10^{11} platelets, respectively) to maintain a platelet count of 15×10^9 to 20×10^9/L. The high and very high platelet dose cohorts had greater platelet-count incremental increases and prolonged time to next transfusion when compared with the standard platelet dose cohort. However, as the platelet dose increased, the ratio of median number of platelets transfused/median transfusion interval decreased, suggesting that lower platelet doses may decrease the overall number of platelets required to maintain a platelet count of 15×10^9 to 20×10^9/L.

Mathematical modeling of platelet survival predicts that lower doses of prophylactic platelet therapy (approximately 2×10^9 vs. 4×10^9) transfused to maintain a platelet count of 10×10^9/L would decrease platelet usage by 22%. To evaluate the effects of low-dose platelet therapy on platelet utilization and risk of hemorrhage, a randomized study in thrombocytopenic patients receiving high-dose chemotherapy or a stem cell transplant compared low-dose (approximately 2×10^{11}) with standard-dose (approximately 4×10^{11}) platelet therapy. Over the course of their hospitalization, patients in the low-dose arm required 25% fewer platelet units and had a comparable number of bleeding events to the standard-dose group. Further studies of platelet-transfusion dosage strategies are needed to determine an optimal dose.

2. Platelet refractoriness. Infusion of an SDP generally results in a platelet rise of 30,000 to 60,000/μL. *Platelet refractoriness* is defined as a reduced or absent rise in platelet count, especially when measured within 1 hour of transfusion. The differential diagnosis of platelet refractoriness in oncology patients includes infection, DIC, thrombotic thrombocytopenia purpura (TTP), splenomegaly, drugs, or antibody-mediated mechanisms. The first step in managing patients who respond poorly to platelet transfusions is to identify the specific cause of platelet refractoriness, which first requires the measurement of a corrected count increment (CCI), which accounts for the dose of platelets and the recipient size. Platelet refractoriness is typically defined as a CCI of less than 5,000 to 7,500 on two occasions when the patient receives ABO-compatible platelets.

$$CCI = \frac{\text{Platelet count increment} / \text{mm}^3 \times \text{Body surface area (m}^2)}{\text{Number of platelets transfused} (\times 10^{11})}$$

Upon diagnosis of platelet refractoriness, the causative factor must be sought. In multiply transfused patients, a poor response to transfusion may be commonly due to anti–HLA-related antibodies. Antibody-mediated accelerated clearance of platelets is supported by a poor increment when the count is obtained within 30 to 60 minutes after transfusion, in contrast to other potential causes like DIC that may result in an initial (30 to 60 minutes) increase in platelet count, followed by accelerated clearance over the next few hours. The formation of antibodies to HLA antigens occurs when there is exposure to foreign HLA molecules through pregnancy or transfusion. As platelets express HLA class I antigens, the presence of these antibodies may result in platelet refractoriness. Leukocytes present in transfused products have been implicated in the formation of HLA antibodies and, therefore, a large, randomized trial was conducted to examine the benefit of leukoreduced blood products in the reduction of platelet alloantibodies. The TRAP study (Trial to Reduce Alloimmunization to Platelets) found that clinical platelet refractoriness associated with HLA antibody seropositivity was reduced from 13% of patients transfused with unprocessed platelet concentrates to 3% to 5% of patients receiving leukoreduced apheresis platelets, leukoreduced platelet concentrates, or psoralen-/UVB-treated platelets. Notably, there was no difference in the rate of hemorrhage or overall mortality between the groups. The authors concluded that leukoreduced blood helped prevent the formation of alloantibodies.

Alloantibodies to HLA antigens can be detected by methods of lymphocytotoxicity, enzyme-linked immunosorbent assay (ELISA), or flow cytometry. If HLA alloantibodies are found, providing matched platelets at the A and B loci can improve platelet increments. Alternatively, if specificity of the HLA antibody can be determined, antigen-negative platelets may be effective. In fact, some centers utilize cross-match procedures to identify platelet units that will improve responsiveness to platelet transfusion. The largest obstacle to providing HLA-matched platelets is a limited donor pool, which can be mitigated through single antigen mismatches with cross-reactive groups (CREGs). CREGs are structurally similar HLA antigens that react with common antisera. Transfusing alloimmunized patients with selectively HLA-mismatched platelets can increase the number of potential donors while improving platelet increments.

Persistent refractoriness to platelet transfusions despite HLA-matched platelets is not uncommon in heavily alloimmunized patients. Although many immunosuppressive medications have been tried in this circumstance, the only therapy that has demonstrated some success is IVIG. Case reports and small series comprise most of this literature and the efficacy of IVIG in the treatment of alloimmunized patients is variable between reports. IVIG should not be used as a first-line therapy for alloimmunized patients; however, it has a role in patients who are persistently refractory to well-matched platelets or who are refractory and have active bleeding.

Although alloantibodies are an important cause of platelet refractoriness, in some cases patient-specific factors can also influence the response to transfusion. In patients undergoing stem cell transplantation, the type of therapy administered and extent of disease are important predictors of platelet increment following a transfusion. A study of stem cell transplant recipients noted that factors usually associated with patient response to platelets (history of previous transfusion, pregnancy, the presence of HLA, or platelet-specific antibodies) did not significantly correlate with CCI. Rather, patient-specific variables such as disease status (advanced rather than early), conditioning regimen (including total body irradiation or not), progenitor cell source (bone marrow rather than peripheral stem cell), and type of transplant (allogeneic vs. autologous) are significant predictors of platelet refractoriness in patients undergoing stem cell transplantation.

F. **Special blood products**
  1. **Washed RBCs** are rarely indicated, except in patients with severe or recurrent idiosyncratic reactions to plasma or platelets, in patients with IgA deficiency or in patients who cannot tolerate potassium loads especially with older RBC units (e.g., end-stage renal disease).
  2. **Irradiation of blood products** eliminates engraftment by immunologically competent donor lymphocytes and is recommended for immunocompromised patients (high-dose chemotherapeutic regimens, immunosuppressive therapy in allogeneic transplantation, or fludarabine therapy), and any patient receiving directed transfusions from a blood relative.
  3. **Leukoreduced blood products** (i.e., defined as 99.9% of white blood cells [WBCs] removed) have been recommended for the following patients: (a) patients with previous febrile transfusion reactions not prevented by acetaminophen and diphenhydramine

therapy; (b) patients undergoing red cell-exchange transfusions; (c) patients for whom cross-match compatible blood is difficult to obtain; (d) patients who are candidates for solid organ (kidney, heart, and lung) or stem cell (aplastic anemia) transplantation; and (e) patients who should receive CMV-negative blood (e.g., platelets) when CMV-seronegative products are unavailable.

III. **APHERESIS.** Apheresis is a procedure that removes a specified component of whole blood. It can be broadly classified into plasmapheresis (removal of plasma) and cytapheresis (removal of cells). Whole blood is continuously (i.e., 50 to 100 mL/min) removed from the patient either through a central venous catheter or a peripheral vein with a large bore needle and enters the pheresis machine through an extracorporeal circuit. Within the machine, the components of blood are separated by centrifugation, the desired portion (plasma, platelets, white cells, or red cells) is removed, and the remainder is then returned to the patient along with replacement solutions (e.g., plasma, albumin, or hetastarch) and donor red cells (i.e., with a red cell exchange). In the case of plasmapheresis, filtration instead of centrifugation can be used and similarly a replacement fluid is necessary, which may be albumin, plasma, or a combination.

A. **Plasmapheresis.** In general, plasmapheresis is used to remove disease-inducing antibodies or antigen-antibody complexes (e.g., vasculitis) and the amount of antibody removed per procedure depends on the vascular distribution of the pathologic antibody. IgG is 45% intravascular and approximately five procedures (i.e., using a 1.5-plasma volume exchange) are necessary to remove 90% of the antibody; in contrast, IgM is 80% to 90% intravascular and requires two to three procedures to remove 90% of the antibody. Plasmapheresis is used to treat many disease states in patients with cancer diagnoses. The frequency of required maintenance procedures also depends on the half-life of the specific immunoglobulin class (i.e., 21 days for IgG vs. 10 days for IgM and IgA).

Waldenstrom's macroglobulinemia (WM) is a low-grade lymphoma often associated with hyperviscosity symptoms due to excess IgM. If patients with WM present with symptoms of hyperviscosity (dizziness, shortness of breath, bleeding, confusion, visual changes) related to high IgM levels, emergent plasmapheresis can markedly improve symptoms. Additionally, patients with WM who cannot tolerate other therapies may be maintained on a chronic program of plasmapheresis to control symptoms. Plasmapheresis is also effective in the treatment of hyperviscosity associated with multiple myeloma; however, IgG or IgA paraproteins may require multiple procedures for symptom resolution. Recently, a randomized, controlled trial investigated the role of plasmapheresis in acute renal failure of multiple myeloma. Patients were randomized to conventional therapy (supportive care plus treatment of multiple myeloma) or to conventional therapy plus five to seven plasma exchange procedures. No significant differences in dialysis dependence, glomerular filtration rate, or death were noted between the plasmapheresis and standard therapy cohorts. Finally, plasmapheresis can be utilized in stem cell transplantation patients who receive a transplant from an ABO-incompatible donor. In the case of a major incompatibility (A donor → O recipient), recipient isohemagglutinins (anti-A) may persist until erythroid engraftment (A cells) occurs, with resultant potentially life-threatening hemolysis. This incompatibility may also lead to a protracted red cell engraftment period. Alternatively, if the donor is O and the recipient is A blood group, a minor incompatibility is present at the time of transplantation. However, donor lymphocytes (which produce anti-A) are delivered along with stem cells, and approximately 10 days after transplantation, synthesize anti-A in quantities sufficient to cause clinically significant hemolysis. This phenomenon is referred to as *passenger lymphocyte syndrome* and can also be seen after solid organ transplantation. Monitoring forward/reverse blood types, blood counts, lactate dehydrogenase (LDH), and direct antigen test results in susceptible patients (e.g., those with anti-A or anti-B titers >1:8) can allow early identification of patients who might require apheresis management for these hemolytic processes. In major or minor incompatibilities, plasmapheresis can effectively remove the isohemagglutinins and help abate hemolysis. However, if hemolysis is related to IgG (anti-A or anti-B), then plasmapheresis may not be immediately effective (i.e., since five procedures are required for a log reduction in IgG levels). In the case of ABO incompatibility and substantial hemolysis, urgent red cell exchange with O units may be indicated to abate hemolysis and reduce hemolytic-related sequelae.

B. Cytapheresis is used to collect peripheral blood stem cells for transplantation as discussed in Chapter 5. Outlined in the Chapter 35 is leukoreduction for hyperviscosity of acute leukemia.

SUGGESTED READINGS

Benjamin RJ, Kline L, Dy BA, et al. Bacterial contamination of whole-blood-derived platelets: the introduction of sample diversion and prestorage pooling with culture testing in the American Red Cross. *Transfusion* 2008;48:2348–2355.

Benjamin RJ, McDonald CP. the international experience of bacterial screen test of platelet components with an automated microbial detection system: a need for consensus testing and reporting guidelines. *Transfusion Med Rev* 2014;28:61–71.

Bernstein SH, Nademanee AP, Vose JM, et al. A multicenter study of platelet recovery and utilization in patients after myeloablative therapy and hematopoietic stem cell transplantation. *Blood* 1998;91:3509–3517.

Bowden RA, Slichter SJ, Sayers M, et al. A comparison of filtered leukocyte-reduced and cytomegalovirus (CMV) seronegative blood products for the prevention of transfusion-associated CMV infection after marrow transplant. *Blood* 1995;86:3598–3603.

Carson JL, Grossman BJ, Kleinman S, et al. Red blood cell transfusions: a clinical practice guideline from the AABB. *Ann Intern Med* 2012;157:49–59.

Carson JL, Terrin ML, Noveck H, et al. Liberal or restrictive transfusion in high-risk patients after hip surgery. *N Engl J Med* 2011;365:2453–2462.

Dorsey KA, Moritz ED, Steele WR, et al. Transfusion 2013;53(6):1250–1256.

Eder AF, Dy BA, Perez JM, et al. The residual risk of transfusion-related acute lung injury at the American Red Cross (2008–2011): limitations of a predominately male-donor plasma mitigation strategy. *Transfusion* 2013;53:1442–1449.

Finch CA, Lenfant C. Oxygen transport in man. *N Engl J Med* 1972;286:407–415.

Goodnough LT, Brecher ME, Kanter MH, et al. Transfusion medicine, part I: blood transfusion. *N Engl J Med* 1999;340:438–447.

Hebert PC, Wells G, Blajchman MA, et al. A multicenter, randomized, controlled clinical trial of transfusion requirements in critical care. *N Engl J Med* 1999;340:409–417.

Holbrook A, Schulman S, Witt DM, et al. Evidence-based management of anticoagulant therapy: antithrombotic therapy and prevention of thrombosis, 9th ed: American College of Chest Physicians Evidence-Based Clinical Practice Guidelines. *Chest* 2012;141:e152S–e184S.

Lane TA, Anderson KC, Goodnough LT, et al. Leukocyte reduction in blood component therapy. *Ann Intern Med* 1992;117:151–162.

Norol F, Bierling P, Roudot-Thoraval F, et al. Platelet transfusion: a dose-response study. *Blood* 1998;92:1448–1453.

Pealer LN, Marfin AA, Petersen LR, et al. Transmission of west Nile virus through blood transfusion in the United States in 2002. *N Engl J Med* 2003;349:1236–1245.

Poole J, Daniels G. Blood group antibodies and their significance in transfusion medicine. *T Med Reviews* 2007;21:58–71.

Shimian Z, Stramer SL, Dodd RY, et al. Donor testing and risk: current prevalence, incidence, and residual risk of transfusion-transmissible agents in US allogeneic donations. *T Med Rev* 2012;26:119–128.

Stramer SL, Fang CT, Foster GA, et al. West Nile virus among blood donors in the United States, 2003 and 2004. *N Engl J Med* 2005;353:451–459.

Stramer SL, Glynn SA, Kleinman SH, et al. Detection of HIV-1 and HCV infections among antibody-negative blood donors by nucleic acid-amplification testing. *N Engl J Med* 2004;351:760–768.

The Trial to Reduce Alloimmunization to Platelets Study Group. Leukocyte reduction and ultraviolet B irradiation of platelets to prevent alloimmunization and refractoriness to platelet transfusions. *N Engl J Med* 1997;337:1861–1869.

Vassallo RR. IgA anaphylactic transfusion reactions, part I: laboratory diagnosis, incidence, and supply of IgA-deficient products [Review]. *Immunohematology* 2004;20:226–233.

Villanueva C, Colomo A, Bosch A, et al. Transfusion strategies for upper intestinal bleeding. *N Engl J Med* 2013;368:11–21.

Wandt H, Frank M, Ehninger G, et al. Safety and cost effectiveness of a 10 × 10(9)/L trigger for prophylactic platelet transfusions compared with the traditional 20 × 10(9)/L trigger: a prospective comparative trial in 105 patients with acute myeloid leukemia. *Blood* 1998;91:3601–3606.

Welch HG, Mehan KR, Goodnough LT. Prudent strategies for elective red blood cell transfusion. *Ann Intern Med* 1992;116:393–402.

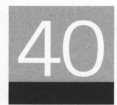

Pain Management

Robert A. Swarm • Rahul Rastogi • Lesley Rao

I. **INTRODUCTION TO CANCER PAIN MANAGEMENT.** Pain remains a common problem in oncology practice largely because standard analgesic therapies are inconsistently applied; the vast majority of patients could receive good cancer pain control from standard pain treatments. In developed countries, up to 30% of people at initial cancer diagnosis, 50% to 70% of those receiving active antitumor therapy, and up to 80% of those with advanced malignant disease suffer inadequately controlled pain. Improving cancer pain management requires: health-care professionals to know and apply pain pathophysiology, epidemiology, and treatment; patients to be more effective self-advocates and better-informed health-care consumers; and a health-care delivery system that requires consistent symptom control as part of individualized, patient-centered goals of therapy for cancer care. Pain control not only improves quality of life for cancer patients but is a major factor in overall symptom control, which may contribute to survival; therefore, optimized pain control is an integral component of comprehensive cancer care. To consistently control cancer pain, each practitioner must insure that every cancer patient under his/her care receives optimized pain control. Factors known to limit optimal cancer pain management must be identified in clinical practice and appropriately managed (Table 40-1).

II. **COMPREHENSIVE PAIN ASSESSMENT.** The starting point for good pain control is a comprehensive pain assessment, including thorough pain history and physical examination. Consider repeating diagnostic evaluations because tumor progression or metastasis is the most common cause of increasing pain in patients with cancer. When feasible, antitumor therapies to control underlying disease may be the most effective pain management therapy.

A. **Pain assessment scales** are used to facilitate measurement of pain intensity and establish a baseline from which to judge the success of pain treatments. A numeric pain scale ("0 = no pain" up to "10 = worst pain imaginable") is easily used by most adults, but the face scale (happy to sad faces) may be more easily used by young children. Measuring pain intensity is only the starting point in understanding the severity and consequence of a patient's pain.

B. **The comprehensive pain evaluation** includes "PQRST" factors: P = provocative factors and palliative factors; Q = quality (characteristics) of pain; R = region, radiation, and referred distribution of pain; S = severity of pain intensity; and T = temporal factors including onset, duration, time of maximum intensity, frequency, and daily variation. Patients should be queried about a previous history of pain and what drugs were effective or ineffective in his or her management.

TABLE 40-1	Barriers to Optimal Cancer Pain Management

Patient-related barriers

1. Poor communication with physicians
2. Reluctance to report pain
3. Misconceptions about pain and available treatments
4. Reluctance to take medications
5. Fear of opioid addiction
6. Fear of medication adverse effects
7. Inability to access therapy, follow plan

Physician-related barriers

1. Inadequate pain assessment of patient
2. Inadequate knowledge, suboptimal use of available techniques
3. Bias limits opioid prescribing specially for female, elderly, minorities, well-functioning patients
4. Reluctance to prescribe opioids

Health-care system–related barriers

1. Reimbursement encourages curative interventions over symptom control
2. Cost of analgesic therapies
3. Administrative burden of opioid regulations
4. Insufficient pain education, training among health-care professionals
5. Poor availability, underutilization of advanced modalities for pain
6. Multiple specialists, fragmented care

Disease- and treatment-related barriers

1. Progressive disease increasing tissue damage and pain
2. Injury, inflammation, nerve damage, opioid tolerance facilitate pain signal processing, increasing pain
3. Coexisting/comorbid diseases may limit use of analgesic therapies
4. Incomplete efficacy of available pain therapies, including opioids

C. **Consider comorbid conditions** that may greatly influence analgesic therapy, especially in elderly or those with advanced disease. Renal and/or hepatic insufficiency will significantly impact analgesic choice. Intractable coagulopathy may preclude the use of interventional pain therapies. Advanced medical illness may increase the risk of analgesic adverse effects.

D. **Assess components of pain.** Nociceptive, neuropathic, affective, behavioral, cognitive, and social. Neuropathic pain may respond best to treatments including anticonvulsant and/or antidepressant therapy. Affect, cognition, and social context may markedly influence selection and/or efficacy of analgesic therapies.

E. **Believe the patient's own report of pain.** It is the most reliable indicator of pain. Malingering is rare in cancer pain management. If you do not (or conclude that you cannot) trust the patient' description of pain, pain will not be controlled.

III. **SYSTEMIC ANALGESICS**

A. **The World Health Organization (WHO) ladder** (Figure 40-1), the most widely used and validated protocol for cancer pain management, is a stepwise approach based on pain intensity. Opioids are the cornerstone of pharmacotherapy for moderate-to-severe cancer pain, but nonopioid and adjuvant analgesics (antidepressants, anticonvulsants) are used to enhance pain relief when needed. Analgesics should be given "*by the mouth*" (the simplest, most effective route of administration); "*by the clock*" (regular dosing schedule rather than sporadic "as-needed" dosing); "*by the ladder*"; and "*for the individual*" (titrate analgesic to effect, monitor for adverse effects). Unrelieved pain can almost always be controlled by reevaluating the patient and reapplying the principles of the WHO ladder. For pain refractory to systemic analgesics, advanced pain therapies (beyond the WHO ladder) should be utilized.

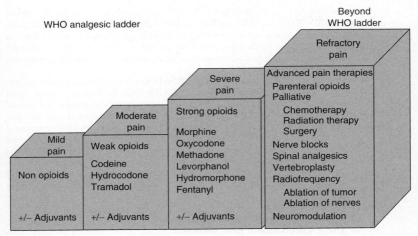

Figure 40-1. Therapy continuum for cancer pain management. The first three steps are based on the World Health Organization (WHO) analgesic ladder and include a wide range of system analgesics (nonopioid, adjuvant, and opioid analgesics). The final step ("Beyond the WHO Ladder") includes additional therapies for pain refractory to systemic analgesics.

B. **Nonopioid analgesics** (Table 40-2) are the principal analgesics for mild pain. In more severe pain, nonopioids are used to supplement opioid to improve pain control and reduce opioid dose (to reduce opioid-related adverse effects and the risk of opioid tolerance).

   1. **Aspirin and the nonacetylated salicylates** are modestly potent analgesics and antipyretics. Aspirin is a uniquely potent inhibitor of platelet function, but the nonacetylated salicylates have no impact on platelet function. The risk of gastrointestinal ulceration, somewhat greater with aspirin than other salicylates, significantly limits the analgesic utility of these agents, especially in medically ill or elderly patients. Salicylate is metabolized in the liver with renal excretion of salicylate and inactive metabolites.

TABLE 40-2	Nonopioid Analgesics		
	Single oral dose (mg)	**Maximum daily dose (mg)**	**Half-life (h)**
Acetaminophen	650–1,000	4,000	2–3
Aspirin	650–1,000	5,000	0.3–0.5[a]
Salsalate	500–1,000	3,000	1[a]
Nonsteroidal anti-inflammatory drugs (NSAIDs)			
Ibuprofen	200–800	3,200	3–4
Celecoxib	100–200	800	10–12
Diclofenac	50	225	1–2
Ketoprofen	50–75	300	2.1
Nabumetone	500–750	2,000	24
Naproxen	220–500	1,500	10–20
Piroxicam	10–20	20	50

[a]Metabolized to salicylic acid that has a half-life of 20–30 h with repeated dosing.

2. **Acetaminophen** is a modestly potent but effective analgesic and antipyretic. Typical doses (650 to 1,000 mg QID, maximum 4,000 mg/day) are well tolerated, but excessive doses may cause severe hepatotoxicity; for added safety margin, consider limiting chronic acetaminophen dosing to 3,000 mg per day. Acetaminophen is available for intravenous, oral, and rectal administration, but intravenous formulation is expensive, and rectal absorption is poor.

C. **Nonsteroidal anti-inflammatory drugs (NSAIDs)** are useful in pain from inflammatory processes and/or boney metastases. NSAIDs limit facilitation of pain signal transmission by inhibiting prostaglandin synthesis in peripheral tissues and central nervous system (CNS). Renal toxicity, gastrointestinal ulceration, and platelet dysfunction limit NSAID utility, especially in medically ill patients. Selective cyclooxygenase 2 (COX-2) inhibitors (celecoxib 200 mg daily or BID) have lower risk of gastrointestinal ulceration and no platelet dysfunction, but increased risk of thromboembolic events limits use. Although NSAIDs are administered orally, intravenous formulations (ketorolac (15 to 30 mg i.v./i.m., QID, maximum 5 days due to gastric ulceration risk) and ibuprofen (400 to 800 mg i.v. q 6 hours) are options when enteral administration is not feasible.

D. **Opioid analgesics**
   1. **General principles for the use of opioid analgesics**
      a. **Use a comprehensive pain assessment** to gather information to guide pain therapy. Repeat/review assessment at each patient contact and whenever pain is not controlled.
      b. **Teach patients** and their families to assess pain by using a numeric score to facilitate communication. Documentation of pain intensity rating, the fifth vital sign, is standard for outpatient and inpatient care.
      c. **Administer analgesics orally** or through the least invasive route that provides effective pain control.
      d. **Document all narcotic prescriptions** in the medical record to aid in the monitoring and adjustment of pain therapy (and to comply with federal and state regulations).
      e. **Individualize opioid dose.** The correct dose is that which adequately controls pain while minimizing adverse effects. Depending on pain severity, degree of opioid tolerance, and comorbid factors, the required daily dose of opioid can range over two to three orders of magnitude.
      f. **Avoid use of combination analgesic preparations,** which contain opioid together with an NSAID or acetaminophen, unless that specific combination of medications is indicated for the specific patient; single agent formulations facilitate analgesic dose titration.
      g. **Anticipate opioid-related adverse effects** and treat promptly (Table 40-3). Almost everyone taking opioid daily will need daily laxatives to prevent constipation.
      h. **Use regularly scheduled, long-acting analgesic preparations** (extended-release preparations of morphine, oxycodone, oxymorphone; fentanyl transdermal patch; and methadone) to improve compliance and provide more consistent pain relief than repeated as-needed dosing of short-acting opioid. Extended-release oral tablets should be swallowed whole and not cut or crushed.
      i. **Prescribe supplemental doses of opioid for "breakthrough pain"** not controlled by the regularly scheduled doses. Use short-acting, immediate-release oral preparations of opioid (morphine, oxycodone, and hydromorphone) at doses of 10% to 15% of total daily opioid dose, as often as every 1 hour as needed.
      j. **Be flexible but aggressive in treating severe, uncontrolled pain.** Hospital admission for parenteral opioids and frequent reassessment of analgesic efficacy may be required. In a pain emergency, opioid should be given intravenously (e.g., morphine 1 to 4 mg i.v., every 10 minutes) and titrated to effect. Once pain is improved, a patient-controlled analgesia (PCA) device may facilitate access to, and documentation of, needed opioid for subsequent conversion to oral formulations.

TABLE 40-3	Managing Common Opioid Side Effects	
Side effects	**Comments and management**	
Constipation	Most common side effect No tolerance Use agents regularly and prophylactically Educate patients Combine agents	Stool softeners (docusate) Stimulants (senna and bisacodyl) Bulk laxatives (psyllium) Osmotic agents (lactulose and polyethylene glycol) Enemas Opioid antagonist (oral naloxone and subcutaneous methylnaltrexone)
Sedation	Avoid confounding medications Lower opioid dose by 25% Use stimulants Opioid substitution Add adjuvant to reduce opioid dose Use neuraxial route of delivery	Dextroamphetamine Methylphenidate Modafinil Donepezil
Nausea and vomiting	Manage constipation Treat with antiemetics Correct metabolic factors Switch to another opioid Tolerance develops slowly	Promethazine Prochlorperazine Olanzapine Ondansetron and dolasetron Scopolamine Hydroxyzine Dexamethasone
Myoclonus	Usually with high dosages Switch to another opioid Lower dose of opioid Avoid meperidine	Lorazepam Clonazepam Diazepam
Pruritus	Treat with antihistamines Consider a different opioid	Diphenhydramine Hydroxyzine Ondansetron Nalbuphine
Withdrawal symptoms	Taper dose by half every other day when discontinuing	Clonidine
Opioid Toxicity Syndrome (OTS)	Risk factors: rapidly increasing, high-dose opioid; dehydration; and renal failure Severe myoclonus may mimic seizures	Opioid rotation, adequate hydration, and opioid dose reduction

Seizures rarely have been reported with high-dose opioid infusion, typically associated with preservative agents. If using high-dose infusion, use preservative-free opioid preparations.

    k. Be aware of equipotent doses of various opioid analgesics to facilitate changes between agents or routes of administration (Table 40-4).

    l. Use naloxone to treat severe respiratory depression related to opioid overdose. About 0.1 to 0.2 mg i.v./i.m. every 1 to 5 minutes as needed; however, opioid antagonism with naloxone may cause extreme pain and other opioid withdrawal symptoms.

TABLE 40-4	Opioid Analgesics for Chronic Pain, with Estimates of Equivalent Doses

	Elimination ($t\frac{1}{2}$) in hours	Dose by injection equivalent to morphine injection 10 mg (single dose)	Dose by mouth equivalent to morphine injection 10 mg (single dose)
Morphine	2–4	10 mg	20–60 mg
Buprenorphine	20–70	0.3 mg	0.4 mg sublingual
Codeine	3	120 mg	200 mg
Fentanyl[a]	4	100 µg	N/A
Hydrocodone	4	N/A	30–40 mg
Hydromorphone	3	2 mg	10 mg
Levorphanol	14	2 mg	4 mg
Meperidine[b]	3	100 mg	300 mg
Methadone[c]	30	—[c]	—[c]
Oxycodone	3	N/A	20–30 mg
Oxymorphone	2	1 mg	10 mg
Tramadol	6	Only the oral formulation of this is available in the United States; limit to 50–100 mg/dose and 400 mg/dose due to seizure risk with higher doses	
Tapentadol	4	NA	100 mg PO

[a]Transdermal fentanyl patch 100 µg/h = morphine 300 mg/day p.o.
[b]CNS toxicity of active metabolites limits use in chronic pain management.
[c]Very long elimination half-life causes methadone to accumulate over many days. Because methadone is eliminated 10 times more slowly than morphine, with repeated dosing methadone is 10 times more potent than morphine and must be dosed with caution. If unfamiliar with methadone dosing, consider consultation with pain specialist or other physician familiar with methadone pharmacology.

2. **Limitations of opioid use in cancer pain management.** Opioids are the principal analgesics for the management of moderate-to-severe cancer pain; however, several factors limit opioid utility, including adverse effects (Table 40-3), limited efficacy, and access-to-care issues (Table 40-1).

   a. **Common opioid adverse effects,** especially constipation and nausea, should be anticipated so that management strategies can be implemented promptly (Table 40-3).

      i. **Respiratory depression**—increased susceptibility with preexisting lung disease, sleep apnea, and cardiac disease; somewhat decreased susceptibility with chronic opioid exposure (tolerance). If significant respiratory depression or opioid-induced sedation develops, consider naloxone administration (0.1 to 0.2 mg i.v./i.m. every 1 to 5 minutes as needed); abrupt naloxone reversal of opioid effect may lead to acute opioid withdrawal syndrome (severe pain exacerbation, hypertension, tachycardia, dyspnea, pulmonary edema, and delirium).

      ii. **Sedation**—typically managed with opioid dose titration, but severe or progressive sedation may signal pending respiratory depression/arrest and necessitate at least temporary opioid discontinuation or even reversal with naloxone. New onset sedation, with stable chronic opioid regimen, may suggest other contributing abnormality: decreased opioid clearance (hepatic and renal insufficiency), CNS pathology, and sepsis.

      iii. **Hypogonadism**—common in chronic opioid therapy, especially higher dose morphine >100 mg daily, due to opioid suppression of hypothalamic–pituitary–gonadal axis. Symptoms, in men and women, may include impaired sexual function, decreased libido, infertility, depression, fatigue, and loss of muscle mass and strength. Opioid endocrine impact may be confounded by consequences of underlying malignancy and/or other medical conditions; management may include opioid titration/discontinuation and/or hormonal replacement therapy, if needed.

   iv. **Immunosuppression**—opioid-induced immunosuppression is readily demonstrated in experimental animals, yet the clinical significance is confounded by comorbid disease pathophysiology and lack of randomized clinical trials.

   v. **Tolerance/hyperalgesia**—essentially all patients receiving chronic opioid therapy develop opioid tolerance, sometimes managed with an increase in opioid dose. Increasingly, opioid tolerance is thought to reflect an induced hyperalgesic state in which chronic opioid still inhibits pain signal transmission, but increasingly facilitates pain signal transmission, resulting in more pain that is more resistant to management. Lack of randomized clinical trials limits clear separation of tolerance from other causes of hyperalgesia; however, people taking opioid chronically generally have significant hyperalgesia. Concern for opioid-induced hyperalgesia has resulted in a marked reduction of opioid use for chronic noncancer pain management and raises concern for chronic opioid use in long-term cancer survivors.

b. **Opioid analgesic efficacy** is best for moderately severe pain that is continuously present. Efficacy may be limited by the following:

   i. **Neuropathic pain,** especially associated with severe sensitivity to light mechanical stimulation, may be relatively resistant to opioid analgesics, but may benefit from adjuvant analgesics (anticonvulsants and antidepressants).

   ii. **Episodically severe pain** may represent a timing challenge for analgesic dosing. Pain episodes may be inadequately controlled while waiting for analgesic effect onset. Conversely, analgesics dosed to control very severe pain episodes may result in relative overdose when the pain episode subsides.

   iii. **Sharp somatic pain** (e.g., wound debridement, pathologic bony fracture) is generally not adequately controlled with opioid except at doses associated with marked sedation. Sharp somatic pain may require "anesthetic" rather than "analgesic" management.

   iv. **Intractable pain,** especially in advanced cancer, may not be adequately controlled despite optimal adjustment of systemic analgesics, and may require interventional pain therapies or other techniques.

3. **Specific opioid analgesics** (Table 40-4)

a. **Morphine** is hepatically metabolized to active metabolites that contribute to analgesic effect and toxicity. Morphine and metabolites undergo combined fecal and renal excretion; morphine should be used with caution in renal insufficiency as metabolites may accumulate and cause toxicity. Although oral administration is preferred for most patients, morphine can be administered through intravenous, intramuscular, subcutaneous, sublingual, rectal, topical (for painful skin ulceration), epidural, and intrathecal routes.

b. **Hydromorphone,** and its active hepatic metabolites, are renally cleared by the kidneys and can accumulate in renal failure, precipitating opioid toxicity. In some individuals, common opioid adverse effects may be less with hydromorphone than with morphine. Hydromorphone can be administered through intravenous, intramuscular, subcutaneous, sublingual, rectal, epidural, and intrathecal routes, although oral absorption is less reliable than with oxycodone or morphine.

c. **Fentanyl** has high lipid solubility and is metabolized by the liver to inactive metabolites that are enterally cleared. Fentanyl is given through intravenous, intramuscular, subcutaneous, transdermal, transoral mucosal, epidural, and intrathecal routes. Long-acting fentanyl transdermal patches may be especially useful when enteral opioids are contraindicated. Typically changed every 72 hours, some patients will require patch replacement every 48 hours. Patients who are cachectic or are experiencing night sweats may have poor absorption of transdermal fentanyl. Short-acting fentanyl transmucosal preparations are partially absorbed through the oral mucosa and may be used for breakthrough pain.

d. Oxycodone is hepatically metabolized to active and inactive metabolites. Oxycodone should be used cautiously in patients with renal and hepatic insufficiency. It is only available for oral administration.

e. Methadone has a remarkably long elimination half-life (30 ± 19 hours). Although equianalgesic to morphine with single-dose administration, methadone accumulates with repeated dosing so that, at steady state, it is fully 10 times more potent than morphine. Methadone must be increased slowly (every 5 to 10 days) and supplemented with as-needed doses of short-acting opioid (morphine and oxycodone) to avoid overdose. Metabolized in the liver by cytochrome P-450 enzymes to inactive metabolites, methadone metabolism is markedly affected by medications that induce or impede P-450 activity. Methadone and metabolites are enterally excreted and do not accumulate in renal failure. Methadone should be avoided in hepatic insufficiency because further prolongation of normally long elimination half-life may preclude safe dose titration. Methadone has nonopioid analgesic effects, through N-methyl D-aspartate (NMDA) receptors, that may add to analgesic effect. Methadone, especially at high doses (greater than 100 mg/day), has been associated with prolongation of QT interval and cardiac arrhythmia. Methadone can be given through oral, rectal, or intravenous routes (local tissue reaction may complicate repeated subcutaneous or intramuscular administration) with high bioavailability.

f. Oxymorphone (parenterally) is approximately 10 times more potent than parenteral morphine, but due to modest oral bioavailability, oral oxymorphone is only three times more potent than oral morphine. Elimination half-life of oxymorphone is 1.3 ± 0.7 hours, with active and inactive oxymorphone metabolites excreted in the urine. Hepatic and/or renal insufficiency greatly influences oxymorphone pharmacokinetics. Oxymorphone is available for oral, parenteral, and rectal administration. Alcohol consumption significantly increases peak oxymorphone absorption from the extended-release oral formulation (Opana ER).

g. Codeine, a prodrug, provides almost no pain relief directly; rather, it undergoes cytochrome P450-2D6 metabolism into active metabolites (morphine and morphine-6-glucuronide) to provide codeine-derived analgesic effect. P450-2D6 polymorphism results in variation of codeine analgesic effect. Approximately 8% Caucasians lack sufficient enzyme activity to derive significant codeine analgesic effect. Conversely, 1% to 10% Caucasians and 3% to 28% of African Americans may be ultrarapid metabolizers at risk for relative opioid overdose from overproduction of active metabolites. Codeine may have higher risk of nausea than hydrocodone or oxycodone. Codeine is available for oral, intramuscular, or subcutaneous administration (intravenous administration should be avoided due to the risk of histamine release and subsequent cardiovascular instability).

h. Hydrocodone, a derivative of codeine, is metabolized by cytochrome P-450 into hydromorphone, which may mediate some of the pharmacologic effects of hydrocodone. It is commonly available for oral administration in preparations combined with nonopioid analgesics, but recently plain hydrocodone long-acting preparations were made available. Patients should be cautioned for rare but nonreversible sensorineural hearing loss with higher dosages of hydrocodone, with most cases reported in context of opioid abuse.

i. Buprenorphine, a mixed agonist-antagonist at μ, δ and κ opioid receptors is a semisynthetic opioid available in sublingual, transdermal, and injectable formulations for management of pain and/or opioid addiction. It is predominately metabolized in liver using cytochrome P450-3A4 enzymes and excreted through bile, with little effect from renal impairment; the active metabolite norbuprenorphine is a potent analgesic. Long buprenorphine half-life of 20 to 70 hour, ceiling effect for both analgesic and euphoric effects, and good safety profile make buprenorphine an alternative to conventional long-acting opioids in chronic and cancer pain.

Concomitant use of buprenorphine with other opioids potentially can precipitate withdrawal syndrome. Buprenorphine should be slowly tapered up to reach desired analgesic effect to prevent these side effects.

    j. Tramadol (50 to 100 mg p.o. QID, maximum 400 mg/day) has modest analgesic efficacy due to weak affinity for μ-opioid receptors. Dose is limited to a maximum of 400 mg/day, due to increased risk of seizures with higher doses. Tramadol is also a norepinephrine, serotonin reuptake inhibitor, similar to some antidepressant medications: it should not be used in individuals receiving full doses of antidepressants, to avoid toxicity (serotonin syndrome). Tramadol undergoes hepatic metabolism by the cytochrome P-450 system. In the United States, it is only available for oral administration.

    k. Tapentadol is a synthetic, centrally acting, opioid with moderate affinity to μ-opioid receptors that also inhibits synaptic norepinephrine reuptake. Dual mechanism provides opioid sparing effects, and potentially fewer opioid-related side effects. Immediate and extended-release dosing is limited to total 600 mg daily. Doses should be reduced in moderate hepatic insufficiency and tapentadol is contraindicated in severe hepatic insufficiency. Tapentadol decreases seizure threshold and raises intracranial pressure, so it is contraindicated in patients with seizures and intracranial pathologies. Caution should be exercised with concomitant use of serotonergic agents due to potential risk of serotonin syndrome.

    l. Meperidine has no utility in pain management. It is metabolized to normeperidine, which accumulates due to a long half-life, and is associated with excitatory effects including tremulousness and seizures. Severe reactions, after even a single dose of meperidine, may occur in patients being treated with monoamine oxidase (MAO) inhibitors, including excitation, delirium, hyperpyrexia, convulsions, and death.

  4. Opioid rotation involves intentionally switching from one opioid analgesic to another, using appropriate guidelines for equianalgesic dosing, to improve pain control and reduce opioid adverse effects. Although individuals tolerant to one opioid will have cross-tolerance to other opioids, the cross-tolerance may be incomplete, such that the effective analgesic dose of the new opioid may be 50% (or less) of the anticipated equianalgesic dose based on the prior opioid requirement. Opioid rotation must be undertaken with caution to avoid overdosing or underdosing, potentially resulting in excess adverse effects, inadequate pain control, or other problems. Although the data are limited to case reports and case series, opioid rotation is widely utilized in clinical practice. Special caution is required when switching to methadone from another systemic opioid, due to the long elimination half-life of methadone.

E. Adjuvant analgesics (Table 40-5)

  1. Anticonvulsants are variably effective analgesics in neuropathic pain. Gabapentin (300 to 1,200 mg p.o. TID) is the most widely used anticonvulsant for pain control, with some analgesic efficacy for acute postoperative pain, as well as for neuropathic pain. Other anticonvulsants (i.e., pregabalin, topiramate, levetiracetam, lamotrigine, and oxcarbazepine) should be considered upon failure/intolerance to gabapentin. Dosing of anticonvulsants must be adjusted in renal and/or hepatic insufficiency. They are only available for oral administration.

  2. Antidepressants, especially tricyclic antidepressants (TCAs), have analgesic efficacy in chronic neuropathic pain. Newer antidepressants (e.g., citalopram, duloxetine, milnacipran, venlafaxine, and fluoxetine) may be less effective analgesics than TCAs but are generally better tolerated. If one antidepressant is poorly tolerated or provides ineffective analgesia, a different antidepressant should be tried. Antidepressants are only available for oral administration.

TABLE 40-5	Adjuvant Analgesics		
	Usual, single oral dose (mg)	Maximum daily dose (mg)	Half-life (h)
Anticonvulsants			
Gabapentin	100–1,200	3,600	5–9
Lamotrigine	50–250	500	15–30
Levetiracetam	250–1,000	3,000	6–8
Pregabalin	50–300	600	10–12
Antidepressants			
Amitriptyline	25–300	300	16–30
Bupropion	50–150	450	14
Citalopram	10–40	40	30–36
Doxepin	25–300	300	16–30
Duloxetine	30–120	60–120	10–14
Milnacipran	25–100	100–200	8–10
Fluoxetine	10–80	80	100
Sertraline	50–200	200	24–60
Trazodone	25–400	400	8
Venlafaxine	25–100	375	5–11

3. **Miscellaneous agents**
   a. **Muscle relaxants** have not been studied in cancer pain, but are commonly used for musculoskeletal pain. Sedation is a common adverse effect. **Baclofen** (10 to 20 mg p.o., three times daily) is widely used for control of spasticity, but also has analgesic efficacy in neuropathic pain. To avoid potentially serious withdrawal, chronic baclofen therapy must be slowly tapered over several days, rather than abruptly discontinued. **Tizanidine** (2 to 8 mg p.o., three to four times daily) is an effective agent for spasticity with limited efficacy in chronic pain. Potential adverse effects include hypotension and hepatotoxicity (periodically monitor liver function, especially during drug initiation). Renally cleared, tizanidine dosing must be reduced in renal insufficiency. Other muscle relaxants (carisoprodol, cyclobenzaprine, metaxalone) have only a limited role in management of cancer-related musculoskeletal pain.
   b. **Local anesthetics.** Lidocaine intravenous infusion (1 to 2 mg i.v./minute, after 25 to 50 mg i.v. loading dose) may be effective for intractable neuropathic pain resistant to systemic opioid. For long-term use, intravenous lidocaine infusion is difficult to maintain and serum level must be checked regularly to avoid toxicity. Oral **mexiletine** (10 mg/kg/day, divided into three doses daily) has modest analgesic efficacy. Lidocaine 5% patch provides pain relief through topical anesthetic action, and is especially indicated where neuropathic pain is associated with markedly increased skin sensitivity (cutaneous mechano-allodynia). With little systemic absorption, lidocaine patch has negligible systemic effects, but the water-based adhesive may cause dermatitis if left in place for more than 12 hours daily.
   c. **Systemic corticosteroids** are used in cancer patients to provide analgesia, improve appetite, prevent nausea and malaise, and improve quality of life. Corticosteroids may be particularly useful in acute pain due to boney metastases, infiltration or compression of neural structures, increased intracranial pressure (headache), obstruction of a hollow viscus or organ capsule distention, or spinal cord compression. Long-term use of steroids may lead to gastrointestinal ulceration, so the use of gastroprotective agents is advised.

    d. Cannabinoids (CBD), the active ingredient of *cannabis sativa*, that is, marijuana, are increasingly used as medicinal agent, as marijuana has gained legal approval in various states. Studies regarding analgesics effect have yielded mixed results: some reports suggest significant analgesia for neuropathic pain; others fail to show benefit over conventional analgesics.

IV. SPECIAL TECHNIQUES FOR THE MANAGEMENT OF RESISTANT CANCER PAIN

    A. Psychological and behavior medicine techniques. Cancer pain is a complex emotional experience, and emotional distress, anxiety, and depression increase pain and suffering. Pharmacologic and nonpharmacologic therapies for the treatment of psychological and psychiatric comorbidities are essential to cancer pain management. **Cognitive behavioral therapies (CBT)** are the most frequently used psychological modalities in chronic pain management. Through CBT, patients learn to control the thoughts, emotions, and behaviors that modulate pain experience. CBT includes hypnosis, relaxation techniques (including progressive muscle relaxation, meditation, and guided imagery), biofeedback, coping skills training, music therapy, cognitive restructuring, supportive and group therapy, and stress management techniques.

    B. Physical and occupational therapies are essential to optimize functional status after prolonged medical illness or surgical intervention. Therapeutic and conditioning exercise programs are essential to successful chronic pain management. Specific therapies such as orthotic bracing and assistive devices may improve pain control and/or function.

    C. Complementary and alternative therapies are widely used, alone or in conjunction with conventional therapies, for pain control by persons with cancer. Patients should be routinely asked about complementary and alternative (CAM) therapies, if only to allow screening for potential adverse interactions between CAM and conventional therapies. Alternative therapies such as acupuncture, massage, healing touch, and many herbal therapies have shown benefits in controlling pain and other symptoms, but comparative trials with other analgesic therapies are lacking.

    D. Interventional techniques for severe cancer pain are important components of comprehensive care for severe cancer pain and should not be relegated to treatments of last resort. Interventional pain therapies should be considered if pain is not adequately controlled with systemic analgesics, or if use of such analgesics is associated with adverse effect (e.g., sedation, constipation, and/or nausea). Interventional pain therapies can potentially improve quality of life by (a) providing more effective pain control and (b) allowing reduction in analgesic dose and/or analgesic adverse effects. Improved pain control and reduced adverse effects through appropriate use of interventional pain therapies may improve life expectancy in patients with terminal disease.

    1. Spinal analgesic administration delivers medication to the spinal cord to enhance analgesic efficacy and minimize systemic (brain) adverse effects of analgesics, especially sedation. Spinal analgesics (opioids, local anesthetics, clonidine, and/or baclofen) are used alone or in combination for intrathecal or epidural administration. Spinal administration of combined opioid, local anesthetic, and clonidine is an especially potent analgesic therapy. Spinal analgesics may be administered by epidural or intrathecal (subarachnoid) systems, but an implanted pump (for intrathecal infusion) is most commonly used.

    a. Spinal opioids (especially morphine and hydromorphone) have significantly increased potency: 100 mg/day parenteral morphine is roughly equivalent to 10 mg/day epidural morphine, which is roughly equivalent to 1 mg/day intrathecal morphine; however, actual doses must be titrated to effect. Fentanyl, because of its high lipid solubility, has rapid systemic absorption after spinal administration; therefore, spinal administration of fentanyl may have little advantage over systemic administration. Spinal opioid adverse effects include sedation, respiratory depression (onset may be delayed for several hours), constipation, nausea, pruritus, peripheral edema, and urinary retention. Exceptionally high doses of spinal opioids may result in myoclonic jerks or even diffuse muscle rigidity.

    b. Spinal local anesthetics (bupivacaine, lidocaine) may markedly decrease pain without sedation or some of the other potential adverse effects associated with opioid analgesics. After spinal administration of low doses of local anesthetic, pain relief is sometimes obtained without significant extremity weakness or numbness. Potential adverse effects include hypotension (especially orthostatic hypotension), extremity weakness, and urinary retention.

    c. Spinal clonidine has analgesic efficacy after epidural or intrathecal administration, through action at spinal α_2-adrenergic receptors. Potential adverse effects include hypotension (especially orthostatic hypotension), bradycardia, congestive heart failure, and sedation.

  2. Electrical stimulation neuromodulation, including spinal cord stimulation (SCS), peripheral nerve stimulation (PNS), and peripheral field stimulation (PFNS), are implanted medical devices that apply electrical current near neural structures to modulate pain signal neural transmission. SCS may be particularly helpful in managing peripheral neuropathic pain in cancer survivors. SCS use was previously limited by device MRI incompatibility; however, MRI-compatible SCS has recently become available, increasing the utility of these devices to include patients who may need periodic MRI imaging.

  3. Vertebral augmentation (vertebroplasty, kyphoplasty, and tumor-ablative vertebroplasty) is a procedure for the percutaneous injection of bone cement (polymethyl methacrylate—PMMA) into vertebral bodies affected by compression fractures due to metastatic tumor, destructive vertebral hemangiomas, or osteoporosis. Kyphoplasty differs from vertebroplasty in that bone cement is injected after a balloon has been used to create a cavity in the vertebral body, in an attempt to restore vertebral body height. Vertebroplasty/kyphoplasty can be highly effective in control of pain from vertebral compression fractures due to osteoporosis and/or tumor. Thorough radiographic evaluation is essential before vertebroplasty/kyphoplasty. Potential adverse effects include spread of unhardened cement beyond the vertebral body, through direct spread to the spinal canal or through vascular embolization.

    In tumor-ablative vertebral augmentation, plasma-mediated radiofrequency ablation is used for metastatic painful vertebral disease to create cavitation within the vertebral body prior to injection of PMMA, to potentially decrease tumor burden and decrease risk of PMMA extravasation beyond vertebral boundaries.

    Vertebroplasty/kyphoplasty need not delay treatment of spinal metastases with radiation therapy, but may provide rapid onset of pain relief, which may facilitate the use of appropriate antitumor therapies.

  4. Neurolytic neural blockade should be considered for patients with terminal disease in whom pain is poorly controlled with less-invasive therapies and pain is localized to a suitable region of the body. If pain recurs after several months, neurolytic blockade may be repeated, but repeated blockade is generally not necessary.

    a. Neurolytic celiac plexus block, the most commonly performed neurolytic technique for cancer pain, is indicated for upper abdominal visceral pain from pancreatic or other upper abdominal malignancy. Up to 85% of appropriately selected patients report good-to-excellent pain relief after neurolytic celiac plexus block. The side effects of orthostatic hypotension and increased frequency of bowel movements (diarrhea) transiently affect most persons after neurolytic celiac plexus block, but only 1% to 2% require long-term medical management of these symptoms. The risk of significant nerve damage or paralysis (0.1% to 0.2%) may cause some cancer patients to decide against celiac plexus block, but to most, the potential for good-to-excellent pain relief (75% to 85%) that may be associated with improvements in constipation, nausea, and a general sense of well-being outweighs procedural risk.

    b. Neurolytic hypogastric plexus block may be effective for visceral pain from pelvic malignancy. Its use is not significantly associated with extremity weakness, but ejaculatory failure/inorgasmia is a potential adverse effect. Neurolytic hypogastric plexus block is not likely to provide good pain control if there is tumor invasion of somatic or neural structures.

5. **Tumor ablation** is a palliative modality using targeted radiofrequency energy, to decrease tumor size to provide analgesia for pain associated with osteolytic bone metastasis, or localized soft tissue solid tumors etc. This can be achieved by image-guided direct application of energy to ablate tissue and/or transarterial embolization to promote cancer devascularization.

E. **Neurosurgical techniques** for pain control, such as cordotomy or cingulotomy, are rarely used but potentially powerful tools for the management of otherwise intractable pain. Especially for unilateral lower body or lower extremity pain, in the setting of terminal illness, cordotomy (percutaneous or open surgical approach) may provide remarkable control of previously intractable pain.

F. **Management of refractory pain and/or other symptoms of terminal illness.** In the last hours to days of life, some dying people develop intractable symptoms such as intractable pain, dyspnea, delirium, and/or emesis (e.g., fecal emesis due to distal bowel obstruction beyond surgical intervention). If such symptoms are intolerable to the dying patient, but would be refractory to further palliative therapy, consideration should be given to alleviation of distress through administration of sedatives. Terminal, palliative sedation should be considered only for those who have requested not to be resuscitated ("no code") in the event of cardiac/respiratory arrest. Midazolam is the most commonly used drug for palliative sedation (1 to 2 mg i.v., i.m., or subcutaneously q1h, p.r.n.; or loading dose of 1 to 2 mg i.v. with infusion 0.5 to 2 mg/hour) but other benzodiazepines (diazepam, 5 to 10 mg p.o., 2 mg i.v. q2h, p.r.n.) can be used instead. Benzodiazepines may worsen agitation in some persons, and they may be better treated with barbiturates (thiopental infusion 0.5 mg/kg i.v. loading dose, followed by 0.25 to 0.5 mg/kg/hour i.v. infusion; pentobarbital infusion 1 to 2 mg/kg/hour), or neuroleptic sedatives (haloperidol, 1 to 4 mg i.v./p.o. q1h, p.r.n.) titrated to effect to ease suffering from otherwise intractable symptoms. These drugs generally have long elimination half-lives and will accumulate to steady-state level over a few days. The use of palliative terminal sedation to provide a dying person relief from intractable, intolerable suffering is firmly within the realm of good, supportive palliative care and should not be confused with euthanasia.

V. SPECIFIC PAIN SYNDROMES

A. **Mucositis** is one of the most debilitating, refractory adverse effects following chemotherapy and/or radiotherapy damage to tissues of the alimentary canal. Mucositis is associated with pain and increased risk of infection, malnutrition, and dehydration. Traditional management of oral mucositis has involved patient education for avoidance of dehydration, oral rinses (saline, hydrogen peroxide diluted 1:1 with saline), topical lidocaine solution, systemic analgesics, nutritional support, and prevention/management of infection.

B. **Bone pain** from cancer, often related to bony metastases, is a common problem. Bone pain management may require various modalities including analgesics, corticosteroids, bisphosphonates, radiation therapy, hormonal and/or chemotherapy, and/or orthopedic surgical intervention.

1. **Bisphosphonates** inhibit osteoclast-mediated bone resorption and have been shown to relieve pain, reduce the number of metastases, prevent osteolysis, and decrease the frequency of fractures. All bisphosphonates can induce gastrointestinal upset, renal damage, and mandibular osteonecrosis. Dose should be adjusted based on renal function.

2. **Denosumab,** a monoclonal antibody against RANKL (receptor activator of nuclear factor kappa-beta ligand), blocks osteoclast activation and thereby reduces bone resorption and lessens skeletal-related events in osseous metastasis of solid tumors and multiple myeloma.

3. **Abiraterone,** an androgen biosynthesis inhibitor acting through selective cytochrome P450 17A1 inhibition, improves survival and bone pain in *castration-resistant prostate cancer.*

4. **Radioisotopes,** through parenteral administration, provide systemic radiation to diminish multifocal painful skeletal metastasis. ^{89}Sr and ^{153}Sm have shown selectivity for bone metastasis and have been found to be effective in reducing pain. High cost, delayed pain relief, and hematologic toxicity limit use.

5. **External-beam radiation** is used in relieving local tumor-related bone pain. Focal lesion can be managed by localized external-beam irradiation (also known as *involved-field irradiation*). Multiple painful sites can be managed by wide-field external-beam irradiation (e.g., hemibody irradiation). Side effects include bone marrow suppression and radiation tissue damage.

C. **Neuropathic pain from tumor invasion of major nerve plexus.** Neuropathic pain may be relatively less responsive to opioid analgesics than nociceptive pain, especially when tumor directly invades a major nerve or plexus. Clinical situations such as tumor invasion of brachial plexus (Pancoast tumor), or retroperitoneal sarcoma invading the lumbosacral plexus, require aggressive pain therapies early in the course of disease. Adjuvant, nonopioid analgesics (anticonvulsants, antidepressant) therapies should be optimized. Although rarely needed, severe neuropathic pain not responding to systemic analgesics is a relatively common indication for spinal analgesics.

D. **Cancer treatment–related pain syndromes/cancer survivors and pain.** Advances in cancer treatment have improved cancer survival, but also increased the prevalence of patients living with chronic, cancer-related pain. It is estimated that chronic posttreatment pain is present in 33% of cancer survivors. The prevalence of pain varies depending on the type and site of cancer, comorbid conditions, treatments used, and pain management techniques employed. Pain in cancer survivors can be the result of tissue damage from the cancer itself or from cancer treatments: chemotherapy, radiation, hormonal therapy, long-term steroid use, and/or surgery. Graft-versus-host disease is another potential source of persistent pain.

Chronic pain management in cancer survivors is complex and frequently requires a multidisciplinary approach. The goals of treatment should focus on functional improvement and management strategies rather than complete elimination of pain. Multimodal analgesia combines analgesics with different mechanisms to provide improved pain relief with fewer medication-related adverse effects. In patients with chronic posttreatment pain, there is increasing concern for potential adverse effects of chronic opioid use, including tolerance/hyperalgesia, hypogonadism, and immunosuppression, in addition to the well-known adverse effects of sedation, respiratory depression, constipation, nausea, etc. Nonopioid and adjuvant analgesics (antidepressants and anticonvulsants), and interventional pain therapies may be utilized to limit opioid use and improve symptom control. Physical and rehabilitation therapies, especially when combined with psychological/behavioral medicine therapies, potentially play an important role in functional restoration.

1. **Chemotherapy-induced peripheral neuropathy (CIPN)** is increasingly seen as a treatment-limiting and potentially disabling complication of some chemotherapy protocols. CIPN most commonly affects large sensory neurons, and therefore may present as a purely sensory disturbance; however, pure motor disturbance or as a mixed sensory-motor disturbance presentation is not uncommon. Typically, paresthesias or dysesthetic sensations follow chemotherapy including platinum compounds, taxanes, vinca alkaloids, thalidomide, ifosfamide, antiganglioside-G-D2 monoclonal antibody, bortezomib, and cytarabine. With no specific treatment of CIPN, effort has been focused on prevention—but with limited success. These strategies include selection of less toxic agents, chemotherapy dose modifications, interruption of dosing (i.e., "stop and go" protocols). Neuroprotective agents that have been used in an attempt to prevent CIPN include various antioxidants (α-lipoic acid, folinic acid, acetyl L-carnitine, glutathione, glutamine, pyridoxine, cyanacobalamin, and fish oil) and various neuroprotectants (GM1 monosialoganglioside, riluzole, minocycline, amifostine, leukemia inhibitory factor, lithium, IGF-1, nimodipine, and calcium–magnesium solution). In lack of proven prevention, various antineuropathic pain medications (gabapentin,

pregabalin, levetiracetam, and topiramate), and/or opioids may be useful analgesics. Acupuncture, electrocutaneous nerve stimulation (scrambler therapy), and SCS have been used in the management of CIPN with varied success.

2. **Radiation neuropathy** presents in patients who have undergone radiation therapy. The incidence is variable and appears to be dose dependent. The most common injuries occur to the brachial plexus (after radiation therapy for breast cancer, lung cancer, or Hodgkin's lymphoma) and the lumbosacral nerves (after radiation for pelvic and abdominal malignancies). Peripheral neuropathy is also seen, but usually is self-limited and less symptomatic. Injury can occur to any nerve in the beam of the radiation therapy device. The common complaints include paresthesias, dysesthesias, allodynia, hyperalgesia, and hyperpathia in the area of nerve injury. Most of these neuropathies present weeks after radiation therapy. Treatment includes anticonvulsants, opioids, NSAIDs, TCAs, and local and topical anesthetics. In very severe cases, SCS or spinal analgesic administration should be considered. Psychological and physical therapy modalities should be utilized as a part of a multidisciplinary pain management program.

3. **Postsurgical pain syndromes**
   a. **Postmastectomy pain syndrome,** involving persistent pain in the anterior chest, axilla, and medial and posterior portions of the arm, occurs after 4% to 30% surgical procedures involving the breast and occurs 2 weeks to 6 months after surgery. The pain is variable but is usually a combination of somatic and neuropathic pain. Treatment includes opioids, anticonvulsants, topical agents (lidocaine patch), physical therapy, and cognitive behavioral therapy.
   b. **Postradical neck dissection pain syndrome** is a combination neuropathic and myofascial pain condition that occurs in as many as 50% of postsurgical patients, typically involving one or more branches of the superficial cervical plexus (SCP). It is usually described as spontaneous, continuous burning pain, shooting pain, or allodynia. Treatment is similar to other postsurgical neuropathic pain syndromes, but myofascial trigger point injections using local anesthetic and/or botulinum toxin may be of benefit.
   c. **Postthoracotomy pain syndrome (PTPS)** is persistent pain in the area of thoracotomy incision scar reflecting intercostal neuralgia. Typically occurring in a small percentage or patients, PTPS can persist indefinitely. Care must be taken not to confuse PTPS with tumor reoccurrence pain. The pain is described as numbness, tingling, burning, itching, or shooting. There is quite often hyperesthesia in the involved dermatome. Treatments include physical therapy, opioids, anticonvulsants, lidocaine patch, transcutaneous electrical nerve stimulation, and/or SCS.

E. **Postherpetic neuralgia**
   1. **Herpes zoster (HZ),** resulting from reactivation of varicella zoster (VZ) infection, is characterized by painful, vesicular cutaneous lesions in a dermatomal pattern. Pain may precede visible lesions by 2 to 3 days. HZ is typically self-limited in normal hosts, but in immunocompromised patients may cause cutaneous dissemination or even potentially fatal systemic and/or CNS infection. Acute HZ pain (acute herpetic neuralgia) typically resolves with healing of cutaneous lesions; however, the risk of persistent postherpetic neuralgia (PHN) increases with age. Even with aggressive therapy, up to 30% of individuals older than 60 years presenting with HZ will experience PHN, and up to 50% of persons with PHN may have pain lasting indefinitely.
   2. **Prevention of postherpetic neuralgia.** The incidence and/or duration of PHN is reduced with oral antiviral agents in adults older than 50 years, if therapy is started within 72 hours of onset of rash. Acyclovir (800 mg every 4 hours, five doses daily, for 7 to 10 days) speeds healing of lesions, decreases pain from acute HZ, and may decrease the incidence of PHN. Newer antivirals famciclovir (500 mg every 8 hours for 7 days) and valacyclovir (1,000 mg every 8 hours for 7 days) have been shown to decrease the incidence of PHN with less frequent dosing, which may improve

compliance. The addition of systemic corticosteroid to antiviral therapy does not further reduce the risk of PHN, but adding TCA (amitriptyline 25 mg orally at bedtime) may be of benefit. Sympathetic nerve blocks and epidural steroid injections provide excellent pain relief in acute HZ and may reduce PHN. High-potency, live-attenuated VZ vaccine has been shown to decrease the incidence of HZ and the severity of PHN in adults 60 years of age and older and will likely be used to prevent HZ and PHN in high-risk populations.

3. **Treatment of established postherpetic neuralgia** is based on the use of systemic analgesics and may include TCAs, anticonvulsants, and/or opioid analgesics. Topical lidocaine 5% patch may be of benefit in PHN associated with cutaneous extra sensitivity (mechano-allodynia).

F. **Opioid toxicity syndrome (OTS)** consists of diffuse hyperalgesia, myoclonus, and altered mental status (agitation/delirium or sedation/confusion). Although rare, it is most often seen when patients are on high doses of opioid (often greater than 100 mg morphine/hour or equivalent), yet inadequate pain control requires further rapid opioid dose escalation. In such settings, increasing opioid dose may not result in improved pain control, but instead worsened pain (hyperalgesia) and deterioration of mental status. In extreme cases, myoclonus may be nearly continuous and resemble seizurelike activity, but patients are generally conscious and conversant (although often delirious). Dehydration and/or renal insufficiency may increase the risk of OTS. OTS has been most frequently described with systemic morphine, but has been reported with other systemic opioids and with spinal opioid. Opioid-induced facilitation of pain signal transmission (opioid-induced hyperalgesia) appears to be one of the principal factors contributing to OTS. Management of OTS requires switching to another opioid (opioid rotation), typically using less than the fully equivalent dose. In extreme cases of OTS, it may be necessary to completely discontinue opioid analgesics temporarily, and rely on nonopioid analgesics (e.g., anticonvulsants or intravenous lidocaine infusion) for pain control. Once OTS symptoms improve, patients may be managed with relatively lower doses of another opioid.

VI. PAIN MANGEMENT IN SPECIFIC POPULATIONS

A. **Cancer pain management in the noncompliant patient.** Pain management therapies are less likely to be successful if not used appropriately and consistently. To manage apparent noncompliance, treating health-care professionals must identify and manage contributing factors such as (a) cognitive impairment (due to underlying disease(s), treatments, and other factors); (b) psychological/psychiatric disorders (depression/anxiety and personality disorders); (c) substance abuse or dependence; and (d) physical ability to obtain, store, and access prescribed treatments.

In chronic illness and/or malignancy, patients often develop tolerance (increasing dose requirement) and physical dependence (withdrawal symptoms with abrupt discontinuation) but rarely develop new substance dependence or addiction. In the context of chronic pain in oncology practice, "drug-seeking" behavior likely reflects inadequate pain control. "Substance dependence" or "addiction" is best characterized by compulsive, continued drug use despite harm, and/or drug craving.

Substance abuse/dependence is rarely newly diagnosed in patients with terminal disease, but can significantly complicate pain management therapies. It is essential to obtain the patient's cooperation in order to get a thorough substance abuse history and find optimal management strategies. Patients with cancer pain and active substance abuse/dependence will require very close monitoring and multidisciplinary care.

1. Involve psychiatrist, addictionologist, especially if substance abuse is recent, ongoing. Encourage participation in a 12-step recovery program (alcoholics anonymous, narcotics anonymous) if feasible.

2. Analgesics filled by only one prescriber.

3. Use one opioid analgesic, preferably a long-acting formulation, given on a regular schedule. As far as possible, limit the use of short-acting or "as-needed" doses of opioid.

4. Optimize the use of nonopioid and nonpharmacologic pain therapies.
5. Utilize pill counts and urine toxicology screens, if needed, to help with monitoring of compliance with prescribed therapies and avoidance of other abuse substances.
6. Limit quantity of controlled substances to weekly supply, if compliance is poor. (In extreme cases, it may be necessary for medication to be dispensed daily by home health nurse or even through a substance abuse program.)
7. Utilization of written opioid analgesic guidelines may help patients to understand what is expected regarding appropriate use of analgesic therapies.

SUGGESTED READINGS

Aghayev K, Papanastassiou ID, Vrionis F. Role of vertebral augmentation procedures in the management of vertebral compression fractures in cancer patients. *Curr Opin Support Palliat Care* 2011;5:222–226.

Angst MS, Clark JD. Opioid-induced hyperalgesia: a qualitative systematic review. *Anesthesiology* 2006;104:570–587.

Bannister K, Dickenson AH. Opioid hyperalgesia. *Cur Opin Support Palliat Care* 2010;4:1–5.

Brack A, Rittner HL, Stein C. Immunosuppressive effects of opioids: clinical relevance. *J Neuroimmune Pharmacol* 2011;6:490–502.

Brennan MJ. The effect of therapy on endocrine function. *Am J Med* 2013;126:S12–S18.

Budd K. Pain management: is opioid immunosuppression a clinical problem? *Biomed Pharmacother* 2006;60:310–317.

Cherny NI. Cancer pain assessment and syndromes. In: McMahon SB, Loltzenburg M, Tracey I, et al. eds. *Wall and Melzack's Textbook of Pain*, 6th ed. Philadelphia, PA: Elsevier, Saunders, 2013:1039–1060.

Deer TR, Prager J, Levy R, et al. Polyanalgesic consensus conference 2012: recommendations for the management of pain by intrathecal (intraspinal) drug delivery: report of an interdisciplinary expert panel. *Neuromodulation* 2012;15:436–464.

Estfan B, LeGrand SB, Walsh D, et al. Opioid rotation in cancer patients: pros and cons. *Oncology* 2005;19:511–516.

Krakauer EL, Thomas EQ. Sedation and palliative medicine. In: Hanks G, Cherny NI, Christakis NA, et al. eds. *Oxford Textbook of Palliative Medicine*, 4th ed. Oxford, UK: Oxford University Press, 2009.

Levy MH, Adolph MD, Back A, et al. Palliative care. *J Natl Compr Canc Netw* 2012;10:1284–1309.

Lo B, Rubenfeld G. Palliative sedation in dying patients: "we turn to it when everything else hasn't worked". *JAMA* 2005;294:1810–1816.

Park N, Patel NK. The role of surgical neuroablation for pain control. In: Hanks G, Cherny NI, Christakis NA, et al. eds. *Oxford Textbook of Palliative Medicine*, 4th ed. Oxford, UK: Oxford University Press, 2009.

Penson RT, Nunn C, Younger J, et al. Trust violated: analgesics for addicts. *Oncologist* 2003;8:199–209.

Smith TJ, Staats PS, Deer T, et al. Randomized clinical trial of an implantable drug delivery system compared with comprehensive medical management for refractory cancer pain: impact on pain, drug-related toxicity, and survival. *J Clin Oncol* 2002;20:4040–4049.

Swarm RA, Abernethy AP, Anghelescu DL, et al. Adult cancer pain. *J Natl Compr Canc Netw* 2013;11:992–1022.

Swarm RA, Karanikolas M, Cousins MJ. Injections, neural blockade, and implant therapies for pain control. In: Doyle D, Hanks G, Cherny NI, et al. eds. *Oxford Textbook of Palliative Medicine*, 4rd ed. Oxford, UK: Oxford University Press, 2009.

Temel JS, Greer JA, Muzikansky A, et al. Early palliative care for patient with metastatic non-small-cell lung cancer. *N Engl J Med* 2010;363:733–742.

Wareham D. Postherpetic neuralgia. *Clin Evid* 2005;15:1–9.

World Health Organization. *Cancer Pain Relief and Palliative Care: Report of a Who Expert Committee*. Geneva, Switzerland: World Health Organization, 1990:804.

Cancer Screening
Megan E. Wren • Aaron M. Goodman

I. GENERAL PRINCIPLES

A. The benefit of screening depends on the prevalence of the disease, the sensitivity and specificity of the screening test, the acceptability of the test to the patient, and, most importantly, the ability to change the natural course of disease with treatment.

B. Studies of the benefits of screening are susceptible to several forms of bias including lead time bias, length bias, overdiagnosis, and volunteer bias.

C. Research evidence has often been inadequate to reach definitive conclusions regarding how, when, whom, and whether to screen for various cancers. The guidelines below are a synthesis of the recommendations of the major organizations (Table 41-1).

II. BREAST CANCER SCREENING

A. Breast cancer is the most commonly diagnosed invasive cancer in US women. About 1 in 8 (12.5%) will develop breast cancer by age 90.

    1. Many women greatly overestimate their risk of breast cancer. In one study (*Patient Educ Couns* 2005;57:294), 89% of women overestimated their risk with an average estimate of 46% lifetime risk.

B. Breast cancer mortality has declined approximately 30% over the past two decades. It is unclear whether it is related to more aggressive screening or improved treatment options.

C. The benefits of screening are best proven for mammography in women aged 50 to 69.

    1. Women aged 40 to 49 have a lower incidence of breast cancer and denser breasts (thus lower sensitivity and specificity of screening), leading to lower predictive values.

        a. The United States Preventive Services Task Force (USPSTF) review stated that "for biennial screening mammography in women aged 40 to 49 years, there is moderate certainty that the net benefit is small." They emphasized the lower incidence in this group and the adverse consequences of screening (*Ann Intern Med* 2009;151:716).

    2. Data are limited for women age 70 and over, and older women have competing causes of mortality, limiting the benefit of cancer screening.

D. Randomized trials have shown that teaching breast self-examination (BSE) does not save lives (*J Natl Cancer Inst* 2002;94:1445), so many now endorse teaching "breast self-awareness" rather than formal BSE.

E. Clinical breast exam (CBE) may modestly improve cancer detection rates if experienced clinicians use very careful technique (*JAMA* 1999;282:1270).

F. Recommendations of some major groups are as follows.

    1. The USPSTF issued updated recommendations in 2009.

        a. Women aged 50 to 74 years should have mammography every 2 years.

        b. Screening mammography should not be done "routinely" for women aged 40 to 49 years. Women and their doctors should base the decision to start mammography before age 50 years on the risk for breast cancer and preferences about the benefits and harms.

        c. Current evidence is insufficient to assess the benefits and harms of the CBE or screening mammography in women 75 years or older.

        d. The USPSTF recommends against teaching patients BSE.

    2. The American Cancer Society (ACS) recommends

        a. Age 20 to 39: CBE every 3 years.

        b. Age 40 and over: annual CBE and annual mammography.

        c. Optional BSEs.

        d. The age to stop screening is not specified but should be individualized based on the potential benefits and risks in the context of overall health status.

TABLE 41-1	Simplified Screening Schedule for Asymptomatic Average-Risk Persons

	Source			
Breast CA		Ages 20–39	Ages 40–49	Ages 50+
	ACS	CBE q 3 yr	CBE q1yr + Mamms q1yr (BSE is an option at all ages)	
	ACOG	CBE q 1 yr	CBE q1yr + Mamms q1yr (BSE is an option at all ages)	
	USPSTF	–	Indiv. decision	50–74: Mamms q2 yrs
Colo-rectal cancer	Joint guideline	Age >50: Acceptable: gFOBT q1 yr, or FIT q1 yr, or stool DNA (interval unkn.) Preferred: FSIG q5 yrs or c'scope q10 yrs or ACBE q 5 yrs or CT c'graphy q5 yrs		
	USPSTF	Age 50–75: FOBT, sigmoidoscopy, or colonoscopy (intervals unspecified)		
Prost CA	ACS	Informed decision making age 50 (at 40–45 in higher-risk men)		
		If screening: PSA q 1–2 yrs; Stop if <10-year life expectancy		
	ACP	Informed decision making 50–69; only test if clear preference for screening		
	AUA	Shared decision making age 55–69 (high risk start age 40); if scr: PSA q2 yrs		
	USPSTF	Do not screen		
Lung cancer	Various	Shared decision making; LDCT if age 55–74, at least 30 pack-years of smoking (current or quit <15 yrs)		
Cerv CA		After age 21:	Age 30+	Stop:
	ACS ACOG USPSTF	Pap q3yr (no HPV test)	Pap + HPV-DNA q5 yrs (or Pap alone q3 yrs)	Age 65+ IF adequate prior screening
		S/P total hysterectomy for benign disease: no cervical cancer screening		
		Continue screening if: hx no/irregular screening, hx abnl Paps or CA, high-risk behavior, or immunocompr (HIV, CA, meds), or hx prenatal DES		
Testic. CA		Routine screening not recommended		
Ovar. CA		Routine screening not recommended		

3. American Congress of Obstetricians and Gynecologists (ACOG) recommends:
   a. Age 20 to 39: CBE every 1 to 3 years.
   b. Age 40 and over: annual CBE and annual mammography.
   c. Over age 75 the decision to screen should be individualized.
   d. "Breast self-awareness should be encouraged and can include BSE."
G. BRCA1 and BRCA2 germline mutations substantially increase the risk that a woman will develop breast cancer over her lifetime (*J Natl Cancer Inst* 2013;11:812).
   1. BRCA 1 carriers have a 60% cumulative risk of breast cancer by age 70.
   2. BRCA2 carriers have a 55% cumulative risk of breast cancer by age 70.
   3. The USPSTF makes no recommendations for screening women at high risk.
   4. The ACS recommends women that very high risk (>20% lifetime risk) or with BRCA1 or BRCA 2 gene mutation should undergo magnetic resonance imaging

(MRI) screening and mammography every year. For most women at high risk, screening with MRI and mammograms should begin at age 30. Women at moderately increased risk (15% to 20% lifetime risk) should talk to their physicians about the benefits and limitations of MRI screening in addition to yearly mammography.

5. ACOG recommends women at very high risk (>20% lifetime risk) should have "enhanced screening" with annual mammography, CBE every 6 to 12 months, instruction in BSE, and possibly MRI.

6. The National Comprehensive Cancer Network (NCCN) recommends the following for BRCA-positive women who have not undergone risk reducing mastectomy:
   a. Consideration of monthly BSE starting at age 18.
   b. CBE every 6 to 12 months beginning at age 25.
   c. Annual mammography and breast MRI beginning at age 25.

III. CERVICAL CANCER SCREENING

A. The effectiveness of cervical cancer screening has never been studied in a randomized trial but is supported by strong epidemiologic evidence. Most cases of cervical cancer occur in unscreened or inadequately screened women.

B. Cervical cytologic screening may be done with the conventional Pap smear or with liquid-based tests (method does not change screening frequency).

C. **HPV vaccination does not change the screening guidelines.**

D. The ACS, USPSTF, and ACOG have similar recommendations, as summarized below.

E. **Do not begin screening until age 21 regardless of sexual history.**
   1. Under age 21, cervical cancer is quite rare (1 to 2 per million), while HPV infection is common and dysplasia may occur, but both usually spontaneously remit.

F. **Women aged 21 to 29 years** should be screened every 3 years with cytology only. (HPV testing would detect many transient infections without carcinogenic potential.)

G. **Women aged 30 and older** may be screened by cytology plus HPV cotesting every 5 years (preferred), or with cytology alone every 3 years.

H. Women who have had a **total hysterectomy** (including removal of the cervix) for benign disease may stop cervical cancer screening.

I. **Screening may be stopped at age 65** in women who have had adequate screening (three consecutive negative Pap tests or two consecutive negative HPV/Pap cotests within past 10 years, and most recent test within 5 years).

J. Risk factors and special cases:
   1. In **women with HIV infection,** the CDC recommends cervical cytology screening twice in the first year after diagnosis and annually thereafter, while ACOG recommends annual cytology starting at age 21.
   2. ACOG recommends that women with a **history of high-grade dysplasia or cancer** should continue routine age-based testing for 20 years, even past age 65.
   3. More frequent screening may be required in women with a history of prenatal exposure to diethylstilbestrol (DES) and women who are immunocompromised (such as organ transplantation).

IV. COLORECTAL CANCER SCREENING

A. Colorectal cancer (CRC) is the second most common cause of cancer deaths in the United States. Screening is associated with decreases in incidence as well as mortality, due to removal of premalignant adenomatous polyps, but only about two-thirds of Americans have been screened adequately (*N Engl J Med* 1993;329:1977).

B. Screening strategies fall into two main categories:
   1. Stool-based tests that primarily detect cancer: guaiac-based fecal occult blood testing (gFOBT), fecal immunochemical test (FIT), or stool DNA testing.
   2. Tests that detect both cancer and adenomatous polyps, thus permitting polyp removal for cancer prevention: flexible sigmoidoscopy (FSIG), colonoscopy, barium enema, or CT colonography.

C. For any test other than colonoscopy, any abnormalities must be followed up with a full colonoscopy, not just repeat testing.

D. A brief summary of screening tests and recommended intervals includes the following:
   1. Annual gFOBT has modest sensitivity and specificity, but has been shown in randomized controlled trials to lower CRC mortality. It should be done with a high-sensitivity test such as Hemoccult SENSA on three specimens collected at home (**in-office rectal exam is not an acceptable stool test for CRC screening**).
   2. Annual FIT that detects human globin from lower GI bleeding (globin from upper GI sources is digested) and is therefore more specific.
   3. Stool DNA test, interval uncertain.
   4. FSIG every 5 years has been shown to lower CRC mortality despite only examining the distal colon. It requires a limited bowel prep, and no sedation is required. Colonic perforation is rare (<1 in 20,000).
   5. Air contrast barium enema (ACBE) every 5 years has only half the sensitivity of colonoscopy. It requires a full bowel prep, no sedation is used, and the test may be uncomfortable.
   6. Computed tomography colonography (CTC) or "virtual colonoscopy" every 5 years.
      a. Requires a full bowel prep and air insufflation.
      b. Sensitivity is probably comparable to colonoscopy.
      c. Patients with large polyps must be referred for colonoscopic resection, but uncertainty exists about management of small (<6 mm) polyps.
   7. Colonoscopy every 10 years.
      a. Requires a full bowel prep and sedation.
      b. Regarded as the gold standard, but may miss 5% to 12% of lesions >1 cm.
      c. Lesions can be resected during the procedure.
      d. Risk of colonic perforation is about 1 in 1,000; can also cause bleeding and cardiovascular complications.

E. Current guidelines were published in 2012 by the American College of Physicians (ACP) (*Annal Intern Med* 2012;156:378), in 2008 by the USPSTF (*Annal Intern Med* 2012;156(5):378), and in 2008 by a joint guideline (*CA Cancer J Clin* 2008;58:130) published by ACS, the United States Multi-Society Task Force on Colorectal Cancer, and the American College of Radiology.

F. The USPSTF recommendations include the following:
   1. Screen adults aged 50 to 75 using annual high-sensitivity gFOBT, or FSIG every 5 years combined with high-sensitivity gFOBT every 3 years, or colonoscopy every 10 years.
   2. Do not routinely screen those aged 76 to 85 years, but there may be considerations that support screening in an individual patient.
   3. Screening is not recommended >85 years of age.

G. The ACP recommends that
   1. Clinicians perform individualized assessment of risk for CRC in all adults.
   2. Average-risk adults should start CRC screening at age 50, using annual gFOBT, annual FIT, FSIG every 5 years, or colonoscopy every 10 years.
   3. High-risk adults should start screening with colonoscopy at age 40 or 10 years younger than the age at which the youngest affected relative was diagnosed with CRC.
   4. Screening should stop at age 75 or if life expectancy is <10 years.

H. The joint guideline recommends that
   1. Screening for CRC in average-risk, asymptomatic adults should begin at age 50.
   2. CRC screening is not appropriate if the patient is not likely to benefit from screening due to life-limiting comorbidity.
   3. Colon cancer prevention should be the primary goal of screening. Preferred tests detect adenomatous polyps and can prevent cancer: FSIG every 5 years, ACBE every 5 years, CT colonography every 5 years, or colonoscopy every 10 years.
   4. Other acceptable screening tests include annual gFOBT with a high-sensitivity test, annual FIT, or stool DNA test, interval uncertain.

I. **High-risk persons** need earlier and/or more frequent screening. These include those with a personal history of CRC or adenomatous polyps, inflammatory bowel disease, endometrial cancer before age 50, a hereditary CRC syndrome, or a strong family history of CRC or polyps.

1. Those with CRC or adenomatous polyps in a first-degree relative <60 years of age or in two first-degree relatives of any age should be screened with colonoscopy every 5 years beginning at age 40, or 10 years before the youngest case in the immediate family, whichever is earlier.

2. For those with CRC or adenomatous polyps in a first-degree relative at 60 or older, or two second-degree relatives with CRC, screening should begin at age 40 with any recommended form of testing at the usual intervals.

V. LUNG CANCER SCREENING

A. Lung cancer is the most common cause of cancer death in the United States.

B. Multiple randomized trials have demonstrated **no mortality benefit to screening with chest X-ray (CXR), with or without sputum cytology.**

C. Observational trials in the late 1990s showed that low-dose single-breath-hold, helical CT (LDCT) scans could detect early stage lung cancers more effectively than CXRs.

D. The National Lung Screening Trial (NLST) published in 2011 was the first randomized trial to show a statistically significant benefit to CT screening for lung cancer (*N Engl J Med* 2011;365:395).

1. The trial compared LDCT to CXR for 3 years in more than 50,000 people aged 55 to 74; participants had at least 30 pack-years of smoking, including current smokers and former smokers who had quit within 15 years.

2. At a median follow-up of 6.5 years, there was a relative mortality reduction of 20% for lung cancer deaths and 6.7% reduction in all-cause mortality in the LDCT group.

3. To prevent one lung cancer death, the number needed to screen with LDCT was 320.

4. Abnormal screening tests occurred in 24% of the LDCT group and 6.9% of the CXR group, >90% of which were false positives. Most only required additional imaging but some required invasive procedures. Complications from the diagnostic workup were uncommon: about 1.5% of the participants who had abnormal screening tests.

E. The USPSTF issued updated guidelines in December of 2013:

1. The USPSTF recommends annual screening for lung cancer with low-dose CT in adults aged 55 to 80 years with a 30 pack-year smoking history and who currently smoke or have quit within the past 15 years.

2. Screening should be discontinued once a person has not smoked for 15 years or develops a health problem that substantially limits life expectancy or the ability or willingness to have curative lung surgery.

F. A number of expert organizations have issued updated guidelines, including the ACS (*CA Cancer J Clin* 2013;63:107), the NCCN, and the American College of Chest Physicians (*Chest* 2013;143(5 Suppl):e78S).

1. They support LDCT screening in individuals similar to those in the NLST:
   a. Age 55 to 74
   b. At least 30 pack-years of smoking.
   c. Current smoker or quit within the past 15 years.

2. Screening is not appropriate for patients with severe comorbidities that limit life expectancy or would preclude potentially curative treatment.

3. The decision to start screening should be preceded by a process of informed and shared decision making, with discussion of the potential benefits, limitations, and harms associated with screening.

VI. PROSTATE CANCER SCREENING

A. Although 17% of men will be diagnosed with prostate cancer, only 2.4% will die of it. Screening for prostate cancer (PrCA) is a controversial topic as trials have shown small or no survival benefit in screened groups and many men die "with" rather than "of" prostate cancer. Treatment has potential harms, including erectile dysfunction, urinary incontinence, and bowel problems.

B. **The USPSTF** (*Annal Intern Med* 2012;157:120) recommends **against PSA testing,** concluding that screening produces more harms than benefits.

C. **The ACS** (*CA Cancer J Clin* 2010;60:70) **stresses the need for informed decision making.**
   1. This information should be provided starting at age 50 (at 40 to 45 in higher-risk men).
   2. Men with <10-year life expectancy should not be offered prostate cancer screening (at age 75, only about half of men have a life expectancy of 10 years or more).
   3. Key discussion points include the following:
      a. Screening may reduce the risk of dying from PrCA, but the evidence is conflicting, and experts disagree about the value of screening.
      b. Not all men whose PrCA is detected through screening require immediate treatment. It is not currently possible to predict which men are likely to benefit from treatment.
      c. Treatment for PrCA can lead to urinary, bowel, sexual, and other health problems.
      d. The PSA and DRE may produce false-positive or -negative results.
      e. Abnormal results require prostate biopsies that can be painful, may lead to complications, and can miss clinically significant cancer.
   4. If screening is elected, the ACS recommends PSA with or without DRE.
      a. Initial PSA <2.5 ng/mL: screen every 2 years.
      b. Initial PSA 2.5 ng/mL or greater: screen annually.
      c. PSA >4.0 ng/mL: refer for biopsy (2.5 to 4.0: individualized assessment).

D. The ACP recommends that PSA testing should only be done in patients with a clear preference for screening (*Annal Intern Med* 2013;158:761).
   1. Clinicians should inform men aged 50 to 69 about the limited potential benefits and substantial harms of screening for prostate cancer.
   2. Screening should not be done in average-risk men aged <50 or >69, nor those with a life expectancy of <10 to 15 years.

E. The American Urological Association (AUA) published its guideline online in 2013 (Carter HB, Albertsen PC, Barry MJ, et al. *Early Detection of Prostate Cancer: AUA Guideline*. 2013. Accessed July 5, 2013 www.auanet.org/education/guidelines/prostate-cancer-detection.cfm).
   1. Men <40 years of age should not be screened.
   2. Average-risk men <55 years of age should not be routinely screened.
      a. For men 40 to 55 years of age who are at higher risk (family history or African American), decisions should be individualized.
   3. For men aged 55 to 69, they strongly recommend shared decision making, based on a man's values and preferences after weighing the benefits against the known potential harms associated with screening and treatment. They estimate that one prostate cancer death is averted for every 1,000 men screened for a decade.
   4. Men should not be routinely screened if they are >70 years of age or have a life expectancy <10 to 15 years.
   5. If men choose screening, an interval of 2 years or more may be preferred over annual screening as this preserves the majority of the benefits and reduces overdiagnosis. Intervals for rescreening can be individualized based on baseline PSA level.
   6. There is **no evidence that DRE is beneficial as a primary screening test.**

VII. OVARIAN CANCER SCREENING

A. Ovarian cancer is uncommon (2% lifetime risk) but often lethal because only 15% are diagnosed while still localized to the ovary (*CA Cancer J Clin* 2013;63:87).

B. Patients at the highest risk for ovarian cancer are those with inherited cancer syndromes: the BRCA1 gene mutation conveys a lifetime risk of about 40%, and the BRCA2 gene mutation conveys a lifetime risk of about 20%.

C. **Pelvic examination is not effective for screening** due to poor sensitivity and specificity.

D. Ovarian cancer is occasionally found incidentally on a Pap smear (sensitivity <30%).

   E. The tumor marker CA125 has limited sensitivity and specificity.
   1. Only about half of early ovarian cancers have elevated levels of CA125.
   2. False positives are too common (about 1%) for an effective screening test. Levels vary with the menstrual cycle, age, ethnicity, and smoking, and CA125 can be increased with endometriosis, uterine leiomyomata, cirrhosis, ascites from any cause, and a variety of cancers.
   F. Transvaginal ultrasound (TVU) has limited sensitivity and specificity for screening.
   G. A large randomized trial in the United States showed that screening with CA125 and TVU did not improve ovarian cancer mortality (relative risk 1.18, screened vs. usual care) (*JAMA* 2011;305:2295). The positive predictive value was only about 1%, and for every screen-detected ovarian cancer about 20 women underwent surgery; 20% of those surgeries resulted in major complications.
   H. Other studies are ongoing.
   I. **No organization recommends screening average-risk women for ovarian cancer.**
   1. The USPSTF specifically recommends against screening due to lack of benefit, and potential harms by leading to unnecessary surgeries (*Annal Intern Med* 2012; 157:900).
   2. ACOG concluded that currently there is no effective strategy for ovarian cancer screening (*Obstet Gynecol* 2011;117:742).
      a. Clinicians should have a high index of suspicion when women present with symptoms commonly associated with ovarian cancer: pelvic or abdominal pain, increase in abdominal size or bloating, and difficulty eating or feeling full.
      b. High-risk women may be offered the combination of pelvic examination, TVU, and CA125 testing.
   3. The NCCN recommends consideration of twice yearly ovarian cancer screening with TVU and serum CA125 levels beginning at age 30, or 5 to 10 years earlier than the earliest age of first diagnosis of ovarian cancer in the family.
   4. Owing to the lack of efficacy of ovarian cancer screening modalities, many organizations recommend bilateral salpingo-oophorectomy for high risk women at age 35 to 40 years or once the patient no longer wishes to bear more children.

VIII. TESTICULAR CANCER
   A. USPSTF recommends against screening for testicular cancer because the incidence is low and testicular germ cell tumors are one of the most curable solid neoplasms. No evidence has shown that routine screening would improve health outcomes.
   B. The AUA recommends monthly testicular self-exams.

IX. SCREENING FOR OTHER CANCERS
   A. Routine population screening is not recommended for the following cancers: endometrial, bladder, thyroid, oral cavity, or skin. Clinicians should be vigilant for early symptoms of possible cancer in those sites.
   B. The ACS recommends that "the cancer-related checkup should include examination for cancers of the thyroid, testicles, ovaries, lymph nodes, oral cavity, and skin, as well as health counseling about tobacco, sun exposure, diet and nutrition, risk factors, sexual practices, and environmental and occupational exposures."

SUGGESTED READINGS

Aberle DR, Adams AM, Berg CD, et al; National Lung Screening Trial Research Team. Reduced lung-cancer mortality with low-dose computed tomographic screening. *N Engl J Med* 2011;365:395–409.

American Cancer Society Screening Guidelines. American Cancer Society recommendations for early breast cancer detection in women without breast symptoms. http://www.cancer.org/cancer/breastcancer/moreinformation/breastcancerearlydetection/breast-cancer-early-detection-acs-recs. Accessed February 7, 2014.

American College of Obstetricians and Gynecologists Committee on Gynecologic Practice. Committee opinion no. 477: the role of the obstetrician gynecologist in the early detection of epithelial ovarian cancer. *Obstet Gynecol* 2011;117:742–746.

American College of Obstetricians-Gynecologists. Practice bulletin no. 122: breast cancer screening. *Obstet Gynecol* 2011;118:372–382.

Barton MB, Harris R, Fletcher SW. Does this patient have breast cancer? *JAMA* 1999;282:1270–1280.

Buys SS, Partridge E, Black A, et al; PLCO Project Team. Effect of screening on ovarian cancer mortality: the prostate, lung, colorectal and ovarian (PLCO) cancer screening randomized controlled trial. *JAMA* 2011;305:2295–2303.

Carter HB, Albertsen PC, Barry MJ, et al. Early detection of prostate cancer: AUA guideline. www.auanet. org. 2013. Accessed July 5, 2013; www.auanet.org/education/guidelines/prostate-cancer-detection.cfm

Detterbeck FC, Mazzone PJ, Naidich DP, et al. Screening for lung cancer: diagnosis and management of lung cancer, 3rd ed: American College of Chest Physicians evidence-based clinical practice guidelines. *Chest* 2013;143(Suppl 5):e78S–e92S.

Fagerlin A, Zikmund-Fisher BJ, Ubel PA. How making a risk estimate can change the feel of that risk: shifting attitudes toward breast cancer risk in a general public survey. *Patient Educ Couns* 2005;57:294–299.

Humphrey LL, Helfand M, Chan BK, et al. Breast cancer screening: a summary of the evidence for the U.S. Preventive Services Task Force. *Ann Intern Med* 2002;137:347–360.

Kaplan JE, Benson C, Holmes KH, et al. Guidelines for prevention and treatment of opportunistic infections in HIV-infected adults and adolescents: recommendations from CDC, the National Institutes of Health, and the HIV Medicine Association of the Infectious Diseases Society of America. Centers for Disease Control and Prevention (CDC); National Institutes of Health; HIV Medicine Association of the Infectious Diseases Society of America. *MMWR Recomm Rep* 2009;58:1–207.

Levin B, Lieberman DA, McFarland B, et al. Screening and surveillance for the early detection of colorectal cancer and adenomatous polyps, 2008: a joint guideline from the American Cancer Society, the US Multi-Society Task Force on Colorectal Cancer, and the American College of Radiology. *CA Cancer J Clin* 2008;58:130–160.

Mavaddat N, Peock S, Frost D et al. Cancer risks for BRCA1 and BRCA2 mutation carriers: results from prospective analysis of EMBRACE. *J Natl Cancer Inst* 2013; 812.

Moyer VA; on behalf of the U.S. Preventive Services Task Force. Screening for prostate cancer: U.S. Preventive Services Task Force Recommendation Statement. *Annal Intern Med* 2012;157:120–134.

Moyer VA; on behalf of the U.S. Preventive Services Task Force. Screening for ovarian cancer: U.S. Preventive Services Task Force Reaffirmation Recommendation Statement. *Annal Intern Med* 2012;157:900–904.

NCCN Clinical Practice Guidelines in Oncology. Breast cancer screening and diagnosis (Version 1.2014). http://www.nccn.org/professionals/physician_gls/pdf/breast-screening.pdf. Accessed February 7, 2014.

NCCN Clinical Practice Guidelines in Oncology. Lung cancer screening (version 1.2014). www.nccn.org/professionals/physician_gls/pdf/lung_screening.pdf. Accessed February 7, 2014.

Qaseem A, Barry MJ, Denberg TD, et al; for the Clinical Guidelines Committee of the American College of Physicians. Screening for prostate cancer: a guidance statement from the clinical guidelines committee of the American College of Physicians. *Annal Intern Med* 2013; 158: 761–9.

Qaseem A, Denberg TD, Hopkins RH, et al; for the Clinical Guidelines Committee of the American College of Physicians. Screening for colorectal cancer: a guidance statement from the American College of Physicians. *Annal Intern Med* 2012;156:378–386.

Screening for Breast Cancer: U.S. Preventive Services Task Force Recommendations. *Annal Intern Med* 2009;151:1–44.

Smith RA, Brooks D, Cokkinides V, et al. Cancer screening in the United States, 2013: a review of current American Cancer Society guidelines, current issues in cancer screening, and new guidance on cervical cancer screening and lung cancer screening. *CA Cancer J Clin* 2013;63:87–105.

Smith RA, Durado Brooks D, Cokkinides V, et al. Cancer screening in the United States, 2013; a review of current American Cancer Society guidelines, current issues in cancer screening, and new guidance on cervical cancer screening and lung cancer screening. *CA Cancer J Clin* 2013;63:88–105.

Thomas DB, Gao DL, Ray RM, et al. Randomized trial of breast self-examination in Shanghai: final results. *J Natl Cancer Inst* 2002;94:1445–1457.

U.S. Preventive Services Task Force. Screening for breast cancer: U.S. Preventive Services Task Force recommendation statement. *Ann Intern Med* 2009;151:716–726.

U.S. Preventive Services Task Force. Screening for colorectal cancer: U.S. Preventive Services Task Force recommendation statement. *Ann Intern Med* 2008;149:627–637.

Wender R, Fontham ET, Barrera E Jr, et al. American Cancer Society lung cancer screening guidelines. *CA Cancer J Clin* 2013;63:107–117.

Winawer SJ, Zauber AG, Ho MN, et al. Prevention of colorectal cancer by colonoscopic polypectomy: The National Polyp Study Workgroup. *N Engl J Med* 1993;329:1977–1981.
Wolf AMD, Wender RC, Etzioni RB, et al. American Cancer Society Guideline for the early detection of prostate cancer: update 2010. *CA Cancer J Clin* 2010;60:70–98.
www.cancer.org/cancer/breastcancer/overviewguide/breast-cancer-overview-key-statistics. Accessed July 27, 2013.

Nutritional Support

Re-I Chin • Amy Glueck • Carolina C. Javier

I. **IDENTIFICATION AND ASSESSMENT OF PATIENTS AT NUTRITIONAL RISK.** Nutrition plays a supportive role in the care of the patient with cancer, whether the goal of therapy is curative or palliative. Nutritional interventions will maintain and preserve body composition and lean body mass, support functional status, and enhance the quality of life. Proactive assessments of nutritional status are essential to assure success in intervention and to improve patient outcome. Treatment modalities may have an impact on the nutritional status of the patient and increase the risk for weight loss and malnutrition. Oncology dietitians play a key role in optimizing nutrition for the cancer patient through counseling and education of patients and their families, and other members of the health-care team. The assessment and nutritional surveillance of the patient with cancer can help meet therapeutic goals.

II. **NUTRITIONAL ASSESSMENT.** Nutritional assessment is an essential component in the nutritional care of the patient with cancer, because it will provide an estimate of body composition, such as fat, skeletal muscle protein, and visceral protein. It will likewise identify patients who are at risk of cancer-induced malnutrition and determine the magnitude of nutritional depletion in patients who are already malnourished.

A. **Patient history and examination.** Information that pertains to the patient's medical history and physical examination will reveal usual body weight, any recent weight change, or inclusion of new or special diets. Unintentional weight loss of 10% or more of body weight within the previous 6 months could mean a significant nutritional deficit and is a good indicator of clinical outcome. Signs of malnutrition such as muscle wasting, loss of muscle strength, and depletion of fat stores may be revealed by a physical examination. However, body weight alone is insufficient as a nutritional assessment tool and will fail to show important changes in disease or therapy-related caloric intake or metabolic rate.

In addition, detailed information should be obtained regarding change in appetite, food intake, gastrointestinal problems, and concomitant disease.

B. **Anthropometric assessment.** Anthropometric measurements are often used in the assessment of nutritional status, particularly when a chronic imbalance occurs between protein and energy intake. Such disturbances change the patterns of physical growth and the relative proportions of body tissues such as fat, muscle, and total body water. The measurement of the triceps skinfold (TSF) is used to calculate an estimation of fat stores, whereas the midarm muscle circumference (MMC) (includes the basic anthropometrics of weight and height) assesses lean body mass MMC (cm) = Arm circumference (cm) − $0.314 \times$ TSF (mm).

Standards for age and gender have been established; however, there are wide variations among individuals, and interobserver measurement variability is considerable.

Anthropometric measurements may be markedly affected by nonnutritional factors and are rarely performed in the routine clinical setting.

C. **Assessment of protein status.** Serum protein concentrations such as retinol-binding protein, transferrin, prealbumin, and albumin can be used to assess the degree of visceral protein depletion.

The relationship between malnutrition and serum protein levels is related to the patient's hydration status and the half-life of the individual protein. Visceral protein status is frequently assessed by the measurement of one or more of the serum proteins. One of the first organs to be affected by protein malnutrition is the liver, which is the main site of synthesis for most of these serum proteins.

The synthesis of serum proteins is impaired by the limited supply of protein substrates, resulting in a decline in serum protein concentrations. Many nonnutritional factors influence the concentration of serum proteins and reduce their specificity and sensitivity. Total serum protein is easily measured and has been used as an index of visceral protein status in several national nutrition surveys; however, it is a rather insensitive index of protein status. Serum albumin reflects changes within the intravascular space and not the total visceral protein pool. Serum albumin is not very sensitive to short-term changes in protein status; it has a long half-life of 14 to 20 days (Table 42-1). Reduced catabolism largely compensates for reductions in hepatic synthesis of serum albumin.

Each transferrin molecule binds with two molecules of iron, and thereby serves as an iron-transport protein. Transferrin responds more rapidly to changes in protein status because of its shorter half-life and smaller body pool than albumin. Like serum albumin concentrations, serum transferrin concentrations are affected by a variety of factors, including gastrointestinal, renal, and liver disease.

The nutritional status of the patient also can be defined by using objective data. The Prognostic Nutritional Index (PNI) has been shown to predict clinical outcome in cancer patients. The PNI is based on serum albumin level, serum transferrin level, delayed cutaneous hypersensitivity, and TSF thickness.

D. **Immune function.** Tests of immunocompetence are sometimes used as functional indices of protein status; however, their sensitivity and specificity are low. Nutritional deficiencies can impair nearly all aspects of the immune system, and no single measurement

TABLE 42-1	**Factors that Decrease or Increase Albumin**	
Albumin	**Factors that decrease albumin**	**Factors that increase albumin**
Normal: 3.5–5.0 g/dL	• Acute-phase response[a]	• Intravascular volume depletion
Depletion: Mild: 3.0–3.4 g/dL Moderate: 2.4–2.9 g/dL Severe: <2.4 g/dL	• Severe liver failure	• Intravenous albumin or plasminate, blood transfusions (temporary rise)
Half-life approximately 14–20 d	• Redistribution: intravascular volume overload, third spacing, pregnancy, minor decrease with recumbency • Increased losses: nephritic syndromes, burns, protein-losing enteropathies, exudates • Severe zinc deficiency	• Anabolic steroids, possibly glucocorticoids

[a]Acute-phase response occurs with inflammation associated with conditions such as infection, injury, surgery, and cancer.

can assess adequacy of the immune response. Examples of immunologic tests include lymphocyte count, measurement of thymus-dependent lymphocytes, and delayed cutaneous hypersensitivity.

  E. Subjective global assessment (SGA). SGA of nutritional status includes relevant history data (dynamic weight loss, dietary intake, specific symptoms, performance status, primary disease, and metabolic demand) as well as clinical data (subjective estimate of fat and protein stores.) The nutritional assessment tools used for clinical routine are summarized in Table 42-2.

III. INTERVENTIONS AND NUTRITIONAL THERAPY.
An estimate of current energy and protein balance is useful in providing nutritional intervention.

  A. Nitrogen metabolism. The measurement of the nitrogen balance can document the effectiveness of nutritional therapy; nitrogen balance is calculated by the following formula:

$$\text{Nitrogen balance} = \frac{\text{protein intake}}{6.25} \text{ (urinary urea nitrogen + 4)}$$

The apparent net protein utilization is generated by using the relationship. The obligatory nitrogen loss is roughly equal to 0.1 g/kg of body weight.

IV. ESTIMATING ENERGY NEEDS IN ADULTS

  A. Harris benedict equation (for healthy adults)
    1. Men: REE = 66 + 13.7W + 5H − 6.8A
    2. Women: REE = 655 + 9.6W + 1.7H − 4.7A
    3. Where REE = resting energy expenditure (kcal/d); W = weight (kg); H = height (cm); and A = age (years).
    4. *Validation studies:* Original studies conducted on healthy volunteers. Note that for obese individuals (BMI > 29.9), formula may overestimate REE by 5% to 15% if actual weight is used.

TABLE 42-2	Synopsis of Nutritional Assessment Parameters

Minimal screening assessment
  Present weight in relation to ideal weight (weight/height index)
  Weight change (percentage weight change/time interval)
  Serum albumin
Complete assessment
  History
    Dietary data (food records, recall methods)
    Concomitant disease
  Physical examination
    Body fat, muscle wasting
    Specific nutritional deficiencies
  Anthropometrics
    Triceps skin fold (caliper method)
    MMC
  Laboratory tests
    Creatinine/height index
    Serum transferrin or albumin
  Immune function
    Total lymphocyte count
    Delayed hypersensitivity skin tests
  Subjective global assessment, clinical experience
Apparative assessment
  Bioelectrical impedance analysis

B. **Mifflin–St Jeor equation (for healthy adults)**
   1. Men: REE = 10W + 6.25H − 5A + 5
   2. Women: REE = 10W + 6.25H − 5A − 161
   3. Where REE = resting energy expenditure (kcal/d); W = weight (kg); H = height (cm); and A = age (years).
   4. *Validation studies:* Equation developed from a sample of obese and nonobese healthy individuals. Some research has indicated that this equation may provide a more accurate estimation of REE than the Harris–Benedict formula in both obese and nonobese individuals, and, therefore, this equation deserves consideration.

C. **Ireton–Jones ((for acutely ill adults)**
   1. Ventilator-dependent patients: EEE = 1784 − 11A + 5W + 244S + 239T + 804B
   2. Spontaneously breathing patients: EEE = 629 − 11A + 25W − 609O
   3. Where EEE = estimated energy expenditure (kcal/d); A = age (y); W = weight (kg); S = sex (male = 1, female = 2); T = diagnosis of trauma (present = 1, absent = 0); B = diagnosis of burn (present = 1, absent = 0); and O = obesity > 30% above ideal body weight from 1959 Metropolitan Life Insurance Tables (present = 1, absent = 0).
   4. *Validation studies:* Equation developed from a sample of hospitalized patients including critically ill patients and patients with burns. Recent research has reported that this equation underestimates energy requirements.

D. **A.S.P.E.N. Energy Expenditure formulas (in calories/kilogram).** These formulas have not been validated using evidence-based information. However, they are used as a baseline in clinical practice and adjusted as needed to meet nutrition goals. Using this method, initial calorie goals usually start with 25 kcal/kg and can be adjusted as high as 40 kcal/kg. See table for more specific estimations.

E. **Protein Needs.** Protein intake is crucial during cancer treatment for the maintenance of lean muscle mass as well as the regeneration and repair of cells. Per the Dietary Reference Intakes, healthy individuals are recommended to consume 0.8g/kg protein. Protein needs can increase for cancer patients, especially those undergoing treatment. A catabolic state can increase protein needs to a range of 1.2g/kg to 2.0g/kg per day.

F. **Assessment of nutritional intake.** Individuals can meet daily energy needs through a variety of ways.
   1. **Oral nutrition.** The preferred method for providing nutrition for patients who are able to eat is by oral diet, which can be modified according to the physiologic and anatomic constraints of their illness. Nutritional support considerations for individuals with daily energy deficits (e.g., patients with anorexia and resulting weight loss, dysphagia) are listed in Table 42-4.
   2. **Dietary supplements.** Nutrients, vitamins, and minerals that are essential for human health as well as a variety of nonessential nutrients such as phytochemicals, hormones, and herbs are used as dietary supplements; however, these should never replace whole foods. The American Cancer Society (ACS) warns against massive doses of any dietary supplement, and recommends supplements that are close to the daily percentage value for most vitamins and minerals. The United States Department of Agriculture

---

TABLE 42-3 A.S.P.E.N. Energy Expenditure Formulas

Medical Condition	Estimated Energy Needs (calories/kg body weight)
Cancer- repletion, weight gain	30–35
Cancer- inactive, non-stressed	25–30
Cancer- hypermetabolic, stressed	35
Sepsis	25–30
Hematopoietic cell transplant	30–35

TABLE 42-4	Nutritional Support Considerations for Individuals with Daily Energy Deficits

Potential problem	Intervention
Anorexia	Small frequent meals seasoned according to individual taste Snacks of nutrient-dense liquids such as instant breakfast, milk shakes, or commercial supplements can provide significant protein and calories and are easily consumed
Dry mouth/thick saliva	Encourage good oral hygiene Artificial saliva and use of a straw may facilitate swallowing Petroleum jelly applied to the lips may help prevent drying Avoid coarse foods; some patients may require a liquid diet
Dysphagia	Encourage a soft, more liquid diet and easy-to-swallow foods Small frequent meals Use liquid nutritional formulas Determine the appropriate consistency of food and fluids or any special swallowing techniques given by the speech therapist
Radiation esophagitis	Soft bland diet, using creamy, lukewarm, or cool foods Avoid coarse, dry, or scratchy textured foods Avoid tart and acidic fruits and juices, alcohol, and irritating spices

(USDA) states that there is no substitute for a well-balanced diet that follows the dietary guidelines for Americans. The daily percentage value (DV) on food labels, formerly known as the recommended daily allowance, is the average daily dietary intake level that is adequate to meet the nutrient requirements of nearly all (97% to 98%) individuals in a specific life stage and gender group. To account for differences in need and ability for absorption, the DV is set considerably higher than the estimated average requirement. Any recommendations for nutritional supplementation at doses higher than twice the DV should be individualized and are dependent on each individual's dietary and disease status. The Academy of Nutrition and Dietetics recommends getting all the nutrients needed from the diet first and then considering supplementation only if it is adequately researched.

3. **Enteral feeding.** Enteral feeding refers to the provision of nutrients, either to supplement oral intake or as the sole source of nutrition, delivered through a catheter or a tube to the gastrointestinal tract for absorption. Enteral feeding is preferred to parenteral feeding because it preserves the gastrointestinal architecture and prevents bacterial translocation from the gut. Enteral feeding has the advantage of delivering nutrients beyond areas of obstruction, at rates that can maximize nutrient absorption. Nutrients should be administered distal to the ligament of Treitz to avoid complications of aspiration pneumonia and gastric ileus. For short-term feeding, a nasogastric or nasoduodenal tube may be used. If there is a need for long-term enteral support, the preferred method is either a gastrostomy or jejunostomy tube, which can be placed either surgically or endoscopically. Nutritionally complete enteral-feeding formulas as well as specialized modular products to meet specific disease-related nutrient requirements are commercially available. Consult with a dietetics professional to determine the most appropriate formula.

4. **Total parenteral nutrition (TPN).** Providing nutritional support by the parenteral route is an important option for patients for whom oral or enteral nutrition is unsuitable. The hyperosmolar TPN solutions require central venous access to reduce complications of venous thrombosis and phlebitis. Inherent complications such as pneumothorax occur infrequently. Parenteral nutrition is more expensive than enteral or oral nutrition, and adherence to specific guidelines is of utmost importance to minimize complications. Some studies on the use of TPN in cancer patients demonstrated improvement in

TABLE 42-5	Common Antioxidants

- Vitamins A, C, and E
- Coenzyme Q10 (ubiquinone)
- Melatonin
- Carotenoids (alpha and beta carotene, astaxanthin, zeaxanthin, lutein, and lycopene)
- Flavonoids
- Isoflavones
- Resveratrol
- Curcumin
- N-acetylcysteine
- Alpha lipoic acid
- Selenium
- Zinc

body weight and total body fat content. Specific minerals, trace elements, and vitamins can be provided with TPN, but TPN does not stop the catabolic process of cancer cachexia, as nitrogen losses continue for patients receiving TPN, or alter the increased protein turnover and the process of lipolysis. When appropriately selected, certain cancer patients receiving TPN have shown significant decreases in morbidity and mortality. This includes patients with severe malnutrition receiving perioperative TPN and bone marrow transplant recipients. The American Society of Parenteral and Enteral Nutrition has recommended TPN supplementation in patients expected to have inadequate oral or enteral nutritional intake for more than 10 to 14 days. TPN can be very beneficial for some patients but the risks must be carefully considered prior to initiation. Complications include but are not limited to: infection at catheter site, sepsis, electrolyte imbalance, hyperlipidemia, hepatic abnormalities and so on. It is important to consult with a dietetics professional to determine the best parenteral nutrition plan prior to feeding.

V. NUTRIENT SUPPLEMENTATION IN ONCOLOGY. Additional nutrients from supplements can help some people meet their nutrient needs as specified by science-based nutrition standards such as the Dietary Reference Intakes. Dietary supplements include things like vitamins, minerals, herbs, or products made from plants. Dietary supplements are also defined to include powdered amino acids, enzymes, energy bars, and liquid food supplements. The use of these dietary supplements is prevalent and growing in the United States. Consumers may not be well informed about the safety and efficacy of supplements and some may have difficulty interpreting product labels. The expertise of dietetics practitioners is needed to help educate consumers on the safe and appropriate selection and use of nutrient supplements to optimize health. Cancer patients commonly use dietary supplements most often without the guidance or expertise of a knowledgeable practitioner, including antioxidants (Table 42-5) and herbs, with the latter associated with potential drug interactions (Table 42-6).

SUGGESTED READINGS

ASPEN Board of Directors and Clinical Guidelines Task Force. A.S.P.E.N. guidelines for the use of parenteral and enteral nutrition in adult and pediatric patients. *J Parenter Enteral Nutr* 2001;26(1) (Suppl):22SA.

Bauer J, Capra S, Ferguson M. Use of the scored patient-generated subjective global assessment (PG-SGA) as a nutrition assessment tool in patients with cancer. *Eur J Clin Nutr* 2002;56:779–785.

Daily Values [Internet]. Office dietary supplements, national institutes of health: strengthening knowledge and understanding of dietary supplements. 2013 [cited November 13, 2013]. http://ods.od.nih.gov/HealthInformation/dailyvalues.aspx.

Dietary Supplements: How to know what is safe [Internet]. *Am Cancer Soc* 2013 [cited November 20, 2013]. http://www.cancer.org/treatment/treatmentsandsideeffects/complementaryandalternativemedicine/dietarysupplements/dietary-supplements-toc.

TABLE 42-6	Common Herb–Drug Interactions and Precautions in Oncology

Botanical product	Common uses	Potential drug interactions and precautions
Ginseng, American or Asian	To improve cognition, immune function, and energy; promotes blood sugar metabolism	None known, but diabetics may need to monitor blood sugars due to a potential hypoglycemic effect
Black Cohosh	Menopausal symptoms	None known
Echinacea	Prevention of colds; used for immune support in cancer patients	None known; no documented interactions with immunosuppressive drugs
Garlic	Hyperlipidemia and atherosclerosis; prevention of colds	May enhance the effect of antiplatelet therapy and warfarin
Ginkgo	To improve cognition; to improve blood flow to the brain and extremities	Contraindicated in bleeding disorders; may enhance the effect of antiplatelet therapy and warfarin
Green tea	Reduce risk of cardiovascular disease and cancer	Can diminish the effect of dipyridamole; possible synergistic effects with sulindac and tamoxifen; large amounts of caffeine may increase the side effects of theophylline; antagonizes the tumoricidal effect of bortezomib
Ginger	Nausea	None known; anecdotal reports of interaction with warfarin but not proven
Kava	Anxiety and sleep	Should not be taken with alcohol, barbiturates, and other drugs with significant CNS effects; large doses may cause scaly ichthyosis
Milk thistle	Liver diseases and "cleansing"	An antioxidant; no known drug interactions
St. John's Wort	Depression	Should not be taken with prescription antidepressants; may interact with oral contraceptives, warfarin, theophylline, Indinavir, cyclosporine, digoxin; avoid alcohol; induces CYP3A4
Saw Palmetto	Prostate health, urinary outlet obstructive symptoms	None known; may cause mild nausea when taken without food

FDA 101: Dietary Supplements [Internet]. U.S. Food Drug Administration: Protecting and Promoting Your Health. 2013 [cited November 19, 2013]. http://www.fda.gov/forconsumers/consumerupdates/ucm050803.htm.

Forchielli ML, Miller SJ. Nutritional goals and requirements. In Merritt R, ed. *A.S.P.E.N Nutrition Support Practice Manual*. 2nd ed. Silver Spring, MD: ASPEN Publishing, 2005;50–51.

Frankenfield D, Smith JS, Cooney RN. Validation of 2 approaches to predicting resting metabolic rate in critically ill patients. *J Parenter Enter Nutr* 2004;28(4):259–264.

Frankenfield DC, Rowe WA, Smith JS, et al. Validation of several established equations for resting metabolic rate in obese and nonobese people. *J Am Diet Assoc* 2003;103(9):1152–1159.

Fuhrman MP. The albumin-nutrition connection: separating myth from fact. *Nutrition* 2002;18(2):199–200.

Halpern-Silveira D, Susin LRO, Borges LR, et al. Body weight and fat-free mass changes in a cohort of patients receiving chemotherapy. *Support Care Cancer* 2010;18(5):617–625.

Health Information: Making Decisions [Internet]. Office dietary supplements, national institutes of health: strengthening knowledge and understanding of dietary supplements. 2013 [cited November 15, 2013]. http://ods.od.nih.gov/HealthInformation/

Hoda D, Jatoi A, Burnes J, et al. Should patients with advanced, incurable cancers ever be sent home with total parenteral nutrition? *Cancer* 2005;103(4):863–868.

Howell WH. Anthropometry and body composition analysis. In: Matarese LE, Gottschlich MM, eds. *Contemporary Nutrition Support Practice*. 2nd ed. Philadelphia, PA: Saunders, 2002: 31–44.

Forchielli ML, Miller SJ. Nutritional goals and requirements. In Merritt R, ed. A.S.P.E.N Nutrition Support Practice Manual. 2nd ed. Silver Spring, MD: ASPEN Publishing, 2005;50-51.

Institute of Medicine of the National Academies. *Dietary Reference Intakes for Energy, Carbohydrate, Fiber, Fat, Fatty Acids, Cholesterol, Protein and Amino Acids*. Washington, DC: The National Academies Press, 2002/2005. Available at: www.nap.edu. Accessed July 2013.

Ireton-Jones C, Jones J. Why use predictive equations for energy expenditure assessment? *J. Am Diet Assoc* 1997;97(9): A44.

Ireton-Jones C, Turner WJ, Liepa G, et al. Status, equations for the estimation of energy expenditures in patients with burns with special reference to ventilatory. *J Burn Care Rehabil* 1992;13(3):330–333.

Isenring E, Bauer J, Capra S. The scored patient-generated subjective global assessment (PG-SGA) and its association with quality of life in ambulatory patients receiving radiotherapy. *Eur J Clin Nutr* 2003;57:305–309.

Kondrup J, Allison SP, Elia M, et al. ESPEN guidelines for nutrition screening 2002. *Clin Nutr* 2003;22(4):415–421.

Laviano A, Meguid M. Nutritional issues in cancer management. *Nutrition* 1996;12(5):358–371.

Loh NH, Griffiths RD. The curse of overfeeding and the blight of underfeeding. In: *Intensive Care Medicine*. New York, NY: Springer-Verlag, 2009:675–682.

Mahan LK, Escott-Stump S. Intervention: enteral and parenteral nutrition support. In: *Krause's Food and Nutrition Therapy*. St. Louis, MO: Saunders, 2008:521–522.

Marra M, Boyar A. Position of the American Dietetic Association: nutrient supplementation. *J Am Diet Assoc* 2009;109(12):2073–2085.

Mifflin MD, St Jeor ST, Hill LA, et al. A new predictive equation for resting energy expenditure in healthy individuals. *Am J Clin Nutr* 1990;51(2):241–247.

Molassiotis A, Xu M. Quality and safety issues of web-based information about herbal medicines in the treatment of cancer. *Complement Ther Med* 2004;12(4):217–227.

Muscaritoli M, Molfino A, Laviano A, et al. Parenteral nutrition in advanced cancer patients. *Crit Rev Oncol Hematol* 2012;84:26–36.

Payne-James J, Grimble GK, Silk DBA. Nutrition support in patients with cancer. *Artif. Nutr. Support Clin. Pract.* 2nd ed. New York, NY: Cambridge University Press; 2012. p. 639–680.

Raykher A, Russo L, Schattner M, et al. Enteral nutrition support of head and neck cancer patients. *Nutr Clin Pr* 2007;22(1):68–73.

Schwartz LM. Complementary and alternative medicine in the older cancer patient. In: Naeim A, Reuben D, Ganz P, eds. *Management of Cancer in the Older Patient*. Philadelphia, PA: Saunders, 2012:195–204.

Schwartz LM. Complementary and alternative medicine in the older cancer patient. In: Dimock K, Crowley K, eds. *Manag. Cancer Older Patient*. Philadelphia, PA: Saunders, 2012:195–204.

Vanitallie T. Frailty in the elderly: contributions of sarcopenia and visceral protein depletion. *Metabolism* 2003;52(10 Suppl 2):22–26.

Walsh D, Mahmoud F, Barna B. Assessment of nutritional status and prognosis in advanced cancer: interleukin-6, C-reactive protein, and the prognostic and inflammatory nutritional index. *Support Care Cancer* 2003;11:60–62.

Genetic Counseling in Oncology

Jennifer Ivanovich

Cancer genetic counseling and risk assessment is the process of identifying and educating individuals and their families who are at increased risk for developing cancer due to their family's cancer history. Cancer genetic counseling addresses the psychosocial issues associated with hereditary disease and identifies mechanisms for adaptation and personal control (*Cancer Genetics Risk Assessment and Counseling (PDQ)*. www.cancer.gov, 2014; *Am J Med Genet C Semin Med Genet* 2006;142C:269; *J Genet Counsel* 2012;21:151; *J Genet Counsel* 2006;15:77).

A genetic counselor is a health-care provider who is specifically trained in clinical genetics, communication, and family-based risk. While the Master's level training is directed at the study of general clinical genetics, many genetic counselors have chosen to specialize in cancer genetics. In most settings, genetic counselors work with clinical geneticists, physicians boarded in clinical genetics. However, as the discipline of cancer genetics continues to expand, many genetic counselors now work independently with medical and surgical oncologists.

The intended goal of the cancer genetic counseling *process* is to *educate* individuals about their family's cancer risk in a manner that is useful to them and utilize this information to guide medical care that is reflective of this risk (Fig. 43-1). This objective remains with or without the use of cancer genetic testing. Ideally, the process of assisting a family extends over several years, as new research discoveries transition to clinical care, the family history changes, or family members in the next generation approach an age when medical management will be altered (*JAMA* 2011;306:172).

Understanding a person's motivations for and expectations from the assessment, knowledge of cancer genetics, decision-making approach, personal experience with cancer, family communication style, family dynamics, as well as general psychological issues, such as cancer worry, is key to tailoring the education to meet his/her unique needs. This phase of the process has been termed *contracting* and, at its core, identifies factors that influence an individual's personal utility of the information to be shared (*Cancer J* 2012;18:287).

It is estimated 5% to 10% of any cancer type has an inherited genetic component. Data from a twin study conducted by Lichtenstein et al. suggest this proportion may be underestimated, at least for three common cancer types (*N Engl J Med* 2000;343:78). The authors evaluated the concordance rates of 28 cancer types among 44,788 monozygotic and dizygotic twin pairs from the Swedish, Danish, and Finnish twin registries. They estimated the effect of heritability, the proportion of disease susceptibility accounted for by inherited genetic abnormalities. Statistically significant effects of heritable factors were identified for cancers of the breast (27%), colon (35%), and prostate (42%) (*N Engl J Med* 2000;343:78). If these data hold true for other populations, the contribution of inherited genetic factors in cancer predisposition may be higher than currently estimated.

Families with hereditary disease have significantly increased cancer risks above the general population. Thorough attention must be directed first to identifying families with increased cancer risks, allowing for intensified surveillance as well as medical and surgical interventions, reflective of their family risk, to be implemented.

I. **ASSESSMENT.** Evaluation of both the personal medical history and the family cancer history is necessary to address the basic question *does this individual/family have features of hereditary cancer?*

For the personal medical history, special attention is paid to any history of benign and malignant tumors, cancer screening history, birth marks or unusual skin lesions, environmental exposures, reproductive history, and major illnesses (*J Genet Counsel* 2012;21:151). At present, physical examination adds limited diagnostic value, with some notable exceptions. Mucosal neuromas of the lips and tongue, which characterize the multiple endocrine neoplasia syndrome, type 2B, or the dark brown macules of the lips, mouth, and digits associated with the Peutz–Jeghers syndrome, are two examples (*Dig Dis Sci* 2007;52:1924; *Genet Med* 2011;13:755).

Family history is often a neglected component of the medical intake, making it challenging, if not nearly impossible, to identify individuals with an increased cancer risk due to their family

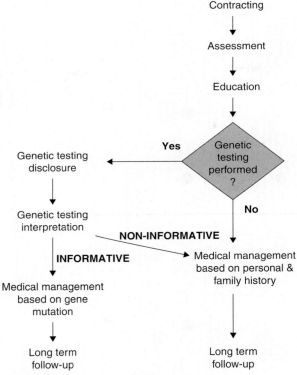

Figure 43-1. Cancer genetic counseling process.

history. It is not unusual to find the following reporting: *family history is not contributory.* What does this statement mean? Does the clinician imply a thorough family history was obtained and there were no features of hereditary disease? Or consider the following reporting: *mother with breast cancer, uncle with lung cancer, cousin with stomach cancer, grandmother with ovarian cancer.* This note is not useful either as the biological relationships are not clarified (are the affected individuals all from the same side of the family?), the ages at diagnosis are not recorded, and exposure history such as tobacco use is not documented. The importance of taking a thorough family cancer history cannot be overstated and requires detailed data regarding the family structure and reported cancer diagnoses.

Clinical genetic providers summarize the family history using a pedigree format. The family history can quickly be constructed, and by its very structure, biological relations are defined and patterns of cancer, and other key clinical characteristics, may be visualized. Three generation histories are typically obtained documenting individual family members, their children, and the family ethnic background. Recording extended relatives allows for the scope of at-risk family members to be recognized. The age at diagnosis, cancer type, as well as key exposure history, are solicited. When feasible, self-reported family histories are completed in advance of the genetics evaluation, allowing for family members to be contacted or medical records obtained. Limited research suggests that family history questionnaires completed in advance provide thorough family history information (*J Genet Counsel* 2009;18:366).

Consider a 28-year-old man diagnosed with colon cancer (Fig. 43-2). There is no reported family cancer history in the first example (Fig. 43-2A), and the genetics assessment is based

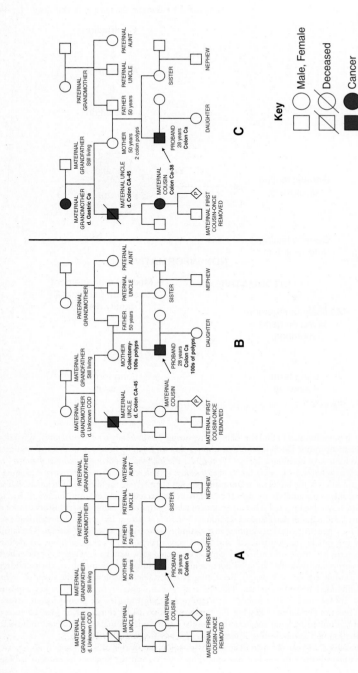

Figure 43-2. Example pedigrees.

solely on the age at diagnosis and tumor characteristics. Minimal changes to the reported family cancer history, as demonstrated in Figure 43-2B, leads to a diagnosis of familial polyposis based on the number of colonic polyps and dominant pattern of inheritance. Slightly different cancer reporting, as noted in Figure 43-2C, also demonstrates dominant inheritance but with a cancer pattern now diagnostic for the Lynch syndrome. Familial polyposis and Lynch syndrome are both hereditary colon cancer predisposition syndromes; however, they result from mutations in different genes, have distinct cancer risks, and consequently the medical recommendations differ. Visualization of the family history provides diagnostic and practical advantages.

There are several personal and family history features suggestive of hereditary disease (Table 43-1). To date, most, but not all, hereditary cancer syndromes are inherited following an autosomal dominant pattern of inheritance. Multiple affected individuals, who are closely related to one another, with more than one generation affected, are characteristics suggestive of any dominant disease. Young age at diagnosis, more than one primary cancer in a single individual, bilaterality of paired organs, the occurrence of rare tumor types, and unusual cancer presentations are key features. Distinct histologic features of specific cancers and specialized tumor genetic studies (e.g., microsatellite instability (MSI) testing) may provide important clues. It is the combination of features, not a single trait, that leads to the suspicion, or diagnosis, of inherited cancer predisposition. More specific clinical criteria, dependent on the predominant cancer in the family, have been developed (*J Med Genet* 2004;41:81). Independent evaluation of the maternal and paternal side of the family is necessary as the two histories are not additive.

Clinical assessment of the family cancer history may be hindered by the level of accuracy of reported cancer history, family structure, and the general age of the family. Overreporting the family cancer history may lead to an overestimation of risk with implementation of inappropriate medical interventions. In contrast, underreporting the family cancer history may result in lower cancer risk estimates with consequential underutilization of potentially beneficial surveillance and or prophylactic medical and surgical interventions.

Several studies have assessed the validity of cancer reporting, using both cancer and general populations, with evaluation of reporting for several different cancer types (*J Med Genet* 1999;36:309; *J Natl Cancer Inst* 2011;103:788; *JAMA* 2004;292:1480; *Am J Prev Med* 2003;24:190). Key findings include the following: (a) cancer reporting for first-degree relatives is more accurate than for second- or third-degree relatives; (b) cancer populations, who may be more motivated to seek family history information and demonstrate higher levels of reporting

---

TABLE 43-1 | **Personal and Family History Features Suggestive of Hereditary Cancer**

- Multiple affected individuals who are closely related to one another
- Cancers occurring in multiple generations
- Clusters of the same type of cancer (e.g., brother, father, paternal uncle with prostate cancer)
- Young age at diagnosis (e.g., colon cancer diagnosed at 35 yr)
- Multiple primary cancers in a single individual (e.g., sarcoma and breast cancer)
- Bilaterality in paired organs or multifocal disease (e.g., bilateral renal clear cell cancer)
- Uncommon presentation (e.g., male breast cancer)
- Rare cancer types (e.g., retinoblastoma, paraganglioma)
- Unusual tumor histology (e.g., renal chromophobe histology)
- Tumor genetic studies designed to screen for specific cancer syndromes (e.g., MSI analysis)
- Presentation of unusual skin lesions (e.g., mucocutaneous hyperpigmentation of mouth and lips)
- Combination of cancers suggestive of a known cancer syndrome
- Ethnic background associated with higher incidence of specific gene mutations

accuracy than general populations; (c) reporting accuracy varies by cancer site with breast and colon cancer consistently being correctly reported among first degree relatives; and (d) younger informants tend to have higher reporting accuracy (*J Med Genet* 1999;36:309; *J Natl Cancer Inst* 2011;103:788; *JAMA* 2004;292:1480; *Am J Prev Med* 2003;24:190).

To verify the reported cancer history, medical records and/or death certificates are collected. Pathology, medical, and surgical records are the most informative; however, these records are not always available given the limited time health-care facilities maintain paper records. Widespread implementation of electronic medical record systems will help to address this issue. Death certificates are inexpensive and readily available through a state's vital statistics office and may confirm a family member's cancer type and age at diagnosis.

Family structure may also impact the evaluation of the family's cancer history. Consider a woman with a pancreatic neuroendocrine tumor. Each parent was an only child with no siblings. This woman has no biological aunts, uncles, or cousins. Simply put, there are a limited number of people or "data" to evaluate the family history. The relative "age" of a family may also lead to a biased assessment. The parents of the proband in Figure 43-2a are only 50 years of age, and nearly 10 years younger than the average age of diagnosis for many common cancer types. It is important to understand that the family's cancer history may not have fully expressed itself yet when evaluating a young adult with cancer or a "young" family.

II. HEREDITARY CANCER PREDISPOSITION SYNDROMES. If the personal and family history features are consistent with hereditary disease, then the question is, *what is the underlying cancer syndrome in the family?*

The number of cancer predisposition syndromes described continues to grow (Table 43-2) (*J Natl Cancer Inst Monogr* 2008:1; *Fam Cancer* 2013;12:1). Overlapping clinical features (cancer risks) may necessitate the consideration of multiple diagnoses for a given family. Diagnostic guidelines have been established for many syndromes to assist in their clinical recognition (*Cancer Res* 1988;48:5358; Genetic/familial high-risk assessment: breast and ovarian. www.nccn.org, 2013; *Gastroenterology* 1999;116:1453).

Most of the cancer syndromes delineated to date are highly penetrant, dominantly inherited disorders. *Penetrance* is the frequency in which a gene or gene combination manifests itself in a gene carrier. *Every* person who carries a gene mutation in a disease with 100% penetrance will develop feature(s) of that disease, whereas only 30% of individuals will develop feature(s) in a syndrome with 30% penetrance. For cancer syndromes, high penetrance translates to high risk for certain cancer types. Expressivity is the term used to describe the clinical variability of a specific disease, and in the case of hereditary cancer is the spectrum of benign and malignant tumors associated with that cancer predisposition syndrome. Much of these data are currently derived from highly selected families, which may represent the extreme end of the disease spectrum. The penetrance and expressivity of a given syndrome will be used to determine screening and medical management.

As the genetic heterogeneity of inherited cancer predisposition is unraveled, more cancer syndromes will be defined, following varying patterns of inheritance, and with low-to-modest penetrance rates. Syndrome recognition will become increasingly more challenging leading to a greater reliance on genetic testing.

III. GENETIC TESTING. Genetic testing may encompass the analysis of gene(s), exomes, or even the entire genome. Genetic testing conducted to identify *germline* (inherited) gene mutations is typically performed on a blood, mouthwash, buccal swab, or banked DNA specimen. The purpose of germline genetic testing in the oncology setting is to identify the underlying genetic basis for the cancer predisposition in the family and subsequently use this information to guide treatment, follow-up, and make genetic testing available to at-risk family members.

In contrast, genetic analysis performed on a malignant tumor is primarily intended to characterize *somatic* (acquired) genetic aberrations for the purpose of identifying potential therapeutic targets. Tumor genetic testing may be used to screen a tumor for characteristics for a specific syndrome. For example, MSI analysis, performed on colon or endometrial malignancies, is used to screen for the Lynch syndrome (*JAMA* 2012;308:1555). Follow-up germline genetic testing is absolutely necessary to distinguish if the positive tumor screen resulted from a germline mutation or somatic events.

TABLE 43-2 Some Hereditary Cancer Predisposition Syndromes

Cancer syndrome gene(s)	Core clinical features	Primary medical recommendations beyond population-based cancer screening guidelines
Familial adenomatous polyposis *APC*	High risk for 100s–1,000s of colon polyps. Without total colectomy, colon cancer will eventually develop	• Consideration of screening for hepatoblastoma with liver ultrasound and serum alpha-fetoprotein concentrations up to 5 yr of age
	Increased risk for small bowel, thyroid, hepatoblastoma, pancreas cancer	• Colonoscopy screening beginning by 10 yr of age
	Desmoid tumors (10%–20%), congenital hypertrophy of retinal pigmentation (CHRPE), gastric polyps, osteomas	• Colonoscopy performed annually once polyps are detected until total colectomy is performed
		• Total colectomy when polyps develop
		• Esophagogastroduodenoscopy (EGD) screening by 25 yr, repeated every 1–3 yr
Hereditary breast and ovarian cancer 1 syndrome *BRCA1*	High risk for breast and ovarian cancer	Females only: • Mammography and breast MRI screening by 25 yr of age, repeated annually • Consideration of prophylactic mastectomy or prophylactic Tamoxifen therapy
	Increased risk for prostate and pancreatic cancer	• Consideration of transvaginal ultrasound and CA125 testing for ovarian cancer by 35 yr of age, repeated annually • Consideration of prophylactic oophorectomy • Annual clinical examinations of the skin and eye
Hereditary breast and ovarian cancer 2 syndrome *BRCA2*	High risk for breast and ovarian cancer	Females only: • Mammography and breast MRI screening by 25 yr of age, repeated annually • Consideration of prophylactic mastectomy or prophylactic Tamoxifen therapy
	Increased risk for prostate, pancreatic, melanoma (including ocular melanoma), male breast cancer, gastric cancer	• Consideration of transvaginal ultrasound and CA125 testing for ovarian cancer by 35 yr of age, repeated annually • Consideration of prophylactic oophorectomy
Hereditary HDGC *E-CADHERIN*	High risk for lobular breast cancer and diffuse gastric cancer	• Consideration of upper gastrointestinal endoscopy screening with random biopsies to begin 5–10 yr prior to earliest cancer diagnosis in family, repeated every year • Prophylactic total gastrectomy
		Females only: • Mammogram and breast MRI starting by 25 yr of age, repeated annually • Consideration of prophylactic bilateral mastectomy

(Continued)

TABLE 43-2 Some Hereditary Cancer Predisposition Syndromes (*Continued*)

Cancer syndrome gene(s)	Core clinical features	Primary medical recommendations beyond population-based cancer screening guidelines
Hereditary Pheochromocytoma/ Paraganglioma syndrome *SDHB, SDHD, SDHC, SDHA, SDHAF2, MAX*	High risk for pheochromocytoma and paragangliomas	• Screening recommendations vary by gene • Biochemical and imaging screening is recommended to begin by 10 yr of age or 10 yr younger than earliest diagnosis in the family • Urine or plasma levels of fractionated metanephrine and catecholamines • MRI or CT scans performed every 1–2 yr in asymptomatic individuals • Consideration of screening for renal cell carcinoma
Li-Fraumeni syndrome *TP53*	High and increased risk for a variety of tumors The classic associated tumors include breast cancer, sarcomas, brain tumors, adrenocortical carcinoma, and leukemias, and a variety of other malignancies may occur	• Avoidance of radiation exposure when possible • Comprehensive physical examination beginning in early childhood, repeated annually • Colonoscopy screening by 25 yr of age, repeated every 2–3 yr • Consideration of organ-targeted surveillance based on family cancer history Females only: • Mammogram and breast MRI starting by 25 yr of age, repeated annually
Lynch syndrome *MLH1, MSH2, MSH6, PMS2, Epcam*	High risk for colon, uterine cancer Increased risk for gastric and ovarian cancer, hepatobiliary tract, urinary tract, and brain tumors, and sebaceous carcinomas	• Colonoscopy surveillance by 20–25 yr of age, or 10 yr younger than earliest diagnosis in family, repeated every 1–2 yr • Upper endoscopy surveillance by 30–35 yr of age, repeated every 2–3 yr • Consideration of endometrial cancer surveillance and annual urine analysis for urinary tract tumors
Multiple endocrine neoplasia, type 1 *MEN1*	Syndrome characterized by multiple endocrine and nonendocrine tumors. Parathyroid tumors are the most common manifestation. Pituitary, gastro-entero-pancreatic tract tumors, including pancreatic neuroendocrine tumors, carcinoid, and adrenocortical tumors are common features Meningiomas, facial angiofibromas, lipomas, and leiomyomas	• Serum concentration of prolactin beginning at 5 yr of age, repeated annually • Serum concentrations of calcium to begin at 8 yr of age, repeated annually • Fasting serum gastrin concentration beginning at 20 yr, repeated annually • Head MRI beginning at 5 yr of age, repeated every 3–5 yr • Abdominal MRI surveillance to begin at 20 yr, repeated every 3–5 yr

Syndrome / Gene	Description	Surveillance/Management
Multiple endocrine neoplasia, type 2A *RET*	High risk for medullary thyroid cancer, pheochromocytoma Hyperparathyroidism	• Prophylactic thyroidectomy with consideration of autotransplantation of the parathyroid glands • Annual measurement of serum calcitonin following thyroidectomy • Biochemical screening for pheochromocytoma with urine or plasma levels of fractionated metanephrine and catecholamines beginning by 10 yr of age
Neurofibromatosis type 1 *NF1*	Increased risk for optic nerve and other central nervous system gliomas, malignant peripheral nerve sheet tumors Neurofibromas, plexiform neurofibromas, Lisch nodules, café-au-lait spots, axillary and inguinal freckling, and scoliosis	• Annual physical and ophthalmologic evaluation including blood pressure monitoring • Regular development assessment of children • Other studies indicated only on the basis of apparent signs or symptoms
Peutz–Jeghers syndrome *STK11.*	High risk for breast, colorectal, pancreatic cancer Increased risk for ovarian cancer, sex cord tumors with annual tubules and adenoma malignum of the cervix in females. Males may develop Sertoli cell tumors of the testes Peutz–Jeghers (PJ) polyps predominantly in small bowel, but found throughout GI tract, GI obstruction, intussusceptions, mucocutaneous hyperpigmentation around the mouth and finger tips	• Upper gastrointestinal endoscopy screening and small bowel examination with capsule endoscopy or MR enterography by 8 yr or earlier if symptomatic, repeated every 3 yr • Colonoscopy screening by 8 yr of age, repeated every 3 yr • MRI-MRCP or endoscopic ultrasound at 25 yr, repeated every 1–2 yr Females only: • Mammogram and breast MRI starting by 25 yr of age, repeated annually • Consider transvaginal ultrasound and serum CA125 by 20 yr of age, repeated annually Males only: • Testicular examination at birth with ultrasound performed if abnormality on exam, repeat annually
PTEN hamartoma syndrome (Cowden syndrome) *PTEN*	High risk for breast cancer Increased risk for thyroid and uterine cancer Lhermitte–Duclos disease is considered pathognomonic. Macrocephaly, fibrocystic breast disease, thyroid nodules, uterine fibroid tumors, trichilemmomas, papillomatous papules, hamartomatous polyps	• Annual skin examination • Baseline thyroid ultrasound at 18 yr • Consider annual thyroid ultrasound Females only: • Mammogram and breast MRI starting by 30–35 yr, repeated annually • Colonoscopy surveillance to begin by 35–40 yr • Consider transvaginal ultrasound and random uterine biopsy by 35–40 yr of age

The efficacy of surveillance or prophylactic interventions on morbidity and mortality has not been evaluated in controlled clinical trials for most of the known hereditary cancer syndromes. Current medical recommendations for families with hereditary cancer are based primarily on expert opinion only. See GeneReviews (www.genereviews.org) and Lindor et al. (2008) for a detailed review of different cancer predisposition syndromes.

Genetic testing is typically performed using both gene sequencing and a second technique such as multiplex ligation-dependent probe amplification (MLPA). This latter laboratory analysis is necessary to identify large gene deletions and duplications, types of mutations that cannot be detected using gene sequencing. Deletions and duplications comprise a significant portion of the total mutation profile for genes associated with cancer risk. Analysis of these mutation types is a required component of any cancer genetic testing protocol (*Hum Mol Genet* 2009;18:1545; *J Med Genet* 2006;43:e18; *Cancer Res* 2008;68:7006; *JAMA* 2006;295:1379). Current testing techniques are descriptive analyses that compare the individual's gene sequence to the reference sequence for a specific gene(s). Functional analyses are often not available and thus interpreting the results of the genetic testing may be challenging.

The most informative approach to genetic testing is to begin with an affected family member, an individual diagnosed with one of the known associated cancers for the suspected cancer syndrome. When possible, begin genetic testing with a family member who was diagnosed at a young age or one who has a double primary cancer, as their genetic testing is more likely to be informative. If an affected family undergoes testing first and if a gene mutation is discovered, *then* the underlying genetic basis for the cancer predisposition in the family has been identified, the testing is *informative, and* other family members may pursue mutation specific analysis. In this same scenario, if a gene mutation is not identified, then the underlying genetic basis for disease has *not* been identified, the testing is *noninformative*, and, consequently, predictive genetic testing is not available for other family members (Fig. 43-3).

Consider a 34-year-old man with a paraganglioma who has a dominant maternal family history of paragangliomas and pheochromocytomas consistent with hereditary disease. His family has hereditary cancer; the question is *can genetic testing identify the underlying gene mutation causative for disease?* He undergoes genetic testing of the six known genes causative for hereditary paraganglioma/pheochromocytoma (SDHB, SDHD, SDHC, SDHA, SDHAF2, and MAX). There are three possible test results from his genetic testing.

First, the testing is positive; a deleterious mutation is identified. This test result is *informative* because the basis for disease predisposition has been identified. At-risk family members may pursue mutation analysis to predict their cancer risk and guide medical follow-up. One example of a deleterious mutation is a truncating mutation that causes a premature stop codon, halting protein synthesis, and inhibiting protein function. The functional consequences are easily predicted from the gene sequence even without functional analysis.

Second, the testing is negative; no mutation is identified in the six genes analyzed. This test result is *noninformative*. The test result is *not* a true negative because the genetic etiology for their cancer predisposition remains unknown. Thus, at-risk family members cannot pursue genetic testing. In this family, all at-risk family members would need to be considered at "high risk" and followed accordingly until a gene mutation is identified and it is possible to use genetic testing to clarify their cancer risk.

Given the vast majority of genes associated with cancer risk have not been identified, negative genetic testing is common, even for families with clearly defined hereditary disease. Breast cancer susceptibility is exemplar. Despite extensive breast cancer susceptibility research, it is estimated only 20% of inherited breast cancer risk has been explained (*Nat Genet* 2008;40:17).

Third, the test result is neither positive nor negative; a variant of unknown clinical significance (VUS) is identified. VUSs are frequently missense gene variants, single nucleotide changes that code for a different amino acid. Given the lack of available functional analyses, prediction of the clinical significance of a VUS, if any, is not possible with the current data sets. This result is *noninformative*. At-risk family members should not pursue genetic testing as the clinical significance of the *presence or absence* of the VUS cannot be determined.

Interpretation of genetic testing should be performed with extreme caution and care. A common mistake is to start genetic testing with an unaffected family member. Incorrect interpretation of noninformative testing or testing that identified a VUS has resulted in misdiagnoses or delays in diagnoses with significant clinical consequences (*Cancer J* 2012;18:303; *N Engl J Med* 1997;336:823). In contrast to other medical testing, genetic testing impacts the clinical care of not just a single individual but an entire family.

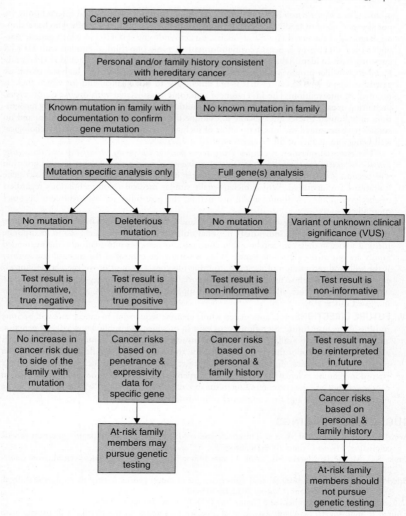

Figure 43-3. Genetic testing for cancer susceptibility. Modified from Cancer Genetics Risk Assessment and counseling (PDQ); Figure 2; National Cancer Institute.

IV. MEDICAL AND LONG-TERM FOLLOW-UP. Medical surveillance and treatment recommendations for families with hereditary cancer are typically based only on expert opinion, given the relatively recent time frame in which these syndromes have been described, and lack of clinical trials to evaluate the efficacy of any screening protocol or medical/surgical intervention.

The recommendations are straightforward for some cancer syndromes based on the extreme nature of disease. The familial adenomatous polyposis syndrome (FAP) presents with 100s–1,000s of colonic polyps beginning in childhood with total colectomy as the only clinical option (*Dis Colon Rectum* 2003;46:1001). Yet the most appropriate clinical interventions are not always evident or readily accepted by individuals at risk. Consider a family who has a clinical diagnosis of the hereditary diffuse gastric cancer syndrome (HDGC) in which genetic testing of the CDH1 gene is negative (noninformative). Only one-third of families with HDGC currently have an identifiable gene mutation (*J Med Genet* 2010;47:436). Should at-risk family members consider prophylactic gastrectomy as a means to reduce their very high risk of diffuse gastric cancer, a type of cancer that is not amendable to surveillance, and for which there is no medical intervention? The Li–Fraumeni syndrome is associated with diverse cancer types, presenting in early childhood and throughout adulthood. Despite the syndrome's early recognition, only limited studies are available to examine the efficacy of a screening regimen, and no studies have examined the long-term effect of such an intensified surveillance on psychological well-being and quality of life (*Lancet Oncol* 2011;12:559).

The essential question is *can we bring about positive change by identifying and instituting intensified medical interventions for families at increased cancer risk?* Answering this question will become even more challenging as a greater number of low-penetrant (low-risk) gene mutations are identified. Will clinicians make similar medical recommendations regardless of the level of risk? Without careful distinction, the possibility for overtreatment becomes more likely.

Ultimately, benefits gained by identifying and educating individuals at increased cancer risk are dependent on an individual's personal utility. How individuals choose to incorporate medical advice in their care and how they communicate complex information to their extended family are out of the clinician's hands. What is within the control of the medical community is the will, and recognition of the need, to bring together a team of providers who are knowledgeable of the dynamic medical and psychosocial aspects of hereditary disease. Building an informed infrastructure affords individuals a supportive environment as they address their increased cancer risk.

V. FUTURE DIRECTIONS. It is anticipated whole genome sequencing in cancer care will become routine in the near future. Significant gaps exist in provider and public knowledge of genetics, and limited funding is available to support the investigation of health communication strategies and the identification of the type of information to be conveyed. Significant cultural shifts in medical/public genetics education and current research funding priorities are necessary to fully transition genomic science to oncology care. Expanded integration of the discipline of clinical cancer genetics and genetic counseling in the care of people with cancer will be necessary as the technology advances and the complexity of information increases.

SUGGESTED READINGS

Armel SR, McCuaig J, Finch A, et al. The effectiveness of family history questionnaires in cancer genetic counseling. *J Genet Counsel* 2009;18:366–378.

Banks KC, Moline JJ, Marvin ML, et al. 10 rare tumors that warrant a genetics referral. *Fam Cancer* 2013;12:1–18.

Brierley KL, Blouch E, Cogswell W, et al. Adverse events in cancer genetic testing: medical, ethical, legal, and financial implications. *Cancer J* 2012;18:303–309.

Cancer Genetics Risk Assessment and Counseling (PDQ). www.cancer.gov, 2014.

Church J, Simmang C, Standards Task F, et al. Practice parameters for the treatment of patients with dominantly inherited colorectal cancer (familial adenomatous polyposis and hereditary nonpolyposis colorectal cancer). *Dis Colon Rectum* 2003;46:1001–1012.

Douglas FS, O'Dair LC, Robinson M, et al. The accuracy of diagnoses as reported in families with cancer: a retrospective study. *J Med Genet* 1999;36:309–312.

Fitzgerald RC, Hardwick R, Huntsman D, et al. Hereditary diffuse gastric cancer: updated consensus guidelines for clinical management and directions for future research. *J Med Genet* 2010;47:436–444.

Genetic/familial high-risk assessment: breast and ovarian. 2013. www.nccn.org.

Giardiello FM, Brensinger JD, Petersen GM, et al. The use and interpretation of commercial APC gene testing for familial adenomatous polyposis. *N Engl J Med* 1997;336:823.

Hampel H, Sweet K, Westman JA, et al. Referral for cancer genetics consultation: a review and compilation of risk assessment criteria. *J Med Genet* 2004;41:81–91.

Li FP, Fraumeni JF Jr., Mulvihill JJ, et al. A cancer family syndrome in twenty-four kindreds. *Cancer Res* 1988;48:5358–5362.

Lichtenstein P, Holm NV, Verkasalo PK, et al. Environmental and heritable factors in the causation of cancer—analyses of cohorts of twins from Sweden, Denmark, and Finland. *N Engl J Med* 2000;343:78–85.

Lindor NM, McMaster ML, Lindor CJ, et al; National Cancer Institute, DoCPCO, Community Oncology and Prevention Trials Research Group. Concise handbook of familial cancer susceptibility syndromes, 2nd ed. *J Natl Cancer Inst Monogr* 2008:1–93.

Mai PL, Garceau AO, Graubard BI, et al. Confirmation of family cancer history reported in a population-based survey. *J Natl Cancer Inst* 2011;103:788–797.

Mehenni H, Resta N, Guanti G, et al. Molecular and clinical characteristics in 46 families affected with Peutz-Jeghers syndrome. *Dig Dis Sci* 2007;52:1924–1933.

Moline J, Eng C. Multiple endocrine neoplasia type 2: an overview. *Genet Med* 2011;13:755–764.

Moreira L, Balaguer F, Lindor N, et al. Identification of Lynch syndrome among patients with colorectal cancer. *JAMA* 2012;308:1555–1565.

Murff HJ, Spigel DR, Syngal S. Does this patient have a family history of cancer? An evidence-based analysis of the accuracy of family cancer history. *JAMA* 2004;292:1480–1489.

O'Daniel JM, Lee K. Whole-genome and whole-exome sequencing in hereditary cancer: impact on genetic testing and counseling. *Cancer J* 2012;18(4):287-292.

Oliveira C, Senz J, Kaurah P, et al. Germline CDH1 deletions in hereditary diffuse gastric cancer families. *Hum Mol Genet* 2009;18:1545–1555.

Palma MD, Domchek SM, Stopfer J, et al. The relative contribution of point mutations and genomic rearrangements in BRCA1 and BRCA2 in high-risk breast cancer families. *Cancer Res* 2008;68:7006–7014.

Resta RG. Defining and redefining the scope and goals of genetic counseling. *Am J Med Genet C Semin Med Genet* 2006;142C:269–275.

Riley BD, Culver JO, Skrzynia C, et al. Essential elements of genetic cancer risk assessment, counseling, and testing: updated recommendations of the National Society of Genetic Counselors. *J Genet Counsel* 2012;21:151–161.

Stratton MR, Rahman N. The emerging landscape of breast cancer susceptibility. *Nat Genet* 2008;40:17–22.

Task F, Resta R, Biesecker BB, et al; National Society of Genetic Counselors' Definition. A new definition of genetic counseling: national society of genetic counselors' task force report. *J Genet Counsel* 2006;15:77–83.

Vasen HF, Watson P, Mecklin JP, et al. New clinical criteria for hereditary nonpolyposis colorectal cancer (HNPCC, Lynch syndrome) proposed by the International Collaborative group on HNPCC. *Gastroenterology* 1999;116:1453–1456.

Villani A, Tabori U, Schiffman J, et al. Biochemical and imaging surveillance in germline TP53 mutation carriers with Li-Fraumeni syndrome: a prospective observational study. *Lancet Oncol* 2011;12:559–567.

Volikos E, Robinson J, Aittomaki K, et al. LKB1 exonic and whole gene deletions are a common cause of Peutz-Jeghers syndrome. *J Med Genet* 2006;43:e18.

Walsh T, Casadei S, Coats KH, et al. Spectrum of mutations in BRCA1, BRCA2, CHEK2, and TP53 in families at high risk of breast cancer. *JAMA* 2006;295:1379–1388.

Ziogas A, Anton-Culver H. Validation of family history data in cancer family registries. *Am J Prev Med* 2003;24:190–198.

Ziogas A, Horick NK, Kinney AY, et al. Clinically relevant changes in family history of cancer over time. *JAMA* 2011;306:172–178.

44 Palliative Care in Oncology

Anna Roshal

"The best care possible does not stop with excellent disease treatments; it includes concern for a person's physical comfort, emotions and spiritual well-being." Ira Byock, *The Best Care Possible*

I. **INTRODUCTION.** The focus of palliative care is to achieve the best possible quality of life (QOL) for patients and their caregivers at any stage of serious illness. Its hallmark is a comprehensive, team-based interdisciplinary approach, emphasizing collaboration and coordination of care with other providers and across settings. According to the most recent WHO definition, "palliative care is an approach that improves quality of life of patients and their families facing problems associated with life-threatening illness, through prevention and relief of suffering by means of early identification and impeccable assessment and treatment of pain and other problems, physical, psychosocial, and spiritual."

II. **HISTORY OF PALLIATIVE CARE.** The wider concept of palliative care began with the establishment of the hospice movement. The term "hospice" (from the same linguistic root as "hospitality") can be traced back to medieval times when it referred to a place of shelter and rest for weary or ill travelers on a long journey. The name was first applied to specialized care for dying patients by social worker and physician Dame Cicely Saunders, who began her work with the terminally ill in 1948 and eventually went on to create the first modern hospice, the St. Christopher's Hospice, in London in 1967.

The first American hospice opened in 1974 in New Haven, Connecticut. In 1979, the National Hospice Organization was formed in the United States, and in 1982, the Health Care Finance Administration established the Medicare Hospice Benefit (MHB). Although at its inception hospice care was most often provided at specialized facilities, today most hospice care in the United States is delivered at home. Hospice care is also available in homelike hospice residences, nursing homes, assisted living facilities, veterans' facilities, hospitals, and prisons. However, availability of hospice care is generally limited by its payments structure (capitated payments) and eligibility criteria, which generally do not allow patients to receive hospice care alongside with disease-modifying or life-prolonging treatments.

Palliative care originated within the hospice movement and shares its philosophy as a well-care model based on interdisciplinary teams emphasizing that patient and family wishes and goals are recognized and respected. The first US hospital-based palliative care programs began in the late 1980s at a handful of institutions such as the Cleveland Clinic and Medical College of Wisconsin. Since then, there has been a marked increase in hospital-based palliative care programs—now numbering over 1,500—as well as recent developments in home-based palliative care and establishment of outpatient centers. In 2001, with the support of the Robert Wood Johnson Foundation, palliative care leaders from across the United States met to discuss the standardization of palliative care across settings with the goal of improving quality. In order to facilitate the discussion, the National Consensus Project was formed, which became a task force in 2003, under the organizational structure of the Coalition of Hospice and Palliative Care, which includes the American Academy of Hospice and Palliative Medicine (AAHPM), the Center to Advance Palliative Care (CAPC), the Hospice and Palliative Nurses Association (HPNA), and the National Palliative Care Research Center (NPCRC). Advanced Palliative Care Certification for hospitals was first offered by Joint Commission in 2011, to promote high standards in quality and adherence to published guidelines. To reflect specialized expertise and training required for the practice of palliative care, the American Board of Medical Specialties (ABMS) approved the creation of Hospice and Palliative Medicine (HPM) as a subspecialty of 10 participating boards. As a result of this approval, the first ABMS-recognized examination was administered in 2008. There are currently close to 200 HPM fellowships in the United States, and the specialty is rapidly growing. Despite this growth, many sources project severe shortages of HPM physicians in the coming years, emphasizing the need for wider education of other specialists, including oncologists, as well as primary care physicians, and midlevel providers in basic palliative care skills.

III. **PALLIATIVE CARE CORE PRINCIPLES** According to the National Consensus Project, the following features characterize palliative care philosophy and delivery:

   A. Care is provided and services are coordinated by an interdisciplinary team consisting of physicians, nurses, social workers, chaplains, and may also include pharmacists, psychologists, physical therapists, nutritionists, as well as other support specialists to meet patient and family physical, psychosocial, and spiritual needs.

   B. Patients, families, and palliative and nonpalliative providers communicate and collaborate about care needs.

   C. Services are provided concurrent with or independent of curative or life-prolonging care.

   D. Patients' and families' hopes for peace and dignity are supported through the course of illness, through the dying process, and after death.

   Like hospice, palliative care aims to relieve suffering in its many forms and improve QOL, but it is applicable to a much broader patient population, including patients living with progressive, chronic conditions (i.e., AIDS, cardiovascular diseases, dementia, neurodegenerative conditions, metabolic diseases, renal or kidney dysfunction, and advanced malignancy), and acute, life-threatening illnesses or injuries (i.e., severe trauma, ICU admission, or acute leukemia) where the disease itself or its treatments pose significant challenges to the QOL and well-being of the patient and family.

IV. **RATIONALE FOR ONCOLOGY PALLIATIVE CARE.** Despite multiple advances in oncology in recent years and decades, patients and caregivers still shoulder significant physical, psychological, spiritual, and financial burdens while dealing with cancer and its treatments. For example, in a recent large systematic review including over 25,000 patients with incurable cancers, including solid tumors and hematologic malignancies, pain was present in 71%, gastrointestinal symptoms (nausea, vomiting, or constipation) in 20% to 37%, dyspnea in 35%, fatigue in 74%, depressed mood in 39%, and anxiety in 24% (*J Pain Symptom Manage* 2007;34:94). These symptoms have a significant negative effect on QOL and are associated with worsened ECOG performance status. Unfortunately, symptom management and adequate control remains a challenge, even for patients with early stage malignancies and cancer survivors. A seminal research published in a recent study of 3,123 ambulatory patients with breast, colorectal, lung, or prostate cancer revealed that 33% were still receiving inadequate analgesic treatments (*J Clin Oncol* 2012;30:1980). Pain rarely occurs in isolation, with most patients experiencing a variety of symptoms that tend to occur at a similar time, a phenomenon recently dubbed symptom cluster (*J Pain Symptom Manage* 2011;42:1). Family caregivers of patients with advanced cancer also experience significant morbidity as a result of their role. In addition to reducing symptom burden and improving QOL for patients with cancer and their caregivers, palliative care clinicians can help bridge a communication gap surrounding prognostic information and documenting patient's wishes and advance directives. Although the majority of advanced cancer patients and their family members report they desire realistic and timely information about the incurable or terminal nature of their disease, available data support that a large proportion does not receive this information until very late in the illness trajectory (*J Clin Oncol* 2010;28:4364). The reasons for this delay include the difficult nature of these discussions, time pressure, lack of training, prognostic uncertainties, and perceived negative effect on patients and families. Unfortunately, this lack of communication leads to an increased resource utilization at the end of life, increase in costs of care, and, most importantly, less good time spent with family and friends (*JAMA* 2008;299:2667).

V. **EVIDENCE BASE FOR PALLIATIVE CANCER CARE MODELS**

   A. **Inpatient consultation service.** Investigators from the MD Anderson Cancer Center described clinical characteristics and outcomes of mobile interdisciplinary palliative consultation team in the setting of a comprehensive cancer center. They demonstrated that 28% of patients evaluated by a consult team showed symptom improvement within 24 hours and 38% within 72 hours after initial consultation. The consult team found an average of eight symptoms per patient, most commonly pain, delirium, and opioid side effects, such as excessive sedation, confusion, and constipation (*J Palliat Med* 2007;10:948). In a randomized multicenter controlled trial of inpatient palliative care team consultation versus usual hospital care for patients admitted with life-limiting illness including 27% of patients had cancer, there were decreased ICU stays, decreased hospital readmissions, and increased number of patients who completed advance directives in the palliative care group, although there were no differences in symptoms or QOL measures (*J Palliat Med* 2008;11:180).

B. Outpatient education and support interventions. The projects ENABLE and ENABLE II (Education, Nurture, Advise, Before Life Ends) investigated a nurse-led educational and support intervention in patients with advanced cancer in a rural NCI-designated comprehensive cancer center (*Palliat Support Care* 2009;7:75). Both demonstration project and subsequent randomized control trial, compared with usual oncology care, combined in-person sessions and telephone-based follow-up (*Palliat Support Care* 2009;7:75). Advance practiced nurses assessed patients utilizing NCCN distress thermometer and provided targeted and problem-solving resources based on identified areas of distress. In addition, with participant permission, nurses contacted their clinical team about issues requiring immediate attention. Patients in the usual care group were allowed to have unrestricted access to all oncology and supportive services available at the institution. Patients receiving intervention had higher scores for QOL ($p = 0.02$), and fewer incidence of depression ($p = 0.02$). Symptom intensity did not change significantly, although a trend toward lower intensity was noted ($p = 0.06$). The intervention did not affect hospitalizations, emergency room visits, or ICU days. Limitations of the study included lack of in-person contact and relatively low baseline symptom intensity reported in both groups of patients. A randomized trial of an innovative educational intervention, COPE (Creativity, Optimism, Planning, and Expert information), administered to patients simultaneously enrolled in phase I, II, and III therapeutic oncology clinical trials, and their caregivers was conducted at the City of Hope (*J Palliat Med* 2011;14:465). Similar to ENABLE model, this intervention focused on couching and guided problem solving around common sources of distress, including physical, psychological, social, and spiritual. Patients and caregivers in an intervention arm participated together in three educational sessions, led by trained instructors, during their first month of clinical trial enrollment, followed by six month follow-up period. Control arm received usual oncology care. Primary outcome measure was global QOL for patients and caregivers. Results indicated significantly slower rate of QOL decline for caregivers in the intervention arm, but no difference in QOL measures for patients. Limitations of this study included group-based intervention, rather than individual patient and caregiver visits. It was also not specifically mentioned how the information gained from the intervention was communicated to the patient's primary oncology team.

C. Palliative home care. Investigators from Kaiser Permananente Medical Group (*J Am Geriatr Soc* 2007;55:993) assigned patients with life-limiting illness and less than one year expected survival, including 47% of patients with cancer, to usual care versus in-home palliative care, provided by interdisciplinary team, with the goals of improving symptom control and overall QOL. Usual care consisted of home health care as deemed appropriate by patient's physicians and Medicare guidelines, including hospice services for patients who met hospice criteria. Although modeled on hospice care, intervention program did not require patients to forgo disease-modifying or potentially curative treatments, and allowed patients with estimated 12-months survival to participate. Palliative care physicians involved in the program took an active role of coordinating care with patient's primary care physician and specialists to develop and implement a treatment plan. The study's primary end points were satisfaction with care, place of death, utilization of acute care services, and overall costs of care. Investigators were able to demonstrate increased satisfaction with care at 30 and 90 days after enrollment ($p < 0.05$). In addition, patients receiving in-home palliative care utilized emergency rooms and acute care hospitals at a significantly lower rate, resulting in 33% overall decreased cost of care for patients enrolled in the intervention arm, versus usual care.

D. **Early integrated outpatient palliative care clinic.** Temel and colleagues (*N Engl J Med* 2010;363:733) conducted a groundbreaking randomized trial (1:1 randomization) of early palliative care integrated into standard oncology care versus standard oncology care alone in patients with metastatic non–small cell lung cancer. Patients were enrolled within 8 weeks from diagnosis, and were evaluated by palliative care team within 3 weeks of enrollment and at least monthly thereafter. Intention to treat analysis included 74 patients in the usual care arm, and 77 patients in the early palliative care arm. Patients in the control team could be referred to the palliative care team at the discretion of the treating oncologist, but did not cross over to the integrated palliative care group. The palliative care team consisted of board-certified physicians and specially trained advance practice nurses. The care was provided according to National Consensus Project for Quality Palliative Care guidelines and included symptom assessment and management, discussions about patient and family coping with the disease, and illness understanding and education. All patients were ambulatory and had ECOG PS 0-2 at the start of the study. Primary outcome was change in the QOL at 12 weeks determined by Functional Assessment of Cancer Therapy-Lung scale. Investigators also collected data on changes in mood, type of end-of-life care received (chemotherapy within 14 days of death, and use and timing of hospice care). Patients receiving early palliative care had significantly better QOL ($p = 0.03$), lower depression scores ($p = 0.01$), were less likely to receive aggressive end-of-life care ($p = 0.05$), and had longer median hospice stay ($p = 0.09$, 11 vs. 4 days) compared with standard oncology care group. In addition, more patients in the early palliative care arm had their resuscitation preferences documented in the ambulatory medical record ($p = 0.05$). In a post hoc analysis, median overall survival was significantly longer for those in the concurrent care arm (11.6 months vs. 8.9 months, $p = 0.02$), despite fewer patients receiving aggressive end-of-life care. Of note, although palliative care consultation was allowed in a control group at the discretion of the oncologist, only a small minority of patients (14%) in that group had any contact with palliative care team. The exact mechanism by which early palliative care leads to apparent improvement in survival remains unclear. Additional analysis of the data revealed that there was no significant difference between the groups with respect to the total number of regimens and time to the administration of second- or third-line chemotherapy. However, patients in the palliative care group were less likely to receive IV chemotherapy in the last 2 months of life, and any chemotherapy in the last 14 days (*J Clin Oncol* 2012;30:394). On the basis of this study and other randomized clinical trials, the American Society of Clinical Oncology published "Provisional Clinical Opinion: the Integration of Palliative Care into Standard Oncology Care" in February 2012 (*J Clin Oncol* 2012;30:880). It states: "it is the Panel's expert consensus that combined standard oncology care and palliative care should be considered early in the course of illness for any patient with metastatic cancer and/or high symptom burden." Muir and colleagues published their experience with a novel service delivery model, consisting of embedding pilot palliative care clinic into high-volume, fast-paced busy private practice oncology clinic (*J Pain Symptom Manage* 2010;40:126). As this was not a randomized trial, results were intended as demonstration of feasibility and potential benefit. Over the first two years of the services, 134 patients were referred for palliative care consultations. Diagnosis distribution was representative of general oncology practice, including 22% of patients with gastrointestinal cancer, 17% breast cancer, 13% with lung cancer, and 13% with hematologic malignancies. Palliative care consultations resulted in a reduction of the symptom burden as measured by ESAS (Edmonton Symptom Assessment System) by 21% over multiple visits. The authors were able to estimate that this model of palliative care delivery was able to provide substantial time saving for oncology practice (over 4 weeks during 2 years).

VI. PRIMARY VERSUS SPECIALTY PALLIATIVE CARE. As the recognition of palliative care needs is increasing, so is the controversy over who should be managing those needs. Multiple models of specialized palliative care have been shown to improve outcomes, but in reality it might be impractical and unnecessary for every patient even with advanced cancer to receive care from a palliative care specialist, in addition to their oncology team. Therefore, certain primary palliative skills, such as basic management of pain, nausea, other symptoms, as well as basic communication and prognostication skills should be able to be delivered by oncologists. Other skills that are more complex and take specialized training to learn and apply, such as negotiating a difficult family meeting, addressing persistent distress, and managing difficult or refractory symptoms, are suited for consultation or comanagement with a palliative care specialist/team (*N Engl J Med* 2013;368:1173).

VII. BARRIERS AND POTENTIAL APPROACHES TO PALLIATIVE CARE INTEGRATION INTO ONCOLOGY PRACTICE. Despite significant advances in palliative care research and practice over the last decade, significant barriers remain for integration of palliative care and cancer care across disease trajectory and in different settings where care might be provided. Many answered questions exist in regard to the feasibility of different models, availability of primary and specialized palliative care, standardization of the interventions, patient selection for inpatient and outpatient palliative care consultations, and financial models. Some of these barriers include physician knowledge and attitude toward their ability to provide symptom management and perception that palliative care is the same as hospice and end-of-life care.

VIII. HOSPICE
   A. Eligibility criteria. Under Medicare, Medicaid, and most private insurance plans, a patient is eligible for hospice if his/her physician and the hospice medical director certify that he/she is terminal and has 6 months or less to live. The patient and caregivers must agree to the philosophy of hospice. That is, they must agree that the focus is on managing symptoms of the disease without the use of life-prolonging measures. The patient needs to have a 24-hour caregiver or be willing to come up with a plan with the hospice team for 24-hour care. The patient could hire 24-hour private-duty nursing care, enter a long-term care facility, arrange for friends or family to take shifts in the patient's own home, or live with a family member. The patient does not have to sign a Do Not Resuscitate (DNR) order to be on hospice. It is the patient's right to choose hospice and still remain full code. The patients may decide after initiating hospice to change their code status. The Medicare eligibility for hospice for patients with diagnosis of cancer is that the disease has distant metastasis at presentation or that the patient has progressed from an earlier stage of metastatic disease, or patient refuses further treatment of the disease. A patient is eligible for hospice with certain cancer diagnosis without evidence of metastasis. This includes small cell lung cancer, brain cancer, and pancreatic cancer. Patients may remain on hospice beyond 180 days (6 months) as long as criteria for hospice care are still met and a face-to-face encounter with a physician or nurse practitioner is performed by hospice team.
   B. Funding. Hospice is covered by a specific MHB (Medicare Hospice Benefit). Most private insurance companies and Medicaid offer a similar benefit. When a patient signs for MHB, he or she is electing to have his or her Medicare Part A (hospital benefit) assigned to a Medicare-certified hospice ("Medicare-Certified Agency" or "MCA"). The hospice is then responsible for the patient's plan of care and cannot bill the patient for services. The MCA receives a per diem rate from Medicare that covers all medications for pain and symptom management, durable medical equipment and supplies, nursing care, social services, chaplain visits, and other needed services. The current per diem rate is about $160 a day.

   The MHB does not cover private-duty nursing or the cost of room and board at a nursing facility. If the patient is dually eligible for Medicare and Medicaid, the hospice is funded by Medicare and the room and board is covered by Medicaid. If the patient is eligible only for Medicare, the family must pay privately for room and board in a nursing facility.

The MHB provides four levels of care for hospice patients:

1. **Routine home care.** Hospice services provided in the patient's home or a nursing facility.
2. **Inpatient respite care.** Short-term inpatient admission (usually limited to five days) to promote caregiver well-being. Owing to the physical and psychological stress and strain experienced by the 24-hour care of the family member, respite care is essential. It may be for a few days or the patient may be transferred to a facility from the hospital setting.
3. **Inpatient symptom management.** Inpatient admission for more intensive palliative measures. Such admissions would be warranted for severe pain, intractable seizures, uncontrolled bleeding, and intractable nausea/vomiting due to gastrointestinal obstruction. Before admission, the medical director, primary physician, patient, and family discuss the purpose of the hospitalization. The hospice is still responsible for the plan of care and needs to be involved daily and at all levels of decision making in collaboration with the inpatient staff.

   The MHB limits how much active treatment a patient can receive and still be on hospice. The patient's primary physician must discuss with the hospice program on a case-by-case basis the types of services that may be provided to a given patient without disqualifying him or her from hospice. Some measures, such as intravenous hydration, blood transfusions, tube feedings, paracentesis, and thoracentesis, may be appropriate for palliation, but must be approved by the hospice medical director first.
4. **Bereavement care.** A very important service for hospice families and caregivers is bereavement care. Bereavement services are provided by hospice programs for at least up to a year after the patient's death. The services are provided by specially trained staff. Depending on the hospice, this service may be provided by the nurse, social worker, chaplain, or specially trained volunteers. Bereavement services include periodic mailings, phone calls, and home visits. Some hospices offer bereavement support groups, and some host annual memorial services. If the family requires additional counseling services, the hospice may choose to provide extended services or refer them to other resources in the community.

SUGGESTED READINGS

Teunissen SC, Wesker W, Kruitwagen C, et al. Symptom prevalence in patients with incurable cancer: a systematic review. *J Pain Symptom Manage* 2007;34:94–104.

Fisch MJ, Lee JW, Weiss M, et al. Prospective, observational study of pain and analgesic prescribing in medical oncology outpatients with breast, colorectal, lung, or prostate cancer. *J Clin Oncol* 2012;30:1980–1988.

Laird BJ, Scott AC, Colvin LA, et al. Pain, depression and fatigue as a symptom cluster in advanced cancer *J Pain Symptom Manage* 2011;42:1–11.

Keating NL, Beth Landrum M, Arora NK, et al. Cancer patients' roles in treatment decisions: do characteristics of the decision influence roles? *J Clin Oncol* 2010;28:4364–4370.

Harrington SE, Smith TJ. The role of chemotherapy at the end of life: "when is enough, enough?" *JAMA* 2008;299:2667–2678.

Temel JS, Greer JP, Muzikansky A, et al. Early palliative care for patients with metastatic non-small-cell lung cancer. *N Engl J Med* 2010;363:733–742.

45 Smoking Cessation and Counseling

Aaron Abramovitz • Mario Castro

I. **INTRODUCTION.** Tobacco products are the number one cause of preventable morbidity and mortality in the United States. An estimated 500,000 people die each year from tobacco-related illness. In 2012, 22% of adults and 6.6% of children 12 to 17 years of age were cigarette smokers. In 1965, the year of the landmark Surgeon General Report on tobacco, the smoking rate in adults was 42%. This decrease is due to efforts in the political, medical, and private spheres to educate the population on the risks of tobacco smoking. Public awareness of the health risks of tobacco in 2012 can be seen in the 69% of daily smokers who were interested in quitting and the 43% of daily smokers with at least one quit attempt in the last year.

II. **SMOKING CESSATION PRACTICE GUIDELINES.** The US Department of Health and Human Services published updated practice guidelines regarding smoking cessation in 2008. The full report is available at www.surgeongeneral.gov/tobacco. Recommendations will be summarized here. The two key questions that every patient must be asked are: "Do you smoke?" and "Do you want to quit?" Following this, the clinician can apply the following guidelines:
   A. Tobacco dependence is a chronic disease that often requires repeated intervention and multiple attempts to quit.
   B. Clinicians and health-care delivery systems must document tobacco status and treat every tobacco user seen in a health-care setting.
   C. Brief tobacco-dependence treatment is effective.
   D. Counseling and medication are effective when used by themselves for treating tobacco dependence. The combination of counseling and medication is more effective than either alone.
   E. Tobacco-dependence treatments are both clinically effective and highly cost effective relative to interventions for other clinical disorders. Providing insurance coverage for these treatments increases quit rates.

III. **SMOKING CESSATION COUNSELING/BEHAVIORAL MODIFICATION.** A template for tobacco cessation counseling in the office setting called the "Five A's" (Table 45-1) is provided in the smoking cessation practice guidelines. This was developed to provide a strategy to engage

TABLE 45-1	The Five A's
Ask about tobacco use	Identify and document tobacco use status for every patient at every visit
Advise to quit	In a clear, strong, and personalized manner, urge every tobacco user to quit
Assess willingness to make a quit attempt	Is the tobacco user willing to make a quit attempt at this time?
Assist in the quit attempt	For the patient willing to make a quit attempt, offer medication and provide or refer for counseling or additional treatment to help the patient quit
	For patients unwilling to quit at the time, provide interventions designed to increase future quit attempts
Arrange follow-up	For the patient willing to make a quit attempt, arrange for follow-up contacts, beginning within the first week after the quit date
	For patients unwilling to make a quit attempt at the time, address tobacco dependence and willingness to quit at the next clinic visit

smokers in a counseling session that takes less than 10 minutes while opening the door to give more detailed information on how to quit.

It is important to take a practical approach to smoking cessation counseling in order to provide each patient with a full range of information. Patients must be counseled to identify triggers for smoking behavior such as smoking cues (e.g., after a meal and while driving), drinking alcohol, and being around other smokers. Coping skills such as avoiding triggers, making lifestyle changes to reduce stress, and limiting access to cigarettes are useful to discuss. In addition, information about the person's lung age based on the current lung function and expected decline of lung function if they continue to smoke has been helpful in increasing cessation rates (Fig. 45-1). Discussing the duration and nature of withdrawal symptoms can help motivate and prepare the patient to quit smoking.

For patients unwilling to make a quit attempt, motivational interviewing strategies can be employed to give the patient further information about smoking cessation. In a nonconfrontational manner, explore how quitting is personally relevant to the patient (e.g., having children in the home or cost). Discuss briefly the risks of tobacco smoking and the rewards of quitting (e.g., feeling better and performing better in physical activities). If the patient is resistant to counseling efforts, readdress tobacco at the next clinic visit. Provide the quitline number (1-800-QUIT-NOW) to every patient.

IV. **MEDICATIONS TO AID SMOKING CESSATION.** All smokers who are trying to quit should be offered medication except when contraindicated. First-line medications include nicotine replacement products, buproprion, and varenicline. These are effective in moderate to heavy smokers (>10 cigarettes daily). Light smokers may be prescribed lower doses of nicotine replacement therapy (NRT), and pregnant patients should be encouraged to quit without medication. The choice of first-line medication should be discussed with each patient and prescribed on an individual basis in conjunction with behavioral modification. NRT can be used in combination with buproprion or varenicline. Table 45-2 provides an overview of medical therapies.

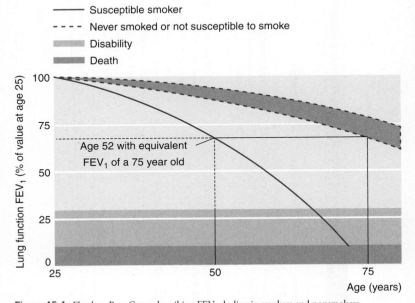

Figure 45-1. Fletcher–Peto Curve describing FEV_1 decline in smokers and nonsmokers.

Reproduced from *BMJ*: Parkes G, Greenhalgh T, Griffin M, et al. Effect on quit rate of telling patients their lung age. *BMJ* 2008;336:598. Adapted from *BMJ*: Fletcher C, Peto R. The natural history of COPD. *BMJ* 1977;1:1645–1648.

TABLE 45-2 Summary of Medical Therapy Available for Smoking Cessation

Medication	Effective dose	Mechanism	Side effects	Contraindications	Abstinence at 6 months
NRT (nicorette, nicoderm, commit lozenge)	Available in gum, patch, lozenge, nasal spray, and inhaler	Reduces nicotine craving by supplying steady dose of nicotine	Irritation at site of administration	Use with caution in patients with recent MI, arrhythmia, unstable angina	Gum 19% Patch 24%–27% Lozenge 24% Spray 27% Inhaler 25%
Buproprion (Zyban, Wellbutrin)	150 mg BID	Dopamine and norepinephrine reuptake inhibitor; alleviates withdrawal symptoms	Dry mouth, insomnia	Do not use in patients with seizures or eating disorders	24%
Varenicline (Chantix)	1 mg BID	Nicotinic receptor partial agonist/antagonist; reduces craving and blocks pleasurable effects of smoking	Nausea, constipation, vivid dreams Monitor for mood changes	Use with caution in patients with psychiatric illness	33%

Adapted from Fiore MC, Jaén CR, Baker TB, et al. Treating Tobacco Use and Dependence: 2008 Update. Clinical Practice Guideline. Rockville, MD: U.S. Department of Health and Human Services. Public Health Service, 2008.

NRT is available in the form of gum, an inhaler, a nasal spray, a lozenge, and a patch. These medications are designed to reduce nicotine craving and alleviate withdrawal symptoms by providing a steady dose of nicotine. The cost and method of administration should be discussed, as this helps the patient decide which product to use. Common side effects include local irritation at the site of administration, which is reported by most patients as mild and improves with duration of use. NRT is not an independent risk factor for cardiovascular events, even in patients with known cardiovascular disease. These medications should be used with caution in patients with recent myocardial infarction (<2 weeks), severe arrhythmias, and unstable angina. Smoking cessation efficacy at 6 months of NRT when used with behavioral modification is 19% to 27%, depending on the method of administration.

Buproprion-sustained release should be administered 2 weeks prior to the quit date. The dose is 150 mg daily for 3 days and then 150 mg twice daily. This medication is a dopamine and norepinephrine reuptake inhibitor. Buproprion works to reduce craving and alleviates withdrawal symptoms such as anxiety, difficulty concentrating, and low mood. It is contraindicated in patients with seizures or eating disorders. Common side effects include dry mouth and insomnia. Smoking cessation efficacy at 6 months of buproprion when used with behavioral modification is 24%.

Varenicline should be administered 1 week prior to the quit date. The dose is 0.5 mg for 3 days, then 0.5 mg twice daily for 4 days, and then 1 mg twice daily. This medication is a nicotinic receptor partial agonist and antagonist and works to reduce craving, alleviate withdrawal symptoms, and block the pleasurable effects of smoking. The dose should be reduced in patients with creatinine clearance less than 30 mL/min or if they experience side effects. Side effects include nausea, constipation, and vivid dreams. A black box warning was issued in 2009 due to postmarketing reports of an increase in depression and suicidal actions in patients taking varenicline. It is important to establish any history of psychiatric illness prior to starting this medication and to monitor the patient for changes in mood and behavior during therapy. Smoking cessation efficacy at 6 months of varenicline when used with behavioral modification is 33%.

V. TOBACCO USE IN CANCER PATIENTS AND SURVIVORS. Many patients are cigarette smokers at the time of cancer diagnosis and continue to use tobacco through treatment and survivorship. In addition to nicotine dependence, efforts to quit may be hampered by depression, nihilism, and the increased stress associated with a cancer diagnosis. It is important to counsel this group of patients about the ongoing risks of tobacco use. In patients with cancer, tobacco use contributes to all-cause mortality, can reduce the efficacy of chemotherapy, and may create a more aggressive tumor phenotype.

All-cause mortality in patients with cancer was assessed in the 2014 Surgeon General's Report on tobacco. The relative risk (RR) all-cause mortality was 1.22 in former smokers and 1.51 in current smokers when compared with never smoked controls. Overall, these studies showed an increase in all-cause and cancer-related mortality in patients with cancer who smoke when compared with patients who do not. Evidence of a dose–response relationship between the number of cigarettes smoked and cancer-related mortality was observed.

The RR of recurrence of primary cancer was 1.15 in former smokers and 1.42 in current smokers. Tobacco use was also shown to increase the risk of developing a second primary cancer associated with smoking (lung, head and neck, esophageal, and bladder).

VI. CONCLUSION. Smoking cessation is an important goal for all patients and one of the most important actions with which a clinician can assist his or her patients. Data from the Surgeon General's Report strongly link continued tobacco use with worse outcomes in cancer patients and survivors. Counseling, behavioral modification, and medications available to treat tobacco dependence are efficacious and cost effective. Counseling should be offered to every patient who smokes and medication to every patient willing to make a quit attempt. These efforts will help many patients who smoke achieve sustained abstinence and improve cancer-related morbidity and mortality.

SUGGESTED READINGS

Aubin HJ, Luquiens A, Berlin I. Pharmacotherapy for smoking cessation: pharmacological principles and clinical practice. *Br J Clin Pharmacol* 2014;77:324.

Fiore MC, Jaén CR, Baker TB, et al. *Treating Tobacco Use and Dependence: 2008 Update. Clinical Practice Guideline.* Rockville, MD: U.S. Department of Health and Human Services. Public Health Service, 2008.

Parkes G, Greenhalgh T, Griffin M, et al. Effect on quit rate of telling patients their lung age. *BMJ* 2008;336:598.

U.S. Department of Health and Human Services. *The Health Consequences of Smoking—50 Years of Progress: A Report of the Surgeon General,* 2014. Rockville, MD: Office of the Surgeon General; 2014.

Warren GW, Kasza KA, Reid ME, et al. Smoking at diagnosis and survival in cancer patients. *Int J Cancer* 2013;132:401.

Dose Adjustments of Commonly Used Chemotherapy Agents in Hepatic Failure and Renal Failure

B. Peters

INTRODUCTION

The clinical decision to dose adjust chemotherapy is often based on multiple factors related to the patient. These factors include, but are not limited to, patient's age, previous treatments, performance status, comorbitities, hematologic parameters, neurologic function, and compromised renal and/or hepatic function.

Renal excretion and biliary excretion represent common routes for the elimination of many frequently used chemotherapy drugs. If either of these routes of excretion becomes impaired, the risk of decreased clearance of certain chemotherapy drugs increases. This decreased clearance can manifest itself as increased toxicity to the patient or may worsen the impaired renal or hepatic function. Thus, in the presence of diminished renal or hepatic function, recommendations may exist to modify dosing of various chemotherapy drugs. While some recommendations are well established, others are not, and variations may be found throughout the published literature. Tables I-1 and I-2 are intended to serve as guidelines for employing dose modifications when renal or hepatic impairment exists in the patient undergoing chemotherapy. The recommendations listed are based on single-agent therapy and do not account for combination therapy. If the patient is receiving combination chemotherapy, the clinician should consider potential additive effects. Guidelines for dialyzing chemotherapy drugs or dosing during dialysis are not included in the tables. Clinical judgment and patient assessment along with recommended dose modifications should dictate the final decision for any dose modification. The tables do not provide a complete list of recommendations, and the reader is cautioned to always refer to the prescribing information for the respective drug before making any treatment or dosing adjustment decision.

| TABLE I-1 | Recommendations for Dose Adjustments of Commonly Used Chemotherapy Agents in Patients with Renal Dysfunction |

Drug	Dose modification (% reduction)	Creatinine clearance (CrCl)	Serum creatinine (SCr)	Proteinuria
Aldesleukin	Hold dose		>4.5 mg/dL	
Alemtuzumab	None			
Amifostine	None			
Arsenic trioxide	Use caution			
L-asparaginase	Hold dose	<60 mL/min		
Azacitidine	Hold dose		Elevated SCr or BUN	
Bendamustine	Hold dose	<40 mL/min		
Bevacizumab	Hold dose			If severe
Bleomycin	25%	10–50 mL/min		
Bleomycin	50%	<10 mL/min		
Bortezomib	None			
Brentuximab	Use caution			
Cabazitaxel	Use caution	<30 mL/min		
Carboplatin	AUC dose based on CrCl			
Carfilzomib	Hold dose	≥2 × baseline		
Carmustine	Hold dose	<60 mL/min		
Cetuximab	None			
Cisplatin	50%	30–60 mL/min		
Cisplatin	Hold dose	<30 mL/min		
Cladribine	Use caution			
Clofarabine	Hold dose		For grade 3 rise	
Cyclophosphamide	25%	10–50 mL/min		
Cyclophosphamide	50%	<10 mL/min		
Cytarabine	Use caution			
Dacarbazine	Use caution			
Dactinomycin	None			
Daunorubicin	50%		SCr >3.0 mg/dL	
Decitabine	Use caution			
Denileukin diftitox	Use caution			
Docetaxel	None			
Doxorubicin	25%	≤10 mL/min		
Doxorubicin liposomal	25%	≤10 mL/min		
Epirubicin	Use caution			
Eribulin	1.1 mg/m^2	30–50 mL/min		
Etoposide	25%	10–50 mL/min		
Etoposide	50%	<10 mL/min		
Etoposide phosphate	25%	10–50 mL/min		
Etoposide phosphate	50%	<10 mL/min		
Floxuridine	None			
Fludarabine	Use caution			
5-Fluorouracil	None			
Fulvestrant	None			

Drug	Dose modification (% reduction)	Creatinine clearance (CrCl)	Serum creatinine (SCr)	Proteinuria
Gemcitabine	Use caution			
Gemtuzumab	None			
Goserelin acetate	None			
Ipilumumab	None			
Idarubicin	Use caution			
Ifosfamide	25%–50%		SCr = 2.1–3.0 mg/dL	
Ifosfamide	Hold dose		SCr >3.0 mg/dL	
Irinotecan	None			
Ixabepilone	Use caution			
Mechlorethamine	None			
Melphalan	15%	≤60 mL/min		
Melphalan	25%	≤45 mL/min		
Melphalan	30%	≤30 mL/min		
Mesna	None			
Methotrexate	50%	10–50 mL/min		
Methotrexate	Hold dose	<10 mL/min		
Mitomycin	25%	<10 mL/min		
Mitomycin	Hold dose		SCr >1.7 mg/dL	
Mitoxantrone	None			
Nelarabine	Use caution	<50 mL/min		
Oxaliplatin	None			
Paclitaxel	None			
Paclitaxel-protein bound	None			
Panitumumab	None			
Pegaspargase	None			
Pemetrexed	Dose adjust/hold	<45 mL/min		
Pentostatin	Dose adjust	30–60 mL/min		
Pertuzumab	None	if ≥30 mL/min		
Rituximab	None			
Sipuleucel-T	None			
Streptozocin	Hold dose	<60 mL/min		
Temsirolimus	None			
Thiotepa	Monitor closely			
Topotecan	50%	20–39 mL/min		
Topotecan	Hold dose	<20 mL/min		
Trastuzumab	None			
Valrubicin	None			
Vinblastine	None			
Vincristine	None			
Vincristine liposome	None			
Vinorelbine	None			
Ziv-afibercept	Hold dose			≥2 Gm/24 h

BUN, blood urea nitrogen.

TABLE I-2	Recommendations for Dose Adjustments of Commonly Used Chemotherapy Agents in Patients with Hepatic Dysfunction

Drug	Dose modification (% reduction)	Bilirubin (mg/dL)	SGOT (mg/dL)	Alkaline phosphatase	AST or ALT
Aldesleukin	Hold if hepatic failure				
Alemtuzumab	None				
Amifostine	None				
Arsenic trioxide	None				
L-Asparaginase	Use caution				
Azacitidine	Monitor liver chemistries				
Bendamustine	Use caution				
Bendamustine	Hold	1.5–3 × ULN			2.5–10 × ULN
Bevacizumab	None				
Bleomycin	None				
Bortezomib	Use caution				
Brentuximab	Use caution				
Busulfan	None				
Cabazitaxel	Use caution				
Carboplatin	None				
Carfilzomib	Hold dose	Grade 3/4 ↑	Grade 3/4 ↑		Grade 3/4 ↑
Carmustine	Use caution				
Cisplatin	None				
Cetuximab	None				
Cladribine	None				
Clofarabine	Hold dose	Grade 3 ↑			
Cyclophosphamide	25%	3.0–5.0	>180		
Cyclophosphamide	Hold dose	>5.0			
Cytarabine	Use caution				
Dacarbazine	Use caution				
Dactinomycin	50%	>3.0			
Daunorubicin	25%	1.2–3.0	60–80		
Daunorubicin	50%	>3.0	>180		
Daunorubicin	Hold dose	>5.0			
Decitabine	Use caution				
Denileukin diftitox	Use caution				
Docetaxel	Hold dose	>1.5	>60	>2.5 × ULN	
Doxorubicin	50%	1.2–3.0	60–80		
Doxorubicin	75%	3.1–5.0	>180		
Doxorubicin	Hold dose	>5.0			
Doxorubicin liposomal	50%	1.2–3.0			
Doxorubicin liposomal	75%	3.1–5.0			
Doxorubicin liposomal	Hold dose	>5.0			
Epirubicin	50%	1.2–3.0	2–4 × ULN		
Epirubicin	75%	>3.0	>4 × ULN		

Drug	Dose modification (% reduction)	Bilirubin (mg/dL)	SGOT (mg/dL)	Alkaline phosphatase	AST or ALT
Eribulin	Reduce dose				
Etoposide	50%	1.5–3.0	60–180		
Etoposide	Hold dose	>3.0	>180		
Etoposide phosphate	50%	1.5–3.0	60–180		
Etoposide phosphate	Hold dose	>3.0	>180		
Floxuridine	Use caution				
Fludarabine	None				
5-Fluorouracil	Hold dose	>5.0			
Fulvestrant	None				
Gemcitabine	None				
Gemtuzumab	None				
Goserelin acetate	None				
Ipilumumab	Use caution				
Idarubicin	25%	1.5–3.0	60–180		
Idarubicin	50%	3.1–5.0	>180		
Idarubicin	Hold dose	>5.0			
Ifosfamide	Use caution				
Irinotecan	Hold dose	>2.0	>3 × ULN		
Ixabepilone	20%–50% dose ↓				
Mechlorethamine	None				
Melphalan	Use caution				
Mesna	None				
Methotrexate	25%	3.1–5.0	>180		
Methotrexate	Hold dose	>5.0			
Mitomycin	None				
Mitoxantrone	25%	>3.0			
Nelarabine	Use caution				
Oxaliplatin	None				
Paclitaxel	Hold dose	>5.0	>180 or 1.5 × ULN		
Paclitaxel protein-bound	Hold dose	>5 × ULN			>10 × ULN
Panitumumab	None				
Pegaspargase	None				
Pemetrexed	Use caution				
Pentostatin	None				
Pertuzumab	None				
Rituximab	None				
Sipuleucel-T	None				
Streptozocin	Use caution				
Temsirolimus	Hold dose	>1.5 × ULN			
Thiotepa	Monitor closely				
Topotecan	None				
Trastuzumab	None				
Valrubicin	None				
Vinblastine	50%	>3.0	>180		

(continued)

TABLE I-2	Recommendations for Dose Adjustments of Commonly Used Chemotherapy Agents in Patients with Hepatic Dysfunction (*Continued*)

Drug	Dose modification (% reduction)	Bilirubin (mg/dL)	SGOT (mg/dL)	Alkaline phosphatase	AST or ALT
Vincristine	50%	1.5–3.0	60–180		
Vincristine	Hold dose	>3.0	>180		
Vincristine liposome	Monitor closely				
Vinorelbine	50%	2.1–3.0			
Vinorelbine	75%	3.1–5.0			
Vinorelbine	Hold dose	>5.0			
Ziv-aflibercept	None				

SGOT, Serum glutamic oxaloacetic transaminase; AST, Aspartate transaminase; ALT, alanine transaminase; ULN, upper limit of normal.

Selected Chemotherapeutic Regimens

Leigh M. Boehmer • Sara K. Butler • Janelle Mann

This appendix, which can be accessed in the electronic version of this book, is a compilation of common chemotherapeutic regimens reported in the literature and national guidelines for the treatment of patients with cancer. It is not an all-inclusive list, and the regimens are sorted alphabetically by cancer. The chemotherapeutic regimens chosen are not meant to infer superiority or priority over other regimens, but rather to serve as a general reference and starting point for making treatment decisions. No liability will be assumed for the use of the appendix, nor for typographic errors. It is highly recommended to refer to the literature, practice guidelines, and package insert for information pertaining to the patient population participating in pertinent clinical trials, confirmation of dosing, administration rates, scheduling, duration of therapy, and need for supportive care medications (e.g., colony stimulating factors). Furthermore, evaluation of the literature and package inserts for dose modification recommendations based on hepatic dysfunction, renal dysfunction, and therapy-related toxicities is encouraged. Alteration in therapy may be necessary, based on good clinical judgment, for the individualization of therapy according to the patient's response and tolerability.

Please register your electronic version of this book, using the instructions on the inside front cover of this book, to access Appendix II.

Index